Manual of Pediatric Nutrition

Sixth Edition

Manual of Pediatric Nutrition

Sixth Edition

Editors

Christopher P. Duggan, MD, MPH

Samuel Meltzer, MD Professor of Pediatrics in the Field of Gastroenterology
Harvard Medical School
Director, Center for Nutrition
Division of Gastroenterology, Hepatology, and Nutrition
Boston Children's Hospital
Professor, Departments of Nutrition and Global Health and Population
Harvard T.H. Chan School of Public Health
Boston, Massachusetts

Kendrin R. Sonneville, ScD, RD

Associate Professor and Associate Chair, Department of Nutritional Sciences
Director, Center of Excellence for Maternal, Child, and Adolescent Health
University of Michigan School of Public Health
Ann Arbor, Michigan
Lecturer on Pediatrics
Harvard Medical School
Division of Adolescent Medicine
Boston Children's Hospital
Boston, Massachusetts

Wolters Kluwer

Philadelphia • Baltimore • New York • London
Buenos Aires • Hong Kong • Sydney • Tokyo

Acquisitions Editor: James Sherman
Development Editor: Cindy Yoo
Editorial Coordinator: Remington Fernando
Editorial Assistant: Kristen Kardoley
Marketing Manager: Janet Feeney
Production Project Manager: Jennifer L. Harper
Manager, Graphic Arts & Design: Stephen Druding
Manufacturing Coordinator: Lisa Bowling
Prepress Vendor: S4Carlisle Publishing Services

Sixth edition

9 8 7 6 5 4 3 2 1

Printed in the United States of America

Library of Congress Cataloging-in-Publication Data

Names: Duggan, Christopher editor | Sonneville, Kendrin editor
Title: Manual of pediatric nutrition / [edited by] Christopher Duggan, Kendrin Sonneville.
Description: Sixth edition. | Philadelphia, PA : Wolters Kluwer Health, [2027] | Includes bibliographical references and index. | Summary: "In nearly every level of treatment and counseling, care providers must take into account the effects of patients' diets. This is true in pediatric cases as well. The Manual of Pediatric Nutrition is a quick and easy to use guide to help health professionals provide well-informed dietary assessment, prescription, and treatment for specific disease states. The updated 6th edition is edited by an internationally recognized gastroenterologist and professor of pediatrics (Dr. Duggan) and a well-respected nutritionist"— Provided by publisher.
Identifiers: LCCN 2026006034 | ISBN 9781975244347 paperback | ISBN 9781975244354 ebook
Subjects: LCSH: Children—Nutrition | Nutrition disorders in children | BISAC: MEDICAL / Pediatrics | MEDICAL / Gastroenterology | LCGFT: Handbooks and manuals
Classification: LCC RJ206 .H42 2027
LC record available at https://lccn.loc.gov/2026006034

shop.lww.com

MPP0526

Contributors

CONTRIBUTING EDITOR

Coral Rudie, MS, RD, LDN, CNSC
Clinical Nutrition Educator
Center for Nutrition
Division of Gastroenterology, Hepatology, and Nutrition
Boston Children's Hospital
Boston, Massachusetts

CONTRIBUTING AUTHORS

Chantelle Arentsen, MS, RD, LDN
Clinical Nutrition Specialist I
Center for Nutrition
Division of Gastroenterology, Hepatology, and Nutrition
Boston Children's Hospital
Boston, Massachusetts

Kimberly H. Barbas, BSN, RN, IBCLC
Program Director, Lactation Support Program
Boston Children's Hospital
Boston, Massachusetts

Lindsay Boland, MS, RD, LDN, CNSC
Clinical Nutrition Specialist II
Center for Nutrition
Division of Gastroenterology, Hepatology, and Nutrition
Boston Children's Hospital
Boston, Massachusetts

Jasper Brezsny-Feldman, MS, RD, LDN
Clinical Nutrition Specialist I
Center for Nutrition
Division of Gastroenterology, Hepatology, and Nutrition
Boston Children's Hospital
Boston, Massachusetts

Ariana Cerro, RD, LDN, CNSC
Clinical Nutrition Specialist II
Center for Nutrition
Division of Gastroenterology, Hepatology, and Nutrition
Boston Children's Hospital
Boston, Massachusetts

Denis Chang, MD, MS
Attending Physician
Center for Nutrition
Division of Gastroenterology, Hepatology, and Nutrition
Boston Children's Hospital
Instructor in Pediatrics
Harvard Medical School
Boston, Massachusetts

Allison Churchill, BSN
Staff Nurse, Home Parenteral Nutrition Program
Center for Nutrition
Division of Gastroenterology, Hepatology, and Nutrition
Boston Children's Hospital
Boston, Massachusetts

Sara Farnan Colleary, MS, RD, LDN
Clinical Nutrition Specialist II
Center for Nutrition
Division of Gastroenterology, Hepatology, and Nutrition
Boston Children's Hospital
Boston, Massachusetts

Melanie V. Connolly, MSc, RD, LDN, CNSC
Clinical Nutrition Specialist II
Center for Nutrition
Division of Gastroenterology, Hepatology, and Nutrition
Boston Children's Hospital
Boston, Massachusetts

Mayra Crespo-Bellido, PhD
Postdoctoral Fellow
WIC Team
Center for Nutrition and Health Impact
Omaha, Nebraska

Paul McGreggor Crowley, MD
Attending Physician
Center for Nutrition
Division of Gastroenterology, Hepatology, and Nutrition
Boston Children's Hospital
Instructor in Pediatrics
Harvard Medical School
Boston, Massachusetts

Brittany DePaula, RD, LDN, CNSC
Senior Clinical Nutrition Specialist
Center for Nutrition
Division of Gastroenterology, Hepatology, and Nutrition
Department of Surgery
Boston Children's Hospital
Boston, Massachusetts

Christopher P. Duggan, MD, MPH
Samuel Meltzer, MD Professor of Pediatrics in the Field of Gastroenterology
Harvard Medical School
Director
Center for Nutrition
Division of Gastroenterology, Hepatology, and Nutrition
Boston Children's Hospital
Professor
Departments of Nutrition and Global Health and Population
Harvard T.H. Chan School of Public Health
Boston, Massachusetts

Daniel R. Duncan, MD, MPH
Attending Physician
Division of Gastroenterology, Hepatology, and Nutrition
Boston Children's Hospital
Assistant Professor of Pediatrics
Harvard Medical School
Boston, Massachusetts

Wendy Elverson, RD, CSP, LDN
Senior Clinical Nutrition Specialist
Center for Nutrition
Division of Gastroenterology, Hepatology, and Nutrition
Boston Children's Hospital
Boston, Massachusetts

Sarah Federoff, RD, LDN, CDCES
Clinical Nutrition Specialist I
Center for Nutrition
Division of Gastroenterology, Hepatology, and Nutrition
Division of Endocrinology
Boston Children's Hospital
Boston, Massachusetts

Emily Finnan, MS, RD, LDN, CNSC
Clinical Nutrition Specialist II
Center for Nutrition
Division of Gastroenterology, Hepatology, and Nutrition
Department of Cardiology
Boston Children's Hospital
Boston, Massachusetts

Sarah Fleet, MD
Attending Physician
Center for Nutrition
Division of Gastroenterology, Hepatology, and Nutrition
Boston Children's Hospital
Assistant Professor of Pediatrics
Harvard Medical School
Boston, Massachusetts

Katharine Garvey, MD, MPH
Clinical Chief for Diabetes
Division of Endocrinology
Boston Children's Hospital
Assistant Professor of Pediatrics
Harvard Medical School
Boston, Massachusetts

Sarah Goldman, MS, RD, LDN, CNSC
Clinical Nutrition Specialist II
Center for Nutrition
Division of Gastroenterology, Hepatology, and Nutrition
Boston Children's Hospital
Boston, Massachusetts

Erin Gordon, MS, RD, LDN, CDCES
Clinical Nutrition Educator
Center for Nutrition
Division of Gastroenterology, Hepatology, and Nutrition
Boston Children's Hospital
Boston, Massachusetts

S. Skylar Griggs, MS, RD, LDN
Clinical Nutrition Specialist II
Center for Nutrition
Division of Gastroenterology, Hepatology, and Nutrition
Boston Children's Hospital
Boston, Massachusetts

Kathleen M. Gura, PharmD, BCNSP
Manager, Pharmacy Clinical Research Program
Department of Pharmacy
Center for Nutrition
Division of Gastroenterology, Hepatology, and Nutrition
Boston Children's Hospital
Assistant Professor of Pediatrics
Harvard Medical School
Boston, Massachusetts

Kayla Hernandez, MS
Speech Language Pathologist
Department of Otolaryngology and Communication Enhancement
Boston Children's Hospital
Boston, Massachusetts

Suzanne Hollander, MS, RD, LDN
Senior Clinical Nutrition Specialist
Center for Nutrition
Division of Gastroenterology, Hepatology, and Nutrition
Division of Genetics and Genomics
Boston Children's Hospital
Boston, Massachusetts

Kayla E. Hope, MPH, RD, CNSC
Clinical Nutrition Specialist II
Center for Nutrition
Division of Gastroenterology, Hepatology, and Nutrition
Boston Children's Hospital
Boston, Massachusetts

Bridget M. Hron, MD, MMSc
Associate Director, Center for Nutrition
Division of Gastroenterology, Hepatology, and Nutrition
Boston Children's Hospital
Assistant Professor of Pediatrics
Harvard Medical School
Boston, Massachusetts

Lissette Jimenez, MD, MPH
Attending Physician
Center for Nutrition
Division of Gastroenterology, Hepatology, and Nutrition
Boston Children's Hospital
Instructor in Pediatrics
Harvard Medical School
Boston, Massachusetts

Daniel Kamin, MD
Attending Physician
Center for Nutrition
Division of Gastroenterology, Hepatology, and Nutrition
Boston Children's Hospital
Assistant Professor of Pediatrics
Harvard Medical School
Boston, Massachusetts

Vanessa Kane-Alves, RD, LDN
Clinical Nutrition Specialist II
Center for Nutrition
Division of Gastroenterology, Hepatology, and Nutrition
Boston Children's Hospital
Boston, Massachusetts

Madeline Keyes, MD
Neonatologist
NICU
Pediatrix Fort Worth Neonatology/Cook Children's Hospital
Assistant Professor of Pediatrics
Texas Christian University
Fort Worth, Texas

Jenny Kinne, MS, RD, LDN, CLC
Clinical Nutrition Specialist II
Center for Nutrition
Division of Gastroenterology, Hepatology, and Nutrition
Boston Children's Hospital
Boston, Massachusetts

Alix Krawcke, MS, RDN, LDN
Clinical Nutrition Specialist II
Center for Nutrition
Division of Gastroenterology, Hepatology, and Nutrition
Department of Adolescent Medicine
Boston Children's Hospital
Boston, Massachusetts

Jessica Leonard, RD, LDN, CSP, CCTD, CACFD
Senior Clinical Nutrition Specialist
Center for Nutrition
Division of Gastroenterology, Hepatology, and Nutrition
Boston Children's Hospital
Boston, Massachusetts

Lisa A. Mancini, MS, RD, LDN, CSP, CEDS
Senior Clinical Nutrition Specialist
Center for Nutrition
Division of Gastroenterology, Hepatology, and Nutrition
Boston Children's Hospital
Boston, Massachusetts

Anna Maynes, RD, LDN
Clinical Nutrition Specialist II
Center for Nutrition
Division of Gastroenterology, Hepatology, and Nutrition
Department of Cardiology
Boston Children's Hospital
Boston, Massachusetts

Jennifer McClelland, MS, FNP-BC
Clinical Coordinator, Home Parenteral Nutrition Program
Center for Nutrition
Division of Gastroenterology, Hepatology, and Nutrition
Boston Children's Hospital
Boston, Massachusetts

Melissa P. McDonnell, RD, CSP, LDN
Clinical Nutrition Manager
Center for Nutrition
Division of Gastroenterology, Hepatology, and Nutrition
Boston Children's Hospital
Boston, Massachusetts

Brianna Mears, RD, LDN
Clinical Nutrition Specialist II
Center for Nutrition
Division of Gastroenterology, Hepatology, and Nutrition
Boston Children's Hospital
Boston, Massachusetts

Nilesh Mehta, MD
Chief
Division of Critical Care Medicine
Department of Anesthesiology, Critical Care, and Pain Medicine
Boston Children's Hospital
Professor of Anesthesia
Harvard Medical School
Boston, Massachusetts

Judy Milliano, MS, RD, LD, CNSC
Clinical Nutrition Specialist II
Center for Nutrition
Division of Gastroenterology, Hepatology, and Nutrition
Department of Cardiology
Boston Children's Hospital
Boston, Massachusetts

Kimberly I. Mills, MD, MPH
Medical Director, Cardiovascular Critical Care Unit
Department of Cardiology
Boston Children's Hospital
Assistant Professor of Pediatrics
Harvard Medical School
Boston, Massachusetts

Margaret Murphy, PharmD, BCNSP
Senior Clinical Pharmacist
Department of Pharmacy
Center for Nutrition
Division of Gastroenterology, Hepatology, and Nutrition
Boston Children's Hospital
Boston, Massachusetts

Julie J. Norton, RD, LDN
Clinical Nutrition Specialist II
Center for Nutrition
Division of Gastroenterology, Hepatology, and Nutrition
Boston Children's Hospital
Boston, Massachusetts

Lauren Oliveira, MS, RD, LDN
Clinical Nutrition Specialist II
Center for Nutrition
Division of Gastroenterology, Hepatology, and Nutrition
Boston Children's Hospital
Boston, Massachusetts

Yvette Penner, MS, RD, LDN, CNSC
Clinical Nutrition Specialist II
Center for Nutrition
Division of Gastroenterology, Hepatology, and Nutrition
Boston Children's Hospital
Boston, Massachusetts

Heidi Pfeifer, RD, LDN, FAND
Senior Clinical Nutrition Specialist
Center for Nutrition
Division of Gastroenterology, Hepatology, and Nutrition
Boston Children's Hospital
Boston, Massachusetts

Daniel Pomerantz, MD
Clinical and Postdoctoral Fellow
Division of Genetics and Genomics
Boston Children's Hospital
Instructor in Pediatrics
Harvard Medical School
Boston, Massachusetts

Rachel Potvin, MS, RD, LDN, CCTD
Senior Clinical Nutrition Specialist
Center for Nutrition
Division of Gastroenterology, Hepatology, and Nutrition
Boston Children's Hospital
Boston, Massachusetts

Heidi Quinn, MS, RD, LDN, CDCES
Clinical Nutrition Specialist II
Center for Nutrition
Division of Gastroenterology, Hepatology, and Nutrition
Boston Children's Hospital
Boston, Massachusetts

Nicolle Quinn, MS, RD, LDN, CSR, CCTD
Senior Clinical Nutrition Specialist
Center for Nutrition
Division of Gastroenterology, Hepatology, and Nutrition
Boston Children's Hospital
Boston, Massachusetts

E. Reese, MPH, RDN, LDN, CNSC
Clinical Nutrition Specialist II
Center for Nutrition
Division of Gastroenterology, Hepatology, and Nutrition
Department of Surgery
Boston Children's Hospital
Boston, Massachusetts

Brennan Rhodes-Bratton, DrPH, MPH
Postdoctoral Associate
Center for Anti-racism, Social Justice, and Public Health
New York University
New York, New York

Tracy Richmond, MD
Director, Eating Disorder Program
Division of Adolescent/Young Adult Medicine, Department of Medicine
Boston Children's Hospital
Associate Professor of Pediatrics
Harvard Medical School
Boston, Massachusetts

Sabina Sabharwal, MD, MPH
Attending Physician
Division of Gastroenterology, Hepatology, and Nutrition
Boston Children's Hospital
Assistant Professor of Pediatrics
Harvard Medical School
Boston, Massachusetts

Annette Schille, MS, RD, LDN
Clinical Nutrition Specialist II
Center for Nutrition
Division of Gastroenterology, Hepatology, and Nutrition
Boston Children's Hospital
Boston, Massachusetts

Leanna Shea, MS, RD, LDN, CNSC
Clinical Nutrition Specialist II
Center for Nutrition
Division of Gastroenterology, Hepatology, and Nutrition
Boston Children's Hospital
Boston, Massachusetts

Desiree Sierra-Velez, MD
Medical Director, Adolescent Bariatric Surgery Program
Center for Nutrition
Division of Gastroenterology, Hepatology, and Nutrition
Boston Children's Hospital
Instructor in Pediatrics
Harvard Medical School
Boston, Massachusetts

Kristen J. Slusher, MS, RD, LDN
Clinical Nutrition Specialist II
Center for Nutrition
Division of Gastroenterology, Hepatology, and Nutrition
Boston Children's Hospital
Boston, Massachusetts

Katrina A.S. Smith, RD, LDN
Clinical Nutrition Specialist II
Center for Nutrition
Division of Gastroenterology, Hepatology, and Nutrition
Boston Children's Hospital
Boston, Massachusetts

Kendrin R. Sonneville, ScD, RD
Associate Professor and Associate Chair, Department of Nutritional Sciences
Director, Center of Excellence for Maternal, Child, and Adolescent Health
University of Michigan School of Public Health
Ann Arbor, Michigan
Lecturer on Pediatrics
Harvard Medical School
Division of Adolescent Medicine
Boston Children's Hospital
Boston, Massachusetts

Fatima Cody Stanford, MD, MPH, MPA, MBA, MACP
Obesity Medicine Physician Scientist
Departments of Medicine and Pediatrics
Massachusetts General Hospital
Associate Professor of Medicine
Harvard Medical School
Boston, Massachusetts

Colleen Stegman, MS, RD, LDN, CNSC
Clinical Nutrition Specialist II
Center for Nutrition
Division of Gastroenterology, Hepatology, and Nutrition
Boston Children's Hospital
Boston, Massachusetts

Heather Stone, RD, LDN
Clinical Nutrition Specialist II
Center for Nutrition
Division of Gastroenterology, Hepatology, and Nutrition
Boston Children's Hospital
Boston, Massachusetts

Mollie Studley, MS, RD, LDN
Clinical Nutrition Specialist II
Center for Nutrition
Division of Gastroenterology, Hepatology, and Nutrition
Boston Children's Hospital
Boston, Massachusetts

Tina Sun, MS, RD, LDN, CCTD
Clinical Nutrition Specialist II
Center for Nutrition
Division of Gastroenterology, Hepatology, and Nutrition
Boston Children's Hospital
Boston, Massachusetts

Erin P. Syverson, MD
Attending Physician
Center for Nutrition
Division of Gastroenterology, Hepatology, and Nutrition
Boston Children's Hospital
Assistant Professor of Pediatrics
Harvard Medical School
Boston, Massachusetts

Stacey Tarrant, RD, LDN
Clinical Nutrition Specialist II
Center for Nutrition
Division of Gastroenterology, Hepatology, and Nutrition
Boston Children's Hospital
Boston, Massachusetts

Amy M. Turner, MD, MSHPEd
Attending Physician
Center for Nutrition
Division of Gastroenterology, Hepatology, and Nutrition
Boston Children's Hospital
Instructor in Pediatrics
Harvard Medical School
Boston, Massachusetts

Maria E. Walazek, RD, LDN, CSSD
Clinical Nutrition Specialist II
Center for Nutrition
Division of Gastroenterology, Hepatology, and Nutrition
Female Athlete Program, Sports Medicine Division
Boston Children's Hospital
Boston, Massachusetts

Andrew Wehrman, MD
Attending Physician
Division of Gastroenterology, Hepatology, and Nutrition
Boston Children's Hospital
Instructor in Pediatrics
Harvard Medical School
Boston, Massachusetts

Sharon Weston, MS, RD, LDN, CSP, FAND
Senior Clinical Nutrition Specialist
Center for Nutrition
Division of Gastroenterology, Hepatology, and Nutrition
Boston Children's Hospital
Boston, Massachusetts

Preface

Twelve years have passed since the publication of the fifth edition of the *Manual of Pediatric Nutrition*, and the appreciation for the critical role of nutrition in promoting the health and well-being of children has only deepened. This growing recognition is reflected in the expanding evidence base in nutrition and dietetics, the increasing understanding of the influence of nutritional status and diet throughout the life course on adult health, and the emergence of innovative technologies that enable personalized nutritional therapies.

This sixth edition of the *Manual of Pediatric Nutrition* continues to provide a practical basis for pediatric nutritional assessment and therapy for dietitians, pediatricians, house officers, fellows, and students. We have maintained the organization of the book into three parts. Part I, "Nutrition and the Well Child," covers the basics of nutritional assessment, nutritional requirements, feeding guidelines for healthy infants, children, and adolescents, and dietary supplements. Part II, "Nutrition and the Hospitalized Child," reviews nutritional assessment in sick children, as well as the use of specialized enteral and parenteral products. Part III, "Nutrition and Specific Disease States," provides updated information on the nutritional management of a wide range of pediatric clinical disorders. This edition also includes new and expanded sections on Health Equity and Cultural Humility, Interdisciplinary Care, and an enteral product formulary. All chapters have been extensively updated by content experts and provide practical guidance for patient assessment and management.

We are grateful to our many colleagues who have reviewed the literature and written concise, practical chapters for this edition. We also acknowledge the excellent editorial assistance of Coral Rudie, MS, RD, LDN, CNSC, in completing this edition, as well as the assistance of Remington Fernando and Cindy Yoo from Wolters Kluwer. Finally, we wish to thank Drs. Kristy Hendricks and W. Allan Walker for their invaluable contribution to previous editions and whose leadership in the field of nutrition helped begin this *Manual of Pediatric Nutrition* nearly 40 years ago.

Christopher P. Duggan, MD, MPH
Kendrin R. Sonneville, ScD, RD

Contents

Appendices

PART I

Nutrition and the Well Child

CHAPTER 1

Nutritional Assessment: Food/Nutrition-Related History

Vanessa Kane-Alves

Nutrition assessment is the first step in the nutrition care process. The data collected as part of a nutrition assessment typically include the following: (1) food/nutrition-related history, (2) anthropometric measurements, (3) biochemical data, (4) medical tests and procedures, (5) nutrition-focused physical findings, and (6) patient history.[1] Pediatric clinicians gather nutrition assessment data through interviews with the patient or caregiver, direct observation and measurement, medical records, and/or input from other members of the care team. This chapter provides a brief overview of foundational data collection by age and caregiver. The chapters that follow cover specific food/nutrition-related history assessment indicators by age, feeding route, and condition.

A major component of the food/nutrition-related history is the assessment of food and nutrient intake. While various methods exist, including advances in technology such as image-assisted and mobile application diet recalls, the 24-hour recall remains the most commonly used method in clinical practice. This method involves recalling the dietary intake of the past 24 hours or a recent typical day.[2-4] It is a practical, cost-effective, and inclusive tool for pediatric clinicians, applicable across different ages, conditions, feeding routes, cultures, care settings, and socioeconomic groups.[5] To improve accuracy and reduce recall bias of the 24-hour recall, clinicians can utilize a multipass approach if time allows, such as the U.S. Department of Agriculture (USDA) five-step multipass method.[6,7] This method includes the following:

1. Quick list: The interviewer asks the respondent to list all the foods and beverages they consumed in the past 24 hours without prompting for details.
2. Forgotten foods: The interviewer probes for commonly forgotten foods and beverages, such as snacks, condiments, or supplements.
3. Time and occasion: The interviewer asks about the time and occasion (e.g., breakfast, lunch, snack) for each food or beverage consumed, helping to structure and clarify the recall.
4. Detailed cycle: The interviewer collects detailed information about each item, including portion sizes, preparation methods, brand names, ingredients, and any accompanying foods or condiments, often using visual aids or measuring tools to help estimate portion sizes.
5. Final review: The interviewer reviews the entire recall with the respondent to confirm accuracy, prompting for any corrections or additions.

Clinicians expect that the accuracy of information may vary depending on the method used, the skill of the interviewer, day-to-day dietary variation, social desirability bias, and the patient or caregiver's recall ability. Tailoring methods to specific care settings and age categories can improve data accuracy. For instance, involving school-aged children (around 8 years old) in diet recall can enhance information quality, as children in this age group are often not with caregivers for the full day.[8,9] Children can typically self-report reliably by around 12 years old, depending on the method used.[10]

Pediatric clinicians also assess feeding behaviors, the emotional and physical feeding environment, and the feeding relationship across various ages and stages of growth.[11,12] Other key data to consider include medication and herbal supplement use, knowledge, beliefs, attitudes, factors affecting access to food and nutrition-related supplies, and physical activity and function.[1] Social determinants of health, drawn from the patient history, are critical in shaping the food/nutrition-related history.[13] Table 1.1 summarizes commonly collected food and nutrition-related data by age and caregiver, as used by pediatric clinicians.

TABLE 1.1 COMMONLY COLLECTED FOOD/NUTRITION-RELATED HISTORY DATA

APPLIES TO ALL STAGES	BIRTH TO 12 MO OLD	6-18 Y OLD
• Early feeding history from birth • Foods accepted by food group • Family and child/adolescent food, fluid, and nutrient intake (diet recall) • Division of responsibility in feeding between parent/caregiver and child[11] • Examples of observed hunger and satiety cues • Cultural or religious beliefs influencing family eating practices • Eating environments (e.g., family meals, foods eaten outside the home, eating at the table, screen use during meals, pace of eating) • Physical activity: daily opportunities for safe and enjoyable participation • Medication, vitamin/mineral, and/or herbal supplement intake • Food/nutrition assistance program participation, access to safe food, meals, water, and related supplies • Caregiver food and nutrition knowledge, attitudes, and beliefs about feeding concerns • Caregiver history related to the child/adolescent's food/nutrition concern	If human milk–fed: • Feeding/pumping frequency, duration, and patterns • Infant formula supplementation of human milk (per manufacturer instructions or health care provider's guidance) • Medication, vitamin/mineral, and/or herbal supplement intake for the baby or mother • Fluid/beverage or food additions (e.g., juice, rice cereal, or water) If formula-fed: • Feeding frequency, duration, and patterns • Infant formula preparation (per manufacturer instructions or health care provider's guidance) and storage (safety and sanitation practices) • Fluid/beverage or food additions (e.g., juice, rice cereal, or water) Additional considerations: • Developmental readiness for solid foods typically at 6 mo	Additional considerations: • Caffeine intake • Dissatisfaction with weight, body image, or appearance; presence of disordered eating behaviors • History of weight/body-related teasing or bullying • Beliefs and attitudes about food, body, and readiness to change nutrition-related behaviors • For children aged 6-13 y, interview all caregivers and include the child's input • For those aged 13 y and older, interview the caregiver and adolescent separately

In clinical documentation, it is best practice to conclude the food and nutrition-related history with a summary statement reflecting the clinician's impression of the overall adequacy of the patient's intake. This typically includes the adequacy of calories, protein, vitamins and minerals, fluids, and food groups, as well as strengths and protective factors. Highlighting strengths—such as a supportive family environment, intake from all major food groups, or the ability to use hunger and fullness cues—helps foster mutual respect, trust, and collaboration between families and the care team. This summary also lays the foundation for care by guiding the comparison of assessment findings to established standards, norms, and criteria to identify nutrition-related concerns and support appropriate recommendations for medical nutrition therapy.

REFERENCES

1. Academy of Nutrition and Dietetics. *International Dietetics and Nutrition Terminology (IDNT) Reference Manual: Standardized Language for the Nutrition Care Process*. 4th ed. Academy of Nutrition and Dietetics; 2013.
2. Burrows T, Goldman S, Rollo M. A systematic review of the validity of dietary assessment methods in children when compared with the method of doubly labelled water. *Eur J Clin Nutr*. 2020;74(5):669-681.
3. Kouvari M, Mamalaki E, Bathrellou E, Poulimeneas D, Yannakoulia M, Panagiotakos DB. The validity of technology-based dietary assessment methods in childhood and adolescence: a systematic review. *Crit Rev Food Sci Nutr*. 2021;61(7):1065-1080.
4. Mehranfar S, Jalilpiran Y, Jafari A, et al. Validity of dietary assessment methods compared with doubly labeled water in children: a systematic review and meta-analysis. *Obes Rev*. 2024;25(9):e13768.
5. de Gooijer FJ, Lasschuijt M, Wit RF, Feskens EJ, Brouwer-Brolsma EM, Camps G. Dietary behavior assessments in children—a mixed-method research exploring the perspective of pediatric dietitians on innovative technologies. *Curr Dev Nutr*. 2023;7(6):100091.
6. Moshfegh AJ, Rhodes DG, Baer DJ, et al. The US Department of Agriculture automated multiple-pass method reduces bias in the collection of energy intakes. *Am J Clin Nutr*. 2008;88(2):324-332.
7. Roe AJ, Sankavaram K, Baker S, et al. 24-hour dietary recall in the Expanded Food and Nutrition Education Program: perspective of the program coordinator. *Nutrients*. 2023;15(19):4147.
8. van der Heijden Z, de Gooijer F, Camps G, et al. User requirements in developing a novel dietary assessment tool for children: mixed methods study. *JMIR Form Res*. 2024;8:e47850.
9. Livingstone MB, Robson PJ. Measurement of dietary intake in children. *Proc Nutr Soc*. 2000;59(2):279-293.
10. Livingstone MB, Robson PJ, Wallace JM. Issues in dietary intake assessment of children and adolescents. *Br J Nutr*. 2004;92(suppl 2):S213-S222.
11. Lohse B, Mitchell DC. Valid and reliable measure of adherence to Satter Division of Responsibility in Feeding. *J Nutr Educ Behav*. 2021;53(3):211-222.
12. Ellyn Satter Institute. Raising a child who is a joy to feed. Accessed February 3, 2026. https://www.ellynsatterinstitute.org/raise-a-healthy-child-who-is-a-joy-to-feed/
13. Office of Disease Prevention and Health Promotion. Social determinants of health—Healthy People 2030. Accessed December 16, 2024. https://health.gov/healthypeople/objectives-and-data/social-determinants-health

CHAPTER 2

Nutrition Assessment: Anthropometrics and Growth

Colleen Stegman

Growth is a complex process influenced by nutrition, environment, and genetics. Anthropometry, the study of human body measurements on a comparative basis, includes the measurement of physical dimensions at different ages and is widely used to monitor growth and health.[1] Comparison with standard references for age and sex helps determine abnormalities in growth and development that may have resulted from nutrient deficiencies or excesses.

Accurate assessment of growth requires the use of an appropriate growth reference, precise measurement techniques, correct age calculation, and proper interpretation of the results.[1] In pediatric populations, growth data are typically interpreted using percentiles, z-scores, and percent of the median. These indicators help assess a child's nutritional status in comparison to reference populations. While serial measurements provide a more comprehensive picture of growth trends over time, single measurements can be used to screen children who may be at nutritional risk and determine the need for a more complete nutrition assessment. However, measurement errors due to inconsistent technique and equipment may affect comparisons between measurements taken at different times.[1] A summary of anthropometric measurement techniques is provided in Table 2.1, while detailed descriptions of standardized techniques and equipment for anthropometry are found in standardized anthropometry resources.[1,2]

TABLE 2.1 MEASUREMENT TECHNIQUES

Weight	The subject stands, lies, or sits in the center of a balance scale platform. Minimal clothing and no shoes should be worn. Weight is taken to the nearest 0.1 kg or 1.0 oz in children and to the nearest 0.01 kg or 0.5 oz in infants.
Length/height	Measurement of length is frequently erroneous because of improper technique or equipment. Children younger than 2 y of age should be measured recumbent on a length board; after this age, standing height should be measured if possible.[1] For standing height measurements, the patient should be standing erect, without shoes, on the scale platform or on the floor. Shoulders should be straight, and the subject should look straight ahead. Measurements should be to the nearest 0.1 cm or 0.125 in.

TABLE 2.1 MEASUREMENT TECHNIQUES (*continued*)

Head circumference	A flexible, narrow tape measure is placed firmly around the head above the supraorbital ridges and over the frontal bulge, where the circumference is greatest. Measurements should be taken to the nearest 0.5 cm or 0.25 in.[1]
Skinfold thickness	Measurement of triceps skinfold thickness is taken at the midpoint between the acromion and olecranon on the relaxed right arm at the same level as the arm circumference. The layer of skin and subcutaneous tissue is pulled away from the underlying muscle and held until measurement with the calipers at the midpoint has been taken. Readings should be taken to 0.5 mm, 3 s after the application of calipers. Other skinfold sites may also be used; techniques are described in the Centers for Disease Control Manual of Anthropometry.[1] High-quality skinfold calipers (Lange or Harpenden) are recommended for accurate measurements.[1]
Arm circumference	Arm circumference is measured at the posterior aspect of the midpoint of the upper arm between the acromion and olecranon on the right arm. The measurement is taken perpendicular to the long axis of the upper arm while the patient is standing upright and relaxed.
Knee height for stature estimation	A knee caliper and a measuring tape are used to obtain the upper leg length measurement. The caliper points should be placed on either side of the patella at the distal end of the femur.[1] The caliper should be as vertical as possible.[1] Mark the proximal border of the patella on the anterior side of the thigh.[1] Then, the distance from the marked line up to the inguinal crease (where the leg meets the rest of the body) should be measured using the measuring tape.[1] The value obtained is then entered into an equation to get an estimation of stature.
Ulnar length for stature estimation	Using a tape measure or calipers, measure the distance between the olecranon (point of the elbow) and the styloid process (the prominent bone of the wrist). The value obtained is then entered into an equation to get an estimation of stature.[2]

GROWTH CHARTS

Growth charts contain a series of percentile graphs, including weight-for-age, length/height-for-age, weight-for-length/height, and body mass index (BMI)-for-age for boys and girls from birth to 20 years. The Centers for Disease Control and Prevention (CDC) and the American Academy of Pediatrics (AAP) recommend the use of the World Health Organization (WHO) growth standards for full-term infants (born >37 weeks gestational age), preterm infants once more than 40 weeks postmenstrual age (PMA), and children up to 24 months of age.[3] The CDC charts should be used for children aged 2 years and older.[4] All charts are available for downloading from the CDC website (www.cdc.gov/growthcharts) and are included in Appendix 3.

For mid-upper arm circumference (MUAC), the WHO growth reference should be used for children aged 3 months to 5 years. For children aged 5 to 18 years, MUAC-for-age curves published by Mramba et al. should be used.[5,6]

There are specific growth charts for assessing the premature infant, which are discussed in Chapter 35 (Prematurity). There are also growth charts for specific conditions, including Down syndrome and cerebral palsy (see Appendix 3 for a referenced list of special growth charts). Caution should be taken with the use of these charts, given the same sample size of data from which they were created. Specialty growth charts should *not* be used when classifying malnutrition.

INDICATORS OF NUTRITIONAL STATUS

Three different classification systems can be used to distinguish *normal* from *abnormal* growth in childhood: percentiles, z-scores, and percent of median.

Percentiles

Percentiles are the standard clinical approach for comparing growth parameters, providing a graphical representation on growth charts of how a child's measurements relate to a reference standard. A percentile reflects the proportion of the reference population that falls below the individual child's measurement.

z-Score

The z-scores offer an alternative way to interpret anthropometrics by indicating the number of standard deviations from the median.[7] They provide a more sensitive and precise measure of change relative to percentile changes, particularly for cases outside the percentile curves (i.e., below the 5th or above the 95th percentile). While percentiles are commonly used in the United States, the WHO recommends using z-scores, especially when describing groups.[7]

Percent of the Median

Anthropometric measures can be calculated as a percentage of the median (the 50th percentile for age and sex),[8,9] also referred to as ***percent standard***, as shown here:

$$\%\ \text{Standard} = \frac{\text{Actual measure} \times 100}{\text{Standard measure (50th percentile)}}$$

CLASSIFICATION OF NUTRITIONAL STATUS AND INDICATORS OF MALNUTRITION

Nutritional status is assessed by comparing growth indicators with established standards or criteria to diagnose and document conditions such as malnutrition or obesity. The WHO growth standards, developed using data from healthy children across multiple countries, provide standardized growth curves and z-score cutoffs used to classify nutritional status (see Table 2.2).[10] For children aged 1 month to 18 years, the most current and recommended criteria for diagnosing malnutrition are those from the 2014 consensus statement by the Academy of Nutrition and Dietetics (AND) and the American Society for Parenteral and Enteral Nutrition (ASPEN).[5] These consensus criteria are based on anthropometric indicators and vary depending on whether data are available from one or multiple time points[5]:

- Single time point: Use z-scores for weight-for-length/height, BMI-for-age, length/height-for-age, or MUAC.

TABLE 2.2 WORLD HEALTH ORGANIZATION CLASSIFICATION OF NUTRITIONAL STATUS OF INFANTS AND CHILDREN[10]

NUTRITIONAL STATUS	AGE: BIRTH TO 5 Y INDICATOR AND CUTOFF VALUE COMPARED WITH THE MEDIAN OF THE "WHO CHILD GROWTH STANDARDS"[a]
Obese	Weight-for-length/height[b] or BMI-for-age >3 standard deviations (SD) of the median
Overweight	Weight-for-length/height[b] or BMI-for-age >2 SD and ≤3 SD of the median
Moderately underweight	Weight-for-age <–2 SD and ≥–3 SD of the median
Severely underweight	Weight-for-age <–3 SD of the median
Moderate acute malnutrition	Weight-for-length/height[b] or BMI-for-age ≤–2 SD and ≥–3 SD of the median or mid-upper arm circumference ≥115 mm and <125 mm
Severe acute malnutrition	Weight-for-length/height[b] or BMI-for-age <–3 SD of the median or mid-upper arm circumference <115 mm or bilateral pitting edema
Moderately stunted (moderate chronic malnutrition)	Length/height-for-age[b] ≤–2 SD and ≥–3 SD of the median
Severely stunted (severe chronic malnutrition)	Length/height-for-age[b] <–3 SD of the median
Moderately wasted	Weight-for-length/height ≤–2 SD and ≥–3 SD of the median
Severely wasted	Weight-for-length/height <–3 SD of the median

BMI, body mass index; WHO, World Health Organization.

[a]WHO child growth standards: methods and development. Length/height-for-age, weight-for-age, weight-for-length, weight-for-height, and body mass index-for-age. World Health Organization. 2006. https://www.who.int/publications/i/item/924154693X

[b]Weight-for-length is used in infants and young children aged 0 to 23 months, and weight-for-height is used for children aged 24 months and older.

- Multiple time points: Additional indicators include weight gain velocity (for children under 2 years), weight loss (for ages 2-20 years), decline in weight-for-length/height z-score, and evidence of inadequate nutrient intake.

A diagnosis of malnutrition can be made if any one of these indicators is present. If multiple indicators are met, the most severe classification should be used.

Of note, separate criteria for neonates and preterm infants were published by AND/ASPEN in 2018, although the supporting evidence remains limited.[11] See Tables 2.3 and 2.4 for detailed criteria used at Boston Children's Hospital, based on both the AND/ASPEN consensus statement and WHO standards.[5,12,13] Malnutrition and growth failure are discussed further in Chapter 27.

The WHO also provides criteria for overweight and obesity using z-scores; however, the AAP recommends using percentile-based guidelines for these classifications (see Table 2.5).[14] Obesity is discussed in more detail in Chapter 33.

TABLE 2.3 MALNUTRITION CRITERIA (SINGLE DATA POINT)

	MILD MALNUTRITION	MODERATE MALNUTRITION	SEVERE MALNUTRITION
Weight-for-length z-score (<2 y of age)	−1 to −1.9	−2 to −2.9	−3 or less
BMI-for-age z-score (2-20 y of age)	−1 to −1.9	−2 to −2.9	−3 or less
Length/height-for-age z-score	No data	−2 to −2.9	−3 or less
MUAC z-score[a] (3 mo to 18 y)	−1 to −1.9	−2 to −2.9	−3 or less
MUAC measurement[a] (6 mo to 5 y)	No data	11.5 to 12.5 cm	<11.5 cm

BMI, body mass index; MUAC, mid-upper arm circumference.
This table was created based on the Academy of Nutrition and Dietetics (AND)/the American Society for Parenteral and Enteral Nutrition (ASPEN) malnutrition consensus statement criteria[5] and the WHO criteria.[12,13] The presence of edema from the WHO criteria was excluded since edema is often not nutritionally related in hospitalized patients.
[a]WHO z-scores for 3 mo to 5 y and Mramba z-scores for 5 to 18 y are available utilizing Peditools.org.[6,10]

TABLE 2.4 MALNUTRITION CRITERIA (MULTIPLE DATA POINTS)

	MILD MALNUTRITION	MODERATE MALNUTRITION	SEVERE MALNUTRITION
Weight gain velocity (<2 y of age)	<75% of the norm expected for weight gain	<50% of the norm expected for weight gain	<25% of the norm expected for weight gain
Weight loss (2-20 y of age)	5% usual body weight	7.5% usual body weight	10% usual body weight
Deceleration in weight-for-length or BMI-for-age z-scores	Decline of 1 z-score	Decline of 2 z-scores	Decline of 3 z-scores
Energy intake is a secondary indicator for diagnosing malnutrition. If anthropometrics are unavailable or unreliable, inadequate intake relative to estimated needs may be used alongside physical findings, based on duration by age: 1 to 12 mo ≥ 3 d, 1 to 10 y ≥ 5 d, >10 y ≥ 7 d.			
Inadequate nutrient intake	51%-75% estimated energy/protein need	26%-50% estimated energy/protein need	<25% estimated energy/protein need

BMI, body mass index.
This table was created based on the Academy of Nutrition and Dietetics (AND)/the American Society for Parenteral and Enteral Nutrition (ASPEN)[5] malnutrition consensus statement criteria.

TABLE 2.5 CLASSIFICATION OF PEDIATRIC OVERWEIGHT AND OBESITY

CLASSIFICATION	BMI
Overweight	>85th to 95th percentile
Class 1: Obesity	≥95th percentile
Class 2: Obesity	≥120% to <140% of the 95th percentile or BMI ≥35 kg/m^2 to <40 kg/m^2, whichever is lower based on age and sex
Class 3: Obesity	≥140% of the 95th percentile or BMI ≥40 kg/m^2, whichever is lower based on age and sex

BMI, body mass index.
Criteria based on the American Academy of Pediatrics (AAP), Clinical Practice Guideline for the Evaluation and Treatment of Children and Adolescents with Obesity.[14]

ANTHROPOMETRIC MEASUREMENTS

Weight

Body weight is a reproducible and reliable growth parameter that can indicate both acute and chronic nutritional status. Accurate age, sex, and reference standards are all necessary for the evaluation of weight.

Interpretation. Weight is evaluated using growth charts as weight-for-age and weight-for-height, as well as BMI (described later). Weight-for-age compares the individual with reference data for weight attained at any given age, whereas weight-for-height evaluates the appropriateness of the individual's weight compared with their own height.

Weight velocity evaluates the change in the rate of weight gain over a specified time period. Reference data for increments of expected/average weight gain velocity for sex from 0 to 24 months of age are shown in Table 2.6.[3,4] Reference data for increments of expected/average weight gain velocity for sex for ages 2 to 20 years are shown in Table 2.7.[4,15,16] Once children born prematurely (<37 weeks gestational age) reach 42 to 44 weeks PMA, their growth should be monitored using the WHO growth standards based on their corrected age until 24 months. Weight gain velocity should also be assessed based on corrected age. When aiming to achieve "catch-up" growth, the goal is for the growth rate to be greater than the expected/average growth velocity. Recent changes in weight (loss or gain) are often indicators of acute nutritional problems and can be noted as *percent weight change*, as shown in the following equation.

$$\text{Percent weight change} = \frac{\text{Usual weight} - \text{Current weight}}{\text{Usual weight}} \times 100$$

See Table 2.4 for details on the classification of malnutrition based on the percent of expected weight gain.[5]

TABLE 2.6 EXPECTED/AVERAGE GROWTH VELOCITY FOR AGE/SEX, 0 TO 24 MONTHS[3,4]

	MALES		FEMALES	
AGE (MO)	WEIGHT (G/D)	LENGTH (CM/MO)	WEIGHT (G/D)	LENGTH (CM/MO)
0-1	37.4	4.8	31.3	4.5
1-2	36.5	3.7	33.7	3.3
2-3	27.1	3.0	23.9	2.7
3-4	20.5	2.5	19.2	2.2
4-5	16.9	2.0	15.8	1.9
5-6	14.0	1.7	13.3	1.7
6-7	11.9	1.5	11.5	1.5
7-8	10.5	1.4	10.3	1.4
8-9	9.5	1.3	9.1	1.3
9-10	8.6	1.3	8.4	1.3
10-11	8.1	1.2	7.8	1.2
11-12	7.8	1.2	7.7	1.2
12-24	6.7	1.1	6.7	1.0

Note: These values correlate with expected growth to maintain the 50th percentile weight-for-age on the WHO growth standard.

TABLE 2.7 EXPECTED/AVERAGE GROWTH VELOCITY FOR AGE/SEX, 2 TO 20 YEARS[4,15,16]

AGE (Y)	WEIGHT (G/D)	HEIGHT (CM/MO)
2-4	4-5	0.5-0.8
4-7	6-7	0.5-0.6
7-9	6-8.5	0.4-0.5
9-11	9-12	0.4-0.5
11-13	11.5-14	0.5-0.7
13-15	Male: 14-15 Female: 7-10	Male: 0.5-0.6 Female: 0.1-0.25
15-17	Male: 10-12.5 Female: 3.5-5	Male: 0.2-0.3 Female: 0.1
17-18	Male: 7 Female: 3	
18-20	Male: 4-5 Female: 2.5-3	

Note: These values correlate with expected growth to maintain the 50th percentile weight-for-age on the CDC growth references.

Length/Height

Measured with appropriate equipment and technique, length/height is a simple and reproducible growth parameter that, in conjunction with weight, provides important information about growth failure and chronic undernutrition, especially in early childhood and adolescence.

Interpretation. Length/height is evaluated using length/height-for-age growth charts. Length/height-for-age below the 5th percentile classifies as stunting, and measurements that range between the 5th and 10th percentiles should be evaluated further. See Table 2.2 for details on classifications of stunting using WHO criteria.[10] Predicted mature height may also be considered when interpreting length/height. Further investigation is warranted if a child stops gaining linear growth or has a plateau or decline in their historic percentiles and z-scores on their length/height-for-age despite accurate measurements. While the rate of linear growth varies, reference data for increments of expected/average weight gain velocity by sex for ages 0 to 24 months and 2 to 20 years are shown in Tables 2.6 and 2.7, respectively.[4,15,16]

Mature height estimation may be helpful in evaluating short stature. Due to genetic influences, some children will be taller or shorter than average. The growth patterns of other family members may also be helpful in determining the correct diagnosis in such instances. Short stature in childhood and adolescence should be evaluated to determine whether it reflects normal variation or an underlying energy deficiency or disease. The corrected *mid-parental height method* (Tanner method) shown here is one of several methods available for the prediction of mature height.[17]

Height (cm) at maturity (male) = (Father's height + Mother's height + 13 cm)/2

Height (cm) at maturity (female) = (Father's height + Mother's height − 13 cm)/2

Alternative measurements for estimating height may be helpful in assessing a child's nutritional status when the child is nonambulatory or acutely ill. Some of the alternative measurements that can be used to estimate height include knee height and ulnar length. Once these measurements are obtained, they are entered into an equation to estimate the child's height (see Table 2.8).[18-23]

Head Circumference

Head circumference can be influenced by nutritional status until age 36 months, although deficiencies typically manifest first in weight and height before affecting brain growth.

Interpretation. Head circumference is also interpreted using growth charts. Measurements below the 5th percentile may indicate chronic undernutrition during fetal life and early childhood.

Weight-for-Length/Height

This ratio more accurately assesses body composition and distinguishes wasting (acute malnutrition) from stunting (chronic malnutrition) compared with weight-for-age or height-for-age alone.

TABLE 2.8 ALTERNATIVE MEASUREMENTS TO ESTIMATE STATURE

	EQUATIONS			CONSIDERATIONS FOR USE
Knee height				
Rumapea method[18]	Males		Stature (cm) = 29.895 + (0.081 × Age [months] + [2.267 × Knee height (cm)])	Equations based on healthy children aged 7-12 y old
	Females		Stature (cm) = 26.297 + (0.110 × Age [months] + [2.278 × Knee height (cm)])	
Chumlea method[19]	Males	White	Stature (cm) = (Knee height [cm] × 2.22) + 40.54	Equations based on healthy children aged 6-18 y old
		Black	Stature (cm) = = (Knee height [cm] × 2.18) + 39.6	
	Females	White	Stature (cm) = = (Knee height [cm] × 2.15) + 43.21	
		Black	Stature (cm) = = (Knee height [cm] × 2.02) + 46.59	
Stevenson method[20]	Stature (cm) = (2.69 × Knee height [cm]) + 24.2			Equation based on children with cerebral palsy up to 12 y of age
Ulnar length				
Gauld method (2004)[21]	Males		Stature (cm) = 4.605 × Ulna length (cm) + 1.308 × Age (y) + 28.003	Equation developed in healthy children aged 5 y 4 mo to 19 y 7 mo
	Females		Stature (cm) = 4.459 × Ulna length (cm) + 1.315 × Age (y) + 31.485	
Gauld method (2014)[22]	Males		Stature (cm) = 4.629 × Ulna length (cm) + 1.340 × Age (y) + 26.974	2004 Gauld equations adjusted for 2-6 y old using data from healthy children
	Females		Stature (cm) = 4.577 × Ulna length (cm) + 1.343 × Age (y) + 28.345	
Rasouli method[23]	Stature (cm) = 0.59 × Ulnar length (mm) + 13.1			Equation developed in ICU population aged 1 mo to 23 y old

ICU, intensive care unit.

Interpretation. Measurements that fall between the 3rd and 97th percentiles indicate appropriate weight-for-length/height; measurements outside this range indicate under- or overnutrition. See Tables 2.3 and 2.4 for malnutrition classification based on weight-for-length/height z-scores or change in z-scores.[5,6,10,12,13]

Body Mass Index

BMI is determined by dividing the person's weight in kilograms by their height in meter squared. In adolescents, BMI-for-age correlates with total body adiposity.[24]

Interpretation. BMI percentiles are available for children older than 2 years and are gender- and age-specific until adulthood.[4] BMI-for-age is the only indicator that allows plotting a measure of weight and height with age on the same chart. It is recommended that percentiles be used rather than an absolute number because BMI is expected to change throughout periods of growth.[25] BMI does not diagnose excess body fat but is a screening tool used to assess weight status and identify the risk of wasting or excess body fat. This can be further confirmed through physical examination and possibly additional body composition assessment. A limitation of BMI is that it does not distinguish lean body mass from fat mass. See Tables 2.3 and 2.4 for malnutrition classification based on BMI-for-age z-scores or change in z-scores over time.[5,6,10,12,13] See Table 2.5 for obesity classifications based on BMI-for-age percentiles.[14]

Mid-Upper Arm Circumference

MUAC is the measurement of the circumference of the upper arm and can be a useful measurement to assess nutritional status when unable to obtain accurate weights and/or heights. MUAC correlates well with more sophisticated measures of body composition, as well as mortality.[6,26] Tracking MUAC over time can be useful in monitoring the nutritional status of children whose weight trends are confounded by fluid status (edema, ascites) or steroids.[5]

Interpretation. The z-scores for MUAC are found in Table 2.9. See Table 2.3 for malnutrition classifications based on MUAC cutoffs and z-scores.

■ BODY COMPOSITION ANALYSIS

A determination of body fat and fat-free mass (lean body mass) is useful for comparison to age- and sex-adjusted reference values[27] and for monitoring changes associated with growth, activity, disease, and treatment. Three more common methods used in clinical practice and research include bioelectrical impedance analysis (BIA), dual-energy x-ray absorptiometry (DEXA), and air displacement plethysmography (ADP). Each method has advantages and disadvantages. Most methods for assessing body fat and fat-free mass in children use constants or age ranges that may not be specific to the individual or group being studied, so careful consideration of the relevant calculations is important.

Skinfold Thickness

Measurements of the subcutaneous layer correlate with total body fat and can be used to estimate fat stores. Skinfold thickness measurements are simple, inexpensive, and portable and, when performed with a reliable technique, can be used to monitor body

TABLE 2.9 Z-SCORE FOR MID-UPPER ARM CIRCUMFERENCE (CM)[3,6]

	MALES							FEMALES						
YEARS	−3	−2	−1	0	+1	+2	+3	−3	−2	−1	0	+1	+2	+3
3-11 (mo)	11.3	12.2	13.2	14.2	15.4	16.5	17.8	10.8	11.7	12.7	13.8	15.0	16.3	17.8
1-1.9	11.8	12.7	13.7	14.8	16.0	17.3	18.7	11.4	12.3	13.4	14.5	15.7	17.1	18.6
2-2.9	12.3	13.2	14.3	15.5	16.7	18.1	19.6	12.0	13.0	14.1	15.3	16.6	18.0	19.6
3-3.9	12.6	13.6	14.7	15.9	17.3	18.8	20.5	12.4	13.5	14.6	15.9	17.4	19.0	20.7
4-4.9	12.8	13.9	15.0	16.3	17.8	19.4	21.3	12.7	13.8	15.1	16.5	18.1	19.9	21.9
5-5.9	13.2	14.2	15.4	16.7	18.4	20.3	22.6	13.1	14.2	15.6	17.1	18.8	20.9	23.3
6-6.9	13.7	14.7	15.9	17.3	19.1	21.5	24.6	13.4	14.6	16.0	17.7	19.6	22.0	24.9
7-7.9	14.2	15.2	16.5	18.0	20.1	22.9	27.2	13.7	15.0	16.5	18.3	20.5	23.2	26.7
8-8.9	14.7	15.7	17.1	18.7	21.0	24.4	30.3	14.1	15.4	17.0	19.0	21.5	24.7	29.0
9-9.9	15.1	16.2	17.7	19.5	22.0	26.0	33.3	14.5	16.0	17.7	19.9	22.7	26.4	31.7
10-10.9	15.6	16.8	18.3	20.3	23.2	27.6	35.8	15.1	16.6	18.4	20.8	23.9	28.1	34.5
11-11.9	16.2	17.5	19.2	21.4	24.4	29.1	37.5	15.8	17.4	19.3	21.8	25.1	29.8	37.1
12-12.9	16.9	18.3	20.2	22.6	25.8	30.6	38.5	16.7	18.2	20.2	22.8	26.3	31.3	39.4
13-13.9	17.7	19.4	21.4	23.9	27.3	32.0	39.2	17.5	19.1	21.1	23.8	27.4	32.6	41.0
14-14.9	18.8	20.5	22.6	25.2	28.7	33.4	40.0	18.2	19.8	21.9	24.6	28.2	33.5	42.2
15-15.9	19.8	21.6	23.8	26.5	30.0	34.6	40.9	18.8	20.4	22.5	25.2	28.9	34.2	43.1
16-16.9	20.9	22.7	24.9	27.6	31.1	35.6	42.1	19.2	20.9	22.9	25.7	29.4	34.8	43.8
17-17.9	21.8	23.6	25.8	28.5	32.0	36.7	43.2	19.4	21.1	23.2	26.0	29.7	35.3	44.6
18-19	22.5	24.3	26.5	29.3	32.8	37.5	44.2	19.6	21.3	23.4	26.2	30.0	35.7	45.6

Chart created by averaging monthly data by year from the following sources.
Data from 3 months to 5 years is based on WHO and 5 to 18 years is based on Mramba et al.; World Health Organization. Child growth standards. http://www.who.int/childgrowth/standards/en/; Mramba L, Ngari M, Nwangome M, et al. A growth reference for mid upper arm circumference for age among school age children and adolescents, and validation for mortality: growth curve construction and longitudinal cohort study. *BMJ*. 2017;358:j3423.

fat changes. These measurements assess current nutritional status and body composition, providing an index of body energy stores. They can be used in conjunction with weight-for-age or height-for-age to determine chronic undernutrition and to better assess the body composition of an athletic child who may have an elevated BMI-for-age but low adipose stores.

Interpretation. An estimate of body fat (BF) can be calculated using one or more skinfold measurements and a variety of tested equations.[28] The Slaughter equation, shown here, has been widely used in the United States.[29]

BF% for children with triceps and subscapular skinfolds <35 mm:

$$\text{Boys} = 1.21\ (\text{Sum of 2 skinfolds}) - 0.008\ (\text{Sum of 2 skinfolds}^2) - 1.7$$

$$\text{Girls} = 1.33\ (\text{Sum of 2 skinfolds}) - 0.013\ (\text{Sum of 2 skinfolds}^2) - 2.5$$

BF% for children with triceps and subscapular skinfolds >35 mm:

$$\text{Boys} = 0.783\ (\text{Sum of 2 skinfolds}) - 1.7$$

$$\text{Girls} = 0.546\ (\text{Sum of 2 skinfolds}) + 9.7$$

Measurements of triceps skinfold from childhood through adult life were compiled by Frisancho using large samples of American children throughout the United States[30] (Table 2.10).

Arm Muscle Circumference, Arm Fat Area, and Arm Muscle Area

In conjunction with triceps skinfold thickness, MUAC can be used to determine cross-sectional mid-arm muscle and fat areas.

Interpretation. Percentiles for arm muscle circumference, arm fat area, and arm muscle area were also compiled by Frisancho[30] (see Tables 2.11 and 2.12). Calculations for mid-arm muscle circumference (MAMC), mid-arm muscle area (MAMA), and arm fat area (AFA) are provided here (Note: units must be converted to centimeters for comparison with Table 2.9).

$$\text{MAMC (cm)} = \text{MUAC (cm)} - [\pi \times \text{TSF (cm)}]$$

$$\text{MAMA (cm}^2) = [\text{MUAC (cm)} - \pi \times \text{TSF (cm)}]^2/4\pi$$

$$\text{AFA (cm}^2) = [\text{MUAC (cm)}]^2/4\pi - \text{MAMA}$$

$$\text{TSF} = \text{triceps skinfold}$$

$$\text{MUAC} = \text{mid-upper arm circumference}$$

■ BONE AGE

Epiphyseal closure is a measure of skeletal maturation. Radiographs of the hand and wrist are generally used for convenient determination of this measure. The percentage of maturity can be used to estimate the potential for "catch-up" growth. Measurements

TABLE 2.10 PERCENTILE FOR TRICEPS SKINFOLD (MM^2)[30]

	MALE								FEMALE							
AGE GROUP (Y)	*N*	5	10	25	50	75	90	95	N	5	10	25	50	75	90	95
1-1.9	228	6	7	8	10	12	14	16	204	6	7	8	10	12	14	16
2-2.9	223	6	7	8	10	12	14	15	208	6	8	9	10	12	15	16
3-3.9	220	6	7	8	10	11	14	15	208	7	8	9	11	12	14	15
4-4.9	230	6	6	8	9	11	12	14	208	7	8	8	10	12	14	16
5-5.9	214	6	6	8	9	11	14	15	219	6	7	8	10	12	15	18
6-6.9	117	5	6	7	8	10	13	16	118	6	6	8	10	12	14	16
7-7.9	122	5	6	7	9	12	15	17	126	6	7	9	11	13	16	18
8-8.9	117	5	6	7	8	10	13	16	118	6	8	9	12	15	18	24
9-9.9	121	6	6	7	10	13	17	18	125	8	8	10	13	16	20	22
10-10.9	146	6	6	8	10	14	18	21	152	7	8	10	12	17	23	27
11-11.9	122	6	6	8	11	16	20	24	117	7	8	10	13	18	24	28
12-12.9	153	6	6	8	11	14	22	28	129	8	9	11	14	18	23	27
13-13.9	134	5	5	7	10	14	22	26	151	8	8	12	15	21	26	30
14-14.9	131	4	5	7	9	14	21	24	141	9	10	13	16	21	26	28
15-15.9	128	4	5	6	8	11	18	24	117	8	10	12	17	21	25	32
16-16.9	131	4	5	6	8	12	16	22	142	10	12	15	18	22	26	31
17-17.9	133	5	5	6	8	12	16	19	114	10	12	13	19	24	30	37
18-18.9	91	4	5	6	9	13	20	24	109	10	12	15	18	22	26	30
19-24.9	531	4	5	7	10	15	20	22	1,060	10	11	14	18	24	30	34

Data collected from Whites in the United States Health and Nutrition Examination Survey 1 (1971-1974).

TABLE 2.11 PERCENTILES FOR ESTIMATED UPPER ARM MUSCLE CIRCUMFERENCE (MM)[30]

	MALES							FEMALES						
AGE GROUPS (Y)	5	10	25	50	75	90	95	5	10	25	50	75	90	95
1-1.9	110	113	119	127	135	144	147	105	111	117	124	132	139	143
2-2.9	111	114	122	130	140	146	150	111	114	119	126	133	142	147
3-3.9	117	123	131	137	143	148	153	113	119	124	132	140	146	152
4-4.9	123	126	133	141	148	156	159	115	121	128	136	144	152	157
5-5.9	128	133	140	147	154	162	169	125	128	134	142	151	159	165
6-6.9	131	135	142	151	161	170	177	130	133	138	145	154	166	171
7-7.9	137	139	151	160	168	177	190	129	135	142	151	160	171	176
8-8.9	140	145	154	162	170	182	187	138	140	151	160	171	183	194
9-9.9	151	154	161	170	183	196	202	147	150	158	167	180	194	198
10-10.9	156	160	166	180	191	209	221	148	150	159	170	180	190	197
11-11.9	159	165	173	183	195	205	230	150	158	171	181	196	217	223
12-12.9	167	171	182	195	210	223	241	162	166	180	191	201	214	220
13-13.9	172	179	196	211	226	238	245	169	175	183	198	211	226	240
14-14.9	189	199	212	223	240	260	264	174	179	190	201	216	232	247
15-15.9	199	204	218	237	254	266	272	175	178	189	202	215	228	244
16-16.9	213	225	234	249	269	287	296	170	180	190	202	216	234	249
17-17.9	224	231	245	258	273	294	312	175	183	194	205	221	239	257
18-18.9	226	237	252	264	283	298	324	174	179	191	202	215	237	245
19-24.9	238	245	257	273	289	309	321	179	185	195	207	221	236	249

TABLE 2.12 PERCENTILES FOR ESTIMATES OF UPPER ARM FAT AREA AND UPPER ARM MUSCLE AREA[30]

AGE GROUP (Y)	ARM MUSCLE AREA PERCENTILES (MM²)							ARM FAT AREA PERCENTILES (MM²)						
	5	10	25	50	75	90	95	5	10	25	50	75	90	95
							Male							
1-1.9	956	1,014	1,133	1,278	1,447	1,644	1,720	452	486	590	741	895	1,036	1,176
2-2.9	973	1,040	1,190	1,345	1,557	1,690	1,787	434	504	578	737	871	1,044	1,148
3-3.9	1,095	1,201	1,357	1,484	1,618	1,750	1,853	464	519	590	736	868	1,071	1,151
4-4.9	1,207	1,264	1,408	1,579	1,747	1,926	2,008	428	494	598	722	859	989	1,085
5-5.9	1,298	1,411	1,550	1,720	1,884	2,089	2,285	446	488	582	713	914	1,176	1,299
6-6.9	1,360	1,447	1,605	1,815	2,056	2,297	2,493	371	446	539	678	896	1,115	1,519
7-7.9	1,497	1,548	1,808	2,027	2,246	2,494	2,886	423	473	574	758	1,011	1,393	1,511
8-8.9	1,550	1,664	1,895	2,089	2,296	2,628	2,788	410	460	588	725	1,003	1,248	1,558
9-9.9	1,181	1,884	2,067	2,288	2,657	3,053	3,257	485	527	635	859	1,252	1,864	2,081
10-10.9	1,930	2,027	2,182	2,575	2,903	3,486	3,882	523	543	738	982	1,376	1,906	2,609
11-11.9	2,016	2,156	2,382	2,670	3,022	3,359	4,226	536	695	754	1,148	1,710	2,348	2,574
12-12.9	2,216	2,339	2,649	3,022	3,496	3,968	4,640	544	650	874	1,172	1,558	2,536	3,580
13-13.9	2,363	2,546	3,044	3,553	4,081	4,502	4,794	475	570	812	1,096	1,702	2,744	3,322
14-14.9	2,830	3,147	3,586	3,963	4,575	5,368	5,530	453	563	786	1,082	1,608	2,746	3,508
15-15.9	3,138	3,317	3,788	4,481	5,134	5,631	5,900	521	595	690	931	1,423	2,434	3,100

16-16.9	3,625	4,044	4,352	4,951	5,753	6,576	6,980	542	593	844	1,078	1,746	2,280	3,041
17-17.9	3,998	4,252	4,777	5,286	5,950	6,886	7,726	598	698	827	1,096	1,636	2,407	2,888
18-18.9	4,070	4,481	5,066	5,552	6,374	7,067	8,355	560	665	860	1,264	1,947	3,302	3,928
19-24.9	4,508	4,777	5,274	5,913	6,660	7,606	8,200	594	743	963	1,406	2,231	3,098	3,652
Female														
1-1.9	885	973	1,084	1,221	1,378	1,535	1,621	401	466	578	706	847	1,022	1,140
2-2.9	973	1,029	1,119	1,269	1,405	1,595	1,727	469	526	642	747	894	1,061	1,173
3-3.9	1,014	1,133	1,227	1,396	1,563	1,690	1,846	473	529	656	822	967	1,106	1,158
4-4.9	1,058	1,171	1,313	1,475	1,644	1,832	1,958	490	541	654	766	907	1,109	1,236
5-5.9	1,238	1,301	1,423	1,598	1,825	2,012	2,159	470	529	647	812	991	1,330	1,536
6-6.9	1,354	1,414	1,513	1,683	1,877	2,182	2,323	464	508	638	827	1,009	1,263	1,436
7-7.9	1,330	1,441	1,602	1,815	2,045	2,332	2,469	491	560	706	920	1,135	1,407	1,644
8-8.9	1,513	1,566	1,808	2,034	2,327	2,657	2,996	527	634	769	1,042	1,383	1,872	2,482
9-9.9	1,723	1,788	1,976	2,227	2,571	2,987	3,112	642	690	933	1,219	1,584	2,171	2,524
10-10.9	1,740	1,784	2,019	2,296	2,583	2,873	3,093	616	702	842	1,141	1,608	2,500	3,005
11-11.9	1,784	1,987	2,316	2,612	3,071	3,739	3,953	707	802	1,015	1,301	1,942	2,730	3,690
12-12.9	2,092	2,182	2,579	2,904	3,225	3,655	3,847	782	854	1,090	1,511	2,056	2,666	3,369
13-13.9	2,269	2,426	2,657	3,130	3,529	4,081	4,568	726	838	1,219	1,625	2,374	3,272	4,150
14-14.9	2,418	2,562	2,874	3,220	3,704	4,294	4,850	981	1,043	1,423	1,818	2,403	3,250	3,765
15-15.9	2,426	2,518	2,847	3,248	3,689	4,123	4,756	839	1,126	1,396	1,886	2,544	3,093	4,195
16-16.9	2,308	2,567	2,865	3,248	3,718	4,353	4,946	1,126	1,351	1,663	2,006	2,598	3,374	4,236
17-17.9	2,442	2,674	2,996	3,336	3,883	4,552	5,251	1,042	1,267	1,463	2,104	2,977	3,864	5,159
18-18.9	2,398	2,538	2,917	3,243	3,694	4,461	4,767	1,003	1,230	1,616	2,104	2,617	3,508	3,733
19-24.9	2,538	2,728	3,026	3,406	3,877	4,439	4,940	1,046	1,198	1,596	2,166	2,959	4,050	4,896

for epiphyseal closure can be found in the Radiographic Atlas of Skeletal Development of the Hand and Wrist by Greulich and Pyle.[31] Skeletal age is typically advanced in cases of overnutrition and delayed in conditions where linear growth is slowed due to malnutrition. The success of "catch-up" growth depends on the duration and age at which slowed growth occurs, as well as the adequacy of nutritional repletion. Appropriate treatment of underlying medical problems may also increase the likelihood of maximum growth potential. During "catch-up" growth, height velocity may be twice the average for age and sex, and weight velocity may be 4 times the average for age and sex; the rate of skeletal maturation also increases.[31]

SEXUAL MATURATION

During adolescence, growth in height and weight accelerates, followed by a rapid deceleration after sexual maturation. Assessing sexual maturation helps determine an adolescent's pubertal progression and provides insight into expected growth velocity and body composition. Tanner's stages of sexual development provide a clinical rating scale (1 = preadolescent, 5 = mature) for comparing development. While the age of these events varies, the sequence remains relatively consistent. Refer to Chapter 8 for further information. Clinical judgment must be used when assessing nonbinary and transgender adolescents.

REFERENCES

1. National Center for Health Statistics. *National Health and Nutrition Examination Survey: Anthropometry Procedures Manual*. Centers for Disease Control and Prevention. https://wwwn.cdc.gov/nchs/data/nhanes/public/2011/manuals/Anthropometry_Procedures_Manual.pdf
2. Weidauer L, Wey H, Slater H, Moyer-Mileur L, Specker B. Estimation of length or height in infants and young children using ulnar and lower leg length with dual-energy X-ray absorptiometry validation. *Dev Med Child Neurol*. 2014;56(10):995-1000.
3. World Health Organization. Child growth standards. http://www.who.int/childgrowth/standards/en/
4. National Center for Health Statistics. 2000 CDC growth charts: United States. http://www.cdc.gov/growthcharts/
5. Becker P, Carney LN, Corkins MR, et al. Consensus statement of the Academy of Nutrition and Dietetics/American Society for Parenteral and Enteral Nutrition: indicators recommended for the identification and documentation of pediatric malnutrition (undernutrition). *J Acad Nutr Diet*. 2014;114(12):1988-2000.
6. Mramba L, Ngari M, Nwangome M, et al. A growth reference for mid upper arm circumference for age among school age children and adolescents, and validation for mortality: growth curve construction and longitudinal cohort study. *BMJ*. 2017;358:j3423.
7. Dibley MJ, Staehling N, Nieburg P, Trowbridge FL. Interpretation of Z-score anthropometric indicators derived from the international growth reference. *Am J Clin Nutr*. 1987;46(5):749-762.
8. Gomez F, Galvan RR, Cravioto J, Frenk S. Malnutrition in infancy and childhood, with special reference to kwashiorkor. *Adv Pediatr*. 1955;7:131-169.
9. Waterlow JC. Classification and definition of protein-calorie malnutrition. *Br Med J*. 1972;3(5826):566-569.
10. World Health Organization. WHO child growth standards: head circumference-for-age, arm circumference-for-age, triceps skinfold-for-age and subscapular skinfold-for-age: methods and development. 2007. https://www.who.int/publications/i/item/9789241547185
11. Goldberg DL, Becker PJ, Brigham K, et al. Identifying malnutrition in preterm and neonatal populations: recommended indicators. *J Acad Nutr Diet*. 2018;118(9):1571-1582.
12. World Health Organization/UNICEF. WHO child growth standards and the identification of severe acute malnutrition in infants and children: a joint statement by the World Health Organization and the United Nations Children's Fund. 2009. https://www.who.int/publications/i/item/9789241598163

13. World Health Organization. *Training Course on Child Growth Assessment: WHO Child Growth Standards*. World Health Organization; 2008.
14. Hampl SE, Hassink SG, Skinner AC, et al. Clinical practice guideline for the evaluation and treatment of children and adolescents with obesity. *Pediatrics*. 2023;151(2):e2022060641.
15. DeTallo C, Freeman H, Klein B, et al. *The Practitioner's Guide to Nutrition-Focused Physical Exam of Infants, Children, and Adolescents*. 1st ed. American Society for Parenteral & Enteral Nutrition; 2019.
16. Delgado NB, Hastings E, Kommes K, et al., eds. *Texas Children's Hospital Pediatric Nutrition Reference Guide*. 13th ed. Texas Children's Hospital; 2022.
17. Tanner JM, Goldstein H, Whitehouse RH. Standards for children's height at ages 2-9 years allowing for heights of parents. *Arch Dis Child*. 1970;45:755-762.
18. Rumapea F, Fadlyana E, Dhamayanti M, Tarigan R, Rahmayani R, Rusmil K. Height prediction using the knee height measurement among Indonesian children. *Food Nutr Bull*. 2021;42(2):247-258.
19. Chumlea WC, Guo SS, Steinbaugh ML. Prediction of stature from knee height for black and white adults and children with application to mobility-impaired or handicapped persons. *J Am Diet Assoc*. 1994;94(12):1385-1388, 1391; quiz 1389-1390.
20. Stevenson RD. Use of segmental measures to estimate stature in children with cerebral palsy. *Arch Pediatr Adolesc Med*. 1995;149(6):658-662.
21. Gauld LM, Kappers J, Carlin JB, Robertson CF. Height prediction from ulna length. *Dev Med Child Neurol*. 2004;46(7):475-480.
22. Gauld L, Keeling L, Sly P, Shakleton C. Predicting height from ulna length in 2-6 year olds. *Eur Respir J*. 2014;42(suppl 57):P1265.
23. Rasouli MA, Newth CJL, Khemani RG, Ross PA. Predicting body height in a pediatric intensive care unit using ulnar length. *Front Pediatr*. 2018;6:187.
24. Freedman DS, Mei Z, Srinivasan SR, Berenson GS, Dietz WH. Cardiovascular risk factors and excess adiposity among overweight children and adolescents: the Bogalusa Heart Study. *J Pediatr*. 2007;150(1):12-17.e2.
25. Kuczmarski RJ, Ogden CL, Grummer-Strawn LM, et al. CDC growth charts: United States. *Adv Data*. 2000;314:1-27.
26. Berkley J, Mwangi I, Griffiths K, Ahmed I, Mithwani S, English M, et al. Assessment of Severe Malnutrition Among Hospitalized Children in Rural Kenya. *JAMA*. 2005;294(5):591-597.
27. Ellis KJ. Human body composition: in vivo methods. *Physiol Rev*. 2000;80(2):649-680.
28. Reilly JJ, Wilson J, Durnin JV. Determination of body composition from skinfold thickness: a validation study. *Arch Dis Child*. 1995;73(4):305-310.
29. Slaughter MH, Lohman TG, Boileau RA, et al. Skinfold equations for estimation of body fatness in children and youth. *Hum Biol*. 1988;60:709-723.
30. Frisancho AR. New norms of upper limb fat and muscle areas for assessment of nutritional status. *Am J Clin Nutr*. 1981;34(11):2540-2545.
31. Greulich WW, Pyle SI. *Radiographic Atlas of Skeletal Development of the Hand and Wrist*. 2nd ed. Stanford University Press; 1959.

CHAPTER 3

Nutrition Assessment: Clinical Evaluation

Sara Farnan Colleary and Amy M. Turner

Assessment of nutritional status is an essential part of clinical evaluation in the pediatric setting, as children are undergoing rapid growth and development.[1] While severe nutritional deficiencies are often easily identified, less severe deficiencies may present with more subtle or nonspecific physical signs. Physical examination findings suggestive of nutrient deficiencies or excesses should be clearly documented in detail and confirmed by biochemical, anthropometric, and dietary evaluation. Table 3.1 provides an overview of essential nutrients, including their major physiologic functions, signs of deficiency, signs of excess, important food sources, potential causes of deficiency, and status assessment. Recommended intakes for all nutrients are detailed in Chapter 5.

TABLE 3.1 CLINICAL EXAMINATION IN NUTRITIONAL DEFICIENCIES AND EXCESSES

	MAJOR PHYSIOLOGIC FUNCTIONS	DEFICIENCY SIGNS	EXCESS SIGNS	IMPORTANT FOOD SOURCES	POTENTIAL CAUSES OF DEFICIENCY	STATUS ASSESSMENT
Macronutrients						
Carbohydrate	• Supplies energy at an average of 4 kcal/g (sparing protein) • Major energy source for CNS function • Helps control blood glucose and insulin metabolism • Unrefined, complex carbohydrates supply fiber, which aids in normal bowel function	Ketosis	Lipid abnormalities, poor metabolic health, weight gain	Fruits, vegetables, legumes, grains (bread, cereal, crackers, rice), sugars (glucose, fructose, lactose, sucrose), milk, breast milk, infant formula	Malabsorption, restriction, metabolic disorders	Blood sugar, OGTT
Fat	• Concentrated calorie source that supplies energy at an average of 9 kcal/g • Constitutes part of the membrane structure of every cell • Protects organs • Supplies essential fatty acids • Produces hormones • Provides and carries fat-soluble vitamins	Dietary fat deficiency can lead to dry, scaly skin, poor wound healing, brittle nails, poor weight gain, and hair loss; essential fatty acid deficiency can lead to adverse effects on brain development/cognition and impaired immune function.	Atherosclerosis, lipid abnormalities, weight gain	Protein-rich foods (meat, dairy, nuts, seeds, fish), oil, butter, margarine, breast milk, infant formula	Cystic fibrosis, biliary disease, short bowel syndrome, hereditary lipoprotein disorders	Total cholesterol, LDL, HDL, triglycerides

(*continued*)

TABLE 3.1 CLINICAL EXAMINATION IN NUTRITIONAL DEFICIENCIES AND EXCESSES (*continued*)

	MAJOR PHYSIOLOGIC FUNCTIONS	DEFICIENCY SIGNS	EXCESS SIGNS	IMPORTANT FOOD SOURCES	POTENTIAL CAUSES OF DEFICIENCY	STATUS ASSESSMENT
Protein	• Supplies energy at an average of 4 kcal/g • Regulates body processes as part of enzymes, hormones, body fluids, and antibodies that increase resistance to infection • Provides nitrogen • Aids in wound healing and tissue regeneration • Constitutes part of the membrane structure of every cell	Dry (depigmented, easily pluckable) hair, dry skin (with pellagroid dermatosis in severe cases), bilateral dependent edema, cirrhosis, fatty liver, decreased visceral proteins	Azotemia, acidosis, hyperammonemia	Meat, poultry, fish, legumes, eggs, cheese, milk and other dairy products, nuts, breast milk, infant formula	Protein-losing enteropathy, liver disease, gastrointestinal disease, renal disease	Albumin, retinol-binding protein, prealbumin
Fat-soluble vitamins						
Vitamin A	• Important in the formation and maintenance of skin and mucous membranes • Precursor to rhodopsin, which is responsible for vision in dim light and in color • Aids in the regulation of membrane structure and function • Necessary for growth and normal immune function	Night blindness, degeneration of the retina, xerophthalmia, keratomalacia, Bitot spots, follicular hyperkeratosis, poor growth, thyroid dysfunction	Fatigue, malaise, lethargy, abdominal pain, dry skin, hepatomegaly, alopecia, headache with increased intracranial pressure	Beta carotene: Carrots, green vegetables, sweet potatoes, apricots, melons, peaches; Retinol: liver, fortified cereal, eggs, butter, breast milk, infant formula	Liver disease, pancreatic disease, cystic fibrosis, short bowel syndrome, inflammatory bowel disease, protein deficiency (alters transport)	Plasma retinol (HPLC), plasma retinol-binding protein, relative dose response, dark adaptation test, liver biopsy concentration

Vitamin D	• Promotes intestinal absorption of calcium and phosphate, and renal conservation of calcium and phosphorus • Essential for bone mineralization	Rickets, osteomalacia, costochondral beading, epiphyseal enlargement, cranial bossing, bowed legs, persistently open anterior fontanel	Hypercalcemia, vomiting, anorexia, diarrhea, convulsions	Fish liver oil, fish (tuna, mackerel, salmon, herring, sardines), eggs, liver, certain fortified foods (milk, soy milk, orange juice, cereal, infant formula), sunlight (activation of 7-dehydrocholesterol in the skin)	Liver disease, cystic fibrosis, short bowel syndrome, renal disease, lack of exposure to sunlight, exclusive breastfeeding (not on supplementation)	Plasma 25-hydroxy vitamin D (HPLC), serum alkaline phosphatase, calcium and phosphate, radiography, bone densitometry
Vitamin E	• Acts as an antioxidant and free radical scavenger to prevent peroxidation of polyunsaturated fatty acids in the body • Aids in neuromuscular function • Assists in immune response	Hemolytic anemia in premature infants and newborns, enhanced fragility of red blood cells, increased peroxidative hemolysis, neurologic symptoms (impaired balance, peripheral neuropathy, muscle weakness, retinopathy)	Impaired blood clotting and increased risk of hemorrhage	Oils high in polyunsaturated fatty acids (olive, safflower, sunflower), tree nuts, peanuts, spinach, *carrots, avocado*, milk, eggs, breast milk, infant formula	Cystic fibrosis, short bowel syndrome, liver disease	Plasma tocopherol (HPLC) (corrected for total or LDL-cholesterol), hydrogen peroxide hemolysis
Vitamin K	• Necessary for prothrombin and the three blood clotting factors VII, IX, and X • Necessary for bone mineralization • Half of the vitamin K in humans is of intestinal origin, synthesized by gut flora	Hemorrhagic manifestations (especially in newborns), prolonged clotting	Hemolytic anemia, nerve palsy, liver toxicity, oxidative damage to cells	Green leafy vegetables, peas, fruits, cereals, cashews, oils (soybean, canola, olive), dairy products, soybeans, naturally fermented foods, breast milk, infant formula	Liver disease, fat malabsorption disorders, antibiotic therapy, medical therapy with vitamin K antagonists	Prothrombin time (prolonged), plasma phylloquinone, clotting factor levels, proteins induced by vitamin K absence or antagonists-II (PIVKA-II)

(*continued*)

TABLE 3.1 CLINICAL EXAMINATION IN NUTRITIONAL DEFICIENCIES AND EXCESSES (*continued*)

	MAJOR PHYSIOLOGIC FUNCTIONS	DEFICIENCY SIGNS	EXCESS SIGNS	IMPORTANT FOOD SOURCES	POTENTIAL CAUSES OF DEFICIENCY	STATUS ASSESSMENT
Water-soluble vitamins						
Ascorbic acid (vitamin C)	• Forms collagen cross-linkage of proline hydroxylase, thus strengthening tissue and improving wound healing and resistance to infection • Aids absorption of iron • Antioxidant in cells and blood • Assists in the production of adrenaline, carnitine, collagen, and serotonin	Joint tenderness, scurvy (capillary hemorrhaging), impaired wound healing, acute periodontal gingivitis, petechiae, purpura, anemia	Chronic high doses of vitamin C may result in "rebound" deficiency symptoms when supplements are stopped	Guava, papaya, orange, mango, grapefruit, strawberries, tomatoes, peppers, potatoes, leafy vegetables, broccoli, breast milk, infant formula	Oxidative stress, iron overload, diarrhea	Plasma level (enzyme assay/HPLC), leukocyte concentration (longer term), whole blood concentration, urine concentration
Biotin (B_7)	• Component of several carboxylating enzymes • Plays an important role in the metabolism of fat and carbohydrates • Assists in glucose production	Anorexia, nausea, vomiting, glossitis, depression, dry scaly dermatitis, thin hair, loss of eyebrows		Liver, kidney, pork, egg yolk, avocado, whole wheat bread, yeast, cheese, breast milk, infant formula	Certain inborn errors of metabolism	Plasma (microbiologic plasma lactate assay), urine organic acids, lymphocyte carboxylase
Cobalamin (B_{12})	• Cobalamin-containing coenzymes function in the degradation of certain odd-chain fatty acids and in the recycling of tetrahydrofolate • Plays a role in nerve function • Assists with red blood cell production • Assists in releasing energy from protein and fat	Megaloblastic anemia, neurologic deterioration		Animal products (meat, fish), milk, cheese, eggs, fortified cereal, breast milk, infant formula	Ileal disease, strict vegetarian diet, lack of intrinsic factor, pernicious anemia, atrophic gastritis	Plasma level (RIA or microbiologic), Schilling test, plasma homocysteine, deoxyuridine suppression test

Folate (B_9)	• Utilized in carbon transfer and nucleotide synthesis • Assists in producing red blood cells • Prevents neural tube defects	Megaloblastic anemia, stomatitis, glossitis, neural tube defects in pregnancy		Liver, chicken, leafy vegetables, asparagus, peas, beans, lentils, fruit, yeast, breast milk, infant formula	Liver disease, alcoholism, celiac disease, inflammatory bowel disease	Plasma level (RIA or microbiologic), red cell level
Niacin (B_3)	• Aids in energy utilization as part of a coenzyme (NAD^+ and $NADP^+$) in fat synthesis, tissue respiration, and carbohydrate utilization • Aids digestion and fosters normal appetite; synthesized from the amino acid tryptophan	Pellagra (dermatitis, diarrhea, dementia, death), cheilosis, angular stomatitis, inflammation of mucous membranes, weakness	Flushing, gastrointestinal disturbances (nausea/vomiting), pruritus, skin rashes, some reports of hypotension	Liver, meat, fish, poultry, peanuts, avocado, mushrooms, fortified cereal products, yeast, breast milk, infant formula	B_6 deficiency (impairs conversion of tryptophan to niacin), chronic alcoholism	Urine ratio of metabolites (*N*-methylnicotinamide/2-pyridone), tryptophan load, red cell NAD or NAD/NADP ratio
Pantothenic acid (B_5)	• Component of coenzyme A • Plays a role in the release of energy from carbohydrates and in the synthesis and degradation of fatty acids • Assists in the synthesis of fat, steroid hormones, cholesterol, and hemoglobin	Slow growth, depression, vomiting, malaise, abdominal stress, numbness of hands and feet, headache, insomnia	Diarrhea, water retention	Meat, fish, poultry, whole grains, legumes, lentils, eggs, sweet potatoes, avocado, broccoli, peas, mushrooms, yogurt, milk, breast milk, infant formula	Severe malnutrition	Urine excretion, whole blood level (RIA/microbiologic)
Pyridoxine (B_6)	• Coenzyme component for many of the enzymes of amino acid metabolism • All compounds implicated as neurotransmitters are synthesized and/or metabolized in B_6-dependent reactions. • Aids in the production of hemoglobin and DNA	Convulsions, weight loss, abdominal distress, vomiting, hyperirritability, depression, confusion, oral ulcers, hypochromic and macrocytic anemia	Neuropathy	Fish, poultry, meat, hazelnuts, walnuts, beans, prunes, bananas, potatoes, wheat, fortified cereal, breast milk, infant formula	High protein intake, alcoholism	Red cell aminotransferase activity, pyridoxal phosphate (HPLC), tryptophan load test, urine 4-pyridoxic acid

(*continued*)

TABLE 3.1 CLINICAL EXAMINATION IN NUTRITIONAL DEFICIENCIES AND EXCESSES (*continued*)

	MAJOR PHYSIOLOGIC FUNCTIONS	DEFICIENCY SIGNS	EXCESS SIGNS	IMPORTANT FOOD SOURCES	POTENTIAL CAUSES OF DEFICIENCY	STATUS ASSESSMENT
Riboflavin (B_2)	• Functions primarily as the reactive portion of flavoproteins concerned with biologic oxidations (cellular metabolism)	Cheilosis, glossitis, photophobia, angular stomatitis, corneal vascularization, scrotal skin changes, seborrhea, magenta tongue, dermatitis		Dairy products, eggs, liver, clams, chicken, beef, lamb, pork, salmon, almonds, broccoli, spinach, asparagus, fortified cereal, bread, breast milk, infant formula	Alcoholism, starvation, chronic diarrhea, malabsorption, lactose intolerance	Red cell glutathione reductase activity (EGR), red cell flavine adenine dinucleotide, urine riboflavin/creatinine ratio
Thiamine (B_1)	• Aids in energy utilization as part of the coenzyme component to promote the utilization of carbohydrates • Promotes normal functioning of the nervous system • Acts as a coenzyme for the oxidative carboxylation of 2-keto acids	Beriberi, neuritis, cardiac failure, anorexia, restlessness, confusion, loss of vibration sense and deep tendon reflexes, calf tenderness, edema, Wernicke encephalopathy		Pork, nuts, sunflower seeds, beans, lentils, peas, cantaloupe, whole grain and fortified bread and cereal products, brown rice, breast milk, infant formula	Alcoholism, refeeding syndrome, prolonged dialysis	Red cell transketolase activity, whole blood level (HPLC), urine thiamine/creatinine ratio, thiamine diphosphate (TDP)
Minerals						
Calcium	• Essential for calcification of bone (matrix formation) • Assists in blood clotting • Functions in normal muscle contraction and relaxation and in normal nerve transmission	Osteomalacia, osteoporosis, neuromuscular excitability (tetany)	Hypercalcemia, vomiting, anorexia, lethargy, renal stones, metabolic bone disease	Dairy products (milk, cheese), grains, sardines, oysters, salmon, herring, greens, breast milk, infant formula	Renal disease, liver disease	Plasma total calcium, plasma free calcium in altered protein binding (e.g., hypoalbuminemia), acidosis, radiographs, CT, photon densitometry

Magnesium	• Essential part of many enzyme systems • Important for maintaining electrical potential in nerves and muscle membranes and for energy turnover	Tremor, convulsions, hyperexcitability (hypocalcemia tetany)	Diarrhea, transient hypocalcemia, muscle weakness	Green leafy vegetables, whole grains, breast milk, infant formula	Protein-calorie malnutrition, refeeding syndrome, calcineurin inhibitors, loop and thiazide diuretics	Plasma total or free magnesium, magnesium loading test
Phosphorus	• Important intracellular anion • Involved in many chemical reactions within the body • Necessary for energy turnover (ATP)	Muscle weakness, anorexia, malaise, bone pain, growth arrest	Altered calcium metabolism	Dairy products, fish, legumes, pork, eggs, breast milk, infant formula	Renal disease, starvation, refeeding syndrome	Plasma concentration, alkaline phosphatase activity, radiography, densitometry, renal tubular excretion threshold
Trace elements						
Chromium	• Important for the maintenance of normal glucose metabolism • Cofactor for insulin	Disturbed glucose metabolism (lower glucose tolerance caused by insulin resistance)		Brewer's yeast, meat products, cheeses	Protein-calorie malnutrition, elderly	Plasma chromium, glucose tolerance
Copper	• Constituent of proteins and enzymes, some of which are essential for the proper utilization of iron • Essential for immunity • Important for skeletal development	Anemia (hemolytic), neutropenia, bone disease	Excess accumulation in the liver, brain, kidney, cornea; Wilson disease; anemia, diarrhea	Oysters, nuts, liver, kidney, corn oil, margarine, dried legumes	Chronic diarrhea, chronic dialysis, preterm infant on prolonged parenteral nutrition, excessive Zn ingestion, parenteral nutrition with insufficient copper, foregut surgery, Menkes disease (kinky hair)	Plasma copper, plasma ceruloplasmin (ferrochelatase), 24-h urine copper, liver biopsy concentration, superoxide dismutase activity

(continued)

TABLE 3.1 CLINICAL EXAMINATION IN NUTRITIONAL DEFICIENCIES AND EXCESSES (*continued*)

	MAJOR PHYSIOLOGIC FUNCTIONS	DEFICIENCY SIGNS	EXCESS SIGNS	IMPORTANT FOOD SOURCES	POTENTIAL CAUSES OF DEFICIENCY	STATUS ASSESSMENT
Fluoride	• Incorporated into the crystalline structure of hydroxyapatite in teeth and bones • Strengthens enamel and increases resistance to dental caries	Poor dentition, dental caries	Acute: Gastrointestinal symptoms; Chronic: fluorosis (mottling, brown staining of teeth)	Fluoridated water, black tea, canned crab, cooked rice; content of most other foods geographically dependent	Unfluoridated water, bottled water	
Iodine	• Component of thyroid hormones triiodothyronine and thyroxine • *Important in the regulation of* cellular oxidation and growth	Goiter, depressed thyroid function, cretinism, developmental delay, growth failure	Thyroid suppression (thyrotoxicosis)	Iodized table salt, saltwater, fish, shellfish, eggs, milk, breast milk, infant formula; content of most other foods geographically dependent	Endemic goiter in low iodine areas	Thyroid hormones, TSH, urinary iodide/creatinine ratio
Iron	• Part of the hemoglobin molecule • Prevents nutritional anemia and fatigue • Increases resistance to infection • Functions as part of enzymes involved in tissue respiration	Anemia, malabsorption, irritability, anorexia, pallor, lethargy	Hemosiderosis, hemochromatosis	Red meats, fish, poultry, liver, dried beans and peas, iron-fortified foods, including infant formula and cereals	Protein-losing enteropathy, malabsorption, acute or chronic blood loss, pica	Plasma iron and ferritin, total iron-binding capacity, transferrin, hemoglobin/hematocrit, red cell indices, RBC zinc protoporphyrin:heme ratio, bone marrow aspirate stain

Manganese	• Essential part of several enzyme systems involved in protein and energy metabolism and in the formation of mucopolysaccharide		In extremely high exposure to contamination: severe psychiatric and neurologic disorders	Nuts, whole grains, dried fruits, fruits, green leafy vegetables		Plasma level, whole blood level, mitochondrial superoxide dismutase
Molybdenum	• Essential for the function of flavin-dependent enzymes involved in the production of uric acid and in the oxidation of aldehydes and sulfites	Very rare and not a concern in humans	Gout-like syndrome associated with elevated blood levels of molybdenum, uric acid, and xanthine oxidase	Meat, grains, legumes; content of most other foods geographically dependent		
Selenium	• Functions as a part of the enzyme glutathione peroxidase, which protects cellular components from oxidative damage	Cardiomyopathy and skeletal muscle dysfunction (likely secondary to oxidative damage)	Nausea, emesis, diarrhea, hair loss, nail changes, mental status changes, visual loss, and peripheral neuropathy	Seafoods, kidney, liver meat, grains (depending on growing environment), nuts	Keshan disease, chronic parenteral nutrition without adequate trace elements	Plasma concentration, glutathione peroxidase activity, nail/hair selenium
Zinc	• Constituent of enzymes involved in most major metabolic pathways (specifically nucleic acid synthesis for growth and repair)	Growth failure, skin changes, delayed wound healing, hypogeusia, sexual immaturity, immune dysfunction, hair loss, diarrhea	Acute gastrointestinal upset, vomiting, sweating, dizziness, copper deficiency	Whole grains, legumes, beef, lamb, pork, poultry, nuts, seeds, shellfish, eggs, some cheeses, breast milk, infant formula	Malabsorption, chronic diarrhea, malnutrition, liver disease, sickle cell disease, prolonged parenteral nutrition, acrodermatitis enteropathica	Plasma concentration, alkaline phosphatase activity, urinary excretion, leukocyte concentration

ATP, adenosine triphosphate; CNS, central nervous system; CT, computed tomography; EGR, erythrocyte glutathione reductase; HDL; high-density lipoprotein; HPLC, high-performance liquid chromatography; LDL, low-density lipoprotein; NAD, nicotinamide adenine dinucleotide; NADP, nicotinamide adenine dinucleotide phosphate; OGTT, oral glucose tolerance test; RIA, radioimmunoassay.

Data from Duggan C, Watkins JB, Koletzko B, et al. Nutrition in Pediatrics: Basic Science and Clinical Applications. 5th ed. People's Medical Publishing House-USA; 2016.

REFERENCE

1. Duggan C, Watkins JB, Koletzko B, Walker WA, eds. *Nutrition in Pediatrics: Basic Science and Clinical Applications*. 5th ed. People's Medical Publishing House; 2016.

CHAPTER 4

Laboratory Assessment of Nutritional Status

Ariana Cerro and Paul McGreggor Crowley

Nutritional assessment in pediatrics largely relies on the food/nutrition-related history and anthropometric measurement methods outlined in the preceding chapters. However, biochemical data, medical tests, and procedures play a complementary role that may be critical in (1) diagnosing subclinical micronutrient deficiencies, (2) confirming nutritional deficiency suggested by clinical assessment, and (3) providing baseline and serial data with which to monitor response to nutritional interventions. Reference ranges of various laboratory nutritional parameters are included in Table 4.1.

PROTEINS

Plasma Proteins

Plasma proteins like albumin, prealbumin, retinol-binding protein (RBP), and transferrin are commonly used as markers to assess nutritional status, particularly in the context of protein-energy malnutrition. Proteins synthesized by the liver are subject to influences other than nutritional status, particularly the presence of an inflammatory state and fluid shifts. The concentrations of positive acute-phase proteins are increased in infectious or other catabolic illnesses due to preferential secretion by the liver. Conversely, negative acute-phase proteins are decreased in these circumstances. The magnitude of a positive acute-phase response is attenuated in protein-energy malnutrition.[1]

Albumin

Albumin has historically been the most used biochemical marker to assess protein status as it is the most abundant protein in blood and the least expensive and easiest to measure. Since more than half of body albumin is extravascular (primarily in skin and muscle), maintenance of normal plasma levels can occur from mobilization of these stores, despite prolonged energy or protein inadequacy. Combined with its long half-life of 20 days, these factors make serum albumin an insensitive marker of nutritional status and an insensitive measure of nutritional recovery.

Hypoalbuminemia is not specific for malnutrition and can also be seen in situations of decreased synthesis (e.g., in people with liver disease or >70 years of age), increased losses (e.g., nephrosis, protein-losing enteropathy, burn injuries), or increased losses to extravascular spaces (e.g., acute catabolic stress with capillary leak). Fluid overload can also dilute albumin concentrations, and bed rest can decrease levels by 0.5 g/dL over several days due to redistribution into tissues.

TABLE 4.1 REFERENCE RANGES OF SELECT NUTRITIONAL LABORATORY VALUES

NUTRIENT	AGE	ALL	MALES	FEMALES
Albumin (g/dL)	<15 d	3.3-4.5		
	15 d-<1 y	2.8-4.7		
	1-<8 y	3.8-4.7		
	8-<15 y	4.1-4.8		
	15-<19 y		4.1-5.1	4.0-4.9
Alkaline phosphatase (U/L)	1-<15 d	90-273		
	15 d-<1 y	134-518		
	1-<10 y	156-369		
	10 to <13 y	141-460		
	13-<15 y		127-517	62-280
	15-<17 y		89-365	54-128
	17-<19 y		59-164	48-95
Ammonia, plasma (µmol/L)	Newborn	<50		
	Child and adult	<35		
Calcium (mg/dL)	1-<1 y	8.5-11		
	1-<19 y	9.2-10.5		
Calcium, ionized whole blood (mmol/L)	0-1 mo	1.0-1.5		
	1-6 mo	0.95-1.5		
	1-17 y	1.22-1.37		
Carnitine, total, fasting (µmol/L)	0-<1 y	23-77		
	1-<12 y	28-61		
	12-<19 y		32-58	25-52
Ceruloplasmin (mg/L)	0-<2 mo	74-237		
	2-<6 mo	135-329		
	6 mo-<3 y		160-370	180-370
	3-<6 y		180-370	180-360
	6-<9 y		200-450	190-400
	9-<12 y		200-440	200-430
	12-<15 y		170-420	200-410
	15-<18 y		170-420	200-510
Cholesterol (mg/dL)	0-1 y	91-205		
	1-<15 y	104-227		
	15-<19 y		95-208	93-233
Copper (µg/dL)	6 mo-2 y	72-178		
	3-4 y	80-160		
	5-6 y	76-167		

TABLE 4.1 REFERENCE RANGES OF SELECT NUTRITIONAL LABORATORY VALUES (*continued*)

NUTRIENT	AGE	ALL	MALES	FEMALES
	7-8 y	79-147		
	9-10 y	84-154		
	11-12 y	73-149		
	13-14 y	66-137		
	15-16 y	60-132		
	17-18 y	59-146		
Ferritin (ng/mL)	0-<2 wk	69.3-527		
	2 wk-<13 y	9.51-75.6		
	13-<19 y		12.5-114	8.28-70
Folic acid (serum) (nmol/L)	5 d-1 y	23.9-45.3		
	1-3 y	8.7-45.3		
	3-6 y	27-45.3		
	6-8 y	29.7-45.3		
	8-12 y	25.9-45.3		
	12-14 y	27-45.3		
	14-<19 y	18-45.3		
Ammonia, plasma (µmol/L)	Outside neonatal period	73-112		
Growth hormone (unstimulated) (µg/L)	0-<3 mo	0.8-33.54		
	3 mo-<2 y	0.14-6.27		
	2-<7 y	0.05-5.11		
	7-<12 y	0.02-4.76		
	12-<14 y	0.01-6.2		
	14-<19 y		0.02-3.81	0.03-5.22
Hemoglobin (g/dL)	1-3 d		12.8-19.7	12.8-19.2
	4-7 d		13.3-19.3	13.0-19.4
	8-14 d		11.0-17.5	12.0-18.3
	15-30 d		9.8-15.4	10.2-15.8
	31-60 d		9.0-12.9	8.9-12.7
	2-6 mo		10.1-13.2	10.0-14.1
	6 mo-2 y		10.1-13.6	10.1-13.7
	2-6 y		10.2-13.7	10.3-13.7
	6-12 y		10.3-14.3	10.6-14.7
	12-18 y		11.2-16.4	10.4-14.6
	>18 y		12.3-16.9	10.5-14.8

(*continued*)

TABLE 4.1 REFERENCE RANGES OF SELECT NUTRITIONAL LABORATORY VALUES (*continued*)

NUTRIENT	AGE	ALL	MALES	FEMALES
Hemoglobin A1c (%)	Nondiabetic	4.0-6.0		
Homocysteine, total (μmol/L)	5 d-1 y	2.87-10		
	1-7 y	2.76-7.62		
	7-12 y	3.43-8.45		
	12-15 y		4.71-10.4	4.07-10.36
	15-<19 y		5.5-13.39	4.92-11.88
Iron (μg/dL)	0-1 y	20-153		
	1-5 y	9-151		
	6-10 y	6-148		
	11-14 y	19-156		
	15-<19 y	14-156		
Iron-binding capacity (μg/dL)	0-90 d		155-330	165-275
	91 d-1 y		150-380	250-455
	1-3 y		215-420	160-415
	4-10 y		185-415	260-385
	11-14 y		265-410	250-420
	15-<19 y		270-415	285-410
Magnesium (mg/dL)	0-90 d		1.4-2.1	1.5-2.0
	91 d-1 y		1.6-2.5	1.6-2.2
	1-3 y		1.6-2.2	1.5-2.2
	4-10 y		1.5-2.2	1.6-2.5
	11-15 y		1.3-2.0	1.6-2.1
	16-<19 y		1.6-2.1	1.5-1.9
Mean corpuscular volume (MCV) (μm^3)	1-3 d		95.7-110.8	96.4-112.4
	4-7 d		93.0-105.4	91.6-104.1
	8-14 d		91.8-103.5	94.0-105.6
	15-30 d		89.5-101.3	90.0-101.7
	31-60 d		86.2-96.8	86.5-97.2
	2-6 mo		68.2-92.2	74.2-96.9
	6 mo-2 y		68.2-88.4	70.5-87.6
	2-6 y		68.1-87.8	67.8-88.6
	6-12 y		70.2-89.9	70.9-92.7
	12-18 y		74.2-93.7	70.7-96.0
	>18 y		77.3-95.6	73.3-96.9

TABLE 4.1 REFERENCE RANGES OF SELECT NUTRITIONAL LABORATORY VALUES (*continued*)

NUTRIENT	AGE	ALL	MALES	FEMALES
Osmolality (plasma) (mOsm/kg)	1 mo-18 y	280-295		
Phosphate (mg/dL)	0-<15 d	5.6-10.5		
	15 d-<1 y	4.8-8.4		
	1-<5 y	4.3-6.8		
	5-<13 y	4.1-5.9		
	13-<16 y		3.5-6.2	3.2-5.5
	16-<19 y	2.9-5.0		
Potassium (mEq/L)	0-<1 y		4.3-6.7	4.2-6.2
	1 y-<19 y	4.0-5.3		
Prothrombin time (seconds)		11-15		
Prealbumin (transthyretin) (mg/dL)	0-<15 d	2-12		
	15 d-<1 y	5-24		
	1-<5 y	12-23		
	5-<13 y	14-26		
	13-<16 y	18-31		
	16-<19 y		20-35	17-33
Protein, total (g/dL)	0-<15 d	5.3-8.3		
	15 d-<1 y	4.4-7.1		
	1-<6 y	6.1-7.5		
	6-<9 y	6.4-7.7		
	9-<19 y	6.5-8.1		
Retinol-binding protein (RBP) (mg/dL)	0-30 d		0.91-5.6	1.01-5.75
	1 mo-18 y		1.09-8.7	0.98-6.76
Selenium (mg/L)	<1 mo	15-106.3		
	1-2 mo	15-100		
	2-4 mo	10.2-92.9		
	4-12 mo	13.4-115.7		
	1-5 y	33.9-128.3		
	5-<19 y	41.7-123.6		
Transferrin (mg/dL)	0-1 y	104-392		
	1-5 y	241-432		
	6-10 y		256-379	209-438
	11-14 y		214-417	236-433
	15-<19 y		216-428	228-497

(*continued*)

TABLE 4.1 REFERENCE RANGES OF SELECT NUTRITIONAL LABORATORY VALUES (*continued*)

NUTRIENT	AGE	ALL	MALES	FEMALES
Transferrin saturation (%)	0-<1 y	4.1-59		
	1-<14 y	6.5-39		
	14-<19 y		9.6-58	5.2-44
Triglycerides (mg/dL)	0-14 d	82-259		
	15 d-<1 y	53-258		
	1-<19 y	44-197		
Urea nitrogen (blood) (mg/dL)	0-15 d	2.8-23		
	15 d-<1 y	3.4-16.8		
	1-<10 y	9-22.1		
	10-<19 y		7.3-21	7.3-19
Vitamin A (retinol) (μg/dL)	0-<1 y	8.6-54.4		
	1-<11 y	28.7-45.8		
	11-<16 y	25.8-54.4		
	16-<19 y	28.7-74.5		
Vitamin B_1 (thiamine) (μg/dL)		1.6-4.0		
Vitamin B_6 (pyridoxine) (μg/L)		3.6-18.0		
Vitamin B_{12} (total) (pmol/L)	5 d-<1 y	191-1163		
	1-<9 y	209-1190		
	9-<14 y	186-830		
	14-<17 y	180-655		
	17-<19 y	150-598		
Vitamin C (ascorbic acid) (μmol/L)		23-114		
Vitamin D (as 25-hydroxy D) (ng/mL)	5-<15 d	2-34		
	15 d-<3 mo	6-40		
	3 mo-<1 y	7-47		
	1 y-<9 y	13-55		
	9-<14 y	13-46		
	14-<19 y	5-42		
Vitamin D (as 1, 25-dihydroxy D) (pg/mL)	0-<1 y	32-196		
	1-<3 y	47-151		
	3-<19 y	45-102		
Vitamin E μmol/L	0-<1 y	5-50		
	1-<19 y	14-33		

TABLE 4.1 REFERENCE RANGES OF SELECT NUTRITIONAL LABORATORY VALUES (*continued*)

NUTRIENT	AGE	ALL	MALES	FEMALES
Zinc (µg/dL)	<1 y		53-89	54-95
	1-2 y		58-97	58-101
	2-3 y		62-109	64-105
	4-6 y		66-118	68-115
	7-9 y		66-121	63-125
	10-14 y		65-119	68-139
	15-19 y		64.1-117	60.1-100.7

Adapted from Wong ECC, Brugnara C, Straseski J, et al. Pediatric Reference Intervals. 8th ed. Elsevier; 2020.

Prealbumin

Prealbumin or transthyretin is a transport molecule for thyroxine. It circulates in plasma in a 1:1 ratio with RBP. Its short half-life (2 days), small body pool, and high ratio of essential to nonessential amino acids make it a good measure of visceral protein status and a more sensitive marker than albumin as a measure of nutritional recovery.

Retinol-Binding Protein

RBP has similar properties to prealbumin in that it has a small body pool, a rapid response to protein-energy depletion and repletion, and a short half-life (12 hours). RBP levels are high in renal failure as the kidneys excrete it. RBP levels decrease in vitamin A deficiency and, as with albumin and prealbumin, with infectious or other catabolic stresses.

Transferrin

Transferrin is another plasma protein sometimes used to assess visceral protein status. It is synthesized primarily in the liver and has a half-life of 8 days. Transferrin concentrations are decreased in all situations that depress serum albumin, as well as with steroid therapy, iron overload, and anemia of chronic disease. Increased concentrations can be seen in pregnancy, oral contraceptive use, and iron deficiency anemia.

Other Biochemical Indicators of Protein Status

Nitrogen Balance

Nitrogen balance can be used to define amino acid requirements, as a deficiency in any essential amino acid will result in a negative nitrogen balance. Children and others who should be actively gaining lean body mass should be in positive nitrogen balance, whereas healthy adults may be said to be in nitrogen equilibrium if nitrogen loss is within 5% of nitrogen intake. Notably, a positive nitrogen balance does not provide information about nitrogen distribution throughout the body, nor about the accumulation of lean body mass.

Urea, which is the main excretory product of nitrogen metabolism, appears in both urine and sweat. Other sources of nitrogen loss include fecal losses, integumental losses (e.g., desquamating skin, sweat, hair, and nail growth), and miscellaneous losses (e.g., tissue fluid, saliva, vomitus, blood drawing, and menstrual losses). Since most proteins contain 16% nitrogen, dietary protein intake is divided by a factor of 6.25 to estimate nitrogen intake. Thus, the equation for calculating nitrogen balance is as follows:

Nitrogen balance = Nitrogen intake − Nitrogen output

= (24-h dietary protein intake in grams/6.25) − 24-h UUN − factor

UUN = urine urea nitrogen (in grams)

Factor = allowance made for uncollected *N loss in stool, skin, and miscellaneous sources; in adults, this factor is 2 to 4 g/d, and in children, an estimate of 10 mg/kg/d may be used*

Negative nitrogen balance can result from inadequate energy intake, inadequate protein intake, or catabolic stress and lean body mass breakdown. Positive nitrogen balance implies adequate energy and/or protein intake.

Amino Acid Profiles

In practice, actual amino acid concentrations in plasma are not as helpful as they might seem since individual amino acids are subject to a wide range of physiologic variation; their levels poorly reflect release or uptake by tissues, or they may be influenced by inherited metabolic disorders.

■ LIPIDS

Essential Fatty Acids

Fatty acids are classified according to carbon chain length and whether they contain any double bonds. Long-chain fatty acids (LCFAs), which have aliphatic tails of 13 to 21 carbon atoms, are the most common fatty acid configuration found in nature. LCFAs are further classified as -9, -6, or -3, depending on the number of carbon atoms between the terminal methyl group and its nearest double bond. Mammals can introduce double bonds in the -9 position only; -6 and -3 fatty acids must be supplied preformed in the diet, and thus, the essential fatty acids (EFA) in humans are linoleic acid ($C_{18:2}$-6) and linolenic acid ($C_{18:3}$-3). Clinical scenarios leading to EFA deficiency include reliance on lipid-free parenteral nutrition, prolonged fasting, extended use of a formula with a predominance of medium-chain fatty acids, and fat malabsorption or excretion disorders. Clinical signs of deficiency include poor growth, a desquamating skin rash, or redness and oozing in skin creases; however, deficiencies of zinc and biotin should also be considered with such skin features. It is much more common to diagnose EFA deficiency by biochemical profile.

When EFA deficiency occurs, the non-EFA eicosatrienoic acid ($C_{20:3}$-9) increases in serum; its three double bonds make it a "triene." Conversely, arachidonic acid ($C_{20:4}$-9, i.e., a "tetraene") is reduced. A triene-to-tetraene ratio of >0.2 is consistent with EFA deficiency. Clinical findings may not be apparent at this level, however, and some laboratories use different cutoffs.

Carnitine

Carnitine is a small water-soluble molecule recognized to play two major physiologic roles: (1) facilitating the transport of LCFAs, as acylcarnitines, into the mitochondrion for the generation of energy and (2) facilitating the removal of short- and medium-chain fatty acids that accumulate inside the mitochondrion.[2] The main dietary sources of carnitine are red meat and dairy products, but it can be synthesized endogenously from peptide-bound lysine and methionine. In strict vegetarians, this latter source provides more than 90% of the total available carnitine. It is stored mainly in muscle (98%); liver stores comprise 1.6%; and a very minor proportion exists in extracellular fluid.

Carnitine is generally considered a conditionally essential nutrient. Acquired carnitine deficiency is most likely to develop where there is reduced intake, reduced synthesis, increased requirements, or increased excretion. Both strict and lacto-ovo vegetarian children have lower plasma carnitine levels than their omnivorous peers, as do newborn infants, who are heavily dependent upon lipids as a concentrated fuel source for rapid growth in early life and whose relatively low plasma and tissue carnitine levels are due to immature synthetic pathways and lower renal excretion thresholds. This may be of particular relevance in preterm infants, whose carnitine stores are very low compared to those of term infants. Critical illness has been reported to cause increased carnitine excretion, and parenteral nutrition formulas do not normally contain carnitine. Thus, the preterm sick infant who is maintained exclusively on intravenous feeding is likely to be at greatest risk for functional carnitine deficiency, which may conceivably manifest with defective energy-dependent processes (e.g., hypoglycemia, respiratory distress, hyperlipidemia, and inadequate growth).[2]

■ MICRONUTRIENTS

Nutritional status tests for micronutrients are shown in Table 4.2; see Table 4.1 for reference ranges. When interpreting plasma micronutrient levels, it is important that care is exercised with results obtained during metabolic stress as acute illness results in the redistribution of vitamins and trace elements for various reasons, including acute-phase response of some carrier molecules.[3-5] Monitoring trends and magnitude of the acute-phase response (e.g., by measuring C-reactive protein concentrations) will facilitate the interpretation of blood micronutrient levels.

TABLE 4.2 NUTRITIONAL STATUS TESTS FOR MICRONUTRIENTS

MICRONUTRIENT	TEST(S)	COMMENTS
Chromium	Serum chromium	May not fully reflect tissue stores
Copper	Serum copper, ceruloplasmin	Positive acute-phase reactants (APR)
Iodine	Urine iodine, serum thyroxine, serum thyroglobulin	Urine iodine may be influenced by recent dietary intake; thyroid-stimulating hormone levels may be in the normal range for older children and adults with marginal iodine deficiency.
Iron	Combination of serum iron, ferritin, transferrin saturation (TS), and total iron-binding capacity (TIBC) with complete blood count (CBC)	Ferritin is a positive APR; iron is a negative APR.
Manganese	Whole blood and urine manganese	There is poor correlation between whole blood or urine manganese levels and dietary intake.
Molybdenum (Mo)	Serum and urine molybdenum	Neither accurately reflect nutritional status; serum Mo may be impacted by inflammation and recent dietary intake.
Selenium (Se)	Serum selenium, erythrocyte selenium concentration, glutathione peroxidase (GPX) activity	Serum Se may be influenced by recent dietary intake; GPX activity assay is not commonly available.
Zinc	Serum zinc, serum alkaline phosphatase	Zinc is a negative APR and is not adequate for assessing zinc status; alkaline phosphatase is not a sensitive indicator of zinc stores.
Fluoride	Serum and urine fluoride	Serum fluoride is a better indicator, though neither is routinely utilized.
B_1	Whole blood thiamine, transketolase enzymatic activity	Serum thiamine is not reflective of thiamine nutritional status; not an APR.
B_2	Pre- and postsupplementation erythrocyte glutathione reductase activity coefficient (EGRAC)	Spot urine riboflavin assays are influenced by recent dietary intake, but 24-h assays may be used if EGRAC cannot be tested; not an APR.
B_3	First morning void or 24-h urine niacin metabolites	Serum niacin does not reflect total body niacin stores; not an APR.
B_5	Urine pantothenic acid level	Very rarely assessed and of limited clinical utility; not an APR
B_6	Plasma pyridoxal-5-phosphate (PLP), erythrocyte aspartic acid transaminase (AST), and alanine transaminase (ALT) activity	Plasma PLP may be influenced by inflammation, hypophosphatasia, and hypoalbuminemia; erythrocyte AST and ALT are not influenced by these factors, but assays may not be widely available; possible negative APR.

TABLE 4.2 NUTRITIONAL STATUS TESTS FOR MICRONUTRIENTS (*continued*)

MICRONUTRIENT	TEST(S)	COMMENTS
B_7	Leukocyte holocarboxylases, urine 3-hydroxyisovaleric acid	Urine biotin does not identify deficiency; urine 3-hydroxyisovaleric acid testing has lower sensitivity than leukocyte holocarboxylase assays, which have limited availability; not an APR.
B_9	Red blood cell folate level, serum folate level	RBC folate may be less influenced by recent dietary folate intake; obtain with B_{12} due to overlap in deficiency symptoms; not an APR.
B_{12}	Active B_{12} level, serum B_{12} level, urine or serum methylmalonic acid (MMA)	Active B_{12} level may be a more specific and sensitive test and may detect early deficiency better than total serum B_{12} level; obtain with folate due to overlap in deficiency symptoms; not an APR.
Vitamin C	Serum ascorbic acid level, leukocyte ascorbic acid concentration	Leukocyte ascorbic acid is a more sensitive indicator of tissue stores; negative APR.
Choline	Serum choline	Serum choline has limited use in assessing choline nutritional status; unknown if APR.
Vitamin A	Retinol-binding protein (RBP) concentration, serum retinol level	RBP is a negative APR and may also be depressed in malnutrition/protein deficiency states.
Vitamin D	25-hydroxyvitamin D (OHD)	Possible negative APR
Vitamin E	Serum tocopherol level, tocopherol/total lipid ratio	Levels of vitamin E/tocopherols fluctuate with plasma lipid concentrations.
Vitamin K	Activated partial thromboplastin time (aPTT) and partial thromboplastin time (PTT), proteins induced in vitamin K absence or antagonism-factor II (PIVKA-II)	Consider evaluating aPTT/PTT pre- and post-vitamin K supplementation to determine therapy efficacy.

Adapted from Frates E, Hivert MF, Duggan C. Essentials of Clinical Nutrition in Healthcare. McGraw-Hill Education; 2024.

REFERENCES

1. Cruickshank AM, Hansell DT, Burns HJ, Shenkin A. Effect of nutritional status on acute phase protein response to elective surgery. *Brit J Surg*. 1989;76(2);165-168.
2. Walter JH. L-carnitine. *Arch Dis Child*. 1996;74:475-478.
3. Duncan A, Talwar D, McMillan DC, Stefanowicz F, O'Reilly DS. Quantitative data on the magnitude of the systemic inflammatory response and its effect on micronutrient status based on plasma measurements. *Am J Clin Nutr*. 2012;95(1):64-71.
4. Shen J, Lai CQ, Mattei J, Ordovas JM, Tucker KL. Association of vitamin B-6 status with inflammation, oxidative stress, and chronic inflammatory conditions: the Boston Puerto Rican Health Study. *Am J Clin Nutr*. 2010;91(2):337-342.
5. Reid D, Toole BJ, Knox S, et al. The relation between acute changes in the systemic inflammatory response and plasma 25-hydroxyvitamin D concentrations after elective knee arthroplasty. *Am J Clin Nutr*. 2011;93(5):1006-1011.

CHAPTER 5

Nutritional Requirements and Recommendations

Judy Milliano and Kendrin R. Sonneville

THE DIETARY GUIDELINES

The U.S. Department of Agriculture's (USDA) Center for Nutrition Policy and Promotion (CNPP), established in 1994, aims to improve the health and well-being of Americans by developing and promoting dietary guidance based on research and consumer nutrition needs. In partnership with the U.S. Department of Health and Human Services (HHS), the CNPP publishes the *Dietary Guidelines for Americans* every 5 years. These guidelines provide science-based, accessible recommendations to help Americans make healthy food and beverage choices (www.dietaryguidelines.gov). The Dietary Guidelines for Americans, 2025–2030 emphasize healthy dietary patterns rich in fruits, vegetables, whole grains, lean proteins, and healthy fats, while limiting added sugars, saturated fat, sodium, and alcohol.

KID'S HEALTHY EATING PLATE

The Kid's Healthy Eating Plate (Figure 5.1) is a visual guide developed by the Harvard T.H. Chan School of Public Health to help educate and encourage children to eat well and keep moving. The graphic features examples of food choices to inspire the selection of healthy meals and snacks and emphasizes physical activity.

NUTRIENT REQUIREMENTS/DIETARY REFERENCE INTAKES

The dietary reference intakes (DRIs) are a comprehensive set of nutrient reference values developed jointly by the U.S. and Canadian governments, under the direction of the National Academies of Sciences, Engineering, and Medicine. The DRIs are used by health professionals, researchers, and policymakers to assess and plan diets, ensuring that individuals receive adequate nutrients while avoiding excessive intake that could lead to adverse health effects. The DRI values are based on current scientific research and vary by age, gender, and life stage.

Most nutrients have several DRI reference values representing values related to meeting nutritional requirements, preventing excessive intake, and reducing the risk of chronic disease.

- The Recommended Dietary Allowance (RDA) is the daily intake level of a nutrient that meets the needs of nearly all healthy individuals in a specific age and sex group, based on extensive scientific evidence.

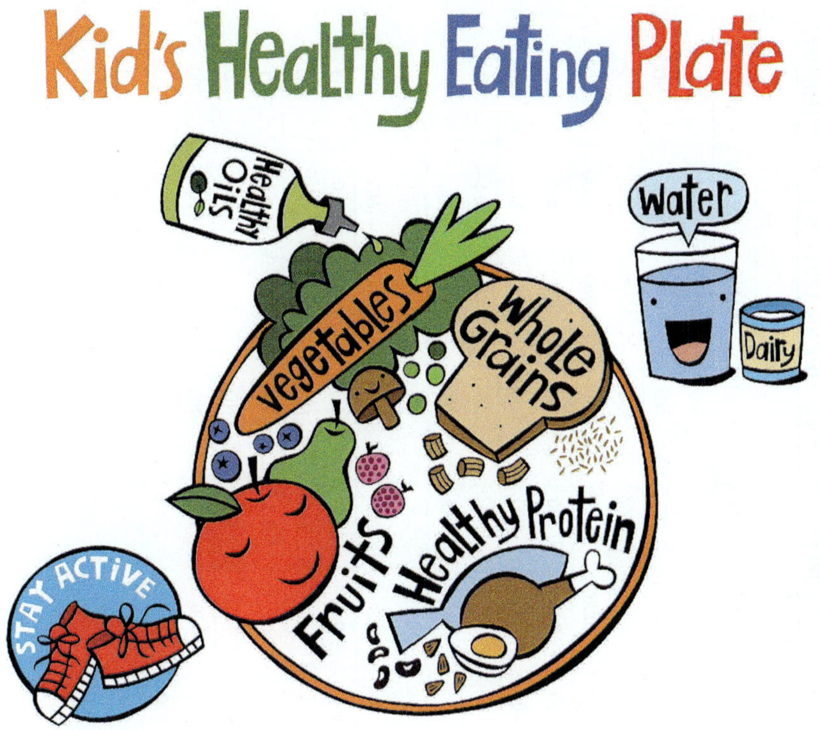

Figure 5.1 Kid's healthy eating plate. The Nutrition Source. https://nutritionsource.hsph.harvard.edu/kids-healthy-eating-plate/

- When sufficient data are unavailable to set an RDA, the Adequate Intake (AI) is used as a best estimate of nutrient requirements.
- The Tolerable Upper Intake Level (UL) represents the maximum daily intake likely to pose no risk of adverse health effects for most individuals.
- The Acceptable Macronutrient Distribution Range (AMDR) is the range of intake for each macronutrient that is associated with a reduced risk of chronic diseases and provides AI of essential nutrients.

DRIs for vitamins,[3-6] elements,[7-9] total water,[7] and macronutrients[10] are summarized in Tables 5.1 to 5.3. Baseline water (i.e., fluid) requirements for children can also be estimated using the Holliday-Segar Method (Table 5.4).[11]

ENERGY REQUIREMENTS

Multiple predictive energy equations have been developed to estimate basal metabolic rate (BMR) using readily available anthropometric data, age, and sex. The oldest and most commonly used of these is the Harris-Benedict equation for adults (Table 5.5).[12] In pediatrics, the World Health Organization (WHO), Schofield weight, and Schofield weight and height equations are commonly used in estimating BMR (Table 5.6).[13,14]

TABLE 5.1 RECOMMENDED DIETARY ALLOWANCES, ADEQUATE INTAKES, AND UPPER LIMITS FOR VITAMINS

		INFANTS		CHILDREN		MALES			FEMALES		
		0-6 MO	7-12 MO	1-3 Y	4-8 Y	9-13 Y	14-18 Y	19-30 Y	9-13 Y	14-18 Y	19-30 Y
Biotin (μg/d)	RDA/AI*	5*	6*	8*	12*	20*	25*	30*	20*	25*	30*
	UL	ND[a]	ND	ND	ND	ND	ND	ND	ND	ND	ND
Choline (mg/d)	RDA/AI*	125*	150*	200*	250*	375*	550*	550*	375*	400*	425*
	UL	ND	ND	1,000	1,000	2,000	3,000	3,500	2,000	3,000	3,500
Folate (μg/d)	RDA/AI*	65*	80*	**150**	**200**	**300**	**400**	**400**	**300**	**400**	**400**
	UL	ND	ND	300	400	600	800	1,000	600	800	1,000
Niacin (mg/d)	RDA/AI*	2*	4*	**6**	**8**	**12**	**16**	**16**	**12**	**14**	**14**
	UL	ND	ND	10	15	20	30	35	20	30	35
Pantothenic acid (mg/d)	RDA/AI*	1.7*	1.8*	2*	3*	4*	5*	5*	4*	5*	5*
	UL	ND	ND	ND	ND	ND	ND	ND	ND	ND	ND
Riboflavin (mg/d)	RDA/AI*	0.3*	0.4*	**0.5**	**0.6**	**0.9**	**1.3**	**1.3**	**0.9**	**1.0**	**1.1**
	UL	ND	ND	ND	ND	ND	ND	ND	ND	ND	ND
Thiamin (mg/d)	RDA/AI*	0.2*	0.3*	**0.5**	**0.6**	**0.9**	**1.2**	**1.2**	**0.9**	**1.0**	**1.1**
	UL	ND	ND	ND	ND	ND	ND	ND	ND	ND	ND
Vitamin A (μg/d)	RDA/AI*	400*	500*	**300**	**400**	**600**	**900**	**900**	**600**	**700**	**700**
	UL	600	600	600	900	1,700	2,800	3,000	1,700	2,800	3,000
Vitamin B_6 (mg/d)	RDA/AI*	0.1*	0.3*	**0.5**	**0.6**	**1.0**	**1.3**	**1.3**	**1.0**	**1.2**	**1.3**
	UL	ND	ND	30	40	60	80	100	60	80	100

Vitamin B_{12} (μg/d)	**RDA**/AI*	0.4*	0.5*	**0.9**	**1.2**	**1.8**	**2.4**	**2.4**	**1.8**	**2.4**	**2.4**
	UL	ND	ND	ND	ND	ND	ND	ND	ND	ND	ND
Vitamin C (mg/d)	**RDA**/AI*	40*	50*	**15**	**25**	**45**	**75**	**90**	**45**	**65**	**75**
	UL	ND	ND	400	650	1,200	1,800	2,000	1,200	1,800	2,000
Vitamin D (μg/d)	**RDA**/AI*	10	10	**15**	**15**	**15**	**15**	**15**	**15**	**15**	**15**
	UL	25	38	63	75	100	100	100	100	100	100
Vitamin E (mg/d)	**RDA**/AI*	4*	5*	**6**	7	**11**	**15**	**15**	**11**	**15**	**15**
	UL	ND	ND	200	300	600	800	1,000	600	800	1,000
Vitamin K (μg/d)	**RDA**/AI*	2.0*	2.5*	30*	55*	60*	75*	120*	60*	75*	90*
	UL	ND	ND	ND	ND	ND	ND	ND	ND	ND	ND

UL, tolerable upper intake level.

Recommended Dietary Allowances (RDAs) are represented *in bold type.*

Adequate Intakes (AIs) are represented in regular type and are followed by an asterisk (*).

[a]ND = Not determinable due to lack of data on adverse effects in this age group and concern regarding the lack of ability to handle excess amounts.

Adapted from DRI reports: 2025 Dietary Guidelines Advisory Committee. *Scientific Report of the 2025 Dietary Guidelines Advisory Committee: Advisory Report to the Secretary of Health and Human Services and Secretary of Agriculture.* U.S. Department of Health and Human Services; 2024; Institute of Medicine. *Dietary Reference Intakes for Calcium, Phosphorus, Magnesium, Vitamin D, and Fluoride.* The National Academies Press; 1997; Institute of Medicine. *Dietary Reference Intakes for Calcium and Vitamin D.* The National Academies Press; 2011; Institute of Medicine. *Dietary Reference Intakes for Thiamin, Riboflavin, Niacin, Vitamin B_6, Folate, Vitamin B_{12}, Pantothenic Acid, Biotin, and Choline.* The National Academies Press; 1998. The complete reports can be accessed at www.nap.edu

TABLE 5.2 RECOMMENDED DIETARY ALLOWANCES, ADEQUATE INTAKES, AND UPPER LIMITS FOR ELEMENTS

		INFANTS		CHILDREN		MALES			FEMALES		
		0-6 MO	7-12 MO	1-3 Y	4-8 Y	9-13 Y	14-18 Y	19-30 Y	9-13 Y	14-18 Y	19-30 Y
Calcium (mg/d)	RDA/AI*	210*	270*	500*	800*	1,300*	1,300*	1,000*	1,300*	1,300*	1,000*
	UL	1,000	1,500	2,500	2,500	3,000	3,000	2,500	3,000	3,000	2,500
Chloride (g/d)	RDA/AI*	0.18*	0.57*	1.5*	1.9*	2.3*	2.3*	2.3*	2.3*	2.3*	2.3*
	UL	ND[a]	ND	2.3	2.9	3.4	3.6	3.6	3.4	3.6	3.6
Chromium (µg/d)	RDA/AI*	0.2*	5.5*	11*	15*	25*	35*	35*	21*	24*	25*
	UL	ND	ND	ND	ND	ND	ND	ND	ND	ND	ND
Copper (µg/d)	RDA/AI*	200*	220*	**340**	**440**	**700**	**890**	**900**	**700**	**890**	**900**
	UL	ND	ND	1,000	3,000	5,000	8,000	10,000	5,000	8,000	10,000
Fluoride (mg/d)	RDA/AI*	0.01*	0.5*	0.7*	1*	2*	3*	4*	2*	3*	3*
	UL	0.7	0.9	1.3	2.2	10	10	10	10	10	10
Iodine (µg/d)	RDA/AI*	110*	130*	**90**	**90**	**120**	**150**	**150**	**120**	**150**	**150**
	UL	ND	ND	200	300	600	900	1,100	600	900	1,100
Iron (mg/d)	RDA/AI*	0.27*	**11**	7	**10**	**8**	**11**	**8**	**8**	**15**	**18**
	UL	40	40	40	40	40	45	45	40	45	45
Magnesium (mg/d)	RDA/AI*	30*	75*	**80**	**130**	**240**	**410**	**400**	**240**	**360**	**310**
	UL	ND	ND	65	110	350	350	350	350	350	350
Manganese (mg/d)	RDA/AI*	0.003*	0.6*	1.2*	1.5*	1.9*	2.2*	2.3*	1.6*	1.6*	1.8*
	UL	ND	ND	2	3	6	9	11	6	9	11

Molybdenum (µg/d)	RDA/AI*	2*	3*	**17**	**22**	**34**	**43**	**45**	**34**	**43**	**45**
	UL	ND	ND	300	600	1,100	1,700	2,000	1,100	1,700	2,000
Phosphorus (mg/d)	RDA/AI*	100*	275*	**460**	**500**	**1,250**	**1,250**	**700**	**1,250**	**1,250**	**700**
	UL	ND	ND	3,000	3,000	4,000	4,000	4,000	4,000	4,000	4,000
Potassium (mg/d)	RDA/AI*	400*	860*	2,000*	2,300*	2,500*	3,000*	3,400*	2,300*	2,300*	2,600*
	UL	No UL[b]	No UL	No UL	No UL	No UL	No UL	No UL	No UL	No UL	No UL
Selenium (µg/d)	RDA/AI*	15*	20*	**20**	**30**	**40**	**55**	**55**	**40**	**55**	**55**
	UL	45	60	90	150	280	400	400	280	400	400
Sodium (mg/d)	RDA/AI*	110*	370*	800*	1,000*	1,200*	1,500*	1,500*	1,200*	1,500*	1,500*
	UL	ND[a]	ND	1.5	1.9	2.2	2.3	2.3	2.2	2.3	2.3
Zinc (mg/d)	RDA/AI*	2*	**3**	**3**	**5**	**8**	**11**	**11**	**8**	**9**	**8**
	UL	4	5	7	12	23	34	40	23	34	40

UL, tolerable upper intake level.
Recommended Dietary Allowances (RDAs) are represented in **bold type**.
Adequate Intakes (AIs) are represented in regular type and are followed by an asterisk (*).
[a]ND = Not determinable due to lack of data on adverse effects in this age group and concern regarding the lack of ability to handle excess amounts.
[b]In the absence of ULs, extra caution may be warranted in consuming levels above recommended intakes.
Adapted from DRI reports: Institute of Medicine. *Dietary Reference Intakes for Vitamin C, Vitamin E, Selenium, and Carotenoids*. The National Academies Press; 2000; Institute of Medicine. *Dietary Reference Intakes for Water, Potassium, Sodium, Chloride, and Sulfate*. The National Academies Press; 2005; National Academies of Sciences, Engineering, and Medicine. *Dietary Reference Intakes for Sodium and Potassium*. The National Academies Press; 2019. The complete reports can be accessed at www.nap.edu

TABLE 5.3 RECOMMENDED DIETARY ALLOWANCES, ADEQUATE INTAKES, AND ACCEPTABLE MACRONUTRIENT DISTRIBUTION RANGES FOR TOTAL WATER AND MACRONUTRIENTS

		INFANTS		CHILDREN		MALES			FEMALES		
		0-6 MO	7-12 MO	1-3 Y	4-8 Y	9-13 Y	14-18 Y	19-30 Y	9-13 Y	14-18 Y	19-30 Y
Water (L/d)	RDA/AI	0.7*	0.8*	1.3*	1.7*	2.4*	3.3*	3.7*	2.1*	2.3*	2.7*
Carbohydrate (g/d)	RDA/AI*	60*	95*	**130**	**130**	**130**	**130**	**130**	**130**	**130**	**130**
	AMDR	ND[a]	ND	45-65	45-65	45-65	45-65	45-65	45-65	45-65	45-65
Total Fiber (g/d)	RDA/AI*	ND	ND	19*	25*	31*	38*	38*	26*	26*	25*
Fat (g/d)	RDA/AI*	31*	30*	ND	ND	ND	ND	ND	ND	ND	ND
	AMDR	ND	ND	30-40	25-35	25-35	25-35	20-35	25-35	25-35	20-35
***n*-6 polyunsaturated fatty acids (linoleic acid) (g/d)**	RDA/AI*	4.4*	4.6*	7*	10*	12*	16*	17*	10*	11*	12*
	AMDR	ND	ND	5-10	5-10	5-10	5-10	5-10	5-10	5-10	5-10
***n*-3 polyunsaturated fatty acids (-Linolenic acid) (g/d)**	RDA/AI*	0.5*	0.5*	0.7*	0.9*	1.2*	1.6*	1.6*	1.0*	1.1*	1.1*
	AMDR	ND	ND	0.6-1.2	0.6-1.2	0.6-1.2	0.6-1.2	0.6-1.2	0.6-1.2	0.6-1.2	0.6-1.2
Protein (g/d)[b]	RDA/AI*	9.1*	**11**	**13**	**19**	**34**	**52**	**56**	**34**	**46**	**46**
	AMDR	ND	ND	5-20	10-30	10-30	10-30	10-35	10-30	10-30	10-35

AMDR, acceptable macronutrient distribution range.
Recommended Dietary Allowances (RDAs) are represented in **bold type**.
Adequate Intakes (AIs) are represented in regular type and are followed by an asterisk (*).
[a]ND = Not determinable due to lack of data on adverse effects in this age group and concern with regard to the lack of ability to handle excess amounts.
[b]Based on 1.5 g/kg/d for infants, 1.1 g/kg/d for 1 to 3 years, 0.95 g/kg/d for 4 to 13 years, 0.85 g/kg/d for 14 to 18 years, and 0.8 g/kg/d for adults.
Adapted from the DRI report: Institute of Medicine. *Dietary Reference Intakes for Vitamin C, Vitamin E, Selenium, and Carotenoids*. The National Academies Press; 2000; Institute of Medicine. *Dietary Reference Intakes for Water, Potassium, Sodium, Chloride, and Sulfate*. The National Academies Press; 2005; National Academies of Sciences, Engineering, and Medicine. *Dietary Reference Intakes for Sodium and Potassium*. The National Academies Press; 2019; Institute of Medicine. *Dietary Reference Intakes for Vitamin A, Vitamin K, Arsenic, Boron, Chromium, Copper, Iodine, Iron, Manganese, Molybdenum, Nickel, Silicon, Vanadium, and Zinc*. The National Academies Press; 2001. The complete report can be accessed at www.nap.edu

TABLE 5.4 BASELINE FLUID REQUIREMENTS: HOLIDAY-SEGAR METHOD

1-10 kg	100 mL/kg
11-20 kg	1000 mL + 50 mL/kg for each kg >10 kg
>20 kg	1500 mL + 20 mL/kg for each kg >20 kg

Data from Holliday MA, Segar WE. The maintenance need for water in parenteral fluid therapy. *Pediatrics.* 1957;19(5):823-832.

The terms BMR and REE (resting energy expenditure) are often used as synonyms but are not. BMR refers to the amount of energy expended at complete rest in a neutrally temperate environment while NPO (nothing by mouth) for 12 hours. REE is the amount of energy required by the body to maintain basic bodily functions at rest but without the strict conditions required for BMR and is therefore ~10% higher than BMR. Indirect calorimetry (see Chapter 14) is commonly used to measure REE.

To calculate total energy expenditure, a physical activity coefficient (see Table 5.7) or stress factor reflecting illness (e.g., sepsis, burns) is applied to the estimated BMR (or measured REE). However, recent studies have raised concerns that the indiscriminate use of predictive energy equations and variable stress factors can be inaccurate, putting patients at risk for underfeeding or overfeeding.[15]

The DRIs also include Estimated Energy Requirement (EER) equations to predict an appropriate energy intake to plan and assess diets for individuals and groups. The EER equations from the 2005[10] and 2023[16] DRIs are included in Tables 5.7 and 5.8. The EER is the average daily energy intake predicted to maintain energy balance in a healthy adult based on their age, sex, weight, height, and physical activity level.[12] These equations may not be appropriate for use in transgender and gender-diverse patients. In 2022, the Academy of Nutrition and Dietetics released practice guidelines with considerations for nutrition and dietetics practitioners working with transgender and gender-diverse individuals.[17] For patients who have not medically transitioned, it is recommended to use the equations corresponding to the sex assigned at birth.[17] For patients who have medically transitioned, it is recommended to use the World Professional Association for Transgender Health guidelines on the expected time of onset and maximum effect to determine which equations to utilize.[17]

TABLE 5.5 HARRIS-BENEDICT EQUATIONS FOR CALCULATING BASAL METABOLIC RATE IN ADULTS[a]

Males	66 + (13.7 × weight) + (5 × height) − (6.8 × age)
Females	665 + (9.6 × weight) + (1.8 × height) − (4.7 × age)

[a]Age is in years, weight is in kilograms, and height is in centimeters.
Data from Harris JA, Benedict FG. *A Biometric Study of Basal Metabolism* (Publication No. 279). Carnegie Institution of Washington; 1919.

TABLE 5.6 CALCULATING RESTING METABOLIC RATE IN CHILDREN USING WEIGHT ± HEIGHT[a]

AGE	GENDER	WHO (WEIGHT ONLY)	SCHOFIELD (WEIGHT ONLY)	SCHOFIELD (HEIGHT AND WEIGHT)
0-3 y	Male	(60.9 × weight) – 54	(59.512 × weight) – 30.4	(0.167 × weight) + (15.174 × height) – 617.6
	Female	(61 × weight) – 51	(58.317 × weight) – 31.1	(16.252 × weight) + (10.232 × height) – 413.5
3-10 y	Male	(22.7 × weight) + 495	(22.706 × weight) + 504.3	(19.59 × weight) + (1.303 × height) + 414.9
	Female	(22.5 × weight) + 499	(20.315 × weight) + 485.9	(16.969 × weight) + (1.618 × height) + 371.2
10-18 y	Male	(17.5 × weight) + 651	(17.686 × weight) + 658.2	(16.25 × weight) + (1.372 × height) + 515.5
	Female	(12.2 × weight) + 746	(13.384 × weight) + 692.6	(8.365 × weight) + (4.65 × height) + 200.0
18-30 y	Male	(15.3 × weight) + 679	(15.057 × weight) + 692.2	(15.057 × weight) + (1.004 × height) + 705.8
	Female	(14.7 × weight) + 496	(14.818 × weight) + 486.6	(13.623 × weight) + (2.83 × height) + 98.2

WHO, World Health Organization.
[a]Weight is in kilograms, and height is in centimeters.
Data from World Health Organization, 1985 and Schofield W, 1985.

TABLE 5.7 ESTIMATED ENERGY REQUIREMENTS (2005 DIETARY REFERENCE INTAKES)[a]

CATEGORY	ESTIMATED ENERGY REQUIREMENTS (KCAL/D)
Infants and Children (0-2 y)	
0-3 mo	(89 × weight − 100) + 175
4-6 mo	(89 × weight − 100) + 56
7-12 mo	(89 × weight − 100) + 22
13-35 mo	(89 × weight − 100) + 20
Males	
3-8 y	88.5 − 61.9 × age + PA[b] × (26.7 × weight + 903 × height) + 20
9-18 y	88.5 − 61.9 × age + PA × (26.7 × weight + 903 × height) + 25
>19 y	662 − 9.53 × age + PA × (15.91 × weight + 539.6 × height)
Females	
3-8 y	135.3 − 30.8 × age + PA × (10.0 × weight + 934 × height) + 20
9-18 y	135.3 − 30.8 × age + PA × (10.0 × weight + 934 × height) + 25
>19 y	354 − 6.91 × age + PA × (9.36 × weight + 726 × height)
Pregnancy	
14-18 y	
First trimester	Adolescent EER
Second trimester	Adolescent EER + 340
Third trimester	Adolescent EER + 452
19-50 y	
First trimester	Adult EER
Second trimester	Adult EER + 340
Third trimester	Adult EER + 452
Lactation	
14-18 y	
First 6 mo	Adolescent EER + 330
Second 6 mo	Adolescent EER + 400
19-50 y	
First 6 mo	Adult EER + 330
Second 6 mo	Adult EER + 400

EER, estimated energy requirement.
[a]Age is in years, weight is in kilograms, and height is in centimeters.
[b]PA = physical activity coefficient based on physical activity level (PAL). PA = 1.00 if PAL is estimated to be >1.0 and <1.4 (sedentary). PA = 1.12 if PAL is estimated to be >1.4 and <1.6 (low active). PA = 1.24 if PAL is estimated to be >1.6 and <1.9 (active). PA = 1.45 if PAL is estimated to be >1.9 and <2.5 (very active).
Adapted from the DRI report: Institute of Medicine. *Dietary Reference Intakes for Energy, Carbohydrate, Fiber, Fat, Fatty Acids, Cholesterol, Protein, and Amino Acids*. The National Academies Press; 2005. The complete report can be accessed at www.nap.edu

TABLE 5.8 ESTIMATED ENERGY REQUIREMENTS (2023 DIETARY REFERENCE INTAKES)[a]

SEX	AGE	ACTIVITY LEVEL	ESTIMATED ENERGY REQUIREMENTS (KCAL/D)
Males	0-2.99 mo	-	−716.45 − (1.00 × age) + (17.82 × height) + (15.06 × weight) + 200
	3-5.99 mo	-	−716.45 − (1.00 × age) + (17.82 × height) + (15.06 × weight) + 50
	6 mo-2.99 y	-	−716.45 − (1.00 × age) + (17.82 × height) + (15.06 × weight) + 20
	3-13.99 y	Inactive	−447.51 + (3.68 × age) + (13.01 × height) + (13.15 × weight) + 20/15/25[b]
		Low active	19.12 + (3.68 × age) + (8.62 × height) + (20.28 × weight) + 20/15/25
		Active	−388.19 + (3.68 × age) + (12.66 × height) + (20.46 × weight) + 20/15/25
		Very active	−671.75 + (3.68 × age) + (15.38 × height) + (23.25 × weight) + 20/15/25
	14-18.99 y	Inactive	−447.51 + (3.68 × age) + (13.01 × height) + (13.15 × weight) + 20
		Low active	19.12 + (3.68 × age) + (8.62 × height) + (20.28 × weight) + 20
		Active	−388.19 + (3.68 × age) + (12.66 × height) + (20.46 × weight) + 20
		Very active	−671.75 + (3.68 × age) + (15.38 × height) + (23.25 × weight) + 20
	19+ y	Inactive	753.07 − (10.83 × age) + (6.50 × height) + (14.10 × weight)
		Low active	581.47 − (10.83 × age) + (8.30 × height) + (14.94 × weight)
		Active	1,004.82 − (10.83 × age) + (6.52 × height) + (15.91 × weight)
		Very active	−517.88 − (10.83 × age) + (15.61 × height) + (19.11 × weight)
Females	0-2.99 mo	-	−69.15 + (80.0 × age) + (2.65 × height) + (54.15 × weight) + 180
	3-5.99 mo	-	−69.15 + (80.0 × age) + (2.65 × height) + (54.15 × weight) + 60
	6 mo-2.99 y	-	−69.15 + (80.0 × age) + (2.65 × height) + (54.15 × weight) + 20/15[c]
	3-13.99 y	Inactive	55.59 − (22.25 × age) + (8.43 × height) + (17.07 × weight) + 15/30[d]

TABLE 5.8 ESTIMATED ENERGY REQUIREMENTS (2023 DIETARY REFERENCE INTAKES)[a] (*continued*)

SEX	AGE	ACTIVITY LEVEL	ESTIMATED ENERGY REQUIREMENTS (KCAL/D)
		Low active	−297.54 − (22.25 × age) + (12.77 × height) + (14.73 × weight) + 15/30
		Active	−189.55 − (22.25 × age) + (11.74 × height) + (18.34 × weight) + 15/30
		Very active	−709.59 − (22.25 × age) + (18.22 × height) + (14.25 × weight) + 15/30
	14-18.99 y	**Inactive**	55.59 − (22.25 × age) + (8.43 × height) + (17.07 × weight) + 20
		Low active	−297.54 − (22.25 × age) + (12.77 × height) + (14.73 × weight) + 20
		Active	−189.55 − (22.25 × age) + (11.74 × height) + (18.34 × weight) + 20
		Very active	−709.59 − (22.25 × age) + (18.22 × height) + (14.25 × weight) + 20
	19+ y	**Inactive**	584.90 − (7.01 × age) + (5.72 × height) + (11.71 × weight)
		Low active	575.77 − (7.01 × age) + (6.60 × height) + (12.14 × weight)
		Active	710.25 − (7.01 × age) + (6.54 × height) + (12.34 × weight)
		Very active	511.83 − (7.01 × age) + (9.07 × height) + (12.56 × weight)

[a]Age is in years, weight is in kilograms, and height is in centimeters.
[b]Energy cost of growth for boys: 3 years: 20 kcal/d; 4 to 8 years: 15 kcal/d; 9 to 13 years: 25 kcal/d.
[c]Energy cost of growth for girls: 6 to 11.99 months: 20 kcal/d; 12 to 35.99 months: 15 kcal/d.
[d]Energy cost of growth for girls: 3 years: 15 kcal/d; 4 to 8 years: 15 kcal/d; 9 to 13 years: 30 kcal/d.
Adapted from DRI report: Institute of Medicine. *Dietary Reference Intakes for Energy, Carbohydrate, Fiber, Fat, Fatty Acids, Cholesterol, Protein, and Amino Acids*. The National Academies Press; 2005. The complete report can be accessed at www.nap.edu

■ REFERENCES

1. U.S. Department of Agriculture & U.S. Department of Health and Human Services. (2026). Dietary Guidelines for Americans, 2025–2030. https://cdn.realfood.gov/DGA.pdf
2. 2025 Dietary Guidelines Advisory Committee. *Scientific Report of the 2025. Dietary Guidelines Advisory Committee: Advisory Report to the Secretary of Health and Human Services and Secretary of Agriculture*. U.S. Department of Health and Human Services; 2024.
3. Institute of Medicine. *Dietary Reference Intakes for Calcium, Phosphorus, Magnesium, Vitamin D, and Fluoride*. The National Academies Press; 1997.
4. Institute of Medicine. *Dietary Reference Intakes for Calcium and Vitamin D*. The National Academies Press; 2011.
5. Institute of Medicine. *Dietary Reference Intakes for Thiamin, Riboflavin, Niacin, Vitamin B6, Folate, Vitamin B12, Pantothenic Acid, Biotin, and Choline*. The National Academies Press; 1998.
6. Institute of Medicine. *Dietary Reference Intakes for Vitamin C, Vitamin E, Selenium, and Carotenoids*. The National Academies Press; 2000.

7. Institute of Medicine. *Dietary Reference Intakes for Water, Potassium, Sodium, Chloride, and Sulfate*. The National Academies Press; 2005.
8. National Academies of Sciences, Engineering, and Medicine. *Dietary Reference Intakes for Sodium and Potassium*. The National Academies Press; 2019.
9. Institute of Medicine. *Dietary Reference Intakes for Vitamin A, Vitamin K, Arsenic, Boron, Chromium, Copper, Iodine, Iron, Manganese, Molybdenum, Nickel, Silicon, Vanadium, and Zinc*. The National Academies Press; 2001.
10. Institute of Medicine. *Dietary Reference Intakes for Energy, Carbohydrate, Fiber, Fat, Fatty Acids, Cholesterol, Protein, and Amino Acids*. The National Academies Press; 2005.
11. Holliday MA, Segar WE. The maintenance need for water in parenteral fluid therapy. *Pediatrics*. 1957;19(5):823-832.
12. Harris JA, Benedict FG. *A Biometric Study of Basal Metabolism* (Publication No. 279). Carnegie Institution of Washington; 1919.
13. Energy and protein requirements. Report of a joint FAO/WHO/UNU expert consultation. *World Health Organ Tech Rep Ser*. 1985;724:1-206.
14. Schofield W. Predicting basal metabolic rate, new standards and review of previous work. *Hum Nutr Clin Nutr*. 1985. 39(suppl 1):5-41.
15. Mehta NM, Compher C; A.S.P.E.N. Board of Directors. A.S.P.E.N. clinical guidelines: nutrition support of the critically ill child. *JPEN J Parenter Enteral Nutr*. 2009;33(3):260-276.
16. National Academies of Sciences, Engineering, and Medicine. *Dietary Reference Intakes for Energy*. The National Academies Press; 2023.
17. Linsenmeyer W, Garwood S, Waters J. An examination of the sex-specific nature of nutrition assessment within the nutrition care process: considerations for nutrition and dietetics practitioners working with transgender and gender diverse clients. *J Acad Nutr Diet*. 2022;122(6):1081-1086.

CHAPTER 6

Human Milk and Breastfeeding/Chestfeeding

Kimberly H. Barbas and Jenny Kinne

Human milk is the preferred primary source of infant nutrition throughout the first year of life, with extensive research supporting its benefits (Table 6.1). Both the World Health Organization and the American Academy of Pediatrics recommend infants receive human milk exclusively through the first 6 months of life, followed by continued breastfeeding/chestfeeding alongside nutritionally adequate and safe complementary foods for at least 2 years.[1,2] Greater than 80% of families initiate breastfeeding/chestfeeding in the United States, but many families fall short of recommendations for exclusivity and duration.

The tables in this chapter provide guidance on various aspects of lactation support. Table 6.2 outlines essential practices for initiating lactation, including components such as positioning, latch, and milk transfer, all critical to successful breastfeeding/chestfeeding. Table 6.3 focuses on breastfeeding/chestfeeding assessment.

Human milk expression may be necessary to maintain milk production whenever the infant is unable to feed directly at the breast due to illness, prematurity, anatomic or neurologic issues, surgery, or if the parent returns to work, needs to travel, or has medical contraindications to breastfeeding. Milk expression may also be used to relieve engorgement from delayed or missed breastfeed/chestfeed or to increase milk supply. Manual hand expression is low cost and ideal for occasional use and milk

TABLE 6.1 HUMAN MILK NUTRITION COMPONENTS AND BENEFITS

MACRONUTRIENTS

- **Protein:** Whey predominant (whey-to-casein ratio of 70:30), easily digestible, high biologic value protein. Supports rapid gastric emptying and provides immunologic defense. Nonprotein nitrogen, such as free amino acids, supports growth and is more concentrated in colostrum.
- **Fat:** Provides 40%-50% of calories. Hind milk may have twice the amount of fat as foremilk, and preterm milk has a 30% higher fat concentration. Essential fatty acids and long-chain fatty acids, including docosahexaenoic acid and arachidonic acid, support vision and cognition. Cholesterol in human milk aids central nervous system development.
- **Carbohydrate:** Lactose, the most abundant carbohydrate, enhances calcium absorption and breaks down into galactose and glucose for energy to the brain. Lactose is important in developing the physiologic function of the gastrointestinal tract and maintaining the composition of the intestinal microbiota. Human milk oligosaccharides (HMOs), complex sugars found in breast milk, also support gut health in the early stages of life. Amylase aids in starch digestion.[5]

(continued)

TABLE 6.1 HUMAN MILK NUTRITION COMPONENTS AND BENEFITS (*continued*)

MICRONUTRIENTS AND SUPPLEMENTS

- **Vitamin D:** Essential for bone health, especially in infants of vitamin D-deficient parents. The American Academy of Pediatrics (AAP) recommends 400 IU/day for all infants starting soon after birth, with higher doses (6,400 IU) for lactating parents to improve milk content.[2]
- **Fluoride:** Human milk has a low fluorine content. Fluoride supplements (0.25 mg) are recommended for infants aged 6 mo to 3 y if the local water fluoride content is deficient. Every child should have a dental visit by 12 mo of age.[6]
- **Iron:** Iron content (0.5-1.0 mg/L) is well absorbed from human milk, sufficient for term infants for the first 6 mo. Preterm infants may need supplementation. Iron supplements are not typically recommended for term infants.
- **Vitamin K:** All infants (human milk-fed or formula-fed) must receive vitamin K at birth to prevent bleeding.
- **Water:** Human milk is 87.5% water, providing adequate hydration with sufficient intake. Supplementing with water is not recommended, even in hot or humid climates, as it may worsen conditions like hyperbilirubinemia in the newborn.
- **Maternal Diet:** The maternal diet affects the micronutrient content of human milk. A balanced intake of fruits, vegetables, whole grains, protein, and heart-healthy fats is encouraged, along with three meals and snacks. If the baby has food intolerances or allergies, an elimination diet may be necessary. Continuing a daily multivitamin during lactation is also recommended.

BENEFITS

- **Protection Against Infection and Allergy:** Human milk provides passive immunologic protection through factors like secretory immunoglobulin A (IgA), lactoferrin, lysozyme, and leukocytes. It reduces the risk and severity of infections such as diarrhea, respiratory tract infections, otitis media, and urinary tract infections. Breastfeeding may also offer protection against conditions like sudden infant death syndrome (SIDS), diabetes, asthma, and chronic digestive diseases.
- **Physiologic and Psychological Benefits:** Human milk supports kidney function, intestinal maturation, and self-regulated infant intake. It changes in composition to meet the infant's needs, from colostrum to mature milk, and varies during each feeding. Psychologically, it promotes bonding between the infant and lactating parent and encourages mutual caregiving.
- **Maternal Health Benefits:** Breastfeeding aids in postpartum recovery, reduces the risk of certain cancers, improves bone health, and lowers the risk of type 2 diabetes.
- **Community and Economic Benefits:** Breastfeeding reduces health care costs, absenteeism, and environmental burdens. It supports workplace productivity through lactation support, providing economic benefits to families and communities.

Adapted in part from Meek JY, Noble L; AAP Section on Breastfeeding. Policy statement: breastfeeding and the use of human milk. *Pediatrics.* 2022;150(1):e2022057988.

relief, while breast pumps are recommended for longer term use (Table 6.4). Best practices for milk storage and handling include labeling expressed milk with infant's name, date, and time and providing fresh milk first, followed by refrigerated, then frozen milk. Milk should be thawed in the refrigerator or a warm water bath but never microwaved to avoid damaging the immune properties of human milk and creating hot spots in the milk. More detailed information about storing and handling human milk is included in Table 6.5.[3]

TABLE 6.2 INITIATING LACTATION

PERINATAL

- Choose a supportive midwife, obstetrician-gynecologist (OB-GYN), and pediatrician who encourage breastfeeding/chestfeeding. Discuss any prior lactation issues and request a breast exam to identify potential anatomic concerns. Request a prenatal referral to a lactation consultant for anticipatory guidance, if needed.
- Select a "baby-friendly" birth center/hospital (Table 6.7) that promotes breastfeeding/chestfeeding as soon as possible after delivery, offers lactation consultant support, and practices rooming-in. Ensure the hospital does not distribute formula unless medically necessary.[7]
- Attend prenatal breastfeeding/chestfeeding classes, observe a successful feeding, and identify support individuals or groups for postbirth guidance.
- If returning to work/school, obtain a quality breast pump.

POSTPARTUM

- Initiate breastfeeding/chestfeeding as soon as possible after birth, preferably within 30 min. Encourage "on-demand" feeding (as frequent as every hour, no more than 4 h between feeds) and observe infant hunger cues (e.g., rooting, sucking on hand, fussiness, awake state; crying is a late cue for hunger).
- Clinical staff should assess latch, suck, swallow, and milk transfer (see Table 6.3). Refer to an International Board Certified Lactation Consultant (IBCLC) if necessary.
- If an infant is unable to feed from the breast/chest (see Table 6.4), begin milk expression within 1-3 h after birth. Teach hand expression of colostrum to provide small volumes in the first several days prior to onset of milk production and to support increased milk production later. The more frequently milk is expressed in the first 5 d, the more milk is available by the second week.
- If the parent is unavailable or the infant has difficulty latching, suggest alternative feeding methods such as a spoon, syringe, cup, or finger feeding. These methods can stimulate hunger and support breastfeeding efforts while preventing nipple confusion.

  Instruct the parent on proper storage and handling techniques for expressed human milk (Table 6.5).

ESTABLISHING MILK PRODUCTION

- Milk supply is dependent upon regular milk removal, either by infant or breast pump.
- Encourage breastfeeding 8-12 times per 24 h (waking newborns if more than 4 h have passed) and alternate breasts to promote equal milk production.
- Express milk during the night and ensure frequent feedings to establish a strong supply.
- Newborn infants initially feed every 1-3 h and may go longer between feedings in later infancy. Human milk-fed infants initially feed more frequently than formula-fed infants.
- Low milk production common causes include ineffective milk removal, insufficient breastfeeding frequency, delayed feeds, or excessive pacifier use. Other factors include stress, dehydration, medications, or previous breast surgeries.

PREMATURE INFANTS

- Colostrum or human milk should be the first feeding for premature infants; consider the use of donor human milk from a human milk bank, if necessary.
- Provide lactation support to initiate and maintain milk supply with long-term pumping.
- Consider fortifying human milk before full feeding volumes are reached and providing higher calorie hindmilk to promote infant growth.
- Encourage skin-to-skin care, early breastfeeding/chestfeeding, and non-nutritive suckling to promote growth and breastfeeding/chestfeeding success; recommend the use of nipple shields, if needed.
- Monitor preterm infants' progress with weight before and after feedings.

TABLE 6.3 ASSESSMENT OF BREASTFEEDING/CHESTFEEDING

POSITIONING

- Parent should be comfortable, supported with pillows and/or a footrest to keep their body position relaxed.
- Infant positioning options include cradle, cross-cradle or modified clutch, side-lying, clutch, or "football" hold or with the infant prone in a semi-reclining or "laid back" position. The infant should be at the level of the breast/chest to prevent neck strain.
- The infant's head should be gently supported but not held and forced toward the breast/chest. The breast may need to be supported using different holds (U-hold, C-hold, etc.).

LATCH

- Elicit rooting reflex (infant opens mouth wide) by tickling the infant's upper lip with the nipple, then bring the infant to the breast in one quick movement.
- Lips should be flanged wide and flipped outward, taking in as much of the nipple and areola into the mouth as possible.
- The latch should be asymmetrical with the infant's chin deep into the breast, and the nose/head slightly tipped back.
- If the latch is painful or uncomfortable, release the latch and try again (place a finger in the corner of the baby's mouth to break the seal). Refer to an International Board Certified Lactation Consultant (IBCLC) if pain, soreness, or cracked nipples occur.

MILK TRANSFER (SWALLOWING)

- Look for deep jaw movements and audible swallowing (soft "puffs" to loud gulps).
- After feeding, the infant should appear relaxed and satiated, and the breasts should feel softer.
- After the onset of milk production and approximately day 5, the infant should have 6 or more wet diapers per day. Urine should be clear to light yellow; not dark, concentrated, or foul smelling.
- Stool will transition from meconium dark to brown to green to yellow over the first several days. After day 5, the infant should have 3 or more yellow, seedy stools that are loose and small in volume. The frequency of stools changes as the infant grows.
- Weight gain should be approximately 5-7 oz per week after initial weight loss in the first days.

SIGNS OF INADEQUATE MILK INTAKE

- Infant may be lethargic, difficult to wake, feed less than 8-12 times per day in the first weeks, or have little-to-no swallowing at the breast.
- Infant may continue to lose weight or have minimal urine or stool output (<3 per day after day 3).

  Parent reports sore or cracked nipples. Breasts become painful and engorged, making latch difficult, and are not relieved (softened) by feeding the baby.
- If *inadequate intake is suspected, supplementation is necessary:*
  - Lactating parent should express milk with a pump to increase or maintain milk supply (see Table 6.4).
  - Provide colostrum or human milk via syringe, cup, or bottle; if milk expression is not possible, use appropriate infant formula (not water or dextrose water).
  - Close follow-up for weight monitoring and breastfeeding/chestfeeding support is essential.

Although human milk is the preferred source for infant feeding, there are circumstances where human milk may need to be temporarily or permanently avoided, as outlined in Table 6.6. Donor milk, when needed, should be pasteurized and sourced from an accredited milk bank. Milk sharing, though popular, poses health risks, especially

TABLE 6.4 HUMAN MILK EXPRESSION VIA PUMPING

TYPES OF BREAST PUMPS

- **Manual Breast Pump:** Low cost ($20-$50), requires no batteries or electricity, effective for short separations and engorgement relief.
- **Battery/Electric Pumps:** Moderate cost ($75-$150), requires batteries or electricity to use, portable, suitable for part-time separation but not long-term milk supply maintenance.
- **Wearable Pumps:** Higher cost ($60-$500), allows for discreet expression, but not for initiation or exclusive pumping.
- **Electric and Hospital-Grade Pumps:** Higher cost ($200-$350), effective for full-time work or long separations, useful after milk supply is established or for hospitalized infants, may be covered by health insurance for medically necessary separation.

BREAST PUMP USE

- **Preparation:** Read instructions, clean equipment, wash hands, and find a clean space for pumping (avoid bathrooms). Use clean bottles or single-use containers.
- **Technique:** Massage breasts to initiate letdown. Choose the correct breast shield size to minimize discomfort; adjust if needed due to nipple tenderness or skin changes. Start with low suction, gradually increasing for comfort and milk flow.
- **Pumping:** Pump for 10-15 min per breast (or both simultaneously). Alternate breasts if pumping one at a time. Double pumping is recommended to maximize supply and save time.
- **Exclusive Pumping:** Pump every 3 h, including overnight, until milk supply is established, then adjust based on needs.

GOALS FOR MILK EXPRESSION[8]

- **Exclusive Pumping:** Pump 6-8 times daily (or more) or at least 100 min total in 24 h.
- **First 5 d:** Pump at least 5 times daily to establish milk production.
- **Milk Volume:** Aim for >500 mL/d after day 7 or when milk volume is established.
- **Part-Time Pumping:** Pump once for every 3 h of separation from the infant (i.e., 2 times in an 8-h workday).

TABLE 6.5 HUMAN MILK STORAGE GUIDELINES

	ROOM TEMPERATURE *77 °F (25 °C) OR BELOW*	REFRIGERATOR *40 °F (4.4 °C) OR BELOW*	FREEZER *0 °F (−18 °C) OR BELOW*
Fresh human milk	Common: Up to 4 h Ideal: Refrigerate immediately if not using for the next feed. Acceptable: 6-8 h Administer continuous enteral tube feedings over 4 h, then replace milk.	Common: 4 d Ideal: <12 h Optimal: <48 h Acceptable: 5-8 d Avoid storing on the refrigerator door.	Common: 6 mo Ideal: <1 mo Optimal: <3 mo Acceptable: ≤12 mo Place milk toward the back of the freezer, not in the door; shorter storage times preserve the fat content of human milk.
Thawed human milk (previously frozen)	Up to 2 h	Common: Up to 24-48 h	Do not refreeze (partially thawed milk with ice crystals may be refrozen).

(continued)

TABLE 6.5 HUMAN MILK STORAGE GUIDELINES (*continued*)

	ROOM TEMPERATURE *77 °F (25 °C) OR BELOW*	REFRIGERATOR *40 °F (4.4 °C) OR BELOW*	FREEZER *0 °F (−18 °C) OR BELOW*
Leftover from a feeding	Use within 2 h of feeding or discard.	Use within 2 h of feeding or discard.	Do not freeze.
Pasteurized donor human milk	Up to 2 h after thawing Preferred: Refrigerate immediately.	Up to 96 h after thawing	Frozen: Up to 12 mo Thawed: Do not refreeze.

Adapted from HMBANA Guidelines 2024[9] and www.cdc.gov[3]

for ill or medically complex infants, if untested and unpasteurized. Tables 6.6 and 6.7 highlight advocacy, equity, and professional resources.

Weaning is the gradual introduction of other foods or fluids to an infant, ultimately replacing human milk feeds. This process is influenced by cultural, social, and individual family factors and typically occurs gradually over weeks, months, or years. Continuing partial breastfeeding/chestfeeding into the second year is common, with weaning spanning 2 to 4 years globally. For infants under 1 year, an alternative milk source, such as iron-fortified infant formula, is necessary. If younger infants still have sucking needs, a bottle, pacifier, or thumb may be offered. For many parents, weaning can be emotionally challenging, often causing feelings of sadness, guilt, or uncertainty. It is best to avoid weaning during stressful times, such as when the child is sick or adjusting to significant changes like a new sibling or daycare.

TABLE 6.6 CONDITIONS FOR WHICH HUMAN MILK MAY BE CONTRAINDICATED

CONDITION	GUIDANCE
Galactosemia	Infants must receive lactose-free formula, not human milk.
Phenylketonuria (PKU)	Provide human milk with prescribed phenylalanine (PHE)-free formula.
Tuberculosis (TB)	Do not breastfeed if untreated, active TB. Pump milk and discard for 2+ weeks of treatment and no longer contagious.
Hepatitis A **Hepatitis B**	Breastfeeding allowed after receiving gamma globulin Breastfeeding allowed after infant receives hepatitis B immunoglobulin (HBIG) and the first dose of the hepatitis B vaccine
Hepatitis C	Breastfeeding allowed; avoid if nipples are cracked or bleeding.
Herpes	Do not breastfeed with active lesions on the breast. Breastfeed from the unaffected side if lesions are covered.
HIV/AIDS	Avoid breastfeeding to eliminate the risk of HIV transmission. If breastfeeding is desired, criteria must be met (e.g., viral suppression, ART adherence).[10]
HTLV-1	Do not breastfeed due to the risk of vertical transmission.
Ebola Disease	Do not breastfeed if confirmed or suspected Ebola or recently recovered.

TABLE 6.6 CONDITIONS FOR WHICH HUMAN MILK MAY BE CONTRAINDICATED (*continued*)

CONDITION	GUIDANCE
Brucellosis	Do not breastfeed if untreated.
COVID-19	Breastfeeding allowed with hygiene precautions, as breast milk does not transmit SARS-CoV-2[11]
Medication Use	Most medications are compatible with breastfeeding. Consult scientific literature and weigh risks to the infant. To minimize infant exposure to medications, administer them after feeding, choose short-acting options, consider alternatives or delay treatment if possible, and pump and discard milk until therapy is complete.[12]
Weight Loss Surgery/ Medication	Encourage breastfeeding with micronutrient supplementation to ensure proper nutrition.[13] Parents taking weight loss medications should talk to their health care providers; there is limited information about the impact on the infant.[14]
Drugs of Misuse	Avoid breastfeeding if using drugs like amphetamines, heroin, cocaine, Phencyclidine (PCP) or marijuana.
Methadone Maintenance	Breastfeeding allowed for parents on methadone, though infants may experience withdrawal symptoms

AIDS, acquired immunodeficiency syndrome; ART, Antiretroviral Therapy HTLV-1, Human T-cell Lymphotropic Virus type 1 HIV, human immunodeficiency virus.

Gradual weaning is the preferred method, as it allows milk supply to decrease while maintaining breast comfort. This process involves reducing feedings by eliminating one feeding every 3 days, starting with the least preferred feeding. Distractions such as activities or walks can help replace breastfeeding/chestfeeding sessions. In contrast, abrupt weaning occurs unexpectedly or due to external influences. If weaning must happen quickly, it is important not to stop all at once, as this can cause breast pain or infection. Parents should pump to relieve fullness but avoid fully draining

TABLE 6.7 ADVOCACY, EQUITY, AND SUPPORT

TOPIC	DETAILS
Ten steps to successful breastfeeding	The Baby-Friendly Hospital Initiative (BFHI) is a global program sponsored by the World Health Organization (WHO) and the United Nations Children's Fund (UNICEF) to promote optimal infant feeding care in hospitals and birthing centers. Institutions can earn the "Baby-Friendly Hospital" designation by implementing these steps (www.babyfriendlyusa.org).
Pumping in the workplace	The Fair Labor Standards Act (FLSA) requires employers to provide reasonable break time and a private, non-bathroom space for employees to pump for up to 1 y after childbirth. Expanded rights include nurses, teachers, home care workers, and others as of the 2022 Consolidated Appropriations Act.[15]
Donor human milk	The Human Milk Banking Association of North America (HMBANA) accredits nonprofit milk banks and sets guidelines for pasteurized donor milk (www.hmbana.org).

the breasts and use cold compresses for swelling. A well-fitting, supportive bra can also reduce discomfort. Milk may persist in the breasts for months after weaning is complete. Parents who wean following the death of their infant can donate expressed milk to a milk bank. More information is available from the Human Milk Banking Association (Table 6.7).

It is the responsibility of every health care provider who cares for families with infants to educate themselves to provide lactation support or to refer to experts such as International Board Certified Lactation Consultants (IBCLC) to help their families meet their breastfeeding/chestfeeding goals. Knowledge about racial, ethnic, and cultural inequities and the care of gender-diverse families is necessary to provide competent care. To be inclusive of varied gender identities, when possible, the language used here is gender neutral, but gendered language is present and is not meant to exclude any persons. Health care providers should ask individual families about their pronouns and preferred language related to their identity, parenting, and lactation to provide inclusive care[4] (Table 6.8).

TABLE 6.8 PROFESSIONAL RESOURCES AND EDUCATION

ORGANIZATION	DESCRIPTION
International Lactation Consultant Association (ILCA) http://www.ILCA.org	The member association for International Board Certified Lactation Consultants (IBCLC) and other health care professionals. Provides educational resources, clinical guidelines, and journal publications
International Board of Lactation Consultant Examiners (IBLCE) http://www.iblce.org	An independent international credentialing body conferring the IBCLC credential and exam requirements. Maintains a list of education providers and an international registry of IBCLCs. Provides oversight of certification requirements, examination development, and related activities
La Leche League International (LLLI) www.llli.org	International breastfeeding peer support and educational resources: volunteer peer counselor and leader training, local chapters, and online support groups
National Lactation Consultant Alliance (NLCA) https://nlca.us/	Supports professionals holding the IBCLC credential and advocates for the clinical lactation consultant profession at the local, state, and national levels. Federal and state policy, legislation, and licensure activity. Continuing education and resources. Center for Lactation Equity
World Alliance for Breastfeeding Action (WABA) http://www.waba.org.my/	Global network dedicated to the protection, promotion, and support of breastfeeding worldwide. Partners with professional organizations and the World Health Organization (WHO)/United Nations Children's Fund (UNICEF). World Breastfeeding Week promotion

REFERENCES

1. World Health Organization. Breastfeeding recommendations. Accessed February 27, 2025. https://www.who.int/health-topics/breastfeeding#tab=tab_1
2. Meek JY, Noble L; AAP Section on Breastfeeding. Policy statement: breastfeeding and the use of human milk. *Pediatrics*. 2022;150(1):e2022057988.
3. Centers for Disease Control and Prevention. Breastfeeding: breast milk storage and preparation. Accessed December 12, 2024. https://www.cdc.gov/breastfeeding/breast-milk-preparation-and-storage/handling-breastmilk.html
4. Bartick M, Stehel EK, Calhoun SL, et al. Academy of Breastfeeding Medicine position statement and guideline: infant feeding and lactation-related language and gender. *Breastfeeding Med*. 2021;16(8):1-4.
5. Ballard O, Morrow AL. Human milk composition: nutrients and bioactive factors. *Pediatr Clin North Am*. 2013;60 (1):49-74.
6. Clark MB, Keels MA, Slayton RL; AAP Section on Oral Health. Clinical report: fluoride use in caries prevention in the primary care setting. *Pediatrics*. 2020;146(6):e2020034637.
7. Massachusetts Breastfeeding Coalition. Hospitals should market health, and nothing else. Accessed February 27, 2025. https://massbreastfeeding.org/ban-the-bags/
8. Hoban R, Medina-Poeliniz C, Signorile M, et al. Early postpartum pumping behaviors, pumped milk volume, and achievement of secretory activation in breast pump-dependent mothers of preterm infants. *J Perinatol*. 2024;44(11):1597-1606.
9. Mannel R, Taylor S. *Best Practice for Expressing, Storing and Handling Human Milk in Hospitals, Homes, and Child Care Settings*. 5th ed. Human Milk Banking Association of North America; 2024.
10. Abuogi L, Noble L, Smith C, et al; American Academy of Pediatrics Committee on Pediatric and Adolescent HIV; Section on Breastfeeding. Infant feeding for persons living with and at risk for HIV in the United States: clinical report. *Pediatrics*. 2024;153(6):e2024066843.
11. Centers for Disease Control and Prevention. Breastfeeding: breast milk storage and preparation. Accessed March 19, 2026. https://www.cdc.gov/breastfeeding/breast-milk-preparation-and-storage/handling-breastmilk.html
12. Hale TW, Krutsch K. *Medications and Mother's Milk™: A Manual of Lactational Pharmacology 2025-2026*. 21st ed. Springer Publishing Company LLC; 2025.
13. Kaska L, Kobiela J, Abacjew-Chmylko A, et al. Nutrition and pregnancy after bariatric surgery. *ISRN Obes*. 2013;2013:492060. Accessed November 1, 2024. https://pmc.ncbi.nlm.nih.gov/articles/PMC3901983/
14. Diab H, Fuquay T, Datta P, Bickel U, Thompson J, Krutsch K. Subcutaneous Semaglutide during Breastfeeding: Infant Safety Regarding Drug Transfer into Human Milk. Nutrients. 2024 Aug 28;16(17):2886. doi: 10.3390/nu16172886. PMID: 39275201; PMCID: PMC11397063.
15. U.S. Department of Labor. FLSA protections to pump at work. The Fair Labor Standards Act Protections to Pump at Work. Accessed November 1, 2024. dol.gov

CHAPTER 7

Feeding Guidelines for Infants, Toddlers, and Children

Annette Schille and Mollie Studley

Proper nutrition is essential for the growth and development of infants, toddlers, and children. Each child grows at a unique rate, so their nutritional needs will vary. This chapter reviews feeding guidelines from infancy through school age, providing general recommendations to support healthy development.

INFANT NUTRITION

As discussed in Chapter 6, breast milk is the ideal food for most infants, offering numerous benefits for both the child and the lactating parent. When breastfeeding/chestfeeding is not possible or not preferred, iron-fortified commercial infant formula is the recommended alternative to human milk. Homemade or imported infant formulas are not recommended. During the first 6 months, human milk or infant formula should be the only source of nutrition. After 6 months, human milk or formula alone may not provide sufficient amounts of certain nutrients, such as iron and zinc. Complementary foods, like iron-fortified cereals or pureed meats, should be introduced to meet the infant's nutritional needs.[1]

Introduction of other foods or fluids typically begins around 6 months of age but should not occur before 4 months. Early introduction of solids before 4 months has been linked to potential health risks, including obesity, celiac disease, type 1 diabetes, and allergies.[2] The introduction of foods should be based on multiple factors, including the infant's developmental readiness. The texture, consistency, type, and amount of solid food offered should align with the infant's feeding skills and development of the gastrointestinal system. See Table 7.1 for an overview of normal sucking and chewing skill development and corresponding feeding recommendations.[3]

Parents can choose between traditional feeding and baby-led weaning (BLW) when introducing solids. In traditional feeding, babies are spoon-fed purees and gradually progress to other textures until they can self-feed. In BLW, babies are not spoon-fed; instead, they are offered pieces of food they can feed themselves. Larger pieces are typically offered during the first few months, progressing to smaller pieces as the infant's self-feeding skills develop. Infants need to be able to sit independently, usually around 6 months of age, to be developmentally ready for BLW. The Academy of Nutrition and Dietetics does not endorse one method over the other. Regardless of the feeding method chosen, they recommend introducing solid foods around 6 months of age,

TABLE 7.1 ORAL MOTOR AND FEEDING DEVELOPMENT

AGE	FEEDING AND ORAL MOTOR DEVELOPMENT	FOOD TYPES AND TEXTURES	TIPS FOR SUCCESSFUL EATING
0-4 mo	• Roots in search of nipple • Sucking and tongue thrusting are reflexes.	• Liquids: Breast milk or formula	• If the baby is gassy, recommend an angled bottle to help reduce air intake.
4-6 mo	• Reflexive suck diminishes • Opens mouth for spoon, but tongue thrust is still present • May gag easily with purees • May put things in mouth to practice biting	• Liquids: Breast milk or formula is generally recommended until 6 mo. • Smooth purees: Infant cereal, stage 1 or 2 purees • BLW not recommended at this stage unless sitting independently	• Use a baby spoon; allow the baby to suck off the spoon instead of placing it directly in their mouth.
6-8 mo	• Spoon feeding improves, and the baby can tolerate thicker purees • Craves a variety of textures, including hard teething foods and dissolvable solids • Tongue moves side to side, and the tongue thrust disappears. • Introduction to cup drinking can begin, using a variety of cups such as open cups, straw cups, or sip cups without no-spill valves.	• Liquids: Breast milk or formula remains primary. • Smooth purees: Infant cereal, stage 1 or 2 purees • Thick purees: Homemade or blenderized purees • Teething biscuits • Crunchy dissolvable solids • BLW: Soft meat patties, large pieces of soft-cooked vegetables, and ripe fruit	• Use long, stick-shaped foods to encourage self-feeding and biting practice. • Early *sippy* cups should allow liquid to flow through the spout easily; the valve can be added once the baby learns to suck from a *sippy* cup.
8-10 mo	• Refines biting and munching • Can eat most soft and dissolvable foods but may gag frequently as the child experiments with more mature foods • Wants to self-feed	• Liquids: Breast milk or formula • Smooth purees • Thick purees • Crunchy dissolvable solids • Soft, well-cooked vegetables • Very well-cooked or ground meat	• Cut solids into an appropriate size (cubed or stick shape) so little fingers and mouths can manipulate them easily. • If the baby gags easily, that particular food may still be too advanced for their skill level.

(*continued*)

TABLE 7.1 ORAL MOTOR AND FEEDING DEVELOPMENT (*continued*)

AGE	FEEDING AND ORAL MOTOR DEVELOPMENT	FOOD TYPES AND TEXTURES	TIPS FOR SUCCESSFUL EATING
10-12 mo	• Eats a variety of table foods • Begins to show more efficient chewing of most soft table foods • Still gags with harder-to-chew foods	• Liquids: Breast milk or formula • Smooth purees • Thick purees • Crunchy dissolvable solids • Soft, well-cooked vegetables • Very well-cooked or ground meat	• Encourage self-feeding as much as possible. • Keep offering the baby new foods even if the baby refuses them. • Baby may spit food out when learning how to eat and chew that food successfully.
12-16 mo	• Refines self-feeding skills, preferring to use utensils • Can drink from a straw cup	• Most table foods, including some raw fruits and vegetables	• Provide utensils with short handles and cups with handles.

BLW, baby-led weaning.
Data from Arvedson JC, Brodsky L, Lefton-Greif MA. *Pediatric Swallowing and Feeding: Assessment and Management*. 3rd ed. Plural Publishing; 2020.

TABLE 7.2 AMERICAN ACADEMY OF PEDIATRICS INFANT FEEDING RECOMMENDATIONS

- Introduce solid foods when the infant is developmentally ready, around 6 mo. Iron, zinc, and protein-rich foods, such as iron-fortified cereals or pureed meats, should be offered as first foods.
- Single-ingredient foods should be offered to observe any adverse reactions. When each single-ingredient food is tolerated, the infant can begin consuming mixed foods that contain only these previously tolerated items. By 7-8 mo, infants should be consuming foods from all food groups.
- To establish healthy eating patterns during childhood, it is important to introduce a variety of foods by the first year of life. It can take 8-15 tries for an infant or child to accept a new food.
- Juices should not be introduced before 12 mo of age. For toddlers aged 1-3 y, juice intake should be limited to 4 oz per day, and for children aged 4-6 y, it should be limited to 4-6 oz per day. Only 100% fruit juice should be offered, and it should be served in a cup, not a bottle, to prevent tooth decay.
- Delay the introduction of cow's milk until 1 y of age; cow's milk should be whole milk during the second year of life.

Data from American Academy of Pediatrics Committee on Nutrition. Complementary feeding. In: Kleinman RE, Greer FR, eds. *Pediatric Nutrition*. 7th ed. American Academy of Pediatrics; 2013:123-139.

offering a variety of safe, age-appropriate foods, and monitoring for potential choking hazards.[4] Studies comparing the two methods have found no significant difference in choking risk.[5]

The American Academy of Pediatrics' (AAP) recommendations for general infant feeding practices are listed in Table 7.2.[1] The volume of solid foods consumed varies by infant; therefore, there are no recommended amounts given but rather general guidelines for feeding solid foods to infants.

Infants should be offered a wide variety of foods to ensure they receive essential nutrients while minimizing risks associated with exposure to contaminants.[6] Contaminants, such as heavy metals like arsenic, occur naturally in the environment and can enter soil and water, impacting our food supply. Rice absorbs more arsenic from groundwater than other crops. While iron-fortified infant rice cereal is a nutritious option, it is recommended to alternate with other infant cereals, including oat, barley, and multigrain. Heavy metals may also be present in fruits and vegetables, impacting both homemade purees and commercially prepared infant foods.

Introduction of peanut and egg around 6 months, but not before 4 months, is recommended to reduce the risk of food allergies in all infants.[7,8] Strategies for introducing allergenic foods can be found in Chapter 24.

■ TODDLER AND CHILDHOOD NUTRITION

Parents and caregivers should be encouraged to offer three scheduled meals and choose whole, nutrient-dense carbohydrate sources, such as whole grains, legumes, fruits, and starchy vegetables, paired with protein (in the form of meat, fish, poultry, eggs, soy, or legumes) and healthy fats at each meal to help support satiety, balanced energy levels, and overall nutrition. Each child's nutritional needs should be balanced with their food preferences and be responsive to their internal hunger and satiety cues. The Division of Responsibility in Feeding[9,10] is a helpful concept to apply throughout childhood. This framework emphasizes that parents are responsible for *what*, *when*, and *where* of feeding, while children decide *how much* and *whether* they eat. See Table 7.3 for feeding recommendations for toddlers.[11]

As children grow, they require adequate amounts of fruits, vegetables, grains, dairy or dairy alternative products, and protein-rich foods. Fruits and vegetables provide vitamins A and C, fiber, and antioxidants. Enriched grains and grain products provide B vitamins, iron, magnesium, and fiber. Whole grains should be prioritized over refined grains and sugars, as they are more filling and nutrient dense. Added sugar should not exceed 10% of total daily calories to ensure sufficient intake of nutrient-dense food choices. Dairy and dairy alternative products, such as cow's milk or soy milk, provide protein and are primary dietary sources of calcium and vitamin D. If a child does not consume cow's milk due to an allergy or family preference, nondairy alternatives should be offered to ensure adequate intake of calcium and vitamin D. Foods from the protein-rich group are good sources of iron and trace elements such as zinc.[12] Fat is an essential part of a child's diet; sources of essential fatty acids should be prioritized over

TABLE 7.3 FEEDING RECOMMENDATIONS FOR TODDLERS

FOOD GROUP	SERVINGS/ DAY	SERVING SIZES AND FOOD SOURCES	IMPORTANT NUTRIENTS
Dairy/dairy alternatives	2-3	½ cup of whole milk or ½ cup of calcium-fortified alternative milk, ½ cup yogurt, ½ oz cheese, ⅓ cup yogurt	Calcium, riboflavin, protein, and vitamin D
Protein rich	2	1 ounce of lean meat, poultry, or fish; 2 tablespoons ground meat; 1 egg; 1 oz or 1-inch cube of cheese; ¼ cup of cooked dried beans, peas, lentils, or tofu; 2 tablespoons peanut butter; ¼ cup cottage cheese; ¼ cup drained tuna; 3 oz is the same as ¼ chicken (½ breast, leg, or thigh); 1 piece of meat or fish the size and thickness of a deck of cards	Protein, iron, zinc
Grains	4-6	½ slice of bread, ¼ cup cooked rice or pasta, ¼ cup cooked cereal, 1-2 crackers, ½ hamburger or hotdog bun, ¼ cup ready-to-eat cereal	B vitamins, iron, fiber
Fruits	2-3	½ pieces of fresh fruit or ½ cup of canned, cooked, or frozen fruit; ¼-½ cup of 100% fruit juice	Vitamins A and C, potassium, fiber
Vegetables	2-3	¼-½ cup of whole, raw, leafy greens, 2-3 tablespoons cooked; ¼-½ cup of fresh, frozen, or canned vegetables	Vitamins A and C, folate, potassium, fiber

Data from U.S. Department of Health and Human Services, U.S. Department of Agriculture. Dietary Guidelines for Americans, 2020-2025. 9th ed. U.S. Government Publishing Office; 2020..

TABLE 7.4 FEEDING RECOMMENDATIONS FOR CHILDREN AGED 6 TO 12 YEARS

FOOD GROUPS	RECOMMENDED FOODS	FOODS TO LIMIT
Grains	Whole grains such as whole wheat bread, brown rice, oatmeal, and quinoa	Refined grains like white bread, pastries, and sugary sweetened cereals
Vegetables	Dark green, orange, red, and legume vegetables; fresh, frozen, or canned without added salt	Vegetables fried or prepared with excessive butter, cream, or cheese sauce
Fruits	Whole fruits, fresh, frozen, or canned fruits in water or 100% juice; unsweetened juice (limit to 4 oz/day)	Fruit canned in syrup; fruit-flavored snacks
Protein rich	Lean meat, poultry, fish, eggs, nuts, nut butters, seeds, beans/legumes	Fried foods (chicken fingers, French fries, fried chicken, mozzarella sticks) Processed meats, bacon, sausage
Dairy/dairy alternatives	Low- or nonfat milk, yogurt, and cheese	Full-fat dairy products, flavored milks with added sugar
Fats and oils	Healthy fats such as olive oil, avocado, nuts, and seeds	Trans fats, hydrogenated oils, and excessive butter or margarine

Data from Satter E. How to get your child to eat...but not too much. Boulder, CO: Bull Publishing Company; 1987. From Satter E. *Child of Mine: Feeding With Love and Good Sense*. Bull Publishing Company; 2000; U.S. Department of Health and Human Services, U.S. Department of Agriculture. Dietary Guidelines for Americans, *2020-2025*. 9th ed. U.S. Government Publishing Office; 2020.

saturated fat, which should be limited to less than 10% of total daily calories.[11] See Table 7.4 for feeding recommendations for children aged 6 to 12 years.[9-11]

Children have higher energy needs, especially during periods of growth, so snacks are an important part of their daily intake. Planned snacks can help prevent grazing, which may disrupt hunger cues and lead to overeating or lack of appetite at meals. Snacks should be chosen based on the child's level of hunger and the time until the next meal. Aim to include at least two of the three macronutrients (carbohydrate, protein, and healthy fats) to promote balance and satiety. See Table 7.5 for nutritious snack ideas.

■ ORAL HEALTH FOR CHILDREN

Good nutrition and oral hygiene are essential for preventing oral diseases and maintaining oral health throughout childhood, with healthy food and drink choices playing a vital role at every stage of a child's development. Tooth decay is the most common chronic disease in children, often caused by prolonged exposure to liquids other than water, such as breast milk, formula, or juice, especially when using a bottle or sippy cup during sleep or frequent sipping throughout the day. Limiting sugary snacks and drinks, offering water as the primary beverage, and promoting balanced meals can help reduce the risk of tooth decay. Routine daily cleaning with a moist cloth or

TABLE 7.5 NUTRITIOUS SNACK IDEAS

- Apple slices with nut butter
- Celery sticks with nut butter and raisins
- Carrot sticks, cucumber slices, and bell pepper strips with hummus
- Fresh fruit kebabs with yogurt dip
- Canned fruit (in juice or water) with cottage cheese
- String cheese with whole-grain crackers
- Low-fat (low sugar) yogurt with granola and berries
- Smoothie made with low-fat milk, frozen fruit, and spinach
- Pudding made with low-fat milk
- Air-popped popcorn with a sprinkle of parmesan cheese or nutritional yeast
- Whole-grain toast with avocado or nut butter
- Whole wheat English muffin pizzas (with marinara and low-fat mozzarella)
- Whole-grain, low-sugar cereal with milk
- Whole-grain crackers with cheese slices or hummus
- Hard-boiled eggs with whole-grain toast
- Lean deli turkey or chicken rolled up with a slice of cheese
- Tuna or chicken salad with whole-grain crackers
- Edamame with a sprinkle of sea salt
- Trail mix (nuts, seeds, dried fruit, dark chocolate, or M&M's)
- Graham crackers with nut butter
- Banana slices with a drizzle of honey and a sprinkle of chia seeds
- Cereal parfait: layer low-fat yogurt, whole-grain cereal, and berries
- Veggie chips: slice sweet potato or zucchini, season to taste, and bake until crisp
- Pizza bites: top whole-grain pita bread with marinara, cheese, and veggie toppings, then toast
- Rabbit bag: prepack prepped fruit and veggies (e.g., carrots, grapes, sliced apple) in bags
- Nachos: top whole-grain tortilla chips with cheese, then heat

infant toothbrush should begin as soon as any tooth erupts, typically by 6 months of age. Children aged 3 years and older should brush their teeth daily with a pea-sized amount of fluoridated toothpaste. All infants should receive an oral health risk assessment by 6 months of age and visit a dentist by 12 months of age.[11,13]

The fluoride content of drinking water varies by community. Parents should contact their local pediatrician, dentist, or town office to determine if fluoride supplementation is necessary. See Table 7.6 for information on fluoride supplementation.[11,13] It is important to note that excessive ingestion of fluoride can cause mottled enamel, a condition known as chronic endemic dental fluorosis.

TABLE 7.6 DIETARY FLUORIDE SUPPLEMENT RECOMMENDATIONS

	FLUORIDE ION LEVEL IN DRINKING WATER		
Age	**<0.3 ppm**	**0.3-0.6 ppm**	**>0.6 ppm**
Birth to 6 mo	0	0	0
6 mo to 3 y	0.25 mg/d	0	0
3-6 y	0.50 mg/d	0.25 mg/d	0
6-16 y	1.0 mg/d	0.50 mg/d	0

Data from U.S. Department of Health and Human Services, U.S. Department of Agriculture. *Dietary Guidelines for Americans, 2020-2025*. 9th ed. U.S. Government Publishing Office; 2020; American Academy of Pediatric Dentistry. Policy on the dental home. *American Academy of Pediatric Dentistry Reference Manual*. Updated 2022.

REFERENCES

1. American Academy of Pediatrics Committee on Nutrition. Complementary feeding. In: Kleinman RE, Greer FR, eds. *Pediatric Nutrition*. 7th ed. American Academy of Pediatrics; 2013:123-139.
2. Woo Baidal JA, Locks LM, Cheng ER, Blake-Lamb TL, Perkins ME, Taveras EM. Risk factors for childhood obesity in the first 1,000 days: a systematic review. *Am J Prev Med*. 2016;50(6):761-779.
3. Arvedson JC, Brodsky L, Lefton-Greif MA. *Pediatric Swallowing and Feeding: Assessment and Management*. 3rd ed. Plural Publishing; 2020.
4. Academy of Nutrition and Dietetics. Position of the Academy of Nutrition and Dietetics: complementary feeding. *J Acad Nutr Diet*. 2019;119(4):731-738.
5. Correia L, Sousa AR, Capitão C, Pedro AR. Complementary feeding approaches and risk of choking: a systematic review. *J Pediatr Gastroenterol Nutr*. 2024;79(5):934-942.
6. American Academy of Pediatrics. 5 Ways to reduce arsenic in your child's diet. HealthyChildren.org. Updated June 2023. https://www.healthychildren.org/English/ages-stages/baby/feeding-nutrition/Pages/reduce-arsenic.aspx
7. American Academy of Pediatrics. Early introduction of allergenic foods may prevent future allergies. *AAP News*. 2018;34(2):13.
8. Fleischer DM, Chan ES, Venter C, et al. A consensus approach to the primary prevention of food allergy through nutrition: guidance from the American Academy of Allergy, Asthma, and Immunology; American College of Allergy, Asthma, and Immunology; and the Canadian Society for Allergy and Clinical Immunology. *J Allergy Clin Immunol Pract*. 2021;9(1):22-43.e4.
9. Satter E. *How to Get Your Child to Eat...But Not Too Much*. Bull Publishing Company; 1987.
10. Satter E. *Child of Mine: Feeding With Love and Good Sense*. Bull Publishing Company; 2000.
11. U.S. Department of Health and Human Services, U.S. Department of Agriculture. *Dietary Guidelines for Americans, 2020–5*. 9th ed. U.S. Government Publishing Office; 2020.
12. Ogata BN, Hayes D. Position of the Academy of Nutrition and Dietetics: nutrition guidance for healthy children ages 2 to 11 years. *J Acad Nutr Diet*. 2014;114(8):1257-1276.
13. American Academy of Pediatric Dentistry. Policy on the dental home. In: *The Reference Manual of Pediatric Dentistry*. American Academy of Pediatric Dentistry; 2022.

CHAPTER 8

Adolescent Nutrition

Julie J. Norton and Lisa A. Mancini

Adolescence is a time of significant biologic, physical, emotional, and cognitive changes. These changes are shaped by factors such as biologic and neurodevelopmental processes, social environments, and the influence of media and cultural norms. These factors, as well as increased nutrient needs, can create unique nutritional challenges and contribute to the risk of a range of health issues, including iron deficiency anemia, poor bone mineralization, micronutrient deficiencies, eating disorders, excess weight gain, and chronic diseases such as type 2 diabetes, heart disease, and osteoporosis later in life. Encouraging autonomy and promoting healthy eating and exercise habits during this stage of development is essential for fostering a positive relationship with food that can carry into adulthood.

Dietary habits formed during adolescence often persist into adulthood,[1] may influence future generations,[2] and are linked to chronic disease risk later in life. Diets low in fruits, vegetables, whole grains, calcium-rich foods, and low-fat dairy, combined with regular consumption of sugar-sweetened beverages and highly processed foods, during adolescence, can result in deficiencies in folate; vitamins A, E, and B_6; calcium; iron; zinc; and magnesium.[4] These patterns are also associated with higher intakes of fat, saturated fat, sodium, cholesterol, and sugar.[5] Adolescents with high intakes of ultra-processed foods are at increased risk of cardiovascular diseases and dental caries.[3]

Body dissatisfaction is also common during this stage due to rapid physical changes and increased media and peer influence. Research shows that up to half of adolescent girls and a quarter of boys engage in dieting behaviors to control their weight, with these behaviors becoming more common as they age. Adolescents who engage in dieting and other unhealthy weight-control methods are at increased risk of weight gain and disordered eating.[1,6]

This chapter will focus on biologic and psychosocial changes, nutrition counseling strategies, bone health, and polycystic ovary syndrome (PCOS). For more detailed information on nutrition assessment, weight management, eating disorders, sports nutrition, and vegetarianism in adolescents, refer to other chapters in this manual.

PUBERTY

Puberty, which occurs during adolescence, profoundly affects and is influenced by nutritional needs and status. During this period, adolescents attain approximately 20% of their final adult height, 50% of their adult weight, and up to 40% of their adult bone mass.[7] However, the age of onset, duration, and rate of puberty vary widely among individuals and can be significantly impacted by nutritional status in childhood. As a result, adolescents of a given chronologic age may show considerable differences in their physiologic development and nutritional needs. A better measure is the Sexual

Maturity Rating (SMR), also known as Tanner Staging, which evaluates growth and developmental age based on the development of secondary sexual characteristics. Tanner Stages range from 1 (prepubertal) to 5 (adult), with girls' stages based on breast maturity and pubic hair development and boys' stages based on the progression of genital and pubic hair development (see Tables 8.1 and 8.2).[8]

Linear growth, which corresponds to peak energy needs, occurs at different periods of development for boys and girls. As noted in Tables 8.1 and 8.2, girls typically begin the linear growth spurt during Tanner Stage 2, with peak height velocity occurring at the end of Tanner Stages 2 through 3 (about 8 cm a year).[8] During this period, girls require between 2,300 and 3,000 calories per day, depending on the amount of physical activity. By the onset of menarche, which typically occurs around Tanner Stage 4, girls will have completed the majority of their growth, adding only about two more inches of height postmenarche. Girls who enter puberty early (before age 11) may experience more linear growth after menarche than girls who enter puberty later. In the United States, the average age for girls to reach menarche is 12.6 years.[7] In boys, peak height velocity occurs between Tanner Stages 3 and 4 (about 7-8 cm and 10 cm/y, respectively), which coincides with peak energy needs.[8] The growth spurt for boys typically occurs between the ages of 12½ and 15. During this period, boys may need between 2,800 and 3,500 calories per day or more, depending on physical activity. In boys, peak weight velocity coincides with peak height velocity, whereas in girls, peak weight velocity occurs 6 to 9 months before peak height velocity.

Adolescents with severely restricted energy intake during this phase are at risk for delayed or slowed linear growth, which could affect the attainment of their full

TABLE 8.1 TANNER STAGES OF DEVELOPMENT IN BOYS

TANNER STAGE	GENITALIA/PUBIC HAIR/OTHER *(MEAN AGE OF PUBERTAL MILESTONES ATTAINMENT)*	GROWTH
1	Prepubescent	About 5-6 cm/y
2	Enlargement of testes and scrotum, reddening of scrotum (11.0 y) First appearance of pubic hair (11.8 y) Increased activity of sweat glands	About 5-6 cm/y
3	Growth of penis, mostly length, further growth of testes/scrotum (12.5 y) Pubic hair darker, covering pubis (13.1 y) Voice beginning to change	About 7-8 cm/y[a]
4	Growth of penis and scrotal skin darker (15.2 y) Adult-type pubic hair, no spread to the thighs (15.1 y) Axillary and facial hair Voice deepening	About 10 cm/y[a]
5	Adult genitalia (16.6 y) Adult-type pubic hair, extending to the thighs.	Deceleration and cessation at about 17 y

[a]Peak energy needs.

Adapted from Tanner JM. *Growth and Adolescence*. 2nd ed. Blackwell Scientific Publications: 1962.

TABLE 8.2 TANNER STAGES OF DEVELOPMENT IN GIRLS

TANNER STAGES	GENITALIA/PUBIC HAIR/OTHER *(MEAN AGE OF PUBERTAL MILESTONES ATTAINMENT)*	GROWTH
1	Prepubescent	About 5-6 cm/y
2	Small breast bud under enlarged areola (10.7 y) Small amount of pubic hair (10.8 y) Increased activity of sweat glands	About 7-8 cm/y[a]
3	Breasts grow larger, no separation of the nipple and the areola (12.5 y) Pubic hair is increased, darker, coarser, and curled (12.2 y) Axillary hair	About 8 cm/y[a]
4	Projection of areola and nipple from secondary mound (14.3 y) Adult-type pubic hair, no spread to medial thighs (14.5 y) Menarche	Deceleration <7 cm/y
5	Adult breast contour (16.1 y) Adult-type pubic hair, extends to medial thighs (16.4 y)	Cessation at about 16 y

[a]Peak energy needs.
Adapted from Tanner JM. *Growth and Adolescence*. 2nd ed. Blackwell Scientific Publications; 1962.

adult height.[9] During the prepubertal period, boys and girls generally have similar proportions of fat and muscle. However, under the influence of testosterone, boys proportionally gain more muscle mass than fat, with muscle mass doubling between the ages of 10 and 17. As a result, boys typically have more lean body mass per unit of height than girls.[9]

■ COGNITIVE AND PSYCHOSOCIAL DEVELOPMENT

Along with the biologic and physical changes, adolescence is a critical period of cognitive and psychosocial development. This development can be divided into three periods, each bringing new emotional, cognitive, and social milestones (Table 8.3). Understanding where an adolescent is in terms of psychosocial development is essential for creating personalized and effective nutritional plans.

Nutritional counseling for adolescents should consider the following strategies[10]:

- Tailor goals and interventions to the adolescent's stage of development.
- Empower adolescents to take control of their health and well-being, focusing on overall wellness rather than weight.
- Explore the impact of media and social relationships on the adolescent's perceptions of health and nutrition.
- Encourage active involvement in food shopping, meal planning, and cooking.

TABLE 8.3 PSYCHOSOCIAL PROCESSES AND THE SUBSTAGES OF ADOLESCENT DEVELOPMENT

SUBSTAGE	EMOTIONALLY RELATED	COGNITIVELY RELATED	SOCIALLY RELATED
Early adolescence (11-14 y)	Adjustment to a new body image, adaptation to emerging sexuality	Concrete thinking, early moral concepts	Strong peer effect
Middle adolescence (15-17 y)	Establishment of emotional separation from parents	Emergence of abstract thinking, expansion of verbal abilities and conventional morality, adjustment to increased school demands	Increased health risk behavior, sexual interests in peers, early vocational plans
Late adolescence (18-21 y)	Establishment of a personal sense of identity; further separation from parents	Development of abstract, complex thinking; emergence of postconventional morality	Increased impulse control, emerging social autonomy, establishment of vocational capability

Adapted from Stang J, Story M, eds. Nutrition needs of adolescents. In: *Guidelines for Adolescent Nutrition Services*. Center for Leadership, Education and Training in Maternal and Child Nutrition, Division of Epidemiology and Community Health, School of Public Health, University of Minnesota; 2005:21-34.

- Set concrete, achievable goals that are realistic for their lifestyle.
- Promote participation in community programs that support health and well-being.
- Discuss the local food environment, exploring available resources and how to navigate them effectively.
- Focus on body-positive, nondiet messaging rather than weight-focused goals to foster a healthier self-image.
- Introduce principles of intuitive eating, which encourage honoring the body's natural hunger cues and food preferences, while avoiding a focus on body weight/shape.
- Encourage family meals at home in a supportive, nonjudgmental environment.
- Educate families about healthy food choices and the importance of modeling desirable behaviors, making healthy food choices available, and avoiding discussions centered on weight.
- Discourage feeding practices that can negatively impact an adolescent's relationship with food and their body, such as restriction or pressure to eat.

BONE HEALTH AND SKELETAL DEVELOPMENT

Bone is a living tissue that undergoes continuous formation and resorption, a process known as bone turnover. During adolescence, bone formation predominates, with the goal of optimizing peak bone mass. Achieving a higher maximum bone density during puberty reduces fracture risk and provides a reserve to delay or prevent osteoporosis later in life.[11] Bone turnover markers peak during mid-puberty (Tanner Stages 2 and 3) and decrease markedly in late puberty (Tanner Stages 4 and 5). Approximately 45% to 50% of total skeletal mass is completed during adolescence. By the age of 18 for girls and 20 for boys, 90% of peak bone mass is attained, with the remaining 10% accrued at a slower rate into the third decade of life.[12]

Estrogen plays a central role in bone growth and maintenance, particularly in girls. Estrogen works alongside growth hormone and insulin-like growth factor in bone modeling. Indirectly, estrogen stimulates the production of $1{,}25(OH)_2D$ from hydroxyvitamin D, which enhances absorption of calcium in the gut and reduces excretion of calcium from the kidneys. Estrogen also supports bone formation by increasing the number of vitamin D receptors on bone cells, especially osteoblasts, and stimulating the secretion of osteocalcin. Girls with early or regular menarche tend to have higher bone mineral density, while late menarche or conditions like anorexia nervosa are associated with lower density and higher fracture risk.

Bone mass is 70% to 80% genetically determined, but 20% to 30% depends on diet and lifestyle factors, such as calcium intake, vitamin D status, weight-bearing activity, and body weight. Calcium is the most abundant mineral in the human body, with 99% found in bones and teeth. Along with phosphorus, calcium contributes to bone strength by being deposited into the porous protein structure of the bone, increasing bone density and strength. Many adolescents do not meet the recommended daily allowance for calcium due to decreased consumption of calcium-rich foods. Puberty is associated with higher rates of dietary calcium absorption, and adolescents experience reduced calcium excretion, thereby enhancing mineral absorption. This increased calcium efficiency during puberty supports bone growth.[13]

Vitamin D is essential for calcium and phosphorus absorption. It enhances calcium absorption by 30% to 40% and phosphorus by 80%. Without sufficient vitamin D, only 10% to 15% of dietary calcium and about 60% of phosphorus are absorbed.[14] Vitamin D deficiency can lead to soft, weak, or brittle bones and can cause rickets in children or osteomalacia and osteoporosis later in life. The primary source of vitamin D is solar exposure, with smaller contributions from dietary intake and fortified foods (see Table 8.4 for food sources of vitamin D). Risk factors for deficiency include darker skin pigmentation, sunscreen use, winter seasons, latitude above 35° north, and inadequate dietary intake. In 2024, the Endocrine Society updated practice guidelines, recommending vitamin D supplementation for children and adolescents aged 1 to 18

TABLE 8.4 FOOD SOURCES OF VITAMIN D

FOOD	MICROGRAMS (μG) PER SERVING	INTERNATIONAL UNITS (IU) PER SERVING
Cod liver oil, 1 tablespoon	34.0	1,360
Trout (rainbow), farmed, cooked, 3 oz	16.2	645
Salmon (sockeye), cooked, 3 oz	14.2	570
Mushrooms, white, raw, sliced, exposed to ultraviolet light, ½ cup	9.2	366
Milk, vitamin D fortified, 1 cup	2.9	120
Soy, almond, and oat milks, vitamin D fortified, various brands, 1 cup	2.5-3.6	120-144
Ready-to-eat cereal, fortified with 10% of the Daily Value for vitamin D, 1 serving	2.0	80

Adapted from Institute of Medicine, Food and Nutrition Board. *Dietary Reference Intakes for Calcium and Vitamin D.* National Academy Press; 2010.

TABLE 8.5 RECOMMENDATIONS FOR VITAMIN D SCREENING IN PATIENTS AT RISK FOR DEFICIENCY

- Bone disease (rickets, osteopenia)
- Hepatic failure
- Malabsorption syndromes (cystic fibrosis, inflammatory bowel disease, Crohn disease, bariatric surgery)
- Chronic kidney disease
- Lymphoma
- Medications (seizure meds, glucocorticoids, human immunodeficiency virus [HIV] medications, antifungals, cholestyramine)

Adapted from Demay MB, Pittas AG, Bikle DD, et al. Vitamin D for the prevention of disease: an Endocrine Society clinical practice guideline. *J Clin Endocrinol Metab*. 2024;109(8):1907-1947.

to prevent rickets. Supplementation can come from fortified foods, multivitamins, or vitamin D supplements.[12] Routine screening for vitamin D deficiency is advised for otherwise healthy adolescents with overweight and obesity and those with dark skin coloring, as supplementation is more cost-effective in these cases. Table 8.5 lists conditions for which vitamin D screening is recommended. Table 8.6 indicates levels of deficiency, adequacy, and toxicity of vitamin D. Table 8.7 includes treatment recommendations for vitamin D deficiency.

■ POLYCYSTIC OVARIAN SYNDROME

PCOS is a complex disorder that impacts 6% to 10% of women of reproductive age. Though its etiology and pathophysiology are not fully understood, the condition is believed to arise from genetic factors and hypothalamic and ovarian dysfunction. Risk factors for PCOS include being born small for gestational age, childhood obesity, premature puberty, and having a mother with PCOS.[16]

PCOS can be classified into four phenotypes[17]:

1. Hypersecretion of androgens, ovarian cysts, and occasional anovulation (most common phenotype)
2. Hypersecretion of androgens and occasional anovulation
3. Hypersecretion of androgens and ovarian cysts
4. Chronic anovulation and polycystic ovaries without clinical or biochemical hyperandrogenism

TABLE 8.6 VITAMIN D (25OHD) THRESHOLDS

Deficiency	<30 nmol/L (<12 ng/mL)
Potential risk for inadequacy	≥30-50 nmol/L (12-<20 ng/mL)
Normal/adequate	>50 nmol/L (≥20 ng/mL)
Risk for adverse effects	>125 nmol/L (≥50 ng/mL)

Adapted from Institute of Medicine, Food and Nutrition Board. *Dietary Reference Intakes for Calcium and Vitamin D*. National Academy Press; 2010.

TABLE 8.7 RECOMMENDATIONS FOR TREATMENT (25OHD: <30 NMOL/L)

- Ergocalciferol (vitamin D_2) 50,000 IU weekly for 6-8 wk
- Calcium per the RDA, divided over the day (see Table 5.3)
  - 9-18 y: 1,300 (UL 3,000 mg)
- Check 25OHD levels approximately 8-10 wk after treatment is initiated
- Maintenance dose of 800-1,000 IU/day once the 25OHD level exceeds 30 ng/mL

25OHD, 25 hydroxyvitamin D; RDA, recommended dietary allowance; UL, tolerable upper intake level.
Adapted from Kaur J, Khare S, Sizar O, et al. Vitamin D deficiency. In: *StatPearls* [Internet]. StatPearls Publishing; 2025. https://www.ncbi.nlm.nih.gov/books/NBK532266/

Common symptoms of PCOS are acne, hirsutism, irregular menstrual cycles (for more than 2 years since menarche), and hyperandrogenism. PCOS may also lead to complications like high blood sugar levels, obesity, metabolic malfunction, and impaired reproductive health.[18]

Treatment for PCOS can include medications, lifestyle changes, and, if needed, weight loss. Medical nutrition therapy plays an important role in managing PCOS by addressing insulin resistance and supporting metabolic and reproductive functions. When counseling adolescents with PCOS, the following dietary and lifestyle modifications should be emphasized:

- Consuming three structured meals daily and one to two snacks as needed
- Increasing fiber intake through complex carbohydrates and low-glycemic foods such as vegetables and whole grains
- Focusing on lean proteins
- Limiting sugary beverages
- Limiting intake of saturated fat while encouraging heart-healthy fats, such as omega-3s
- Recommending moderate-to-vigorous exercise most days of the week, aiming for at least 150 min/wk

Dietary interventions should include specific goals that improve quality of life and meet the patient's needs. While weight loss of 5% to 15% has been shown to improve insulin resistance and reproductive health, care must be taken to promote a positive body image in adolescents with PCOS to prevent negative effects on self-esteem.[19] Weight loss medications, such as glucagon-like peptide-1 (GLP-1) agonists, may support weight loss in adolescents with comorbidities but should be monitored closely by a medical provider.

REFERENCES

1. Neumark-Sztainer D, Wall M, Larson NI, Eisenberg ME, Loth K. Dieting and disordered eating behaviors from adolescence to young adulthood: findings from a 10-year longitudinal study. *J Am Diet Assoc.* 2011;111:1004-1011.
2. Patton GC, Neufeld LM, Dogra S, et al. Nourishing our future: the Lancet Series on adolescent nutrition. *Lancet.* 2022;399(10320):123-125.
3. Larson N, Neumark-Sztainer D. Adolescent nutrition. *Pediatr Rev.* 2009;30:494-496.

4. Stang J, Story M, eds. Nutrition needs of adolescents. In: *Guidelines for Adolescent Nutrition Services*. Center for Leadership, Education and Training in Maternal and Child Nutrition, Division of Epidemiology and Community Health, School of Public Health, University of Minnesota; 2005:21-34.
5. Mescoloto SB, Pongiluppi G, Domene SMÁ. Ultra-processed food consumption and children and adolescents' health. *J Pediatr (Rio J)*. 2024;100(Suppl 1):S18-S30.
6. Solmi F, Sharpe H, Gage SH, Maddock J, Lewis G, Patalay P. Changes in the prevalence and correlates of weight-control behaviors and weight perception in adolescents in the UK, 1986-2015. *JAMA Pediatr*. 2021;175(3):267-275.
7. Norris SA, Frongillo EA, Black MM, et al. Nutrition in adolescent growth and development. *Lancet*. 2022;399(10320):172-184.
8. Tanner JM. *Growth and Adolescence*. 2nd ed. Blackwell Scientific Publications; 1962.
9. Spear B. Adolescent growth and development. *J Am Diet Assoc*. 2002;102(3):S23-S29.
10. Hargreaves D, Mates E, Menon P, et al. Strategies and interventions for healthy adolescent growth, nutrition, and development. *Lancet*. 2022;399(10320):198-210.
11. Giustina A, Bilezikian JP, Adler RA, et al. Consensus statement on vitamin D status assessment and supplementation: whys, whens, and hows. *Endocr Rev*. 2024;45(5):625-654.
12. Benjamin RM. Bone health: preventing osteoporosis. *Public Health Rep*. 2010;125(3):368-370.
13. Mesias M, Seiquer I, Navarro MP. Calcium nutrition in adolescence. *Crit Rev Food Sci Nutr*. 2011;51(3): 195-209.
14. Akimbekov NS, Digel I, Sherelkhan DK, Razzaque MS. Vitamin D and phosphate interactions in health and disease. *Adv Exp Med Biol*. 2022;1362:37-46.
15. Demay MB, Pittas AG, Bikle DD, et al. Vitamin D for the prevention of disease: an Endocrine Society clinical practice guideline. *J Clin Endocrinol Metab*. 2024;109(8):1907-1947.
16. Adone A, Fulmali DG. Polycystic ovarian syndrome in adolescents. *Cureus*. 2023;15(1):e34183.
17. Guastella E, Longo RA, Carmina E. Clinical and endocrine characteristics of the main polycystic ovary syndrome phenotypes. *Fertil Steril*. 2010;94(6):2197-2201.
18. Mumusoglu S, Yildiz BO. Polycystic ovary syndrome phenotypes and prevalence: differential impact of diagnostic criteria and clinical versus unselected populations. *Curr Opin Endocrine Metab Res*. 2020; 12:66-71.
19. Calcaterra V, Verduci E, Cena H, et al. Polycystic ovary syndrome in insulin-resistant adolescents with obesity: the role of nutrition therapy and food supplements as a strategy to protect fertility. *Nutrients*. 2021;13(6):1848.
20. Institute of Medicine, Food and Nutrition Board. *Dietary Reference Intakes for Calcium and Vitamin D*. National Academy Press; 2010.
21. Kaur J, Khare S, Sizar O, et al. Vitamin D deficiency. In: *StatPearls* [Internet]. StatPearls Publishing; 2025. https://www.ncbi.nlm.nih.gov/books/NBK532266/

CHAPTER 9

Vegetarian Diets

Jasper Brezsny-Feldman and Daniel Kamin

Vegetarian diets have long been part of human tradition, appearing in the foundational texts of Hinduism and Buddhism, as well as in ancient Greek and Roman literature.[1] Vegetarian diets do not include meat, fish, or poultry and typically focus on fruits, vegetables, grains, legumes, nuts, and seeds. Lacto-ovo vegetarians consume eggs and dairy products. Lacto-vegetarians exclude eggs but consume dairy products. Vegans avoid all animal-derived foods, including eggs, dairy products, and honey.[2-4] Even within defined types of vegetarian diets, eating patterns can vary widely based on personal health concerns, religious, ethical, and environmental motivations.[3] Interest in vegetarian diets has grown in recent years, particularly in high-income countries, partly due to concerns about the environmental impact of meat and dairy production, which contributes to greenhouse gas emissions.[5]

Well-planned vegetarian diets can be healthful, nutritionally adequate, and beneficial for disease prevention and treatment.[2-4] Vegetarian children and adolescents have lower intakes of cholesterol, saturated fat, and total fat and higher intakes of fruits, vegetables, and fiber than nonvegetarians.[2,3] For children and adolescents, vegetarian diets are associated with lower serum cholesterol levels[2,3] and can foster the development of lifelong healthy eating habits.[1] Vegetarian diets are appropriate for all stages of the life cycle, though proper menu planning and potential supplement considerations are needed, depending on the type of vegetarian diet followed.

While vegetarian diets can provide the necessary nutrients for infants and children, caregivers must select appropriate food alternatives to ensure proper nutrition to support growth and development. Vegetarian infants should be fed human milk or given a commercial infant formula. For vegan infants, soy-based formulas regulated by the U.S. Food and Drug Administration (FDA) are recommended. Infants receiving human milk from a parent following a vegan diet may need a B_{12} supplement, as well as docosahexaenoic acid (DHA)-fortified foods or supplements to meet higher DHA requirements.[2,3] Vitamin D supplementation is also recommended for all infants receiving human milk. Guidelines for the introduction of solid foods to vegetarian infants are similar to those for nonvegetarian infants, though the types of protein-rich foods offered, such as pureed tofu, legumes, dairy or plant-based yogurt, cooked egg, cottage cheese, cubed tofu, cheese or plant-based cheese, and bite-size pieces of veggie burgers, will differ.

See Table 9.1 for selected foods rich in macro- and micronutrients relevant for vegetarian diets.

■ PROTEIN

Plant-based proteins can meet dietary requirements when a variety of plant foods are consumed and energy needs are met.[2,3] It was once believed that vegetarians needed to carefully combine certain plant-based foods to achieve a complete amino acid profile.

TABLE 9.1 VEGETARIAN FOOD SOURCES OF SELECT NUTRIENTS[7]

NUTRIENT	VEGETARIAN FOOD SOURCES
Protein[a]	Eggs, milk, cheese (cottage, ricotta, natural), yogurt, kefir, soy milk or plant milk with added protein, soy yogurt or plant-based yogurt with added protein, tofu, beans and legumes, nuts and seeds, nut and seed butter, tempeh, vegetarian meat substitutes made with textured vegetable protein
Iron[b]	Edamame, tofu, beans (pinto, lima, navy, kidney, garbanzo, lentils), cashews, almonds, pumpkin seeds, sunflower seeds, sesame tahini, fortified cereal,[c] cream of wheat,[c] dried fruit, prune juice/puree, potatoes, blackstrap molasses, green leafy vegetables (spinach, collard greens, kale, Swiss chard)
Calcium[b]	Milk,[c] fortified plant milk,[c] cheese (cottage, ricotta, natural), yogurt, fortified plant-based yogurts, soybeans, tofu (processed with calcium), tempeh, beans (black, garbanzo, navy, pinto), blackstrap molasses, almonds, almond butter, tahini, fortified cereal,[c] figs, and green leafy vegetables (kale, broccoli, turnip greens, mustard greens, collard greens, bok choy), calcium-fortified juice[c,d]
Vitamin D[b]	Mushrooms exposed to ultraviolet light,[c] milk, fortified plant milk, and fortified cereals
Vitamin B_{12}[b]	Eggs,[c] milk,[c] fortified plant milk,[c] fortified cereal,[c] nutritional yeast,[c] and fortified vegetarian meat substitutes[c]
n-3 Fatty acids	Ground flaxseeds, flaxseed oil, canola oil, walnuts, walnut oil, hemp seeds, chia seeds, tofu, soybeans, and soybean oil

[a]Foods that contain at least 5 to 7 g of protein per serving; specific amounts may vary.
[b]Provide 5% or more of the Daily Value for each nutrient per serving for children over 4 years of age, which is the threshold used by the U.S. Food and Drug Administration to define a low source of these nutrients.
[c]Provide 20% or more of the Daily Value for each nutrient per serving for children over 4 years of age, which is the threshold used by the U.S. Food and Drug Administration to define a high source of these nutrients.
[d]Consider general guidelines for total juice consumption in children's diets.

However, research indicates that a diet consisting of a variety of plant foods eaten over the course of a day can provide all essential amino acids and support adequate nitrogen retention.[2]

■ IRON

Iron from plant foods is nonheme iron, which is more affected by inhibitors and enhancers of iron absorption than heme iron.[2,3] Inhibitors of iron absorption include phytates, calcium, and the polyphenolics in tea, coffee, herbal tea, and cocoa.[2] Vitamin C and other organic acids found in fruits and vegetables substantially enhance iron absorption and can counteract the effects of phytates.[2,4] Nonheme iron absorption is significantly affected by an individual's iron status, with iron-deficient individuals absorbing nonheme iron at 10 times the rate of iron-replete individuals.[3] Vegetarians were previously advised to consume 1.8 times the amount of iron recommended for nonvegetarians due to the lower bioavailability of nonheme iron, but current evidence suggests that individuals can adapt to diets low in iron bioavailability by increasing absorption and reducing losses to maintain iron status.[3] While iron stores may be lower in vegetarian individuals, the prevalence of iron-deficiency anemia remains similar to that of nonvegetarians.[2-4]

CALCIUM

Calcium is found in many plant-based and fortified foods, but its absorption can be hindered by oxalates, which are found in some vegetables such as spinach, beet greens, and Swiss chard.[2] Vegetables low in oxalates, such as kale, turnip greens, bok choy, broccoli, Chinese cabbage, and collards, have good calcium bioavailability.[2-4] Dairy products are considered good sources of bioavailable calcium. Dairy alternatives such as plant-based milk or yogurt that are fortified with calcium and tofu set with calcium have comparable calcium bioavailability to dairy products.[3] Calcium intake of lacto-ovo vegetarians is comparable to or higher than that of nonvegetarians, but vegans tend to have lower intake than both groups.[2-4] Vegans may need to consume fortified foods or low-dose calcium supplements to meet their calcium needs.

VITAMIN D

Vitamin D is crucial for maintaining bone health and supporting immune function. Some vegetarian and vegan populations have shown low vitamin D levels and reduced bone mass.[2-4] Vitamin D status is influenced by sunlight exposure and intake of vitamin D-fortified foods or supplements. The effectiveness of sunlight exposure depends on several factors, including time of day, season, latitude, pollution, skin melanin content, sunscreen application, amount of uncovered skin, and age.[3] Fortified food sources of vitamin D are cow's milk, some plant-based milks, fruit juices, and breakfast cereals. Mushrooms exposed to ultraviolet light and eggs may also contain some vitamin D.[3] When sun exposure and intake of fortified foods are insufficient, vitamin D supplements are recommended. Both vitamin D_2 (ergocalciferol) and vitamin D_3 (cholecalciferol) are effective, though vitamin D_3 is generally more effective in raising and maintaining vitamin D levels.[3] Vitamin D_2 is plant-sourced, whereas D_3 is commonly derived from lanolin (sheep's wool), though vegan-friendly sources like lichen are available. Dietary supplements do not always specify the source of vitamin D, so it may be necessary to contact the manufacturer.

VITAMIN B_{12}

Vitamin B_{12} is not naturally found in plant foods, except in cases of contamination. Vegans and most vegetarians should include reliable sources of B_{12} through fortified foods (such as cereals, meat alternatives, plant-based milk, or nutritional yeast) or a daily supplement. For best absorption when supplementing, B_{12} supplements should be taken at two separate times per day.[2-4]

N-3 FATTY ACIDS

Vegetarian diets are typically rich in n-6 fatty acids but may be low in n-3 fatty acids, which are important for cardiovascular health and infant brain development.[2,4] The conversion of alpha-linolenic acid (ALA), a plant-based n-3 fatty acid, to eicosapentaenoic acid (EPA) is generally less than 10% in humans, and the bioconversion of ALA to DHA is substantially less.[2-4] Excessive intake of n-6 fatty acids can further inhibit the conversion of ALA.[2,4] Studies have shown that vegetarians, particularly vegans, have lower blood levels of EPA and DHA.[2] While the conversion process is inefficient, adequate intake of ALA can sustain this system and provide adequate n-3 levels in healthy individuals.[3] Vegetarians should include good sources of ALA in their diets in an effort to promote conversion.[3] Concentrated sources of n-3 fatty acids include flax, chia, canola, hemp, walnuts, and their oils.[3] For individuals needing additional n-3 fatty acids, certain microalgae and fortified foods provide DHA, and oil from brown algae (kelp) provides EPA. For ovo-vegetarians, chickens fed n-3 fatty acids provide a source of EPA and DHA.

■ ZINC

Zinc bioavailability is lower in vegetarian diets compared with nonvegetarian diets, mainly due to the high phytate content of plant foods.[2,4] Studies indicate that zinc intake among vegetarians can vary from marginal to inadequate.[2,4] Vegetarians with high phytate intake may require more zinc than the recommended dietary allowance.[2,4] To improve zinc absorption, vegetarians can use organic acids, such as citric acid, and food preparation techniques, such as soaking and sprouting beans, grains, and seeds, as well as leavening bread.[2-4] Vegetarian food sources of zinc include cashews, pecans, walnuts, pumpkin seeds, chia seeds, sunflower seeds, and hemp seeds. Grains, legumes, cheeses, and other nuts and seeds also contain zinc in lower concentrations.[3,7]

■ IODINE

Plant-based diets are typically low in iodine, and some vegans may be at risk for iodine deficiency.[2,3] Key sources of iodine include iodized salt and sea vegetables. Sea salt, kosher salt, pink Himalayan salt, and tamari are often not iodized, so it is important to ensure adequate iodine intake through iodized salt or iodine-rich foods.

■ SOY

Soy, a staple in traditional Asian diets, has faced controversy due to its high content of isoflavones, an estrogen-like molecule naturally occurring in the plant. Isoflavones were once thought to be endocrine disruptors, raising concerns about the safety of soy consumption.[8] Recent evidence shows that isoflavones confer multiple health benefits, including promoting bone health and cognitive function.[8] Studies have shown no adverse effects on thyroid hormone, testosterone, or estrogen levels from moderate soy consumption, nor have they been shown to affect puberty onset.[8] Concerns about the processing and high n-6 content of some soy products, such as soy oil and soy protein, are similar to those about other ultra-processed foods.

■ ORGANIC FOODS

Many vegetarians also prioritize the consumption of organic foods due to concerns about exposure to antibiotic-resistant bacteria, synthetic fertilizers, and pesticide residues.[9] While the macronutrient composition of organic and nonorganic foods is similar, organic foods tend to have higher concentrations of antioxidants and n-3 fatty acids.[9] Though the long-term health impacts of low-level pesticide exposure remain unclear, consuming organic foods can minimize exposure to pesticides and herbicides classified as "probably carcinogenic" by the World Health Organization.[9] Organic foods can be costly, and current evidence suggests that the variety of whole plant foods consumed is more important than whether the foods are organic or nonorganic.

REFERENCES

1. Leitzmann C. Vegetarian nutrition: past, present, future. *Am J Clin Nutr*. 2014;100(suppl 1):496S-502S.
2. Craig WJ, Mangels AR; American Dietetic Association. Position of the American Dietetic Association: vegetarian diets. *J Am Diet Assoc*. 2009;109(7):1266-1282.
3. Melina V, Craig W, Levin S. Position of the Academy of Nutrition and Dietetics: vegetarian diets. *J Acad Nutr Diet*. 2016;116(12):1970-1980.
4. Craig WJ. Nutrition concerns and health effects of vegetarian diets. *Nutr Clin Pract*. 2010;25(6):613-620.
5. Desmond MA, Fewtrell MS, Wells JCK. Plant-based diets in children: secular trends, health outcomes, and a roadmap for urgent practice recommendations and research—a systematic review. *Nutrients*. 2024;16(5):723.
6. U.S. Department of Agriculture. MyPlate. Accessed February 14, 2026. https://www.myplate.gov/tip-sheet/enjoy-vegetarian-meals
7. U.S. Department of Agriculture. FoodData Central. https://fdc.nal.usda.gov
8. Messina M, Duncan A, Messina V, Lynch H, Kiel J, Erdman JW Jr. The health effects of soy: a reference guide for health professionals. *Front Nutr*. 2022;9:970364.
9. Vigar V, Myers S, Oliver C, Arellano J, Robinson S, Leifert C. A systematic review of organic versus conventional food consumption: is there a measurable benefit on human health? *Nutrients*. 2020;12(1):7.

CHAPTER 10

Sports Nutrition

Alix Krawcke and Maria E. Walazek

Sports participation offers significant benefits for children and adolescents, including improved fitness, greater bone density, lower blood pressure, and reduced risk of cardiovascular disease later in life. Sports participation enhances self-esteem and emotional well-being and is associated with lower levels of anxiety and depression.[1] While young athletes have similar nutrient needs to nonathletes, the combined demands of training, competition, and growth may impact some nutritional requirements, such as energy and fluid needs. This chapter aims to provide guidelines for assessing and supporting the nutritional needs of young athletes.

NUTRIENT NEEDS

Energy Needs

The four major components of energy needs include basal metabolic rate, thermic effect of food, thermic effect of physical activity, and the energy requirements of growth.[2,3] While athletes typically need more calories than nonathletes due to increased physical activity, the exact requirements depend on the individual's sport and training schedule, as well as their developmental stage. Refer to Chapter 5 for energy need equations that can be applied to young athletes based on their estimated activity level. These equations should be considered in conjunction with weight and growth trends, length and intensity of training, history of injury, and symptoms such as fatigue and weakness.

Macronutrient Needs

The recommended macronutrient distribution for young athletes is generally similar to that for nonathletes, although it may vary depending on the athlete's sport, training phase, or specific goals, such as preparing for training, competing, or recovering. Portion sizes of food groups at meals can best be estimated using the performance plate method based on training intensity, as in Figure 10.1.

At rest, fat contributes 85% of adenosine triphosphate (ATP) production, and carbohydrates contribute the remaining 15%. Because energy demands are relatively low at rest, ATP does not need to be produced quickly. There is also ample time for the respiratory and cardiovascular systems to deliver oxygen to the muscles and for lipolysis/beta-oxidation to take place.

As physical activity increases, energy demands rise, and the body shifts toward greater use of carbohydrates, as glycolysis is faster than lipolysis and beta-oxidation. During moderate-intensity exercise, energy production is roughly balanced between carbohydrates and fat, with each contributing about 50% to ATP generation. However, during high-intensity activities, carbohydrates become the dominant fuel source, as

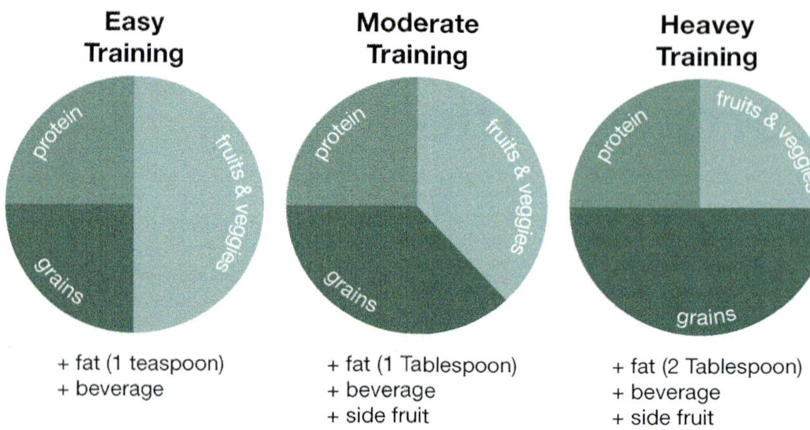

■ **Figure 10.1** Performance plates individualized for training intensity. (Adapted from American Sports and Performance Dietitians Association. https://sportsrd.org/)

they are the fastest and most immediate source of energy and can produce ATP both aerobically and anaerobically (Figure 10.2).[3]

To support these changing energy needs, dietary patterns should be adjusted accordingly. As the duration and intensity of activity increase, grains should make up a larger portion of the plate, while fruits and vegetables make up a smaller portion. Protein intake typically remains consistent regardless of activity level (Figure 10.1).

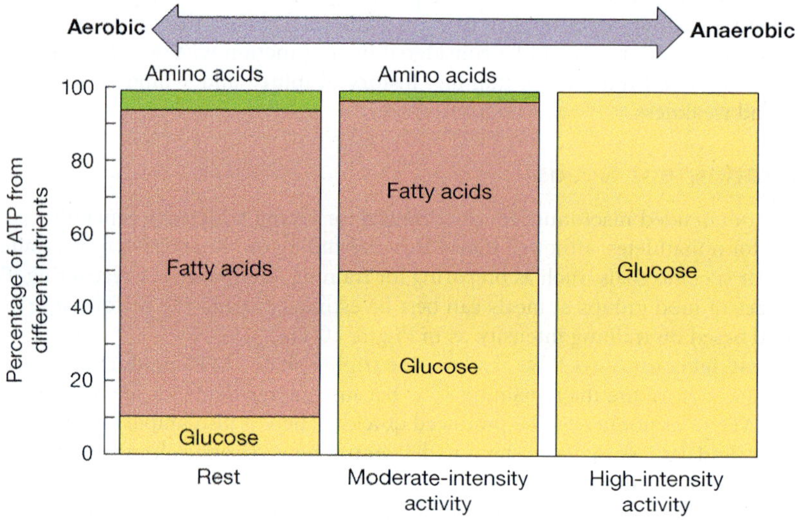

■ **Figure 10.2** Substrate utilization. At rest, our primary fuel source is from fatty acids, with minimal contributions from amino acids and glucose. As the duration and intensity of activity increase, the percentage of glucose as the fuel source becomes greater. ATP, adenosine triphosphate. (From University of Hawaii at Manoa Food Science and Human Nutrition Program; Titchenal A, Hara S, Caacbay NA, et al. Human Nutrition: 2020 Edition. University of Hawaii at Manoa; 2020.)

Carbohydrates: Carbohydrate is the primary source of energy the body uses for physical activity, and carbohydrate intake must increase as training time and intensity increase.[4] Carbohydrate intake should be the majority of the source of increased caloric intake for young athletes, making up 50% of total calories or 3 to 8 g/kg body weight, with the higher end of the range recommended for exercise with higher intensity or longer duration.[4] Carbohydrate intake should occur throughout the day, as well as during lengthy training periods to provide energy and restore glycogen stores in muscle.

Protein: Active individuals require more protein than nonactive individuals due to the breakdown of muscle and the use of protein as a source of energy during activity. The recommended protein intake for most young athletes is between 1.35 and 1.6 g/kg body weight.[5] Athletes participating in strength or resistance training may need to consume protein on the higher end of the range. Excessive protein intake is not shown to have any benefit for performance and may increase the risk of kidney damage.[5,6,7] Protein intake should primarily come from food, with intake spread throughout meals and snacks.[8]

Fat: Dietary fat supports several essential body functions, including the absorption of fat-soluble vitamins and the synthesis of cholesterol and sex hormones.[4] It also serves as an energy source when carbohydrates are unavailable. Restricting fat intake can disrupt the menstrual cycle in female endurance athletes and is associated with lower dietary variety, which increases the risk of nutritional deficiencies.[2,5] The recommended fat intake for children and adolescents is 25% to 35% of calories coming from fat, with 10% or less from saturated fat (see Chapter 5).[2,5] Fat is the most calorie-dense macronutrient, so quality fat sources may be beneficial for athletes who struggle to meet their energy needs. Quality sources of fat are those that are low in saturated fat, which may raise low-density lipoprotein (LDL) cholesterol, and high in unsaturated fat, which may help lower LDL cholesterol. Quality sources of fat include olive oil, nuts, fatty fish, avocado, flaxseeds, and vegetable oils. Some fatty acids, such as omega-3 fatty acids (eicosapentaenoic acid [EPA] and docosahexaenoic acid [DHA]), have been linked to reduced inflammation and improved brain function but do not appear to enhance athletic performance.[4,5] Food sources of DHA are limited primarily to fish, as well as some nuts and seeds. Due to limited food sources, supplementation may be considered for young people who struggle to meet recommendations.[5]

Despite the benefits of including fat in the diet, high-fat and ketogenic diets are not recommended due to insufficient research on their safety and effectiveness in young athletes.[5] To prevent gastrointestinal discomfort, athletes should limit fat consumption immediately before physical activity, instead spreading it throughout other meals and postactivity snacks.[5]

Micronutrient Needs

Micronutrient needs for athletes are similar to those of nonathletes. However, special attention should be given to calcium, vitamin D, and iron, as deficiencies can impact performance and injury risk (see Chapters 4 and 9). Iron status should be monitored, especially in vegetarians, vegans, and athletes with heavy menstrual bleeding, as poor iron stores are related to a decline in athletic performance, especially in endurance athletes.[2,4] Iron status may be assessed by looking at hemoglobin and hematocrit, as well as ferritin and transferrin levels. Iron supplementation should be considered if deficiencies are present (Chapter 9).[7]

Fluid and Electrolyte Needs

Adequate hydration is essential for performance. Even a small amount of dehydration (1% loss of body weight) can negatively impact performance.[4] Intake of fluids should occur throughout the day, before, during, and after exercise to maintain adequate hydration status.[2,4,5] Drinking to thirst may not be adequate, especially if exercising in a warm environment or at a high intensity.[4] Recommendations for fluid intake vary based on activity level, age, size, and the environment, but a general guideline is to drink 8 to 20 oz in the hour prior to starting exercise, along with periodic breaks for water (even when not thirsty), and to consume 1.25 to 1.5 L for every kilogram of body weight lost after activity.[5,7] Daily fluid intake can be in the form of beverages such as water, juice, milk, and sports drinks, as well as from foods like fruits and vegetables.[5] Caffeinated energy drinks, 100% juice, and carbonated beverages are not recommended due to their association with gastrointestinal discomfort.[2,7]

Electrolytes are minerals, including sodium, chloride, and potassium, that are essential for body functions, including the function of cardiac muscles. Electrolytes are lost in sweat and urine, and in situations with high heat or long and intense exercise lasting more than 90 minutes, the repletion of sodium and chloride may be necessary due to the amount lost in sweat. Although sports drinks may not be necessary for the average young athlete, a sports drink containing electrolytes and carbohydrates may be beneficial during and in recovery from settings of profuse sweating to reduce the risk of muscle cramps and hyponatremia.[2,5] The addition of salt to postexercise snacks and meals may also support the restoration of electrolyte balance.[5]

■ COMMON CHALLENGES AND CONCERNS FOR YOUNG ATHLETES

Navigating School and Training Schedules

Young athletes often struggle to balance meals and snack times around school and training. To meet nutritional needs, young athletes should eat every 3 hours, with snacks incorporated throughout the day.[6] Eating prior to exercise can increase energy stores in the liver and muscle to provide consistent energy during periods of competition or training.[6] Highly structured meal plans should be discouraged for youth athletes unless needed due to a specific health condition.

Relative Energy Deficiency in Sport

Relative energy deficiency in sport (REDs) is a syndrome that describes the adverse health and performance outcomes seen in athletes (male and female) in the setting of low energy availability (LEA) or inadequate energy intake in relation to energy expenditure.[9] Signs of REDs include a decline or stagnation in performance, an increase in injuries, impaired bone, and gastrointestinal and neurologic function, as well as impaired growth and development, which is especially concerning in young athletes who are still in the process of growing and establishing peak bone density.[8] Symptoms can also include mental health issues such as depression and anxiety, as well as disordered eating and eating disorders, which can lead to or exacerbate LEA.[9]

Sports Specialization

Early sports specialization in youth athletes should be discouraged due to the increased risk of overuse injuries and burnout.[10] Sports participation should be limited to fewer hours per week than the child's age, and intense participation in a single sport should be limited to less than or equal to 8 months per year.[10] A balanced approach with both free playtime and multisport participation offers greater physical and psychological benefits.[10]

Supplements

Many athletes are drawn to dietary supplements in the pursuit of improved performance or recovery. While certain supplements, such as caffeine and creatine, have shown benefits in adult athletes, the safety and efficacy of supplements in young athletes are not well studied, and the risks should be carefully considered.[5,6,7] Both the American Medical Association (AMA) and the American Academy of Pediatrics (AAP) recommend obtaining nutrients, such as protein, vitamins, and minerals, from food sources rather than supplements, particularly for otherwise healthy children.[2]

Dietary supplements do not require U.S. Food and Drug Administration (FDA) approval before they are sold, and it is the responsibility of the manufacturer to prove that the supplements are safe. Supplements may contain substances that are prohibited by the World Anti-Doping Agency and other sports regulatory agencies due to contamination or mislabeling,[2,5] and energy drinks are at risk of similar issues.[1] Independent organizations, such as ConsumerLab, NSF International, and U.S. Pharmacopeia, may test supplements for quality and contamination, but their seal does not guarantee the safety or effectiveness of the product.

■ NUTRITION ASSESSMENT

A comprehensive nutrition assessment for young athletes involves reviewing all available nutritional, medical, biochemical, clinical, and psychosocial data and can be used to identify areas where education or additional monitoring is needed, including the risk of REDs and disordered eating. The assessment should include a dietary recall to understand meal timing, nutrient intake, and recent dietary changes, as well as an evaluation of energy needs. The assessment should consider the athlete's training pattern, hydration habits, and supplement use, as well as any gastrointestinal issues or sleep disturbances. It is important to conduct a detailed assessment of menstrual status for female athletes, as many athletes are unaware of what is considered normal (see Table 10.1).

■ SUMMARY

Proper nutrition and hydration are essential for supporting growth, training, and performance in young athletes. While supplements are widely available, food should be encouraged as the optimal fuel for exercise and recovery. For athletes struggling to fuel adequately or for those considering the use of supplements or restrictive diets, registered dietitians can create personalized nutrition and hydration plans, provide education around food and fueling, guide supplement use, assess growth, and identify athletes at risk for or experiencing disordered eating.

TABLE 10.1 SPORTS-SPECIFIC NUTRITION ASSESSMENT QUESTIONS

Training

- How many hours per week do you train (in season and off-season)?
- How many hours per week do you compete?
- Do you do any additional recreational activities?
- How much walking do you do per day?

Hydration

- How much water do you drink per day?
- Do you add any electrolyte supplements to your water?
- Do you consume other beverages (i.e., juice, milk, sports drinks, or soda)?
- Do you consume any caffeinated beverages (i.e., coffee, tea, or energy drinks)?

Supplements

- Do you take any vitamins or mineral supplements?
- Do you take any dietary supplements?

Gastrointestinal issues

- How often do you have a bowel movement?
- Do you experience any stomach issues when training or competing (i.e., reflux, nausea, diarrhea)?

Sleep

- What time do you go to bed, and what time do you wake up?
- Do you have any trouble falling or staying asleep?

Menstrual status

- How often do you get your period?
- How many days does your period last?
- What is the flow like?

REFERENCES

1. Logan K, Cuff S; Council on Sports Medicine and Fitness, et al. Organized sports for children, preadolescents, and adolescents. *Pediatrics*. 2019;143(6):e20190997.
2. Desbrow B, McCormack J, Burke LM, et al. Sports Dietitians Australia position statement: sports nutrition for the adolescent athlete. *Int J Sport Nutr Exerc Metab*. 2014;24(5):570-584.
3. Mul JD, Stanford KI, Hirshman MF, Goodyear LJ. Exercise and regulation of carbohydrate metabolism. *Prog Mol Biol Transl Sci*. 2015;135:17-37.
4. Smith JW, Holmes ME, McAllister MJ. Nutritional considerations for performance in young athletes. *J Sports Med (Hindawi Publ Corp)*. 2015;2015:734649.
5. Karpinski C, Rosenbloom C. *Sports Nutrition: A Handbook for Professionals*. Academy of Nutrition and Dietetics; 2017.
6. Firmansyah A, Prasetya MRA. The nutrition needs of adolescent athletes: a systematic review. *J SPORTIF*. 2021;7(3):400-418.
7. Hecht C, Bank N, Cook B, Mistovich RJ. Nutritional recommendations for the young athlete: current concept review. *J Pediatr Orthop Soc North Am*. 2023;5(1):599.
8. Berg EK. Performance nutrition for the adolescent athlete: a realistic approach. *Clin J Sport Med*. 2019; 29(5):345-352.
9. Mountjoy M, Ackerman KE, Bailey DM, et al. 2023 International Olympic Committee's (IOC) consensus statement on Relative Energy Deficiency in Sport (REDs). *Br J Sports Med*. 2023;57:1073-1098.
10. Jayanthi NA, Post EG, Laury TC, Fabricant PD. Health consequences of youth sport specialization. *J Athl Train*. 2019;54(10):1040-1049.

CHAPTER 11

Dietary Supplements

E. Reese

Dietary supplements are products that include vitamins, minerals, prebiotics, probiotics, herbs or botanicals, amino acids, or other ingredients intended to supplement the diet. Supplements often include multiple nutrients and come in various forms, such as tablets, capsules, liquids, powders, lozenges, and candy-like products.[1] For cases of significant malabsorption, some nutrients are available in intravenous or intramuscular forms.

Supplementation of vitamins and minerals is generally not necessary if a child is eating a wide variety of foods. However, supplementation may be indicated if a child is not eating well (e.g., pediatric feeding disorder), is on a medically restricted diet (e.g., food allergies, celiac disease), or has a chronic illness that increases the risk of nutrient losses (e.g., cystic fibrosis, inflammatory bowel disease, intestinal failure). The decision to use a single nutrient supplement or a complete multivitamin with minerals should be based on the child's individual needs.[2]

Supplement dosing should meet science-based standards such as the Dietary Reference Intake (DRI), while not exceeding tolerable upper intake levels (UL, see Chapter 5).[3] In some cases of deficiency, published repletion dosing algorithms should be used. It is generally recommended that vitamins and minerals be taken with meals to improve absorption and to minimize gastric upset. Children who require complex supplementation regimens consisting of multiple nutrients or products should be counseled on the proper timing of supplement doses to maximize absorption.

Prebiotics are nutrients that promote the growth of healthy intestinal bacteria. For example, fructooligosaccharides (FOS) are a prebiotic fiber that stimulates the growth of healthy bacteria in the colon, producing short-chain fatty acids (SCFAs) that fuel colonic cells, maintain gut integrity, inhibit the growth of harmful bacteria, and may reduce diarrhea.[4]

Probiotics are monocultures or mixed cultures of live bacteria or yeast that may improve the properties of indigenous flora in the gut. Probiotics are available as supplements, may be added to foods such as yogurt, or may be naturally present in fermented foods like kimchi, miso, or kombucha.[5] Studies show that probiotics may help optimize healthy gut flora, improve immunity, minimize food allergy risk, manage irritable bowel syndrome and inflammatory bowel disease, control diarrhea or constipation, facilitate clearance of *Helicobacter pylori*, and prevent recurrence of *Clostridioides difficile* infection.[5-10] Because probiotics contain live cultures, it is important to monitor the stability of the product. Most probiotics should be taken with meals. Probiotics should not be given within 2 hours of antibiotic doses, with the exception of *Saccharomyces boulardii*, which is not inhibited by antibiotics and should be taken between meals.[6]

Herbal supplements originate from the bark, roots, leaves, seeds, flowers, and fruit of trees, shrubs, and woody vines of herbaceous plants. They are available in a variety of forms, such as fresh or dried herbs, tablets, capsules, herbal teas, essential oils, and extracts. Many medications originate from plant extracts, and herbs have been used for health purposes across cultures for thousands of years.[11] Herbal remedies may interact with other medications, so health care providers should ask patients about herbal supplement use to prevent potential interactions. Many herbal supplements are not recommended for use by adults during pregnancy or nursing due to risks (known or potential) to the fetus or infant.[1]

Supplements marketed for exercise or athletic performance, improved sleep, mental focus, and weight loss often lack clinical evidence to support their claims. Some products may contain ingredients known to be harmful, especially for pediatric patients. Adolescents, athletes, and those seeking a more "natural" approach to health care are more likely to use these products.[12]

Safety concerns with the use of any type of dietary supplement include inaccurate or misleading labels, issues with purity (e.g., presence of contaminants, drugs, or other harmful substances), and the risk of interactions between supplements and pharmaceuticals, foods, or enteral and formula feeds. Although the Food and Drug Administration (FDA) has established Good Manufacturing Practices that supplement companies must follow to ensure quality, dietary supplements are regulated as food and do not undergo the same rigorous testing process required of pharmaceuticals. Health care providers should recommend products that are third party (e.g., US Pharmacopeia, NSF International) tested for purity. Patients and caregivers should be encouraged to disclose the use or desired use of any dietary supplement to their health care providers, so they can make informed decisions for their safety.[1]

The tables that follow summarize the composition of dietary supplement products commonly used in pediatrics. It is important to confirm the composition of the listed products before use because the composition and ingredients of products, as well as general product availability, change frequently due to discontinuation, shortages, and new product development. Table 11.1 lists vitamin and mineral supplements, as well as any inactive ingredients and miscellaneous information that may be of value to the practitioner. When taken according to the manufacturer's guidelines, the agents in these tables provide or exceed the DRI for most of the nutrients listed. Each table notes the dose for the appropriate age group. Table 11.2 lists common enteral electrolyte and mineral supplementation products. Information regarding the composition of parenteral multivitamin, mineral, and trace element products may be found in Chapter 17 (Parenteral Nutrition). Table 11.3 lists common probiotics, potential benefits of these products, and some commercially available products. Table 11.4 lists information regarding herbal supplements.[11,13-16] Table 11.5 summarizes the different vitamin D analogues and metabolites.

TABLE 11.1 VITAMIN AND MINERAL SUPPLEMENTS

	LIQUID										
	CENTRUM® ADULT LIQUID (PER 15 ML/1 TBSP)	FLORIVA PLUS LIQUID DROPS™ (PER 1 ML)	KIRKMAN® SUPER NU-THERA® LIQUID (PER 5 ML/1 TSP)	MYKIDZ IRON™ (PER 2 ML)	MYKIDZ IRON FL™ (PER 2 ML)	NATURESPLUS® ANIMAL PARADE® BABY PLEX® MULTIVITAMIN DROPS (PER 1 ML)	NATURESPLUS® ANIMAL PARADE® MULTIVITAMIN CHILDREN'S LIQUID (PER 15 ML/1 TBSP)	NATURESPLUS® ANIMAL PARADE® GOLD MULTIVITAMIN CHILDREN'S LIQUID (PER 15 ML/1 TBSP)	POLY-VI-SOL® (PER 1 ML)	POLY-VI-SOL® WITH IRON (PER 1 ML)	TRI-VI-SOL® (PER 1 ML)
Vitamin A	390 μg	345 μg	750 μg	450 μg	450 μg	400 μg	1,500 μg	1,500 μg	250 μg	250 μg	250 μg
Vitamin C	60 mg	32 mg	200 mg	35 mg	35 mg	44 mg			50 mg	50 mg	50 mg
Vitamin D	10 μg	10 μg	2.5 μg	10 μg	10 μg	10 μg	10 μg	12.5 μg	10 μg	10 μg	10 μg
Vitamin E	13.5 mg	2.3 mg	1.7 mg			3.4 mg	20 mg	20 mg	5 mg	5 mg	
Vitamin K								40 μg			
Thiamin (B_1)	1.1 mg	0.5 mg	7.5 mg			0.6 mg	1.4 mg	1.5 mg	0.3 mg	0.3 mg	
Riboflavin (B_2)	1.7 mg	0.6 mg	7.5 mg			0.8 mg	1.7 mg	1.7 mg	0.4 mg	0.4 mg	
Niacin	20 mg	2 mg	12.5 mg			4 mg	20 mg	20 mg	4 mg	4 mg	
Folic acid		29.7 μg					17 μg DFE	17 μg DFE			
Vitamin B_6	2 mg	0.4 mg	200 mg			0.3 mg	2 mg	2 mg	0.3 mg	0.3 mg	
Vitamin B_{12}	6 μg	2 μg	5 μg				6 μg	6 μg	0.5 μg		

(continued)

TABLE 11.1 VITAMIN AND MINERAL SUPPLEMENTS (*continued*)

	LIQUID										
	CENTRUM® ADULT LIQUID (PER 15 ML/1 TBSP)	FLORIVA PLUS LIQUID DROPS™ (PER 1 ML)	KIRKMAN® SUPER NU-THERA® LIQUID (PER 5 ML/1 TSP)	MYKIDZ IRON™ (PER 2 ML)	MYKIDZ IRON FL™ (PER 2 ML)	NATURESPLUS® ANIMAL PARADE® BABY PLEX® MULTIVITAMIN DROPS (PER 1 ML)	NATURESPLUS® ANIMAL PARADE® MULTIVITAMIN CHILDREN'S LIQUID (PER 15 ML/1 TBSP)	NATURESPLUS® ANIMAL PARADE® GOLD MULTIVITAMIN CHILDREN'S LIQUID (PER 15 ML/1 TBSP)	POLY-VI-SOL® (PER 1 ML)	POLY-VI-SOL® WITH IRON (PER 1 ML)	TRI-VI-SOL® (PER 1 ML)
Biotin	300 µg		25 µg			25 µg	50 µg	50 µg			
Pantothenic acid	10 mg		10 mg			1.7 mg		10 mg			
Calcium							20 mg	50 mg			
Iron	9 mg			10 mg	10 mg		2.5 mg	5 mg		11 mg	
Phosphorus											
Iodine	150 µg						100 µg	100 µg			
Magnesium			75 mg				10 mg				
Zinc	3 mg		5 mg				3 mg	3 mg			
Selenium			25 µg					35 µg			
Copper											
Manganese	2 mg		0.75 mg				0.05 mg	1 mg			
Chromium	25 µg							60 µg			
Molybdenum	25 µg										

Potassium												
Sodium												
Coenzyme Q_{10}												
Choline												
Fluoride		0.25 mg			0.25 mg							
Inositol							10 µg	10 mg				
Manufacturer	Haleon	BonGeo Pharmaceuticals	Kirkman	Tris Pharma	Tris Pharma	Nature's Plus	Nature's Plus	Nature's Plus	Mead Johnson	Mead Johnson	Mead Johnson	
Comments	Formulated for adults Contains sucrose and 6% ethyl alcohol	Requires prescription Contains sucralose Free from sugar, saccharin, gluten, and artificial colors or flavors	Contains sorbitol and sucralose Free of the top 9 allergens	Free of alcohol, sugar, gluten, and dyes	Free of alcohol, sugar, gluten, and dyes	Contains fructose	Contains fructose Folate and B_{12} are methylated Free from the top 9 allergens	Also provides lemon bioflavonoid complex and fatty acid complex Contains xylitol Folate and B_{12} are methylated Free from synthetic colors and preservatives and the top 9 allergens	Gluten free	Gluten free	Gluten free	

(continued)

TABLE 11.1 VITAMIN AND MINERAL SUPPLEMENTS (*continued*)

	POWDER					
	KIRKMAN® SUPER NU-THERA® POWDER (PER 2 SCOOPS/2.5 G)	NANOVM® 1-3 Y (PER 2 LEVEL SCOOPS)	NANOVM® 4-8 Y (PER 2 LEVEL SCOOPS)	NANOVM® 9-18 Y (PER 4 LEVEL SCOOPS)	NANOVM® T/F (PER 2 LEVEL SCOOPS)	PHLEXY VITS® (PER 7 G PACKET)
Vitamin A	750 µg	300 µg	400 µg	650 µg	350 µg	800 µg
Vitamin C	250 mg	15 mg	25 mg	49 mg	33 mg	50 mg
Vitamin D	2.5 µg	15 µg	15 µg	16.2 µg	8 µg	10 µg
Vitamin E	6.75 mg	5 mg	7 mg	7.6 mg	7 mg	9 mg
Vitamin K		30 µg	55 µg	65 µg	38 µg	70 µg
Thiamin (B_1)	7.5 mg	0.5 mg	0.6 mg	0.97 mg	0.5 mg	1.2 mg
Riboflavin (B_2)	7.5 mg	0.5 mg	0.6 mg	0.97 mg	0.5 mg	1.4 mg
Niacin	15 mg	6 mg	8 mg	13 mg	7 mg	20 mg
Folic acid	333 µg DFE	150 µg	200 µg	325 µg	200 µg DFE	700 µg
Vitamin B_6	250 mg	0.5 mg	0.6 mg	1.08 mg	0.6 mg	1.6 mg
Vitamin B_{12}	5 µg	0.9 µg	1.2 µg	1.94 µg	1.2 µg	5 µg
Biotin	50 µg	8 µg	12 µg	21.6 µg	13 µg	150 µg
Pantothenic acid	10 mg	2 mg	3 mg	4.3 mg	3 mg	5 mg
Calcium		700 mg	1,000 mg	1,400 mg	650 mg	1,000 mg
Iron		7 mg	10 mg	8.6 mg	6 mg	15.1 mg
Phosphorus		530 mg	540 mg	1,060 mg	500 mg	775 mg
Iodine	50 µg	90 µg	90 µg	130 µg	75 µg	150 µg
Magnesium	125 mg	65 mg	110 mg	260 mg	175 mg	300 mg

Zinc	5 mg	3 mg	5 mg	8.6 mg	5 mg	11.1 mg
Selenium	25 μg	20 μg	30 μg	43 μg	28 μg	75 μg
Copper		0.3 mg	0.4 mg	0.76 mg	0.5 mg	1.5 mg
Manganese	0.8 mg	1.2 mg	1.5 mg	2.05 mg	0.8 mg	1.5 mg
Chromium		11 μg	15 μg	27 μg	12 μg	30 μg
Molybdenum		17 μg	22 μg	36.7 μg	22 μg	70 μg
Potassium		575 mg	780 mg	1,710 mg	1,170 mg	<1.4 mg
Sodium						8.8 mg
Coenzyme Q_{10}						
Choline		50 mg	80 mg	160 mg	150 mg	
Fluoride						
Inositol						
Manufacturer	Kirkman	Solace Nutrition	Solace Nutrition	Solace Nutrition	Solace Nutrition	Nutricia
Comments	Contains fructose Folic acid is methylated Free of the top 9 allergens	Folic acid and B_{12} are methylated Contains both vitamin K_1 and K_2 Free of carbohydrate, egg, dairy, fish, crustacean, soy, gluten, corn, tree nuts, and peanuts	Folic acid and B_{12} are methylated Contains both vitamin K_1 and K_2 Free of carbohydrate, egg, dairy, fish, crustacean, soy, gluten, corn, tree nuts, and peanuts	B_{12} is methylated Contains both vitamin K_1 and K_2 Free of carbohydrate, egg, dairy, fish, crustacean, soy, gluten, corn, tree nuts, and peanuts	For individuals who are exclusively tube-fed B_{12} is methylated Contains both vitamin K_1 and K_2 Free of carbohydrate, egg, dairy, fish, crustacean, soy, gluten, corn, tree nuts, and peanuts	Free of dairy, artificial colors, flavors, or sweeteners Carbohydrate free (0.04 g) Indicated for individuals 11 y and older who have restricted therapeutic diets

(*continued*)

TABLE 11.1 VITAMIN AND MINERAL SUPPLEMENTS (*continued*)

	CHEWABLE TABLET									
	CVS HEALTH™ CHILDREN'S CHEWABLE MULTIVITAMIN (PER TABLET)	EQUATE™ CHILDREN'S CHEWABLE COMPLETE MULTIVITAMIN (PER TABLET)	FLINTSTONES™ COMPLETE (PER TABLET)	FLINTSTONES™ PLUS IMMUNITY SUPPORT (PER TABLET)	FLINTSTONES™ PLUS EXTRA IRON (PER TABLET)	KIRKMAN® CHILDREN'S CHEWABLE MULTIVITAMIN & MINERAL W/5-MTHF (PER 2 TABLETS)	NATURESPLUS® ANIMAL PARADE® MULTIVITAMIN CHILDREN'S CHEWABLES (PER 2 TABLETS)	NATURESPLUS® ANIMAL PARADE® GOLD MULTIVITAMIN CHILDREN'S CHEWABLES (PER 2 TABLETS)	RENZO'S® PICKY EATER MULTI WITH IRON (PER TABLET)	RUGBY® CEROVITE® JR. CHILDREN'S CHEWABLE MULTIVITAMIN WITH MINERALS (PER TABLET)	UP&UP™ KIDS' MULTIVITAMIN COMPLETE (PER TABLET)
Vitamin A	400 µg	900 µg	400 µg	400 µg	400 µg	750 µg	1,500 µg	1,500 µg	400 µg	1,074 µg	900 µg
Vitamin C	90 mg	60 mg	90 mg	140 mg	25 mg	150 mg	60 mg	60 mg	33.75 mg	60 mg	60 mg
Vitamin D	20 µg	15 µg	20 µg	25 µg	15 µg	10 µg	10 µg	13 µg	7.5 µg	10 µg	15 µg
Vitamin E	7.5 mg	13.5 mg	7.5 mg	12 mg	7 mg	15 mg	20 mg	20 mg	7.5 mg	13.5 mg	13.5 mg
Vitamin K	60 µg	55 µg	60 µg					40 µg	45 µg	10 µg	55 µg
Thiamin (B_1)	1.2 mg	1.5 mg	1.2 mg	0.6 mg	0.6 mg	3 mg	1.5 mg	1.5 mg	0.3 mg	1.5 mg	1.5 mg
Riboflavin (B_2)	1.3 mg	1.7 mg	1.3 mg	0.6 mg	0.6 mg	3.4 mg	1.7 mg	1.7 mg	0.65 mg	1.7 mg	1.7 mg
Niacin	12 mg	15 mg	12 mg	8 mg	8 mg	18 mg	20 mg	20 mg	4 mg	20 mg	15 mg
Folic acid	408 µg DFE	680 µg DFE	240 µg	120 µg	120 µg	667 µg DFE	17 µg DFE	17 µg DFE	200 µg DFE	680 µg DFE	680 µg DFE
Vitamin B_6	1.7 mg	2 mg	1.7 mg	0.6 mg	0.6 mg	4 mg	2 mg	2 mg	0.64 mg	2 mg	2 mg
Vitamin B_{12}	2.4 µg	6 µg	2.4 µg	1.2 µg	1.2 µg	24 µg	6 µg	6 µg	1.2 µg	6 µg	6 µg

Biotin	30 µg	40 µg	30 µg	12 µg	12 µg	300 µg	50 µg	50 µg	15 µg	45 µg	40 µg
Pantothenic acid	5 mg	10 mg	5 mg	3 mg	3 mg	10 mg	10 mg	10 mg	2.5 mg	10 mg	10 mg
Calcium	140 mg	100 mg	140 mg				20 mg	25 mg		108 mg	100 mg
Iron	10 mg	18 mg	10 mg	10 mg	18 mg		5 mg	5 mg	6.82 mg	18 mg	18 mg
Phosphorus										50 mg	
Iodine	150 µg	150 µg	150 µg	90 µg	90 µg	150 µg	100 µg	100 µg	75 µg	150 µg	150 µg
Magnesium						40 mg	10 mg	10 mg		40 mg	
Zinc	5 mg	12 mg	5 mg	5 mg	5 mg	15 mg	3 mg	3 mg	4.13 mg	15 mg	12 mg
Selenium						50 µg			27.5 µg		
Copper	0.44 mg	2 mg	0.44 mg				0.02 mg			2 mg	2 mg
Manganese						2 mg	0.05 mg			1 mg	
Chromium						25 µg			17.5 µg	20 µg	
Molybdenum						50 µg				20 µg	
Potassium											
Sodium	10 mg	10 mg	15 mg	15 mg							10 mg
Coenzyme Q_{10}						10 mg					
Choline											

(continued)

TABLE 11.1 VITAMIN AND MINERAL SUPPLEMENTS (*continued*)

	CHEWABLE TABLET										
	CVS HEALTH™ CHILDREN'S CHEWABLE MULTIVITAMIN (PER TABLET)	EQUATE™ CHILDREN'S CHEWABLE COMPLETE MULTIVITAMIN (PER TABLET)	FLINTSTONES™ COMPLETE (PER TABLET)	FLINTSTONES™ PLUS IMMUNITY SUPPORT (PER TABLET)	FLINTSTONES™ PLUS EXTRA IRON (PER TABLET)	KIRKMAN® CHILDREN'S CHEWABLE MULTIVITAMIN & MINERAL W/5-MTHF (PER 2 TABLETS)	NATURESPLUS® ANIMAL PARADE® MULTIVITAMIN CHILDREN'S CHEWABLES (PER 2 TABLETS)	NATURESPLUS® ANIMAL PARADE® GOLD MULTIVITAMIN CHILDREN'S CHEWABLES (PER 2 TABLETS)	RENZO'S® PICKY EATER MULTI WITH IRON (PER TABLET)	RUGBY® CEROVITE® JR. CHILDREN'S CHEWABLE MULTIVITAMIN WITH MINERALS (PER TABLET)	UP&UP™ KIDS' MULTIVITAMIN COMPLETE (PER TABLET)
Fluoride											
Inositol											
Manufacturer	CVS Health	Walmart	Bayer	Bayer	Bayer	Kirkman	Nature's Plus	Nature's Plus	Renzo's Vitamins	Major Rugby	Target
Comments	10% of vitamin A as beta carotene Gluten free	Contains phenylalanine Gluten and lactose free	Contains wheat, soy, sorbitol, mannitol, sucralose, dyes, and gelatin	Contains wheat	Contains wheat	Contains xylitol and stevia Folic acid is methylated Free of the top 9 allergens	Also provides lemon bioflavonoid complex and PABA Folate and B_{12} are methylated Free from synthetic colors and preservatives, milk, eggs, tree nuts, peanuts, wheat, soy, and sesame	Contains xylitol Folate and B_{12} are methylated Free from synthetic colors and preservatives and the top 9 allergens	Contains sugar alcohols and monk fruit extract Folic acid is methylated	Contains phenylalanine Often dispensed by pharmacy as a generic equivalent to the tablet children's complete multivitamin	33% of vitamin A as beta carotene Contains gelatin and sucralose Gluten and lactose free

	GUMMY								
	FLINTSTONES™ COMPLETE AND COMPLETE SOUR GUMMIES (PER 2 GUMMIES)	FLINTSTONES™ PLUS IMMUNITY SUPPORT GUMMIES (PER 2 GUMMIES)	L'IL CRITTERS® GUMMY VITES (PER 1 GUMMY)	NATURE MADE® KIDS FIRST® MULTIVITAMIN + OMEGA-3 GUMMIES (PER GUMMY)	ONE A DAY VITACRAVES® TEEN FOR HER (PER 2 GUMMIES)	ONE A DAY VITACRAVES® TEEN FOR HIM (PER 2 GUMMIES)	RAINBOW LIGHT® KID'S MULTIVITAMIN + BRAIN & EYE SUPPORT (PER 4 GUMMIES)	YUMMI BEARS® SUGAR FREE COMPLETE MULTI (PER 2 BEARS)	YUMMI BEARS® VEGETARIAN COMPLETE MULTI (PER 3 BEARS)
Vitamin A	400 µg	600 µg	225 µg	375 µg	750 µg	750 µg	450 µg	600 µg	600 µg
Vitamin C	30 mg	90 mg	10 mg	25 mg	65 mg	75 mg	90 mg	60 mg	60 mg
Vitamin D	15 µg	15 µg	10 µg	25 µg	15 µg	15 µg	20 µg	3.8 µg	3.8 µg
Vitamin E	7 mg	6.7 mg	6 mg	4.5 mg	13.5 mg	13.5 mg	15 mg	6.8 mg	6.8 mg
Vitamin K					75 µg	75 µg			
Thiamin (B_1)							1.2 mg		
Riboflavin (B_2)							1.3 mg		
Niacin				10 mg	14 mg	16 mg	8 mg	2.5 mg	2.5 mg
Folic acid	120 µg	24 µg	100 µg DFE	200 µg DFE	330 µg DFE	330 µg DFE		150 µg DFE	150 µg DFE
Vitamin B_6	0.6 mg	1 mg	0.9 mg	0.9 mg	1.2 mg	1.3 mg	2.5 mg	1 mg	1 mg
Vitamin B_{12}	1.2 µg	2.4 µg	1.2 µg	3 µg	2.4 µg	2.4 µg	3 µg	3 µg	3 µg
Biotin	12 µg	30 µg	8 µg		30 µg	30 µg		70 µg	70 µg
Pantothenic acid	3 mg	5 mg	1.5 mg					5 mg	5 mg

(continued)

TABLE 11.1 VITAMIN AND MINERAL SUPPLEMENTS (*continued*)

	GUMMY								
	FLINTSTONES™ COMPLETE AND COMPLETE SOUR GUMMIES (PER 2 GUMMIES)	FLINTSTONES™ PLUS IMMUNITY SUPPORT GUMMIES (PER 2 GUMMIES)	L'IL CRITTERS® GUMMY VITES (PER 1 GUMMY)	NATURE MADE® KIDS FIRST® MULTIVITAMIN + OMEGA-3 GUMMIES (PER GUMMY)	ONE A DAY VITACRAVES® TEEN FOR HER (PER 2 GUMMIES)	ONE A DAY VITACRAVES® TEEN FOR HIM (PER 2 GUMMIES)	RAINBOW LIGHT® KID'S MULTIVITAMIN + BRAIN & EYE SUPPORT (PER 4 GUMMIES)	YUMMI BEARS® SUGAR FREE COMPLETE MULTI (PER 2 BEARS)	YUMMI BEARS® VEGETARIAN COMPLETE MULTI (PER 3 BEARS)
Calcium					100 mg	100 mg		9 mg	9 mg
Iron									
Phosphorus					40 mg	40 mg			
Iodine	90 µg	90 µg	21 µg				150 µg	75 µg	75 µg
Magnesium								8 mg	8 mg
Zinc	5 mg	3 mg	1.4 mg	1.9 mg			2 mg	6 mg	6 mg
Selenium									
Copper									
Manganese									
Chromium									
Molybdenum									

Potassium									
Sodium				5 mg					
Coenzyme Q_{10}									
Choline							55 mg	15 µg	15 µg
Fluoride									
Inositol			20 µg					15 µg	15 µg
Manufacturer	Bayer	Bayer	Northwest Natural Products	Nature Made	Bayer	Bayer	Rainbow Light	Hero Nutritionals	Hero Nutritionals
Comments	Contains wheat and gelatin	Contains wheat	Also contains lutein Also available in a no-sugar-added version Free of gluten, dairy, and synthetic dyes	Also provides fish oil (113.5 mg per serving) Free from gluten and synthetic flavors, dyes, and sweeteners	Contains wheat and gelatin	Contains wheat and gelatin	Also contains fruit and vegetable blend, *Bacillus coagulans*, and lutein Contains bovine gelatin Free of wheat, milk, tree nuts, peanuts, soy, eggs, fish, or shellfish	Sweetened with chicory root (2 g fiber per serving) Free from gluten and dairy	Free from gelatin, gluten, and dairy

(continued)

TABLE 11.1 VITAMIN AND MINERAL SUPPLEMENTS (*continued*)

	SWALLOWED TABLET	
	RAINBOW LIGHT® ACTIVE HEALTH™ TEEN (PER 3 TABLETS)	ONE A DAY® WOMEN'S PRENATAL 1 (PER SOFTGEL)
Vitamin A	3,000 μg	650 μg
Vitamin C	300 mg	85 mg
Vitamin D	10 μg	15 μg
Vitamin E	20.1 mg	19 mg
Vitamin K	150 μg	
Thiamin (B_1)	30 mg	1.4 mg
Riboflavin (B_2)	30 mg	1.6 mg
Niacin	30 mg	18 mg
Folic acid	680 μg DFE	1,330 μg DFE
Vitamin B_6	30 mg	2 mg
Vitamin B_{12}	30 μg	2.8 μg
Biotin	300 μg	35 μg
Pantothenic acid	30 mg	7 mg
Calcium	300 mg	150 mg
Iron	9 mg	27 mg
Phosphorus		
Iodine		150 μg

Magnesium	300 mg	40 mg
Zinc	10 mg	13 mg
Selenium	50 µg	
Copper	1 mg	1.3 mg
Manganese	3 mg	
Chromium	200 µg	
Molybdenum	252 µg	
Potassium		
Sodium		
Coenzyme Q_{10}		
Choline	30 mg	
Fluoride		
Inositol	30 mg	
Manufacturer	Rainbow Light	Bayer
Comments	Also contains herbal extract blend; ginger, enzyme, and probiotic blend; spirulina and vegetable complex; citrus extract; hesperidin; rutin; PABA	Also contains fish and soy; provides 235 mg omega-3 fatty acids 50% vitamin A is beta carotene

(*continued*)

TABLE 11.1 VITAMIN AND MINERAL SUPPLEMENTS (*continued*)

	CONDITION-SPECIFIC PRODUCTS							
	DEKAS PLUS™ CHEWABLE TABLETS (PER TABLET)	DEKAS PLUS™ PEDIATRIC LIQUID (PER ML)	DEKAS PLUS™ SOFTGELS (PER SOFTGEL)	MVW COMPLETE FORMULATION® PEDIATRIC DROPS (PER 1 ML)	MVW COMPLETE FORMULATION® CHEWABLE TABLETS (PER TABLET)	MVW COMPLETE FORMULATION® SOFTGELS (PER SOFTGEL)	NEPHRONEX® (PER 5 ML)	DIALYVITE® (PER TABLET)
Vitamin A	5,450 µg	1,727 µg	5,450 µg	2,777 µg	4,800 µg	4,800 µg		
Vitamin C	70 mg	45 mg	75 mg	90 mg	100 mg	100 mg	60 mg	100 mg
Vitamin D	50 µg	18.8 µg	75 µg	38 µg	37.5 µg	37.5 µg		
Vitamin E	67 mg	33.6 mg	100.6 mg	67 mg	134 mg	134 mg		
Vitamin K	1,000 µg	500 µg	1,000 µg	1,000 µg	1,000 µg	800 µg		
Thiamin (B_1)	1.5 mg	0.6 mg	1.5 mg	1 mg	1.5 mg	1.5 mg	1.5 mg	1.5 mg
Riboflavin (B_2)	1.7 mg	0.6 mg	1.7 mg	1.2 mg	1.7 mg	1.7 mg	1.7 mg	1.7 mg
Niacin	10 mg	6 mg	10 mg	12 mg	10 mg	20 mg	20 mg	20 mg
Folic acid	200 µg		200 µg		340 µg DFE	340 µg DFE	900 µg	1,000 µg
Vitamin B_6	1.9 mg	0.6 mg	1.9 mg	1.2 mg	1.9 mg	1.9 mg	10 mg	10 mg
Vitamin B_{12}	12 µg		12 µg		6 µg	6 µg	10 mg	6 µg
Biotin	100 µg	15 µg	100 µg	30 µg	100 µg	100 µg	30 µg	300 µg
Pantothenic acid	12 mg	3 mg	12 mg	6 mg	12 mg	12 mg	5 mg	10 mg
Calcium								
Iron								
Phosphorus								
Iodine								
Magnesium								

Zinc	10 mg	5 mg	10 mg	10 mg	15 mg	10 mg		
Selenium		10 µg	75 µg					
Copper								
Manganese								
Chromium								
Molybdenum								
Potassium								
Sodium	15 mg							
Coenzyme Q_{10}	10 mg	2 mg	10 mg					
Choline								
Fluoride								
Inositol								
Manufacturer	Callion Pharma	Callion Pharma	Callion Pharma	MVW Nutritionals	MVW Nutritionals	MVW Nutritionals	Llorens Pharmaceuticals	Hillestad Pharmaceuticals
Comments	Formulated for fat malabsorption 92% of vitamin A is beta carotene Contains sucralose and sorbitol	Formulated for fat malabsorption 87% of vitamin A is beta carotene Contains sucralose	Formulated for fat malabsorption 92% of vitamin A is beta carotene Contains bovine gelatin and sorbitol	Formulated for fat malabsorption 75% of vitamin A is beta carotene Contains xylitol and sucralose Also available as Hi-D drops, containing 76 µg D3 per 1 mL	Formulated for fat malabsorption 88% of vitamin A is beta carotene Contains sucrose, sorbitol, and sucralose Also available as D3000, containing 75 µg D3 per tablet and D5000, containing 125 µg D3 per tablet	Formulated for fat malabsorption 88% of vitamin A as beta carotene Contains soy and sucralose Also available as D3000, containing 75 µg D3 per softgel and D5000, containing 125 µg D3 per softgel	Vitamin B complex formulated for patients undergoing dialysis treatment	Vitamin B complex formulated for patients undergoing dialysis treatment B_{12} is methylated Also available in varieties with added folic acid, D3, and/or minerals

Data from UpToDate® Lexidrug. Lexi-Drug™ and product-specific websites. *UpToDate*. Accessed December 13, 2024. https://online.lexi.com/lco/action/home and product-specific websites. Its accuracy is to the best of the authors' knowledge at the time of publishing. Due to frequent manufacturer changes to composition, please review product labels for the most up-to-date information.

TABLE 11.2 COMPARISON OF ENTERAL MINERAL AND ELECTROLYTE PRODUCTS

MINERAL	SALT FORM	% CATION	DOSE CONVERSION	REPRESENTATIVE PRODUCTS *LISTED AS NAME, ELEMENTAL DOSE (SALT DOSE)*	COMMENTS
Calcium	Acetate	25	1 g calcium acetate = 250 mg elemental calcium = 12.7 mEq calcium	• PhosLo® gelcaps, 169 mg (667 mg) • Eliphos™ tablets, 169 mg (667 mg) • Phoslrya™ liquid, 169 mg (667 mg) per 5 mL	Primarily used as a phosphate binder May cause constipation or dry mouth
	Carbonate	40	1 g calcium carbonate = 400 mg elemental calcium = 20 mEq calcium	• Calci-Mix® capsule, 500 mg (1,250 mg) • Caltrate® 600 + D3 tablet, 600 mg (1,500 mg); also contains 20 µg vitamin D_3 • Florical® capsule, 145 mg (364 mg); also contains 3.75 mg fluoride • Oyster shell tablet, 500 mg (1,250 mg) • Children's Pepto chewable tablet, 160 mg (400 mg) • TUMS® tablet, 200 mg (500 mg) • TUMS® extra strength tablet, 300 mg (750 mg) • TUMS® ultra-strength tablet, 400 mg (1,000 mg) • Viactiv® calcium chew, 650 mg; also contains 12.5 µg vitamin D and 40 µg vitamin K	Recommended to take with meals or a glass of acidic (e.g., orange) juice May cause gas or constipation Oyster shell sources may be contaminated with lead or other metals
	Citrate	21	1 g calcium citrate = 211 mg elemental calcium = 10.6 mEq calcium	• Cal-Citrate™ capsule, 150 mg • Tablet, 200 and 250 mg • Granules, 760 mg per 3.5 g	Most easily absorbed and most expensive form of oral calcium supplement
	Glubionate	6.5	1 g calcium glubionate = 64 mg elemental calcium = 3.2 mEq calcium	• Calcionate syrup, 115 mg (1,800 mg) per 5 mL	Syrup is a hyperosmolar solution
	Gluconate	9	1 g calcium gluconate = 93 mg elemental calcium = 4.65 mEq calcium	• Tablet, 50 mg	Also available as an intravenous solution (see Chapter 17)

	Lactate	13	1 g calcium lactate = 130 mg elemental calcium = 6.5 mEq calcium	• Tablet, 84 mg (648 mg)	Accumulation may occur with renal impairment
	Phosphate	39	1 g calcium phosphate, tribasic = 390 mg elemental calcium = 19.3 mEq calcium	• Caltrate® gummy bites, 500 mg per 2 chews; also contains 230 mg phosphorus and 20 µg vitamin D_3 • Nature-made® gummies calcium with D_3, 500 mg per 2 chews; also contains 230 mg phosphorus and 25 µg vitamin D_3	Easily absorbed Does not cause gas or constipation More expensive than calcium carbonate salts
Iron	Carbonyl iron	100	1 g carbonyl iron = 1,000 mg elemental iron	• Icar® pediatric suspension, 12 mg per 1 mL	Not an iron salt
	Fumarate	33	1 g ferrous fumarate = 330 mg elemental iron	• Ferrocite™ and Hemocyte® tablet, 106 mg (324 mg) • Ferro-Sequels® timed-release tablet, 65 mg (200 mg); also contains 25 mg vitamin C • Tablet, 106 mg (324 mg)	Timed-release preparations may be poorly absorbed
	Gluconate	11.6	1 g ferrous gluconate = ~115 mg elemental iron	• Ferate tablet, 27 mg (240 mg) • Tablet, 27 mg (240 mg) and 38 mg (324 mg)	Ferate is free of corn, dairy, egg, gluten, sodium, soy Also available as an intravenous solution; see Chapter 17
	Polysaccharide iron complex	100	1 g iron polysaccharide = 1,000 mg elemental iron	• Capsule, 150 mg • Ferrex™, Ferric X-150, iFEREX 150, Nu-Iron 150®, and Poly-Iron 150 capsule, 150 mg • NovaFerrum® 50 capsule, 50 mg • NovaFerrum® high-potency liquid, 125 mg per 5 mL • NovaFerrum® pediatric drops liquid, 15 mg per 1 mL	Not an iron salt

(continued)

TABLE 11.2 COMPARISON OF ENTERAL MINERAL AND ELECTROLYTE PRODUCTS (*continued*)

MINERAL	SALT FORM	% CATION	DOSE CONVERSION	REPRESENTATIVE PRODUCTS *LISTED AS NAME, ELEMENTAL DOSE (SALT DOSE)*	COMMENTS
	Sulfate	20	1 g ferrous sulfate = 200 mg elemental iron	• Fe-Vite, Fer-In-Sol®, and Pedia Iron Drops liquid, 15 mg (75 mg) per 1 mL • One-Vite liquid, 44 mg (220 mg) per 5 mL • Liquid, 15 mg (75 mg) per 1 mL, 44 mg (220 mg) per 5 mL, and 60 mg (300 mg) per 5 mL • Feosol and FeroSul tablet, 65 mg (325 mg) • Tablet, 65 mg (325 mg) • Delayed-release tablet, 65 mg (324 mg and 325 mg) • Slow Fe® slow-release tablet, 45 mg (137 mg)	Every other day (rather than daily) dosing may improve absorption but may negatively impact adherence Enteric-coated and slow-release preparations may be poorly absorbed
Magnesium	Carbonate	28	1 g magnesium carbonate = 280 mg elemental magnesium = 23.4 mEq Mg	• Magonate® liquid, 54 mg per 5 mL • Powder, 250 mg per 1,000 mg	
	Chloride	11.8	1 g magnesium chloride = 120 mg elemental magnesium = 9.85 mEq magnesium	• Nu-Mag® and Slow-Mag™ delayed-release tablet, 71.5 mg; also contains 199 mg calcium	
	Gluconate	5.9	1 g magnesium gluconate = 54 mg elemental magnesium = 4.44 mEq magnesium	• Mag-G tablet, 27 mg (500 mg) • Tablet, 27.5 mg	
	Oxide	60	1 g magnesium oxide = 604 mg elemental magnesium = 49.6 mEq magnesium	• Mag 440 tablet, 265.3 mg (440 mg) • Mag-Ox® tablet, 241.3 mg • Mg Plus Protein tablet, 133 mg; also contains a negligible amount (26 mg) of soy protein • Tablet, 60 mg (100 mg), 120 mg (200 mg), 240 mg (400 mg), 252 mg (420 mg), and 300 mg (500 mg)	May cause diarrhea without improving serum levels (except Mg Plus Protein); consider another salt to treat hypomagnesemia

Potassium	Bicarbonate	39.1	1 g potassium bicarbonate = 391 mg elemental potassium = 9.99 mEq potassium	• Effer-K® effervescent tablet for solution, 10 mEq/390 mg, 20 mEq/780 mg, and 25 mEq/975 mg	Consider using in cases of hypokalemia with concurrent acid-base imbalance
	Chloride	52.4	1 g potassium chloride = 524 mg elemental potassium = 13.4 mEq potassium	• Klor-Con® and K-Tab® extended-release tablet, 8 mEq/312 mg, 10 mEq/390 mg, and 20 mEq/780 mg • Klor-Con® M15 extended-release tablet, 15 mEq/585 mg • Liquid, 20 mEq/780 mg per 15 mL and 40 mEq/1,560 mg per 15 mL • Morton Lite Salt 1 teaspoon, 35.9 mEq/1,400 mg; also provides 1,160 mg sodium	Corrects hypokalemia faster than other potassium salts
	Citrate	38.3	1 g potassium citrate = 383 mg elemental potassium = 9.26 mEq potassium	• Urocit®-K extended-release tablet, 5 mEq/540 mg, 10 mEq/1,080 mg, and 15 mEq/1,620 mg	May cause hypochloremia when used to treat hypokalemia May be used to alkalinize urine for kidney stone management
	Gluconate	16.7	1 g potassium gluconate = 167 mg elemental potassium = 4.3 mEq potassium	• K-99™ capsule, 2.55 mEq/99 mg (595 mg) • Tablet, 2 mEq/78 mg and 2.5 mEq/97.5 mg	Can be used to treat hypokalemia when potassium chloride is not readily available
Sodium	Bicarbonate	27.4	1 g sodium bicarbonate = 274 mg elemental sodium = 12 mEq sodium	• Baking soda 1 teaspoon, 54.8 mEq/1,260 mg; also provides 56 mEq bicarbonate • Tablet, 3.9 mEq/89 mg (325 mg) and 7.7 mEq/178 mg (650 mg)	Dilute baking soda in 120 mL of water for every ½ teaspoon of powder
	Chloride	39.3	1 g sodium chloride = 393 mg elemental sodium = 17.1 mEq sodium	• Liquid, 4 mEq/92 mg per 1 mL • Tablet, 17 mEq/393 mg (1,000 mg) • Table salt 1 teaspoon, 100 mEq/2,300 mg • Morton lite salt 1 teaspoon, 50.4 mEq/1,160 mg; also provides 1,400 mg potassium	

Adapted from UpToDate Lexidrug™. Lexi-Drugs. *UpToDate*. Accessed December 13, 2024. https://online.lexi.com/lco/action/home

TABLE 11.3 RECOMMENDED PROBIOTICS AND SUGGESTED DOSES

	USES	BRAND NAMES, PRODUCT INFORMATION, AND RECOMMENDED DOSAGE
SINGLE STRAIN		

Lactobacillus
 	
(Best studied are strains of *Lactobacillus acidophilus*, *Lactobacillus bulgaricus*, *Lactobacillus reuteri*, and *Lactobacillus rhamnosus* GG)
	• May reduce the risk of antibiotic-associated diarrhea when administered with an antibiotic course
	• May reduce symptoms of irritable bowel syndrome (IBS)
	• May promote clearance of *Helicobacter pylori* in conjunction with standard therapy
	• *L. reuteri* may improve symptoms of colic in infants, especially those fed human milk
	• *L. acidophilus* and *L. rhamnosus* GG may reduce the risk of necrotizing enterocolitis in infants
		Lactinex™: *L. acidophilus*
		• Tablets can be chewed or swallowed, followed by milk, water, or juice
		• The granules can be added to cereal, food, or milk
		• All products are gluten-free
		• All products contain milk, whey, lactose, and soy
		• Keep products refrigerated
		• *Dosage*:
		  • Children and adults: Take 4 tablets or 1 packet of granules 3 to 4 times daily
		
		Biogaia®: *L. reuteri*
		• Drops should be taken by spoon or syringe
		• Chewable tablets and capsules should be followed by water, milk, or juice
		• Lozenges should be dissolved fully in the mouth
		• Some products also contain cholecalciferol
		• Products are dairy- and gluten-free
		• *Dosage*:
		  • Infants: Take 5 drops daily by spoon or syringe
		  • Children: Take 5 drops, 1 chewable tablet, or 1 lozenge daily
		  • Adults: Take 1 capsule, 1 chewable tablet, or 1 lozenge daily

		Culturelle®: *L. rhamnosus GG* • Packets or contents of opened capsules can be added to cool (not warm or hot) beverages and foods; mix until dissolved • "Baby" products also contain *Bifidobacterium animalis* and cholecalciferol • Some products also contain inulin • Some products are free of gluten, dairy, peanut, tree nut, and/or soy

		• *Dosage*:
		  • Infants: Take 5 drops or 1 packet daily
		  • Children: Take 1 packet or 1 capsule daily
		  • Adults: Take 1 to 2 capsules daily

Bifidobacterium
 	
(Best studied are strains of *Bifidobacterium breve*, *Bifidobacterium infantis*, and *Bifidobacterium longum*)
	• May improve quality of life in patients with IBS and help manage symptoms associated with IBS, including diarrhea, abdominal pain, and bloating or distension	**Align®**: *B. longum*
		• Can be taken with or without food
		• All products are gluten-free
		• Products in capsules contain milk protein (sodium caseinate) and trace lactose
		• Some products contain digestive enzymes, inulin, and/or supplemental vitamins
		• Children's products are a different strain (*Bacillus coagulans*)
		• *Dosage*:
		  • Adults and children: Take 1-2 capsules daily
		  • See label instructions for children's products

Saccharomyces (*Saccharomyces boulardii*)	• May reduce the risk of antibiotic-associated diarrhea when administered with an antibiotic course and may reduce the risk of traveler's diarrhea
	• May promote the clearance of *H. pylori* in conjunction with standard therapy
	• May help prevent *Clostridioides difficile* infection
		Florastor®:
		• Swallow capsules with at least 4 oz of water or juice
		• Packets or contents of opened capsules can be sprinkled over semisolid food or dissolved in a cool, noncarbonated liquid
		• Can be taken with or without food though it may be most effective between meals
		• Can be taken at the same time as antibiotics
		• Products contain lactose but may stimulate the production of lactase
		• Products are free from the top 9 allergens; adult products are also corn free
		• Store at room temperature
		• *Dosage*:
		  • Children >2 mo of age and adults:
		    • To maintain intestinal flora balance: Take 1 capsule or packet by mouth twice daily.
		    • To promote intestinal health: Take 2 capsules or packets by mouth twice daily for 30 d

(*continued*)

TABLE 11.3 RECOMMENDED PROBIOTICS AND SUGGESTED DOSES (*continued*)

	USES	BRAND NAMES, PRODUCT INFORMATION, AND RECOMMENDED DOSAGE
MULTIPLE STRAINS		
Visbiome® (*L. acidophilus, Lactobacillus plantarum, Lactobacillus paracasei, L. bulgaricus, Streptococcus thermophilus, B. longum, B. breve,* and *B. infantis*[a])	• May improve response and remission rates of mild-to-moderate ulcerative colitis (UC) in conjunction with standard therapy • May help prevent acute pouchitis and maintain remission following antibiotic treatment for recurrent pouchitis	• Swallow capsules with cold, noncarbonated beverages. Mix powders with a cold, noncarbonated beverage or cold food. • Can be taken with or without food • Available in multiple potencies: 112.5 (capsule) or 450 (powder) billion CFUs • Products are Kosher certified. • Products are gluten and lactose free but not dairy free (contain trace amounts of milk protein).

	• May help improve clinical symptoms such as *abdominal pain in IBS*	• Keep products refrigerated. Can be left unrefrigerated for up to 7 d
		• *Dosage:*
		  • Children 3-11 y of age: Take 1 packet daily.
		  • Children 12 y of age and older: Take 1-2 packets daily.
		  • Adults:
		    • IBS: ½ to 1 packet or 2-4 capsules daily
		    • Pouchitis: 2-4 packets daily
		    • UC (active): 4-8 packets daily
		    • UC (maintenance): 4-8 capsules or 1-2 packets daily

Disclaimer: These statements have not been evaluated by the Food and Drug Administration. These products are not intended to diagnose, treat, cure, or prevent any disease. Some probiotic usage information in the table is transcribed from company websites. Its accuracy is to the best of the authors' knowledge at the time of publishing.

CFU, colony forming unit.

[a]This blend was previously found in VSL #3®, which was reformulated in 2016; results from previous research studies on this blend labeled as VSL #3® now apply to Visbiome®.

Adapted from Office of Dietary Supplements. Probiotics: fact sheet for health professionals. National Institutes of Health. Updated November 3, 2023. Accessed November 22, 2024. https://ods.od.nih.gov/factsheets/Probiotics-HealthProfessional/; UpToDate Lexidrug. Lexi-Drugs. *UpToDate*. Accessed December 13, 2024. https://online.lexi.com/lco/action/home; Goodman C, Keating G, Georgousopoulou E, Hespe C, Levett K. Probiotics for the prevention of antibiotic-associated diarrhoea: a systematic review and meta-analysis. *BMJ Open*. 2021;11(8):43-54; Shi X, Zhang J, Mo L, Shi J, Qin M, Huang X. Efficacy and safety of probiotics in eradicating Helicobacter pylori: a network meta-analysis. *Medicine*. 2019;98(15):e15180; Sung V, D'Amico F, Cabana MD, et al. Lactobacillus reuteri to treat infant colic: a meta-analysis. *Pediatrics*. 2018;141(1):e20171811; Kelesidis T, Pothoulakis C. Efficacy and safety of the probiotic Saccharomyces boulardii for the prevention and therapy of gastrointestinal disorders. *Therap Adv Gastroenterol*. 2012;5(2):111-125.

TABLE 11.4 HERBAL PRODUCTS CONTRAINDICATED IN CHILDREN

HERBAL PRODUCT	RISKS WITH USE OR REASONS FOR CONTRAINDICATION
Aloe (oral)	Abdominal pain, cramping, acute hepatitis; may increase the risk of adverse effects from digoxin
European buckthorn	Stomach cramps, diarrhea, acute kidney injury, heart problems
Cajeput oil	Inhalation may cause or worsen breathing problems
Camphor	Tonic-clonic seizures, nausea, vomiting, agitation
Cascara sagrada bark	Dehydration and hypokalemia as a result of gastrointestinal side effects, especially when used for more than 1 wk
Eucalyptus oil	Seizure and nervous system disorders; can be fatal, even in small amounts (3.5 mL)
Fennel	May pass through human milk, causing emesis, weakness, lethargy, and feeding difficulties in infants
Gingko (raw or roasted seeds; unprocessed leaves)	Allergic skin reaction, convulsions, serotonin syndrome; increased risk of bleeding, especially for those who are on blood thinners
Horseradish	Digestive tract and skin irritant
Rhubarb leaf	High in oxalic acid, which in large quantities can cause kidney stones or other kidney damage, abdominal pain, vomiting, and seizures
Senna leaf	Limit use to 1 wk and use age-recommended doses; side effects include abdominal discomfort, cramping, and diarrhea
St. John's wort	Can weaken the effects of medications, including cyclosporine, digoxin, indinavir, imatinib, warfarin, statins, antidepressants, and contraceptives; may pass through human milk and is associated with colic, drowsiness, and fussiness in nursing infants
Valerian	Sedative effects, headache, dizziness, pruritus, and gastrointestinal disturbances
Watercress	Small amounts (food or garnish) are safe; medicinal quantities are not recommended for ages < 4 y; high in oxalate, which can cause kidney stones

Adapted from Office of Dietary Supplements. Botanical dietary supplements background information. National Institutes of Health. Updated December 11, 2020. Accessed November 22, 2024. https://ods.od.nih.gov/factsheets/BotanicalBackground-Consumer/; Office of Dietary Supplements. Dietary supplement fact sheets. National Institutes of Health. Accessed November 6, 2024. https://ods.od.nih.gov/factsheets/list-all/; National Library of Medicine. *Drugs and Lactation Database (LactMed®)*. National Institutes of Health. Accessed November 22, 2024. https://www.ncbi.nlm.nih.gov/books/NBK501922/; Meuninck J. *Medicinal Plants of North America: A Field Guide*. The Globe Pequot Press; 2008; Blumenthal M, Busse WR, eds. *The Complete German Commission E Monographs: Therapeutic Guide to Herbal Medicines*. American Botanical Council; 1998.

TABLE 11.5 COMPARISON OF VITAMIN D ANALOGUES/METABOLITES

	VITAMIN D_2	VITAMIN D_3	1,25-DIHYDROXYVITAMIN D_3
Generic Name	Ergocalciferol	Cholecalciferol	Calcitriol
Brand name(s)	Calcidol, Calciferol™, Drisdol®, Ergocal	Enfamil® D-Vi-Sol, D-Vite Pediatric, Dialyvite 5000, Delta® D3, aqueous vitamin D, Weekly-D	Rocaltrol®
Notes	1 μg = 40 USP international units	1 μg = 40 USP international units The preferred therapeutic form for single-dose therapy due to its longer half-life	
Dosage	**Prevention of vitamin deficiency:** Premature neonates: • Birth weight ≤1.5 kg: 5 μg daily • Increase to 10 μg daily when weight ≤1.5 kg; up to 20-25 μg daily Breastfed term neonates (fully or partially): • 10 μg daily beginning in the first few days of life • Continue supplementation until the infant is weaned to ≥1,000 mL/d or 1 qt/d of vitamin D-fortified formula. Formula-fed term neonates: • If ingesting <1,000 mL/d of vitamin D-fortified formula: 10 μg daily	**Prevention of vitamin deficiency:** Premature neonates: • Birth weight ≤ 1.5 kg: 5 μg daily • Increase to 10 μg daily when weight ≤1.5 kg; up to 20-25 μg daily Breastfed term neonates (fully or partially): • 10 μg daily beginning in the first few days of life • Continue supplementation until the infant is weaned to ≥1,000 mL/d or 1 qt/d of vitamin D-fortified formula Formula-fed term neonates: • If ingesting <1,000 mL/d of vitamin D-fortified formula: 10 μg daily	**Hypocalcemia:** Oral: • 0.25-1 μg once daily **Hypocalcemic tetany:** Oral or Intravenous: • 0.25 μg once daily • OR 0.01-0.1 μg/kg/d divided into 2 doses (max 2 μg/d) **Management of hypocalcemia in children and adolescents with CKD:** CKD stages 3a-4: Oral: • <10 kg: 0.05 μg every other day

Chronic kidney disease (CKD)-associated vitamin D insufficiency or deficiency:

Serum 25(OH)D 16-30 ng/mL:

- 50 µg/d for 3 mo
- OR 1,250 µg every month for 3 mo

Serum 25(OH)D 5-15 ng/mL:

- 100 µg/d for 12 wk
- OR 1,250 µg every other week for 12 wk

Serum 25(OH)D <5 ng/mL:

- 200 µg/d for 4 wk then 100 µg/d for 2 mo (3 mo total therapy)
- OR 1,250 µg/wk for 4 wk then 1,250 µg 2 times/mo (3 mo total therapy)

Maintenance dose, (following repletion) serum 25(OH)D > 30 ng/mL:

- 5-25 µg/d

Hypoparathyroidism:

Children:

- 1,250-5,000 µg/d with calcium supplementation

Children and adolescents:

- If dietary intake is inadequate, 15 µg daily

Treatment of vitamin D deficiency and/or rickets:

Full-term infants:

- 25-50 µg daily for 6 wk until serum 25(OH)D > 20 ng/mL
- Then reduce to 10-25 µg daily
- Include calcium supplementation

Children and adolescents:

- 50 µg daily for 6-8 wk
- Then reduce the dose to 15-25 µg daily
- Consider single-dose therapy: loading dose, then initiate daily maintenance therapy after 3 mo.

CKD-associated vitamin D insufficiency or deficiency:

- Serum 25(OH)D 16-30 ng/mL:
  - 50 µg/d for 3 mo
  - OR 1,250 µg every month for 3 mo

Serum 25(OH)D 5-15 ng/mL:

- 100 µg/d for 12 wk
- OR 1,250 µg every other week for 12 wk

- 10-20 kg: 0.1-0.15 µg daily
- >20 kg: 0.25 µg daily
- Adjust doses based on intact PTH (iPTH), serum total corrected calcium, and serum phosphorus

CKD stage 5 requiring dialysis:

Oral or IV:

- iPTH 300-500 pg/mL: 0.0075 µg/kg per dialysis session (3 times/wk); not to exceed 0.25 µg daily
- iPTH > 500-1,000 pg/mL: 0.015 µg/kg per dialysis session (3 times/wk); not to exceed 0.5 µg daily
- iPTH >1,000 pg/mL: 0.025 µg/kg per dialysis session (3 times/wk); not to exceed 1 µg daily
- Adjust doses based on patient response and concomitant therapies

(continued)

TABLE 11.5 COMPARISON OF VITAMIN D ANALOGUES/METABOLITES (*continued*)

	VITAMIN D_2	VITAMIN D_3	1,25-DIHYDROXYVITAMIN D_3
	Nutritional rickets and osteomalacia: Infants 1-12 mo: • 50 μg daily for ≥3 mo • Once radiologic evidence of healing is observed, reduce to a maintenance dose of 10 μg daily Children >12 mo: • 75-150 μg daily for >3 mo • Once radiologic evidence of healing is observed, reduce the dose to 15 μg daily • Consider single-dose therapy: Loading dose, then initiate daily maintenance therapy after 3 mo (cholecalciferol recommended for this) **Familial hypophosphatemia:** Initial: • 1,000-2,000 μg/d with phosphate supplements At 3 to 4-mo intervals: • Increase daily dosage in 250-500 μg increments as needed	Serum 25(OH)D < 5 ng/mL: • 200 μg/d for 4 wk then 100 μg/d for 2 mo (3 mo total therapy) • OR 1,250 μg/wk for 4 wk then 1,250 μg 2 times/mo (3 mo total therapy) Maintenance dose, (following repletion) serum 25(OH)D > 30 ng/mL: • 5-25 μg/d **Prevention and treatment of vitamin D deficiency in cystic fibrosis:** *Prevention and Maintenance*: Infants: • 10-12.5 μg/d Children 1-10 y: • 20-25 μg/d Adolescents >10 y: • 20-50 μg/d *Treatment*: Infants: • 20-25 up to max 50 μg/d	**Hypoparathyroidism/ pseudo-hypoparathyroidism:** Oral • Infants <1 y: 0.02-0.06 μg/kg once daily • Children 1-5 y: 0.25-0.75 μg once daily • Children > 6 y and adolescents: 0.5-2 μg once daily **Vitamin D-dependent rickets:** • 0.25-2 μg once daily • *Adjust dose based on clinical* response • Reduce the dose once healed

	Special considerations: • Patients with chronic malabsorption, obesity, or who are maintained on chronic antiseizure, human immunodeficiency virus (HIV), glucocorticoid, or antifungal medications may require higher doses	Children 1-10 y: • 40-75 up to max 100 μg/d Adolescents >10 y: • 40-150 μg up to max 250 μg/d • Alternative weekly dosing protocols are available	
Onset of maximal effect	30 d	Specific data are unavailable, but the initial response takes 10-14 d	Oral: 3-6 h Injection: 5 min
Preparations	**Capsule**: 1,250 μg (50,000 IU) **Tablet**: 10 μg (400 IU) **Solution**: 200 μg (8,000 IU)/mL	**Capsule**: 25 μg (1,000 IU); 50 μg (2,000 IU); 125 μg (5,000 IU); 250 μg (10,000 IU); 1,250 μg (50,000 IU) **Tablet**: 10 μg (400 IU); 25 μg (1,000 IU) **Solution**: 10 μg (400 IU)/drop; 50 μg (2,000 IU)/drop; 10 μg (400 IU)/mL	**Capsule**: 0.25 μg, 0.5 μg **Solution for injection**: 1 μg/mL Topical form (Vectical) available for treatment of plaque psoriasis
Monitoring parameters	• Serum 25(OH)D, calcium, creatinine/blood urea nitrogen (BUN), phosphate, parathyroid hormone (PTH) • Bone mineral status (dual-energy x-ray absorptiometry [DXA] scan)	• Serum 25(OH)D, calcium, creatinine/BUN, phosphate, PTH • Bone mineral status (DXA scan)	• Serum 25(OH)D, calcium, creatinine/BUN, phosphate, iPTH concentrations

Other vitamin D analogues:

- Calcifediol (Rayaldee): For treatment of secondary hyperparathyroidism in adults with CKD stage 3 or 4 and serum 25-hydroxyvitamin D <30 ng/mL. Available as an extended-release capsule (30 μg each)
- Dihydrotachysterol (DHT™): For treatment of hypoparathyroidism, nutritional rickets, or renal osteodystrophy. Available as an oral concentrate solution (Intensol™; 0.2 mg/mL) or oral tablet (0.125 mg each)

Adapted from UpToDate Lexidrug. Lexi-Drugs™. *UpToDate*®. Accessed December 13, 2024. https://online.lexi.com/lco/action/home

REFERENCES

1. Office of Dietary Supplements. Dietary supplements: what you need to know. National Institutes of Health. Updated January 4, 2023. Accessed November 6, 2024. https://ods.od.nih.gov/factsheets/WYNTK-Consumer/
2. Muth ND, Tanaka M. Vitamins. In: *The Clinician's Guide to Pediatric Nutrition*. American Academy of Pediatrics; 2023. Accessed November 6, 2024. https://publications.aap.org/aapbooks/monograph/734/chapter/11477482/Vitamins
3. Dwyer JT, Saldanha LG, Bailen RA, et al. Do multivitamin/mineral supplements for young children fill critical nutrient gaps? *J Acad Nutr Diet*. 2021;122(3):525-532.
4. Davani-Davari D, Negahdaripour M, Karimzadeh I, et al. Prebiotics: definition, types, sources, mechanisms, and clinical applications. *Foods*. 2019;8(3):92.
5. Office of Dietary Supplements. Probiotics: fact sheet for health professionals. National Institutes of Health. Updated November 3, 2023. Accessed November 22, 2024. https://ods.od.nih.gov/factsheets/Probiotics-HealthProfessional/
6. UpToDate Lexidrug. Lexi-Drugs. *UpToDate*. Accessed 13 December 2024. https://online.lexi.com/lco/action/home
7. Goodman C, Keating G, Georgousopoulou E, Hespe C, Levett K. Probiotics for the prevention of antibiotic-associated diarrhoea: a systematic review and meta-analysis. *BMJ Open*. 2021;11(8):43-54.
8. Shi X, Zhang J, Mo L, Shi J, Qin M, Huang X. Efficacy and safety of probiotics in eradicating Helicobacter pylori: a network meta-analysis. *Medicine*. 2019;98(15):e15180.
9. Sung V, D'Amico F, Cabana MD, et al. *Lactobacillus reuteri* to treat infant colic: a meta-analysis. *Pediatrics*. 2018;141(1):e20171811.
10. Kelesidis T, Pothoulakis C. Efficacy and safety of the probiotic *Saccharomyces boulardii* for the prevention and therapy of gastrointestinal disorders. *Therap Adv Gastroenterol*. 2012;5(2):111-125.
11. Office of Dietary Supplements. Botanical dietary supplements background information. National Institutes of Health. Updated December 11, 2020. Accessed November 22, 2024. https://ods.od.nih.gov/factsheets/BotanicalBackground-Consumer/
12. Office of Dietary Supplements. Dietary supplements for exercise and athletic performance: fact sheet for health professionals. National Institutes of Health. Updated April 1, 2024. Accessed November 22, 2024. https://ods.od.nih.gov/factsheets/ExerciseAndAthleticPerformance-HealthProfessional/
13. Office of Dietary Supplements. Dietary supplement fact sheets. National Institutes of Health. Accessed November 6, 2024. https://ods.od.nih.gov/factsheets/list-all/
14. National Library of Medicine. *Drugs and Lactation Database (LactMed®)*. National Institutes of Health. Accessed November 22, 2024. https://www.ncbi.nlm.nih.gov/books/NBK501922/
15. Meuninck J. *Medicinal Plants of North America: A Field Guide*. The Globe Pequot Press; 2008.
16. Blumenthal M, Busse WR, eds. *The Complete German Commission E Monographs: Therapeutic Guide to Herbal Medicines*. American Botanical Council; 1998.

CHAPTER 12

Community Nutrition Programs

Melissa P. McDonnell

Effective feeding practices and dietary recommendations cannot be implemented unless a caregiver has access to food, financial resources to purchase it, or the resources to find assistance. Food assistance programs and resources, many federally funded, provide critical support in this area. The United States Department of Agriculture (USDA) offers Nutrition Assistance Program and Child Nutrition Programs through the Food and Nutrition Service (https://www. fns.usda.gov/programs; see Table 12.1).[1] The USDA also provides valuable nutrition and health educational materials on topics such as food safety, food labeling, and nutrition guidance for all life stages through its Food and Nutrition Information Center (https://www.nal.usda.gov/programs/fnic).[2]

In addition to USDA programs, other federal initiatives support the nutrition and overall well-being of children, adolescents, and families. For example, the Centers for Disease Control and Prevention (CDC) offers Early Intervention programs in all states (https://www.cdc.gov/act-early/early-intervention/contact-information-by-state.html).[3] These programs assist babies and young children with developmental delays and disabilities, providing services that may include speech therapy, physical therapy, and nutrition support. Through its Head Start Program, the U.S. Department of Health and Human Services delivers services centered around early learning and development, health, and well-being to children ages 3 to 5 years and provides breakfast, lunch, and snacks (https://acf.gov/ohs/about/head-start).[4] The Social Security Administration (SSA) also offers financial assistance through Supplemental Security Income for eligible individuals (see Table 12.2).

Beyond federal programs, many state and local agencies, health centers, and schools provide additional resources to promote the nutritional health of children and families, including those with special care needs. Local food assistance programs can be found in neighborhood health centers, community centers, or churches and other places of worship, and may be listed online under food pantries, food assistance, food banks, or social and human services. Nationwide organizations such as Feeding America (www.feedingamerica.org) or the Food Research and Action Center (www.frac.org) offer information on regional programs throughout the country.

Share Our Strength (https://shareourstrength.org) is a national organization working to end childhood hunger and poverty in the United States. No Kid Hungry (nokidhungry.org) is a national campaign run by Share Our Strength that supports multiple nutrition programs including the school breakfast program and the national summer meals program.

TABLE 12.1 USDA FOOD AND NUTRITION SERVICE PROGRAMS

PROGRAM	DESCRIPTION	ELIGIBILITY COMPONENTS[a]
Supplemental Nutrition Assistance Program (SNAP) https://www.fns.usda.gov/	Provides electronic benefit cards to buy food in approved stores	Gross income must be at or below 130% of federal poverty income guidelines Residency requirement: Applicant must live in the state in which they apply
Special Supplemental Nutrition Program for Women, Infants and Children (WIC) https://www.fns.usda.gov/wic	Provides free healthy foods, breastfeeding support, nutrition education, and referrals to health and community resources to low-income women, infants, and children Caregivers including fathers, grandparents, and foster parents may apply for children <5 y in their care	Categorical requirement: Pregnant or postpartum women and children <5 y of age at nutritional risk Residency requirement: Applicant must live in the state in which they apply Income requirement: Gross income must be at or below 185% of federal poverty income guidelines
WIC Farmers Market Nutrition Program (FMNP) https://www.fns.usda.gov/FMNP	FMNP is associated with the WIC Program; eligible WIC participants are issued FMNP coupons in addition to their regular WIC benefits; coupons can be used to buy locally grown fruits and vegetables from farmers, farmers' markets	Pregnant or postpartum women, infants over 4 mo old, and children 1-5 y of age
National School Lunch Program https://www.fns.usda.gov/nslp	Provides low-cost or free lunches to children in public and nonprofit schools and residential childcare institutions Schools are given reimbursement for meals meeting Federal nutrition requirement	Children from families with incomes at or below 130% of the Federal poverty level are eligible for free meals Those with incomes between 130% and 185% of the Federal poverty level are eligible for reduced price meals
National School Breakfast Program https://www.fns.usda.gov/sbp	Provides low-cost or free breakfasts to children in public and nonprofit schools and residential childcare institutions Schools are given reimbursement for meals meeting Federal nutrition requirement	Children from families with incomes at or below 130% of the Federal poverty level are eligible for free meals
Special Milk Program https://www.fns.usda.gov/smp	Provides milk to children in schools and childcare institutions that do not participate in other federal meals service programs	Schools in the National School Lunch or School Breakfast Program may participate in the Special Milk Program
Fresh Fruit and Vegetable Program (FFVP) https://www.fns.usda.gov/ffvp	Provides a variety of free, fresh fruit and vegetable snacks to children at eligible elementary schools	Schools must operate the National School Lunch Program in order to operate the FFVP

TABLE 12.1 USDA FOOD AND NUTRITION SERVICE PROGRAMS (*continued*)

PROGRAM	DESCRIPTION	ELIGIBILITY COMPONENTS[a]
SUN Program https://www.fns.usda.gov/summer	Provides free nutritious meals to low-income children during the summer at schools, parks, and other neighborhood locations	SUN Meals are available to any child aged 18 and under, no application needed
Child and Adult Care Food Program (CACFP) https://www.fns.usda.gov/cacfp	Provides reimbursement for nutritious meals and snacks to eligible children and adults who are enrolled for care at participating childcare centers, day care homes, and adult day care centers	Children and youth participating in afterschool care programs, or children residing in emergency shelters
Food Distribution Program Indian Reservations (FDPIR) https://www.fns.usda.gov/fdpir	Provides a monthly package of USDA foods to low-income households on Indian reservations and to low-income Native American living near Indian reservations	Income-eligible American Indian and non-Indian households that reside on a reservation are eligible for FDPIR Households living in approved areas near a reservation that contain at least one person who is a member of a federally recognized Tribe are also eligible

[a]Refer to USDA guidelines for more detailed eligibility requirements.

TABLE 12.2 SUPPLEMENTAL SECURITY INCOME

- Child is under 18 or is under age 22 and is a student regularly attending school.
- May be eligible for Supplemental Security Income (SSI) disability beginning as early at the date of birth; no minimum age requirement.
- Child must have chronic illness, blindness, disabling condition, or special medical needs.
- In most states, a child who gets SSI benefits can get Medicaid.
- For more information about Medicaid, visit http://www.medicaid.gov.

Adapted from Social Security Administration. *Understanding Supplemental Security Income SSI for children—2025 edition.* https://www.ssa.gov/ssi/text-child-ussi.htm

REFERENCES

1. U.S. Department of Agriculture, Food and Nutrition Service (FNS). https://www.fns.usda.gov/programs
2. Food and Nutrition Information Center (FNIC), National Agricultural Library. https://www.nal.usda.gov/programs/fnic
3. Centers for Disease Control and Prevention (CDC), Early Intervention Contact Information. https://www.cdc.gov/act-early/early-intervention/contact-information-by-state.html
4. U.S. Department of Health & Human Services (HHS), Office of Head Start (OHS), Administration for Children and Families (ACF). https://acf.gov/ohs/about/head-start

CHAPTER 13

Inclusive Nutrition: Advancing Health Equity in Pediatric Care

Brennan Rhodes-Bratton, Mayra Crespo-Bellido, and Fatima Cody Stanford

This chapter provides an overview of key concepts and tools related to cultural humility and health equity within the context of pediatric nutrition. It is designed to guide health care providers in recognizing how cultural identity and social drivers of health influence nutrition-related outcomes for children and families. The goal is to equip providers with the knowledge necessary to incorporate inclusive nutrition practices into pediatric care, fostering stronger patient-provider relationships and improving nutritional outcomes.

By engaging with the principles of cultural competence, cultural humility, and reflexivity, health care providers can lay the foundation for more equitable, respectful, and effective patient care. This chapter introduces essential terminology and theoretical frameworks that support inclusive care practices. Strategies for recognizing and addressing bias are also explored. A glossary of terms is included at the end of the chapter, along with a curated list of resources to deepen understanding and promote continued learning.

HEALTH EQUITY

While efforts for equality and equity in pediatric nutrition aim to provide fair access to resources and improve health outcomes, the two concepts differ. Health equality gives everyone the same opportunities, care, and services. In contrast, health equity describes a state where everyone can reach their full health potential. Achieving health equity involves a continuous societal commitment to (1) value everyone equally, (2) address preventable inequalities, (3) confront historical and present-day injustices, and (4) eliminate health disparities in health outcomes and health care access. By focusing on health equity rather than equality (see Table 13.1), pediatric nutrition programs can more effectively address the diverse needs of children and families, ultimately leading to better health outcomes and reduced disparities.[1]

SOCIAL DRIVERS OF HEALTH

Nonmedical factors play a significant role in shaping health outcomes. The public health and medical community recognize the conditions in which people are born, grow, work, live, worship, and age as social drivers of health. These drivers are embedded in

TABLE 13.1 AN EXAMPLE OF HEALTH EQUALITY VERSUS HEALTH EQUITY IN EARLY CHILDHOOD NUTRITION PROGRAMS

HEALTH EQUALITY	HEALTH EQUITY
All children in a day care center receive the same meals and snacks	Children in the day care center receive meals and snacks to accommodate their individual needs, offering: • Allergen-free options for children with food allergies • Specialized meals for children with developmental disabilities • Additional nutritional support for children from food-insecure households

political systems, economic policies, infrastructure, and social norms. Social drivers of health can be grouped into five domains: (1) economic stability, (2) education access and quality, (3) health care access and quality, (4) neighborhood and built environment, and (5) social and community context.[2] Recognizing the complex interplay of these structural factors allows for a deeper understanding of the root causes of health inequities. Socioeconomic factors such as income, wealth, and education are fundamental causes of numerous health outcomes.

Achieving health equity in nutrition requires a multifaceted approach that extends beyond providing clinical care.

Frameworks such as the Fundamental Cause Theory, the Socioecological Model (SEM), the Food Lifestyle Theory, and the concept of intersectionality are valuable tools in identifying how social drivers of health shape nutritional status (see Table 13.2). The Fundamental Cause Theory emphasizes addressing underlying social and economic conditions to improve population health rather than focusing solely on individual behaviors or medical interventions.[3,4] The SEM identifies spheres of influence at the individual, interpersonal, organizational, community/environment, and society/public policy levels.[5] Intersectionality refers to the unique experiences of privilege and discrimination created by how our social and political identities interact.[6] The Food Lifestyle Theory complements these perspectives by emphasizing how food choices are shaped by social, economic, and environmental factors, including access, affordability, and cultural norms, which influence those structural drivers.[7] Together, these frameworks broaden a clinician's understanding of what influences dietary intake. For example, applying the SEM to a pediatric nutrition issue (e.g., breastfeeding, diet-related chronic disease, food insecurity, etc.) can enhance the recognition of relevant social drivers of health.

The concept of food habitus, which refers to ingrained patterns of behavior formed through lived experience, further illustrates how social, economic, and environmental influences become internalized, reflecting both what is available and what is culturally and socially accepted.[7] Additionally, the concept of food habitus serves as a crucial link that can be represented in each of these frameworks. The role of stigma in food inequities demonstrates how understanding food habitus can help alleviate these inequities.[6] Stigma, defined as harmful and unfair beliefs or attitudes toward individuals based on weight, food security, or cultural food practices, operates structurally and individually to influence food lifestyles. Structural stigma restricts food chances by limiting access, affordability, and availability of healthy options in marginalized

TABLE 13.2 TOOLS/FRAMEWORKS FOR RECOGNIZING AND ADDRESSING SOCIAL DRIVERS OF HEALTH

TOOLS	MAIN CONCEPTS	IN ACTION
Fundamental Cause Theory	Addresses underlying social and economic conditions to improve population health rather than focusing solely on individual behaviors or medical interventions	Increasing SNAP benefits during COVID pandemic
Socioecological Model	Intersecting spheres of influences: • Individual • Interpersonal • Organizational • Community • Policy	People receiving SNAP benefits may desire to purchase fresh ingredients to prepare dinner. Still, they must leave their neighborhood to find quality groceries because the district's zoning recently changed to allow for more industrious companies instead of commercial businesses like grocery stores.
Food Lifestyle Theory	Food Lifestyle Theory explains how a complex mix of social, economic, and environmental factors, including access and affordability, shapes our food choices, influencing those structural factors. Central to this theory is food habitus.	The person receiving SNAP benefits feels uncomfortable and stigmatized using SNAP benefits at the newly built grocery store in their neighborhood. They continue to shop at a familiar store where they do not feel judged.
Intersectionality	The interaction of our social and political identities creates unique experiences of privilege and discrimination.	The person receiving Supplemental Nutrition Assistance Program (SNAP) benefits may practice a religion that requires meats prepared in a particular way unavailable through neighborhood grocery stores or local food pantries.

communities. In contrast, individual stigma internalizes shame and biases that shape food choices, often alienating people from their cultural traditions or discouraging the use of food assistance. This interplay creates a cycle where limited opportunities and stigmatizing attitudes reinforce unhealthy dietary patterns and health disparities. Understanding this dynamic is essential for health care professionals and policymakers to design culturally sensitive, equitable interventions that dismantle stigma, expand access, and honor diverse foodways, ultimately improving nutrition and well-being for stigmatized populations.

Health equity in nutrition involves addressing the broader social drivers of health and social conditions disproportionately affecting specific populations. A crucial aspect of this process is acknowledging and actively contesting racism, which has been recognized as a significant threat to public health.[8] Confronting the historical legacy of unethical health care and public health practices that have led to inequitable health outcomes among different populations is essential for building trust and addressing historical harms. This includes advocating for structural changes that support equitable nutrition outcomes for all children.

LANGUAGE AND TERMINOLOGY

Language plays a powerful role in shaping health care interaction and perceptions. In the United States, dominant discourse has historically centered the perspectives of white, heterosexual, and cisgender individuals as the default, implicitly portraying other experiences as deviations from the norm. Inclusive language shifts this norm by valuing and reflecting diverse lived experiences.

Inclusive language empowers individuals to define their own identities. Although general principles and guidelines for inclusive language exist (see Suggested Readings and Resources), inclusive communication is not about enforcing a fixed list of "correct" terms. Instead, inclusive communication is guided by respect, accuracy, and responsiveness to patient preferences.

An equity-focused approach to language emphasizes person-first language, which describes individuals as having a condition or circumstance rather than being defined by it.[9] For instance, rather than "a diabetic," one could say "a person living with diabetes." Similarly, phrases that imply victimhood or a deficit can lead to unintentional negative assumptions, stereotyping, stigmatization, or blame. For example, the phrase "people who do not use nutrition services" could be rephrased to "people with limited access to nutrition services" to acknowledge structural barriers.

The term "minoritized" is preferred over "minority" to emphasize the active and ongoing process of marginalization that certain groups face. Rather than simply describing a numerical minority, it highlights how systemic inequalities and power structures perpetuate these groups' placement in lower social positions. This terminology acknowledges that the status of these groups is not merely a demographic fact but a result of deliberate social and political processes that create and maintain their marginalized status. Health care providers are encouraged to reflect on the language used in practice, remain open to change, and take cues from patients regarding terminology. Thoughtful and inclusive communication is a critical step toward building trust, promoting respect, and advancing equity in care.

IMPLICIT BIAS

Implicit bias refers to attitudes or stereotypes that unconsciously influence understanding, actions, and decisions.[10] Unlike explicit bias, implicit bias operates automatically and is often rooted in cultural conditioning and personal experiences. These biases can subtly shape behaviors and judgments without conscious awareness, often perpetuating inequitable outcomes. In health care, implicit bias among providers can impact patient care and clinical decision-making, creating disparities in outcomes.

Common implicit biases in health care include those based on race, gender, weight, and socioeconomic status. For example, children living in under-resourced households may be less likely to receive comprehensive developmental screenings because of assumptions about parental engagement or resource availability. Similarly, children who speak a primary language other than English may face delayed diagnoses due to biases about communication challenges or misinterpretations of symptoms. Research has shown that nutrition professionals may harbor biases toward individuals based on body size or dietary patterns. Children with higher body weight may face assumptions about laziness or lack of willpower, leading to stigmatizing interactions and inadequate support for sustainable health changes.

Recognizing and addressing implicit biases is essential for promoting equitable and patient-centered care. Health care professionals can mitigate bias by acknowledging its presence through ongoing self-reflection, utilizing structured decision-making processes, seeking diverse perspectives, and practicing mindfulness and active listening.

CULTURAL COMPETENCY AND HUMILITY

Training in cultural competency has been proposed as a critical strategy to address health disparities affecting minoritized groups. Josepha Campinha-Bacote defines cultural competence as "a process in which the health care provider continuously strives to achieve the ability to effectively work within the cultural context of a client/individual, or family or community." Josepha Campinha-Bacote's Cultural Competency Continuum Model (CCCM)[11] emphasizes a dynamic and evolving process for achieving cultural competency using five stages: cultural awareness, cultural knowledge, cultural skill, cultural encounter, and cultural desire.

- **Cultural awareness** occurs when the practitioner learns about and appreciates "the values, beliefs, lifeways, practices, and problem-solving strategies of a client's culture."
- **Cultural knowledge** is the information-seeking process of the health professional to learn about diverse cultural and ethnic groups. The practitioner can initiate this process by seeking published works (e.g., books, essays, documentaries) on the traditions, life perspectives, and challenges groups they serve may experience.
- **Cultural skill** refers to successfully collecting cultural information in the health assessment process and performing cultural and physical assessments.
- **Cultural encounter** addresses engagement and application of cultural knowledge and skills during practitioner-patient interactions.
- **Cultural desire** refers to the health practitioner's motivation to learn more and adapt their beliefs about other groups and cultures.

Campinha-Bacote's model encourages health care providers to immerse themselves in the ongoing process of cultural competence by engaging firsthand with the populations they serve.

Cultural Humility in Practice

Cultural humility is a lifelong, reflective process that emphasizes understanding one's limitations in comprehending the cultural backgrounds of others. This concept extends beyond acquiring knowledge and prioritizes openness, active listening, and a willingness to learn from patients. Practitioners engage in this process with a heightened awareness of their biases and the cultural lenses through which they view the world. Practitioners are encouraged to:

- **Engage in active listening:** Cultural humility requires health care providers to attentively listen to patients, demonstrating respect for their experiences, knowledge, and beliefs.

- **Remain accountable:** The process is unending, requiring constant reflection and a commitment to improvement. Practitioners must acknowledge their biases and take steps to address them.

Becoming a Culturally Humble Practitioner Through Motivational Interviewing

Motivational interviewing (MI) supports culturally responsive care by fostering a meaningful dialogue incorporating a patient's values, beliefs, and lived experiences.[12] MI is a strengths-based, patient-centered approach that elicits an individual's own motivations and strengths, reinforces collaboration between provider and patient, and supports patient autonomy in health-related decision-making.

MI promotes trust and rapport by centering core principles such as partnership, acceptance, and compassion. The practice of MI involves active listening, which includes attending to both verbal and nonverbal communication, paraphrasing patient responses, and encouraging further elaboration. Providers are encouraged to mirror the patient's body language to support engagement and mutual understanding. Key MI skills to build collaboration include:

- Using open-ended questions to elicit detailed responses
- Reflecting on the speaker's feelings and clarifying the meaning to ensure accurate understanding
- Affirming patients' strengths and efforts to promote confidence and self-efficacy
- Summarizing key points to confirm shared understanding and ensure alignment in goals

■ REFLEXIVITY

Reflexivity critically examines one's beliefs, assumptions, decisions, actions, interactions, and assumptions within a broader context.[13,14] By fostering self-awareness and critical thinking, reflexivity enables health care providers to recognize and address the biases and assumptions that may influence their professional practice and potentially have unintended consequences for patients.[15] This is particularly important in pediatric nutrition, where cultural values, personal experiences, and societal norms may shape care delivery and outcomes.

Reflexivity supports providers in:

- **Understanding how identities shape worldview:** Clinicians' identities, including race, gender, socioeconomic status, and professional role, influence how they perceive patients and interpret information. Reflexivity may help a clinician explore how their values around food and body image may unconsciously shape how the way they provide dietary advice or assess nutritional status.
- **Acknowledging and addressing biases:** Reflexivity enables practitioners to identify and mitigate biases that might lead to inequitable or ineffective care. Recognizing stereotypes or assumptions about certain populations helps providers focus on individualized care.
- **Improving patient-provider relationships:** Reflecting on how communication style, body language, and cultural assumptions affect interactions can improve trust and rapport with patients and families.

- **Providing holistic, culturally responsive care:** By reflecting on their own health-related values and beliefs, providers can better appreciate and adapt to their families' diverse cultural and nutritional practices.

To practice reflexivity, health care providers must reflect on their identities and cultural backgrounds. Questions for self-reflection include: What assumptions are you making about patients with identities different from your own? *How might these assumptions and comments make counseling more difficult or less effective? How might your personal health-related values, beliefs, and practices affect the way you provide medical nutrition care and education?*

Health care professionals may utilize tools and activities such as:

- **Journaling:** Documenting reflections on patient interactions, focusing on moments of discomfort, misunderstanding, or insight
- **Peer Discussion Groups:** Creating spaces for health care professionals to share experiences and discuss potential biases
- **Cultural Self-Assessments:** Using structured assessments to explore how personal background influences clinical decision-making
- **Case Studies:** Analyzing real-life scenarios to identify assumptions, reflect on alternative perspectives, and consider more inclusive approaches

GLOSSARY OF TERMS

- **Bias:** A tendency to lean in a particular direction, often based on stereotypes or incomplete information
- **Cultural Competency:** The process of effectively working within the cultural context of a client
- **Cultural Humility:** A reflexive and ongoing practice to address limitations in understanding others' cultural backgrounds
- **Discrimination:** Unjust treatment of different categories of people, often arising from bias or prejudice
- **Food Habitus:** Patterned food and drink preferences, dispositions, and values developed through the interplay of social conditions (like culture and resources) and individual choices, guiding how people access, choose, and eat.
- **Food Lifestyle:** Maintenance of collective patterns of nutrition-related behaviors that promote or demote health based on food choices from the available food chances
- **Food Stigma:** The learned and reinforced social messages that certain foods (often cultural or traditional foods or those obtained through assistance programs) are "less than" or "not normal," leading people to feel judged, embarrassed, or ashamed about what they eat
- **Health Equity:** A state where everyone can reach their full health potential
- **Holistic Care:** An approach to health care that considers the physical, emotional, social, and cultural needs of the patient
- **Implicit Bias:** Unconscious attitudes or stereotypes that affect understanding, actions, and decisions
- **Intersectionality:** The interaction of our social and political identities creates unique experiences of privilege and discrimination
- **Motivational Interviewing:** A communication technique emphasizing empathy and collaboration to elicit behavior change

- **Prejudice:** Preconceived opinions that are not based on reason or experience
- **Reflexivity:** The practice of examining one's own beliefs, assumptions, and actions to identify their impact on others
- **Social Divers of Health:** The nonmedical factors related to the conditions in which people are born, grow, work, live, worship, and age influence health outcomes
- **Stigma:** The negative and often unfair beliefs or attitudes toward individuals or groups because of specific traits, circumstances, or health conditions
- **Worldview:** The overall perspective through which an individual sees and interprets the world

REFERENCES

1. Braveman P, Arkin E, Orleans T, Proctor D, Plough A. *What Is Health Equity? And What Difference Does a Definition Make?* Robert Wood Johnson Foundation; 2017.
2. Braveman P, Gottlieb L. The social determinants of health: it's time to consider the causes of the causes. *Public Health Rep*. 2014;129(suppl 2):19-31.
3. Phelan JC, Link BG. *Fundamental Cause Theory*. Springer Netherlands; 2013:105-125.
4. Phelan JC, Link BG. Controlling disease and creating disparities: a fundamental cause perspective. *J Gerontol B Psychol Sci Soc Sci*. 2005;60(special_issue_2):S27-S33.
5. Bronfenbrenner U. Ecological models of human development. *International encyclopedia of education*. 1994;3(2):37-43.
6. Bauer GR. Incorporating intersectionality theory into population health research methodology: challenges and the potential to advance health equity. *Soc Sci Med*. 2014;110:10-17.
7. Rhodes-Bratton B. *Can a Changing Food Environment Tip the Scale? A Mixed-Methods Study of Food Habitus and Obesity in a Neighborhood Undergoing Gentrification*. Dissertation. Sociomedical Sciences, Columbia University; 2023.
8. Phelan JC, Link BG. Is racism a fundamental cause of inequalities in health? *Annu Rev Sociol*. 2015;41(1):311-330.
9. American Medical Association; Association of American Medical Colleges. *Advancing Health Equity: A Guide to Language, Narrative, and Concepts*. American Medical Association; 2021.
10. Banaji MR, Greenwald AG. *Blindspot: Hidden Biases of Good People*. Bantam; 2016.
11. Campinha-Bacote J. The process of cultural competence in the delivery of healthcare services: a model of care. *J Transcult Nurs*. 2002;13(3):181-184.
12. Miller WR, Rollnick S. *Motivational Interviewing: Helping People Change*. Guilford Press; 2012.
13. May T, Perry B. *Reflexivity: The Essential Guide*. SAGE Publications Ltd; 2017. Accessed June 19, 2025. https://methods.sagepub.com/book/mono/reflexivity/toc
14. Olmos-Vega FM, Stalmeijer RE, Varpio L, Kahlke R. A practical guide to reflexivity in qualitative research: AMEE guide no. 149. *Med Teach*. 2023;45(3):241-251.
15. Brown JV, Spicer KJ, French E. Exploring the inclusion of cultural competence, cultural humility, and diversity concepts as learning objectives or outcomes in healthcare curricula. *J Best Pract Health Prof Divers*. 2021;14(1):63-81.

SUGGESTED READINGS AND RESOURCES

SOCIAL DRIVERS OF HEALTH

1. UConn Rudd Center for Food Policy and Health. Supportive obesity care. https://supportiveobesitycare.rudd.center.uconn.edu/
2. Community Links Evidence to Action Research Collaboration (CLEAR) Toolkit: https://www.mcgill.ca/clear/files/clear/clear_toolkit_2015_-_english_1.pdf
3. Center for Nutrition & Health Impact. Nutrition security and related measures: nutrition security, healthfulness choice and dietary choice. https://www.centerfornutrition.org/nutrition-security

LANGUAGE AND TERMINOLOGY

1. American Medical Association, Association of American Medical Colleges. *Advancing Health Equity: A Guide to Language, Narrative and Concepts*. American Medical Association. https://www.ama-assn.org/system/files/ama-aamc-equity-guide.pdf
2. Black C, Cerdeñaa JP, Vanessa Spearman-McCarthyd E. I am not your minority. *Lancet Reg Health Am*. 2023;19:100464.
3. Centers for Disease Control and Prevention. Why is addressing SDOH important? https://www.cdc.gov/about/priorities/why-is-addressing-sdoh-important.html
4. Kendrick KN, Bode Padron KJ, Bomani NZ, et al. Equity in obesity review. *Endocrinol Metab Clin North Am*. 2023;52(4):617-627.
5. Nutter S, Eggerichs LA, Nagpal TS, et al. Changing the global obesity narrative to recognize and reduce weight stigma: a position statement from the World Obesity Federation. *Obes Rev*. 2024;25(1):e13642.
6. Oregon Health & Science University. Inclusive language guide. https://www.ohsu.edu/inclusive-language-guide#section-1615846
7. Pearl RL, Donze LF, Rosas LG, et al. Ending weight stigma to advance health equity. *Am J Prev Med*. 2024;67(5):785-791.
8. UConn Rudd Center for Food Policy and Health. https://uconnruddcenter.org
9. Westbrooks J. My experience as a Black RDN in a White-dominated field. Eat Right Pro. https://www.eatrightpro.org/news-center/inspirational-highlights/my-experience-as-a-black-rdn-in-a-white-dominated-field

IMPLICIT BIAS

1. American Medical Association. Resources on combating implicit bias in healthcare: https://www.ama-assn.org
2. Banaji MR, Greenwald AG. *Blindspot: Hidden Biases of Good People*. Delacorte Press; 2016.
3. Kirwan Institute for the Study of Race and Ethnicity. State of the science: implicit bias review. 2020. https://offices.depaul.edu/academic-affairs/academic-diversity/Documents/State%20of%20Science%20Implicit%20Bias%20Review.pdf
4. Project Implicit. https://implicit.harvard.edu
5. Rubino F, Cummings DE, Eckel RH, et al. Definition and diagnostic criteria of clinical obesity. *Lancet Diabetes Endocrinol*. 2025;19:100464.
6. Waldrop SW, Wang D, Kancherla V. Current status of weight bias and stigma in pediatrics and the need for greater focus on populations at risk. *Curr Opin Pediatr*. 2024;36(1):42-48.

MOTIVATIONAL INTERVIEWING

1. Miller WR, Rollnick S. *Motivational Interviewing: Helping People Change and Grow*. 4th ed. Guilford Press; 2023.
2. UConn Rudd Center for Food Policy and Health. Motivational interviewing: example scripts. https://uconnruddcenter.org/wp-content/uploads/sites/2909/2020/07/Motivational-Interviewing-Example-Scripts-1-1.pdf

REFLEXIVITY

1. Alexander SA, Jones CM, Tremblay M-CC. Reflexivity in health promotion: a typology for training. *Health Promot Pract*. 2020;21(4):499-509.
2. Brown JV, Spicer KJ, French E. Exploring the inclusion of cultural competence, cultural humility, and diversity concepts as learning objectives or outcomes in healthcare curricula. *J Best Pract Health Prof Divers*. 2021;14(1):63-81.
3. Rachel L, Cathy C, Anson A, et al. Educational strategies to enhance reflexivity among clinicians and health professional students: a scoping study educational strategies to enhance reflexivity among clinicians and health professional students: a scoping study. *Forum Qual Soc Res*. 2016;17(3).
4. Tremblay M-C, Garceau L, Diouf NT, et al. Improving understanding of reflexivity in family medicine: development of an educational tool based on a rapid review. *MedEdPublish*. 2021;10:181.

5. Olmos-Vega FM, Stalmeijer RE, Varpio L, Kahlke R. A practical guide to reflexivity in qualitative research: AMEE guide no. 149. *Med Teach*. 2022;45(3):241-251.
6. May T, Perry B. *Reflexivity: The Essential Guide*. SAGE Publications Ltd; 2017.
7. National Socio-Environmental Synthesis Center. Practicing reflexivity and appreciating diverse perspectives lesson. https://www.sesync.org/resources/practicing-reflexivity-and-appreciating-diverse-perspectives-lesson

PART II

Nutrition and the Hospitalized Child

CHAPTER 14

Nutritional Assessment in Sick or Hospitalized Children

Brianna Mears, Coral Rudie, and
Christopher P. Duggan

Hospitalized children experience profound metabolic changes associated with acute and chronic illness, which place them at an increased risk of malnutrition.[1] Malnutrition in hospitalized children is associated with complications such as physiologic instability, organ dysfunction, increased infection risk, and longer hospital stays, all of which lead to greater resource use and poorer clinical outcomes.[2] Unfortunately, practices within hospital settings, such as failing to record and accurately track anthropometric data, can further exacerbate malnutrition risk. Table 14.1 outlines practices that enhance nutritional care in hospitalized patients.

A comprehensive nutrition assessment, including screening for malnutrition, is essential for effective nutrition interventions (Chapters 1-4). Table 14.2 outlines

TABLE 14.1 DESIRABLE PRACTICES TO ENHANCE NUTRITION CARE IN HOSPITALIZED PEDIATRIC PATIENTS

- Conduct early nutrition risk screening using a validated tool.
- Obtain accurate weight and height on admission and at regular intervals.
- Ensure timely nutrition assessment and interventions and routine reassessment by a Registered Dietitian, including:
  - Development of individualized nutrition care plans
  - Ongoing monitoring of growth parameters
  - Promotion of oral feeding when appropriate
  - Early initiation of nutrition support when indicated
- Minimize preoperative or procedural NPO duration to the shortest safe period.
- Offer meals that are age-appropriate and visually appealing.
- Provide feeding assistance as needed (e.g., cutting food, spoon-feeding).
- Ensure detailed documentation of intake, including food, fluids, and supplements, in I/O records.
- Clearly document and communicate nutrition goals across the care team.
- Implement multidisciplinary nutrition care planning and coordination.
- Provide nutrition education to patients and caregivers.
- Planning for postdischarge nutrition continuity.
- Utilize nutrition-focused quality improvement initiatives.

I/O, intake/output; NPO, nothing by mouth.
Adapted from Tappenden KA, Quatrara B, Parkhurst ML, Malone AM, Fanjiang G, Ziegler TR. Critical role of nutrition in improving quality of care: an interdisciplinary call to action to address adult hospital malnutrition. *J Acad Nutr Diet*. 2013;113(9):1219-1237.

TABLE 14.2 CHALLENGES WITH ASSESSMENT OF NUTRITIONAL STATUS IN HOSPITALIZED PATIENTS

VALUE ASSESSED	USUAL INDICATION	DIFFICULTY IN APPLYING TO HOSPITALIZED PATIENT
Weight	Standard growth reference	Can be difficult to obtain accurate measurement (scale differences, bed scale used, etc.) falsely affected by acute hydration changes
Height/length	Standard growth reference	Often not obtained/updated, value reported vs. measured on admission, difficult to measure (especially in infants)
Weight-for-length/BMI	Standard growth reference	Value determined by weight and height/length, can be artificially low or high pending accuracy of anthropometric data
Micronutrient labs	Assess for deficiency/adequacy of intake.	Acute phase respondent and thus serum levels can be unreliable when inflammation is present. Recommend to check c-reactive protein (CRP) to help assess presence/degree of inflammation.
Nutrition intake	Assess for adequate intake of nutrition and hydration.	Normal or historical intake subject to recall bias, poor or limited documentation of current intake in medical record, or can be dependent on accurate reporting from patient/caregiver if not visualized by nursing

BMI, body mass index.

standard assessment methods and the difficulties in interpreting them in hospitalized patients. Due to these challenges, additional steps are recommended to assess a patient's nutritional status. A thorough physical examination is crucial for identifying evidence of edema or dehydration, as changes in body water distribution can affect body weight and can skew measurements of body composition, such as triceps skinfold thickness. Along with physical exam, laboratory data play a key role in accurately assessing a patient's nutritional status. In particular, evaluating for gastrointestinal and hepatic disease, as well as considering the acute-phase response (e.g., serum C-reactive protein, erythrocyte sedimentation rate), can help guide the interpretation of specific micronutrient levels. Additionally, it is important to consider an individual patient's nutritional history, underlying diseases, and medication therapy when interpreting biochemical markers.[3]

ENERGY REQUIREMENTS OF HOSPITALIZED PATIENTS

The pediatric metabolic response during critical illness is proportional to the severity of the illness or injury, leading to increased turnover of proteins, fats, and carbohydrates. As a result, protein-energy malnutrition can occur if nutritional requirements are not accurately assessed and met.[4] This metabolic response is highly variable, and the degree of hypermetabolism is unpredictable and unlikely to be sustained during prolonged hospital stays.[5] Factors that affect nutritional requirements during critical illness include anorexia associated with infection, decreased absorption of consumed nutrients, increased energy and protein requirements associated with the severity of illness or injury, drug-nutrient interactions, reduced energy requirements related to the transient absence of growth during illness, and certain medical therapies. These factors contribute to the significant differences in nutritional requirements of hospitalized pediatric patients relative to healthy children. Importantly, the majority of predictive energy equations available are derived from measurements of energy expenditure in healthy children[6] (Chapter 5). Recent studies recommend against using the US Recommended Dietary Allowances (RDAs) to estimate a hospitalized patient's nutritional requirements, as they may overestimate energy requirements in the ICU setting.[7]

The Schofield equation is commonly used in assessing nutritional requirements in pediatrics; however, studies have suggested that the use of predictive energy equations with the indiscriminate use of variable stress factors may be inaccurate and place patients at risk for underfeeding or overfeeding.[8] It is also widely accepted that these calculations are not accurate in estimating the energy needs of critically ill children.[9] Predictive equations are also unable to account for variability of caloric needs throughout hospitalization and likelihood of increased metabolic rates, dependent on phase of critical illness.[4]

ENERGY EXPENDITURE COMPONENTS

To understand energy requirements in both healthy and hospitalized patient, it is helpful to review the components of Total Energy Expenditure (TEE):

$$\text{TEE} = \text{BMR} + \text{SDA} + E_{\text{activity}} + E_{\text{growth}} + E_{\text{losses}}$$

where:

- BMR = basal metabolic rate, which is the largest component of TEE (energy required by the body at rest while fasted, 60%-70%)
- SDA = specific dynamic action of food or thermic effect of food (energy produced as heat during digestion and metabolism of food, 8%-10%)
- E_{activity} = energy required for physical activity
- E_{growth} = energy required for somatic growth
- E_{losses} = obligatory energy lost in urine and stool due to inefficiencies of absorption and metabolism

In healthy children, significant age-related changes in TEE components are seen (Figure 14.1). For example, a 1-month-old infant has relatively low energy requirements for activity (10 kcal/kg/d) but has significant needs to support age-appropriate growth (40-50 kcal/kg/d). In comparison, a 6-month-old infant's energy requirements are distributed differently, with a higher proportion used for activity and lower energy needed for growth.

Hospitalized pediatric patients generally have reduced total energy requirements when compared to healthy children. In critically ill patients, four of the five components of TEE are often significantly reduced. Energy needed for physical activity is minimal in hospitalized patients due to bedrest and use of sedative and paralytic agents. Energy required for growth is often reduced because the catabolic response following severe injury or illness results in a temporary halt to anabolism (accretion of lean body mass). The thermic effect of food is reduced in patients receiving parenteral

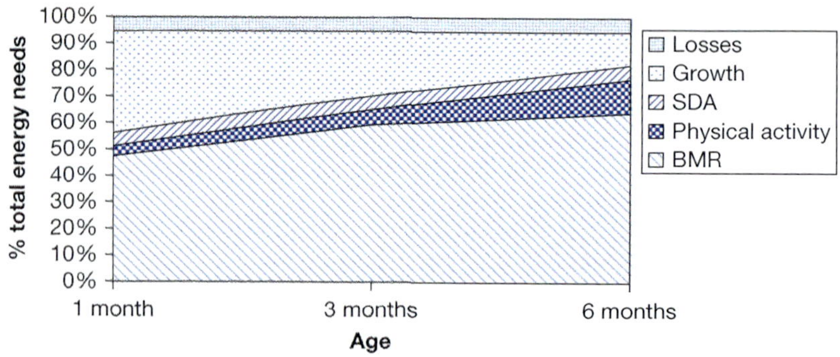

Figure 14.1 Factorial estimates of energy requirements. BMR, basal metabolic rate; SDA, specific dynamic action. (Adapted from Tsang RC, Nichols BL, eds. *Nutrition During Infancy*. CV Mosby Company; 1988.)

nutrition support compared to those receiving enteral nutrition, and obligatory gastrointestinal losses of nutrients are minimized in patients receiving PN.

However, specific clinical circumstances in hospitalized pediatric patients, such as thermal injuries and nutritional rehabilitation (i.e., catch-up growth or weight restoration), may lead to substantially higher energy needs than predicted.[2] For instance, adolescents recovering from malnutrition due to disordered eating may require upward of 4,000 kcal/day to promote weight restoration after prolonged calorie and protein restriction. It remains unclear why rebound hypermetabolism occurs following initial stages of nutritional rehabilitation.[10] Nutritional therapy for burn patients is discussed in Chapter 18, and for patients recovering from malnutrition/growth failure in Chapter 27.

The nutritional needs of hospitalized patients can be estimated by calculating basal metabolic rate (BMR) using a predictive energy equation (see Chapter 5) or by measuring resting energy expenditure (REE) via indirect calorimetry (see below) and then multiplying it by a stress factor to estimate total energy expenditure (TEE). Stress factors are highly variable, ranging from 0.9 to 2.0, depending on the disease process and are subjectively based on the clinician's judgment.[8] Serial monitoring of body weight is the most effective measure for assessing whether nutritional needs are being met during hospitalization.

INDIRECT CALORIMETRY

Indirect calorimetry is the gold standard for measuring a patient's REE and establishing energy goals to avoid the complications associated with both underfeeding and overfeeding. A nutrition plan guided by indirect calorimetry matches a patient's specific needs in that moment, capturing variations to metabolic rate sustained during prolonged admission.[9] As the name implies (*calor* is the Latin word for heat), indirect calorimetry determines the heat production of a biochemical reaction by measuring uptake of oxygen and liberation of carbon dioxide. This contrasts with direct calorimetry, which measures heat produced by the body at rest. Oxygen consumption (VO_2) and carbon dioxide production (VCO_2) measured by the calorimeter are entered into the Weir equation to calculate REE[11]:

$$REE = (3.94 \times VO_2) + (1.06 \times VCO_2) - (2.17 \times UUN)$$

where:

- UUN = urinary N excretion, used as a correction factor for protein oxidation

By calculating the ratio of VCO_2 to VO_2, known as the Respiratory Quotient (RQ), indirect calorimetry can also be used to estimate substrate oxidation and assist in determining whether a patient is being overfed. The RQ in a fasted state is normally 0.70 to 1.00, with RQ in this range representing a mixed substrate oxidation. An RQ significantly greater than 1.0 is consistent with energy intake in excess of nutritional requirements. Other reasons for this occurrence may include hyperventilation (wherein CO_2 is excreted at high rates) or failure to achieve steady state in gas measurement. Although not yet fully supported based on research available, the lower RQ seen for lipid oxidation relative to glucose oxidation has been used as a rationale for use of a higher fat and lower carbohydrate diet in patients with advanced lung disease to avoid an increased carbon dioxide load to emit.

Current critical care nutrition guidelines recommend that energy prescription in children should be guided by accurate measurement of energy expenditure using indirect calorimetry when possible.[9] An alternative to indirect calorimetry is to calculate REE using a modified Fick equation[12]:

$$REE = CO \times Hgb \times (Sao_2 - Svo_2) \times 95.18$$

where:

- CO = cardiac output (L/min) as measured with a thermodilution pulmonary catheter
- Hgb = hemoglobin concentration (g/dL)
- Sao_2 = oxygen saturation in arterial blood
- Svo_2 = oxygen saturation in mixed venous blood

The Fick equation can only be applied to patients whose cardiac output is measured with a pulmonary artery catheter, which is not always a routine pediatric ICU procedure. Although REE measurements are usually taken to approximate BMR, REE actually includes BMR, plus nonshivering thermogenesis and stress hypermetabolism. The difference between REE and BMR is estimated to be 10%.

Even in the presence of an accurate nutrition prescription, critically ill children in the ICU frequently receive inadequate nutrition provisions, resulting in changes to body composition (including loss of adipose tissue and/or skeletal muscle). Sufficient nutrition is often compromised in ICU setting due to hemodynamic instability, feeding intolerance, interruptions of enteral infusions, and absence of clear nutrition intervention plan.[13] Inadequate enteral infusion remains a problem in hospitalized children; it is estimated that fewer than 40% of patients receiving sufficient energy intake while in intensive care.[7] Further, intestinal dysmotility and delayed gastric emptying can promote enteral intolerance, in some cases preventing step-wise increases to goal calories and protein.[4]

PROTEIN REQUIREMENTS OF HOSPITALIZED PATIENTS

Protein requirements in disease and critical illness are typically higher than in health due to the increased urinary nitrogen losses characteristic of the catabolic state, gastrointestinal and skin losses, and the increased requirement for protein synthesis.[14] Hypermetabolic responses mobilize endogenous body stores, prioritizing protein breakdown to aid in tissue repair, wound healing, and inflammatory responses.[2] Children have limited protein reserves available to account for increased protein catabolism following illness.[8] Protein catabolism is the highest in the early phases of critical illness; even if protein intake seems adequate, hospitalized patients may experience net negative protein balance.[4] Enteral protein intake is the preferred route to replenish protein losses, aimed to prevent further degradation of lean body mass, growth failure, malnutrition, and poor clinical outcomes.[14]

Nitrogen balance remains the most direct and objective method for evaluating protein adequacy (see Chapter 4). While serum albumin and prealbumin are frequently used in clinical practice, their role in monitoring the adequacy and effectiveness of nutrition support is not clearly defined. Normalization of these markers may reflect the resolution of inflammation, a reduction in nutrition risk, a shift toward an anabolic state, as well as improved nutritional status.[3]

In general, serum albumin and prealbumin are not reliable indicators of total body protein stores or skeletal muscle mass and should not be used in isolation to assess nutritional status. Instead, they function more accurately as negative acute-phase reactants, inflammatory markers that can provide context within a comprehensive nutrition assessment.[3] It is critical to recognize that protein catabolism and muscle wasting may still occur even when serum levels of visceral proteins are within normal ranges, as these proteins do not reflect changes in lean body mass.[14]

Additionally, the metabolic response to stress and illness must be considered. In states of simple starvation, the body enters a hypometabolic state and primarily utilizes fat stores for energy (after exhausting hepatic glycogen stores). However, during critical illness and catabolic stress, protein, as well as fat and carbohydrate, are used as fuel sources, leading to accelerated muscle breakdown and nitrogen loss, further complicating the assessment of protein status through serum biomarkers alone.[5]

Protein should not serve as a primary energy source, but as amino acid substrates for enzyme synthesis and lean body mass accretion. When nutrition regimens provide significantly less than the REE for energy, protein is used for energy, which is not ideal. Some institutions therefore do not include protein in the calculating energy intake but instead assess adequacy of energy and protein intake be measuring the ratio of non-protein energy to protein intake (grams of N), which acceptable ratios between 150 and 250:1. Refer to Chapter 18 for protein recommendations for critically ill, injured children.

■ REFEEDING SYNDROME

Refeeding syndrome is a serious condition characterized by a constellation of fluid, electrolyte, and metabolic abnormalities that are the result of a rapid reintroduction of nutrition in malnourished patients.[15] During chronic malnutrition, lean body mass and fat stores are broken down and total body stores of nitrogen, phosphorus, magnesium, and potassium are depleted. Despite these changes, serum levels of phosphorus, magnesium, and potassium are usually maintained within the normal range. Upon reintroduction of nutrition (primarily carbohydrates), insulin secretion increases, leading to a rapid shift of glucose and electrolytes (phosphate, potassium, and magnesium) into the intracellular space. These shifts can result in acute drops in serum levels to critically low concentrations, triggering clinical complications. The clinical manifestations of hypophosphatemia include hemolytic anemia, muscle weakness

TABLE 14.3 RISK FACTORS FOR REFEEDING SYNDROME IN PEDIATRIC PATIENTS

Malnutrition indicators	• Weight-for-length z-score (for children <24 mo) or BMI z-score (ages 2-20 y) that meets malnutrition criteria and represents a significant change from baseline (see Chapter 2 for classification details) • Inadequate weight gain relative to expected growth for age or percentile
Inadequate nutritional intake	• Protein or energy intake consistently below 75% of estimated energy requirements over several consecutive days
Abnormal baseline electrolytes	• Prefeeding serum levels of potassium, phosphorus, or magnesium below normal reference ranges
Comorbid conditions affecting intake or nutritional status	• Presence of illnesses such as cancer, malabsorptive disorders, hyperemesis, eating disorders, or other causes of underlying malnutrition
Loss of body reserves	• Evidence of subcutaneous fat or muscle wasting assessed by: • Nutrition-focused physical exam or • Mid-upper arm circumference (MUAC) z-score indicating muscle mass loss

BMI, body mass index.
Adapted from da Silva JSV, Seres DS, Sabino K, et al. ASPEN consensus recommendations for refeeding syndrome. *Nutr Clin Pract.* 2020;35(2):178-195.

(especially diaphragmatic muscle), impaired oxygen delivery, and heart failure. Hypokalemia and hypomagnesemia can result in fluid overload, cardiac arrhythmias, seizures, and cardiac failure.[16]

Pediatric patients at highest risk of refeeding syndrome include those with severe weight loss (e.g., anorexia nervosa, cancer cachexia, and other cases of severe malnutrition), as well as patients who have been maintained on prolonged intravenous hydration in place of enteral or parenteral nutrition. Table 14.3 outlines risk factors for refeeding syndrome in pediatric patients. Initiation of parenteral or enteral nutrition can cause hyperglycemia and exacerbate refeeding syndrome; thus close monitoring is warranted, as onset of refeeding can occur up to 5 days after achieving goal calories. Thiamine (Vitamin B_1) is also rapidly depleted during nutrition rehabilitation and should be supplemented for approximately 1 week. Table 14.4 provides guidelines for the management of refeeding syndrome.

MICRONUTRIENTS AND OTHER ESSENTIAL AND CONDITIONALLY ESSENTIAL NUTRIENTS

The concept that certain nutrients, synthesized endogenously in adequate amounts while healthy, may become essential during illness continues to be widely studied. "Pharmaconutrition" and "Immunonutrition" describe current terminology used to

TABLE 14.4 MANAGEMENT OF REFEEDING SYNDROME IN CHILDREN

Baseline evaluation and preparation	• Measure serum electrolytes (phosphorus, potassium, magnesium, calcium) prior to initiating nutrition support. • Replete any electrolyte deficiencies to within normal limits before starting nutrition, based on established standards of care. • Obtain baseline vital signs, weight, and intake/output measurements.

Initiation of nutrition support	• Start thiamine at 2 mg/kg/d (maximum 100-200 mg/d) before initiating nutrition or IV dextrose, in patients at risk.
	  • Routine thiamine levels are not recommended, as they are unlikely to guide management.
	  • Continue thiamine supplementation for 5-7 d, or longer if, nutrition has not yet advanced to full goal, signs of deficiency are present, or the patient has severe malnutrition.
	• Begin nutrition at no more than 40%-50% of BMR or REE.
	• Calories from IV dextrose (PN or IV Fluids) should be introduced cautiously in high-risk patients.
	  • If a patient has already been receiving IV dextrose or medication in dextrose solution without electrolyte instability or symptoms, nutrition may be cautiously advanced.
	• It is not recommended to restrict protein, fluids, or sodium.
	• No recommendation can be made for whether prophylactic dosing of electrolytes should be given if prefeeding levels are normal.
	• If the nutrition regimen (oral, EN) does not meet full micronutrient needs, provide a complete pediatric multivitamin supplement daily as able.

Advancement of nutrition support	• Advance feeding slowly over 4-7 d, increasing calories by 10%-25% every 1-2 d, as tolerated to goal calories.
	• If serum electrolytes drop precipitously or become difficult to replete:
	  • Hold advancement or reduce caloric intake to the last well-tolerated level.
	  • Focus on electrolyte correction and stabilization before resuming advancement.
	  • Temporary cessation of nutrition may be considered in cases of severe or life-threatening electrolyte derangements, based on clinical judgment.

Monitoring during nutrition advancement	• Monitor serum phosphorus, potassium, and magnesium every 12-24 h until nutrition is advanced to goal and electrolytes are stable.
	• Check daily weights, with strict intake and output monitoring to detect fluid overload or dehydration.
	• Recommend vital signs every 4 h for the first 24 h after initiation in those at risk.
	  • Cardiorespiratory monitoring is recommended for unstable patients or those with severe deficiencies, based on established standards of care.
	• Evaluate short- and long-term nutrition care goals daily during the initial phase.
	  • Patients are considered stabilized once electrolyte supplementation has not been required for at least 48 h.
	  • After stabilization, follow institutional standards of care for ongoing monitoring.

BMR, basal metabolic rate; EN, enteral nutrition; IV, intravenous; PN, parenteral nutrition; REE, resting energy expenditure.

Adapted from da Silva JSV, Seres DS, Sabino K, et al. ASPEN consensus recommendations for refeeding syndrome. *Nutr Clin Pract*. 2020;35(2):178-195.

describe how certain nutrients, perhaps in pharmacologic doses or with certain immunologically active components, may benefit hospitalized patients. Nutrients like glutamine, arginine, antioxidants, zinc, and omega-3 fatty acids are some examples of the nutrients studied for their role in modifying the inflammatory response. Further research is needed in this area to determine the efficacy and safety of these interventions in the pediatric population. Selenium, cholecalciferol, and thiamine are also of special importance in ICU level care, as patients are more prone to depleting these micronutrients when critically ill. It is not uncommon for children to not meet DRI for these nutrients despite receiving enteral formulas, priming them for deficiencies.[17]

REFERENCES

1. De Cosmi V, Milani GP, Mazzocchi A, et al. The metabolic response to stress and infection in critically ill children: the opportunity of an individualized approach. *Nutrients*. 2017;9(9):1032.
2. Mehta NM. Energy expenditure: how much does it matter in infant and pediatric chronic disorders? *Pediatr Res*. 2015;77(1-2):168-172.
3. Evans DC, Corkins MR, Malone A, et al. The use of visceral proteins as nutrition markers: an ASPEN position paper. *Nutr Clin Pract*. 2021;36(1):22-28.
4. Al-Dorzi HM, Arabi YM. Nutrition support for critically ill patients. *JPEN J Parenter Enteral Nutr*. 2021;45(S2):47-59.
5. Sharma K, Mogensen KM, Robinson MK. Pathophysiology of critical illness and role of nutrition. *Nutr Clin Pract*. 2019;34(1):12-22.
6. Jotterand Chaparro C, Pabion C, Tume L, Mehta NM, Valla FV, Moullet C. Determining energy and protein needs in critically ill pediatric patients: a scoping review. *Nutr Clin Pract*. 2023;38(suppl 2):S103-S124.
7. Tume LN, Bickerdike A, Latten L, et al. Routine gastric residual volume measurement and energy target achievement in the PICU: a comparison study. *Eur J Pediatr*. 2017;176(12):1637-1644.
8. van Zanten ARH, De Waele E, Wischmeyer PE. Nutrition therapy and critical illness: practical guidance for the ICU, post-ICU, and long-term convalescence phases. *Crit Care*. 2019;23(1):368.
9. Duan JY, Zheng WH, Zhou H, Xu Y, Huang HB. Energy delivery guided by indirect calorimetry in critically ill patients: a systematic review and meta-analysis. *Crit Care*. 2021;25(1):88.
10. Reed KK, Silverman AE, Abbaspour A, Burger KS, Bulik CM, Carroll IM. Energy expenditure during nutritional rehabilitation: a scoping review to investigate hypermetabolism in individuals with anorexia nervosa. *J Eat Disord*. 2024;12(1):63.
11. Weir JB. New methods for calculating metabolic rate with special reference to protein metabolism. *J Physiol*. 1949;109(1-2):1-9.
12. Liggett SB, St John RE, Lefrak SS. Determination of resting energy expenditure utilizing the thermodilution pulmonary artery catheter. *Chest*. 1987;91(4):562-566.
13. Zhang Y, Fang Z, Zhao X, Zhu X, Zhu Y, Feng Y. Monitoring MUAC reflects the adequacy of nutrition support in critically ill children with a longer intensive care unit stay: a single-center prospective cohort study. *Nutr Clin Pract*. 2025;40(3):679-689.
14. Coss-Bu JA, Hamilton-Reeves J, Patel JJ, Morris CR, Hurt RT. Protein requirements of the critically ill pediatric patient. *Nutr Clin Pract*. 2017;32(1_suppl):128s-141s.
15. Olthof LE, Koekkoek W, van Setten C, Kars JCN, van Blokland D, van Zanten ARH. Impact of caloric intake in critically ill patients with, and without, refeeding syndrome: a retrospective study. *Clin Nutr*. 2018;37(5):1609-1617.
16. Corsello A, Trovato CM, Dipasquale V, et al. Refeeding syndrome in pediatric age, an unknown disease: a narrative review. *J Pediatr Gastroenterol Nutr*. 2023;77(6):e75-e83.
17. Dos Reis Santos M, Leite HP, Luiz Pereira AM, Dell'Acqua Cassão B, de Oliveira Iglesias SB. Factors associated with not meeting the recommendations for micronutrient intake in critically ill children. *Nutrition*. 2016;32(11-12):1217-1222.

CHAPTER 15

Interdisciplinary Care in Pediatric Nutrition

Christopher P. Duggan, Jennifer McClelland, Kayla E. Hope, Coral Rudie, Allison Churchill, Kathleen M. Gura, and Bridget M. Hron

Technologic advances in the 1960s made enteral and parenteral nutrition possible, and by the 1970s, growing recognition of the high prevalence of malnutrition among hospitalized patients led to the development of multidisciplinary nutrition support teams (NSTs). As reviewed by Barrocas et al.,[1] these teams first emerged in academic medical centers where specialized expertise in the provision of these therapies existed, including experts in surgery, gastroenterology, nutrition, nursing, and pharmacy.

This model of "multidisciplinary" care was instrumental in the formation of the American Society of Parenteral and Enteral Nutrition (ASPEN) and similar organizations globally. These groups acknowledged the importance of collaborative models of care, including expertise from the perspective of multiple disciplines in the delivery of safe and effective nutrition support. More recently, ASPEN has advocated for an "interdisciplinary" approach, highlighting that input from different disciplines must go beyond consultation to involve mutual collaboration and shared decision-making.[1] Some experts have further proposed a "transdisciplinary" model in which different team members perform similar roles, thus transcending traditional disciplinary lines.

RATIONALE FOR NUTRITION SUPPORT TEAMS

NSTs aim "to provide safe up to date appropriate nutritional support to an individual patient, who is malnourished or at risk of malnutrition in a coordinated fashion."[2] There is a broad medical literature supporting the rationale for the establishment of NSTs. Early justification for NSTs focused on the avoidance of errors in the administration of specialized nutrition, as well as the reduction of metabolic, infectious, and mechanical complications of central venous catheters and enteral feeding tubes.[3] Studies have since demonstrated the efficacy of these teams in reducing costs and improving nutritional delivery. While the impact of NSTs on mortality and length of stay remains less well documented, perhaps due to the complex and primarily supportive nature of nutrition in many hospitalized patients, NSTs remain integral to improving the overall quality of care. See Table 15.1 for a summary of metrics that have been examined in the medical literature to support the establishment and maintenance of pediatric NSTs.

TABLE 15.1 METRICS THAT SUPPORT THE UTILITY OF INTERDISCIPLINARY NUTRITION SUPPORT TEAMS

OUTCOME	REFERENCE(S)
More appropriate use of parenteral nutrition	11
Fewer central line-related complications	19
Safer provision of parenteral nutrition	20
Higher intake of protein	21
Improved quality of care and outcomes	20,22
Cost savings	23
Increased use of enteral nutrition	20,22
Reduced order errors	24
Shorter length of hospital stay	25

COMPOSITION OF PEDIATRIC NUTRITION SUPPORT TEAMS

The structure of NSTs that care for adult patients has been described,[2] and analogous proposals have also been noted for NSTs caring for pediatric patients.[4]

Medical and/or Surgical Clinician

Pediatric NSTs are typically led by a physician trained in nutrition (i.e., a physician nutrition specialist).[5] These physicians may include various specialists, including gastroenterologists (who have special training in gastrointestinal physiology, malnutrition, and obesity, as well as skills in gastrointestinal (GI) endoscopy, enteral tube placement, indirect calorimetry, and other advanced methods), surgeons (who have training in nutrition, critical care, venous access, GI surgery, stoma care, and other advanced methods), or sometimes endocrinologists, obesity medicine specialists, critical care physicians, or general pediatricians/hospitalists.

The physician team lead is ultimately responsible for the recommendations of the NST, coordination of care, communication with families and consulting services, overseeing quality improvement metrics, leading regulatory-mandated nutrition advisory committees, and interfacing with hospital leadership. Physician members of the NST are also responsible for the detailed physical examination of the patient, confirming findings such as muscle wasting, micronutrient deficiencies, hydration status, and obesity morbidities (see ref[6]). Physicians may also lead the interpretation of advanced body composition methods, assessment of complex x-ray findings of venous access, and interpretation of indirect calorimetry data for the assessment of resting energy expenditure and energy balance.

Registered Dietitian

Pediatric registered dietitians are critical members of the NST. They are responsible for the nutritional assessment of the patient (see Chapters 1-4), including an assessment of underlying nutritional status/risk for malnutrition (undernutrition and obesity) and indications for enteral or parenteral nutrition (see Chapters 16 and 17). As the frontline team members in the clinic or as part of unit-based teams, dietitians are often the first point of contact for nutrition-related issues and may act as a liaison between unit-based teams and the NST. Once the decision has been made to initiate nutrition support, dietitians are usually responsible for designing the composition (macro- and micronutrients), volume, and administration specifics of enteral or parenteral nutrition. In Massachusetts, licensed dietitians can legally order parenteral nutrition for patients, provided that the solution does not contain medications (e.g., heparin, famotidine, insulin), which must be ordered by physicians or other licensed providers. Dietitians are also tasked with interpreting serum vitamin and mineral assays and giving recommendations for repletion or monitoring as needed, often in conjunction with nurse practitioner (NP) and medical doctor (physician) team members.

Pharmacist

Licensed pharmacists play a critical role in NSTs by closely reviewing orders for parenteral nutrition, including the solution's composition, osmolarity (and safety for central vein infusion), calcium and phosphorus solubility, fat source, electrolytes and trace element dosing, and monitoring drug-nutrient interactions. Regular pharmacist attendance at NST walk rounds can streamline communication and ensure timely and safe ordering. Pharmacy staff are also responsible for overseeing the compounding of parenteral solutions, supervising pharmacy technicians, and maintaining adequate stocks of components, an important and dynamic task in the era of recurrent shortages. Pharmacists may also collaborate with informatics teams to build and maintain the databases used to prescribe and compound nutrition solutions and often serve as a conduit for working with home care companies to ensure a seamless transition from hospital to home and vice versa.

Registered Nurse

Inpatient and clinic nurses provide important expertise in the interdisciplinary care of NST patients. Their tasks include ongoing assessment and care of enteral and parenteral devices, hands-on skin and ostomy care, implementing nutrition regimens at the bedside, and monitoring the efficacy and safety of these regimens. Nursing staff also administer medication and nutritional supplements, including parenteral vitamins such as vitamin K and B_{12}, and monitor nutrition safety by obtaining blood and urine samples for various assays. Nurses often triage urgent calls from families at home, review clinical signs and symptoms of dehydration with caregivers, and liaise with community care providers (e.g., school-based providers). A key component of their role is family education about the importance of safe central line care, as well as the management of parenteral and enteral feeding pumps, tubes, and other devices.

Nurse Practitioner

Nurse practitioners can take on a variety of roles and responsibilities on NSTs, such as the assessment of patients receiving specialized home nutritional therapies. This includes patient assessment and physical examination, review of infusion practices, troubleshooting enteral and parenteral infusion devices, repairing fractured central venous catheters, and composing and ordering the parenteral solutions indicated by growth and laboratory results in collaboration with other team members. Nurse practitioners may also be involved in maintaining important relationships with home care companies whose clients include NST patients once they are discharged on parenteral or enteral nutrition. Nurse practitioners also routinely communicate with home care nurses, school nurses, and primary care providers.

Other Team Members

Comprehensive interdisciplinary nutrition care relies on collaboration with additional team members, including speech and language pathologists, social workers, administrative professionals, behavioral psychologists, data quality experts, and trainees in these and many other fields. Comprehensive in- and outpatient nutrition support is made possible by the contributions of and collaboration among these and the aforementioned team members.

CERTIFICATION

Despite growing attention to the importance of nutrition education in medical schools,[7-9] board certification of physicians via sub-boards in nutrition is not currently available from the American Board of Internal Medicine or Pediatrics. Physician NST leaders are therefore commonly certified in their relevant specialty, including gastroenterology, critical care, endocrinology, pediatrics, or surgery. NST members may pursue the following credentials:

- Certified Nutrition Support Clinician (CNSC) examination, sponsored by ASPEN, for multiple disciplines
- Physician Nutrition Specialist (PNS) certification, sponsored by the American Society for Nutrition
- Pharmacist certification in nutrition support, overseen by the Board of Pharmaceutical Specialties (BPS)
- Certification in Obesity Medicine, offered by the American Board of Obesity Medicine

OTHER OUTCOMES OF PEDIATRIC NUTRITION SUPPORT TEAMS

The impact of NSTs extends beyond direct patient care. For example, the collaborative efforts of NSTs can contribute to quality improvement initiatives to improve nutrition assessment metrics,[10] research efforts, the development of policies and protocols for institutional and national use,[11-13] professional development of all team members, advocacy for patient access to lifesaving medical and nutritional therapies,[14,15] training of many different colleagues (e.g., medical, nursing, and pharmacy students; dietetic interns; gastroenterology fellows; surgery residents; advanced practice providers), and collaboration across countries to foster global progress in nutrition interventions.[16,17]

CONCLUSION

More than 50 years have passed since the creation of the first NSTs, and advances in medicine, nutrition, and technology will certainly impact the evolution of these teams.[1] While tools such as the use of artificial intelligence to propose parenteral nutrition (PN) orders in the neonatal intensive care unit[18] are emerging, expert human input into medical and nutrition decision-making remains essential. With the increasing recognition of nutrition's central role in preventing chronic disease and the long-standing appreciation for the critical nature of growth and dietary intake in optimizing child health and development, interdisciplinary NSTs are essential to the delivery of safe and effective nutrition care.

REFERENCES

1. Barrocas A, Schwartz DB, Bistrian BR, et al. Nutrition support teams: institution, evolution, and innovation. *Nutr Clin Pract*. 2023;38(1):10-26.
2. Nightingale J. Nutrition support teams: how they work, are set up and maintained. *Frontline Gastroenterol*. 2010;1(3):171-177.
3. Wesley J. Nutrition support teams: past, present and future. *Nutr Clin Pract*. 1995;10:219-228.
4. Agostoni C, Axelson I, Colomb V, et al. The need for nutrition support teams in pediatric units: a commentary by the ESPGHAN committee on nutrition. *J Pediatr Gastroenterol Nutr*. 2005;41(1):8-11.
5. Lenders CM, Deen DD, Bistrian B, et al. Residency and specialties training in nutrition: a call for action. *Am J Clin Nutr*. 2014;99(5 suppl):1174S-1183S.
6. Waldrop SW, Krebs NF. A perfect storm in a pandemic-a child with complex medical history and special diet encounters COVID. *Am J Clin Nutr*. 2024;119(2):255-261.
7. Kushner RF, Van Horn L, Rock CL, et al. Nutrition education in medical school: a time of opportunity. *Am J Clin Nutr*. 2014;99(5):1167S-1173S.
8. Hitchell KS, Holton L, Surdyk PM, Combes JR. Advancing nutrition knowledge, skills, and attitudes in medical education and training: key themes and recommendations from the 2023 Summit. *Am J Clin Nutr*. 2024;120(3):746-748.
9. McGovern CJP. As White House conference approaches, now is the time for a national plan to address the link between hunger, nutrition education, and health. *Am J Clin Nutr*. 2022;116(4):841-842.
10. Persaud S, Hron BM, Rudie C, et al. Improving anthropometric measurements in hospitalized children: a quality-improvement project. *Nutr Clin Pract*. 2024;39(3):685-695.
11. Duggan C, Rizzo C, Cooper A, et al. Effectiveness of a clinical practice guideline for parenteral nutrition: a 5-year follow-up study in a pediatric teaching hospital. *JPEN J Parenter Enteral Nutr*. 2002;26(6):377-381.
12. Mehta NM, Bechard LJ, Leavitt K, Duggan C. Cumulative energy imbalance in the pediatric intensive care unit: role of targeted indirect calorimetry. *JPEN J Parenter Enteral Nutr*. 2009;33(3):336-344.
13. Mehta NM, Compher C; A.S.P.E.N. Board of Directors. A.S.P.E.N. clinical guidelines: nutrition support of the critically ill child. *JPEN J Parenter Enteral Nutr*. 2009;33(3):260-276.
14. Locks LM, Stewart CP, Hoffman DJ, Duggan CP. A shock to the global nutrition system: Why nutrition scientists should challenge the dismantling of the US Agency for International Development and US withdrawal from the World Health Organization. *Am J Clin Nutr*. 2025;121(5):951-955.
15. Duggan C, Bhutta Z. "Putting America First"—undermining health for populations at home and abroad. *New Engl J Med*. 2025;392(18):1769-1771.
16. Young LS, Huong PT, Lam NT, et al. Nutritional status and feeding practices in gastrointestinal surgery patients at Bach Mai Hospital, Hanoi, Vietnam. *Asia Pac J Clin Nutr*. 2016;25(3):513-520.
17. Dhingra U, Kisenge R, Sudfeld CR, et al. Lower-dose zinc for childhood diarrhea—a randomized, multicenter trial. *N Engl J Med*. 2020;383(13):1231-1241.
18. Phongpreecha T, Ghanem M, Reiss JD, et al. AI-guided precision parenteral nutrition for neonatal intensive care units. *Nat Med*. 2025;31(6):1882-1894.
19. Dalton MJ, Schepers G, Gee JP, Alberts CC, Eckhauser FE, Kirking DM. Consultative total parenteral nutrition teams: the effect on the incidence of total parenteral nutrition-related complications. *JPEN J Parenter Enteral Nutr*. 1984;8(2):146-152.
20. Reber E, Strahm R, Bally L, Schuetz P, Stanga Z. Efficacy and efficiency of nutritional support teams. *J Clin Med*. 2019;8(9):1281.
21. Mehta NM, Bechard LJ, Zurakowski D, Duggan CP, Heyland DK. Adequate enteral protein intake is inversely associated with 60-d mortality in critically ill children: a multicenter, prospective, cohort study. *Am J Clin Nutr*. 2015;102(1):199-206.
22. Hvas CL, Farrer K, Donaldson E, et al. Quality and safety impact on the provision of parenteral nutrition through introduction of a nutrition support team. *Eur J Clin Nutr*. 2014;68(12):1294-1299.

23. Goldstein M, Braitman LE, Levine GM. The medical and financial costs associated with termination of a nutrition support nurse. *JPEN J Parenter Enteral Nutr*. 2000;24(6):323-327.
24. Mitchell KA, Jones EA, Meguid MM, Curtas S. Standardized TPN order form reduces staff time and potential for error. *Nutrition*. 1990;6(6):457-460.
25. Jeong E, Jung YH, Shin SH, et al. The successful accomplishment of nutritional and clinical outcomes via the implementation of a multidisciplinary nutrition support team in the neonatal intensive care unit. *BMC Pediatr*. 2016;16:113.

CHAPTER 16

Enteral Nutrition

Jenny Kinne, Brianna Mears, Colleen Driscoll Stegman, and Bridget M. Hron

Enteral nutrition is the provision of nutrients through the gastrointestinal (GI) tract, either orally or through the use of a feeding tube to ensure that energy, macro-, and micronutrient needs are being met. A feeding tube for the provision of enteral nutrition is indicated when an infant or child is unable to meet estimated nutritional needs orally (Table 16.1). It can provide total or supplemental nutrition and can be used for short- or long-term nutritional management. The GI tract should be the first choice for nutritional support, since enteral nutrition is safer and more physiologic (Table 16.2).

■ ROUTES AND EQUIPMENT

Nasogastric (NG) tubes are easily placed and often the first consideration for short-term enteral nutrition therapy. Small bore silicone or polyurethane tubes can be placed nasally for anticipated usage of 3 months or less.[1] When an NG tube is placed, it is critically important to confirm the placement of the tube to avoid complications of malposition. This is often performed by pH measurement of gastric aspirate, and a pH value of less than or equal to 5.5 suggests intragastric location.[1] Radiographic confirmation must be done when the pH is greater than 5.5, when an aspirate cannot be obtained, when the patient has a high risk clinical condition, or when a patient's condition changes during the insertion procedure.[1] Reconfirmation of the NG tube placement is required if the tube migrates, the patient vomits, or the patient is transferred from an outside facility.

Long-term enteral nutrition can be provided by surgically placed gastric or postpyloric tubes. Choosing between these two methods depends on the function of the GI tract and risk for aspiration. Methods of gastric and postpyloric feedings are described in Tables 16.3 and 16.4. Gastric feeding is preferred, as it easier to position the gastric tubes and is more physiologic.[2] Gastric feedings allow the use of bolus feedings. Bolus feedings into the stomach can mimic typical meal patterns, and allow for periods of time where a patient can be disconnected from the feeding pump. Nocturnal continuous feedings can supplement oral intake or provide additional calories.

Postpyloric feeding may be indicated for patients with severe gastroesophageal reflux, gastric dysmotility, or are at high risk of aspiration, to name a few indications.[3] These feedings must be provided as a continuous feed only since the small intestine cannot expand to accommodate a bolus feeding.[2] Contraindications for small bowel feeding include nonfunctioning GI tract or inability to access the intestine.

TABLE 16.1 INDICATIONS FOR ENTERAL NUTRITION

INABILITY TO MEET FULL NUTRIENT NEEDS ORALLY

- Anatomic abnormalities
- Congenital anomalies (tracheoesophageal fistula [TEF])
    - Facial trauma
- Tumor or other mass
- Anorexia
- Acute or chronic infection (pneumonia, diarrhea)
- Cancer
- Cyanotic heart disease
- Endocrine disease
- Micronutrient deficiency (vitamin B_{12}, iron, zine)
- Pregnancy
- Psychosocial (chronic mental/emotional stress, depression, neglect/misuse)
- Increased metabolic needs
- Brain injury
- Bronchopulmonary dysplasia
    - Burns
    - Chronic renal disease
    - Congenital heart disease
- Cystic fibrosis
- Sepsis
- Trauma
- Neurologic disorders
- Cerebral palsy affecting oral motor skills
- Coma
- Dysphagia
- Severe mental retardation
- Prematurity
- Psychosocial disorders
- Anorexia nervosa
    - Nonorganic growth failure
- Severe food aversion

ALTERED ABSORPTION OR METABOLISM REQUIRING MODIFICATION OF DIET

- Acquired Immunodeficiency Syndrome (AIDS)
- Amino or organic acidopathies
- Chronic diarrhea
    - Chronic intestinal pseudo-obstruction
    - Chronic liver disease, i.e., biliary atresia

(continued)

TABLE 16.1 INDICATIONS FOR ENTERAL NUTRITION (*continued*)

INABILITY TO MEET FULL NUTRIENT NEEDS ORALLY

Glycogen storage disease (types I and III)

Inflammatory bowel disease

Pancreatitis

Short bowel syndrome

Solid organ transplant

Adapted from Davis A. Indications and techniques for enteral feeds. In: Baker SB, Baker RD, Davis A, eds. *Pediatric enteral nutrition*. Chapman and Hall; 1994:68.

TABLE 16.2 ADVANTAGES OF ENTERAL VERSUS PARENTERAL NUTRITION

- Reduced risk of infection and metabolic abnormalities
- Low volume enteral feeds may promote gastrointestinal (GI) maturation in premature infants
- Maintains and can help restore the integrity of gastrointestinal mucosa
- May facilitate restoration of digestive enzymes
- Less expensive than parenteral nutrition
- Mimics standard human nutrition

TABLE 16.3 GASTRIC FEEDING

	ADVANTAGES	DISADVANTAGES
Orogastric	Avoids nasal passage obstruction Appropriate for infants <34 wk gestational age	Not appropriate for patients with gag reflex
Nasogastric	Easy intubation	Nasal or esophageal irritation Easily dislodged
Percutaneous endoscopic gastrostomy (PEG)	Fewer occlusions with larger bore tube Appearance can be hidden under clothing Open surgery not required	Invasive technique for placement Site at risk for infection Appropriate anatomy required Requires repeat sedated procedure for initial exchange
Surgical gastrostomy	Endoscopy not required for placement Procedure directly accesses stomach	Risks of anesthesia/surgery Open surgical wound at risk for infection

TABLE 16.4 POSTPYLORIC/SMALL BOWEL FEEDING

	ADVANTAGES	DISADVANTAGES
Nasoduodenal/ nasojejunal	Temporary access for small bowel feeding pH-guided placement available	Easily dislocated; may require radiographic evidence of appropriate placement
Gastrostomy-jejunostomy	Transpyloric tube may be passed through existing gastrostomy Intestinal access for feeding and gastric access for decompression and medications	If not primary placement, requires healing of gastrostomy tract prior to jejunostomy tube placement Meticulous care of both ports necessary Jejunal port can occlude.
Jejunostomy	Direct access to small bowel	Easily occluded Leakage of intestinal contents

To reduce the risk of serious errors resulting from misconnections between enteral tubes and other medical lines and devices, enteral connectors have been standardized to improve patient safety globally through the International Organization of Standardization process.[4,5] The standardized connector that has been adopted globally is called EnFit and was first implemented in 2015.[4] Flow rates with EnFit devices may be slower due to its smaller effective internal diameter.[4]

FORMULA SELECTION

It is important to perform a nutritional evaluation to ensure the proper formula is selected to determine an appropriate, nutritionally complete formula for enteral feeding. Assessment of the following is necessary: energy and protein requirements, fluid and electrolyte status, growth history, functional status of the gastrointestinal tract (including presence of malabsorption and dysmotility), other medical comorbidities, any food allergies, previous formula intolerance, or macronutrient sensitivities.[6] Age is an important consideration in formula selection since certain formulas are designed to meet the needs of children at specific ages (e.g., preterm for infants <34 weeks gestation, infant [0-12 months], pediatric [1-13 years], and adult [14+]). Tables 16.5 and 16.6 outline the different categories and features of these products. These formulas may differ in their nutrient composition and vitamin and mineral content. For children over the age of 1 year (or over 12 months corrected gestational age), a pediatric formula should be used. "Toddler" formulas are not recommended, as they are not required to—and often do not—meet specific protein or micronutrient requirements set by the U.S. Food and Drug Administration (FDA) and are lower in caloric density than pediatric formulas.[7]

An important clinical practice point is to be on the lookout for "look alike, sound alike" formulas. Many formula companies make a variety of different infant and pediatric formula products with different ingredients, calorie concentrations, and indications, though these different products often have similar names. To avoid potentially harmful medical errors, the full formula name including caloric density must be confirmed with the patient or caregivers and clearly documented in the medical record.

TABLE 16.5 ENTERAL PRODUCT REFERENCES: ENERGY, MACRONUTRIENT, AND OTHER CONTENTS FOR INFANTS

PRODUCT (MANUFACTURER)	KCAL/ML	PROTEIN	FAT	CARBOHYDRATE	GENERAL COMMENTS
Human milk, Term, mature	0.67	Human milk whey and casein IgA, lysozyme, lactoferrin, antibodies, free amino acids	Long-chain fatty acids high in palmitic, oleic, linoleic and linolenic	Lactose and human milk oligosaccharides	Preferred nutrition for human infants; unique macronutrient and immune components not provided by commercial products
Bobbie (organic) (Bobbie Baby)	0.67	Nonfat cow milk, whey protein concentrate	Sunflower oil, canola oil, coconut oil Contains DHA	Lactose	Routine formula for full-term infants
Bobbie Gentle (organic) (Bobbie Baby)	0.67	Partially hydrolyzed whey	Safflower and/or sunflower oil, canola oil, and coconut oil	Lactose	Routine formula for full-term infants Partially hydrolyzed proteins
Bobbie Whole Milk (organic) (Bobbie Baby)	0.67	Whole cow milk, whey protein concentrate, nonfat milk	High-oleic (safflower or sunflower) oil, low erucic acid rapeseed oil, coconut oil Contains DHA and ARA	Lactose	Routine formula for full-term infants Contains higher percentage of fat from milk fats vs oils
EleCare Infant (Abbott)	0.67	Free L-amino acids	High-oleic safflower oil, MCT oil, soy oil	Corn syrup solids	Elemental formula 33% fat as MCT oil
Enfamil A.R. (Mead Johnson)	0.67	Nonfat cow milk	Palm olein, soy oil, coconut oil, high-oleic sunflower oil,	Lactose, rice starch, maltodextrin	Thickened with rice cereal Should not be concentrated above 24 cal/oz Viscosity 10× higher than routine formulas when exposed to stomach acid

Enfamil Enfacare 22 cal/oz (Mead Johnson)	0.74	Whey protein concentrate and nonfat cow milk	High-oleic vegetable oil, soy oil, MCT oil, coconut oil	Liquid: maltodextrin lactose Powder: lactose, corn syrup solids	Designed for former premature infants now >2 kg or 40 wk corrected age Contains additional Ca, P, vit A, vit D, folate, Zn Standard dilution is 22 cal/oz.
Enfamil Gentlease (Mead Johnson)	0.67	Partially hydrolyzed nonfat cow milk and whey protein concentrate solids (60:40 whey:casein)	Palm olein, soy, coconut, and high-oleic sunflower oils	Corn syrup solids	80% reduced lactose compared to standard formulas
Enfamil NeuroPro Infant (Mead Johnson)	0.67	65:35 whey:casein nonfat cow milk	Palm olein, soy, coconut, high-oleic sunflower oils Contains DHA and ARA	Lactose, galactooligosaccharides, polydextrose	Routine formula for full-term infants Contains prebiotics
Enfamil Optimum (Mead Johnson)	0.67	Whey protein concentrate and nonfat coq milk	Palm olein, coconut, soy, and high-oleic sunflower oils	Lactose, galactooligosaccharides, polydextrose	Routine formula for full-term infants Contains prebiotics Contains lactoferrin
Enfamil Premature Infant (Mead Johnson)	0.67	Whey protein concentrate Nonfat cow milk	MCT, soy and high-oleic vegetable oils, single-cell oil blend rich in DHA and ARA	Corn syrup solids, lactose	Designed for low birth weight and premature infants, additional Ca, P, vit A, vit D, folate, Zn High in protein Available in 20, 24, 24 HP, 30 Designed for in hospital use only
Enfamil Prosobee Simply Plant-Based (Mead Johnson)	0.67	Soy protein isolate	Palm olein, soy, coconut, and high-oleic sunflower oils, single-cell oil blend rich in DHA and ARA	Corn syrup solids	Lactose free

(continued)

TABLE 16.5 ENTERAL PRODUCT REFERENCES: ENERGY, MACRONUTRIENT, AND OTHER CONTENTS FOR INFANTS (*continued*)

PRODUCT (MANUFACTURER)	KCAL/ML	PROTEIN	FAT	CARBOHYDRATE	GENERAL COMMENTS
Enfaport (Mead Johnson)	1.01	Nonfat cow milk Whey protein concentrate	MCT oil, soy oil, DHA and ARA	Corn syrup solids	Ready to feed 30 cal/oz formula that can be modified to as low as 20 cal/oz 84% fat as MCT oil Includes all essential fatty acids
Fortini 30 cal/oz (Nutricia)	1.0	Nonfat cow milk and whey protein	Canola oil, modified coconut oil, high-oleic sunflower oil, corn oil, MCT from palm kernel and/or coconut oil, *anhydrous milk fat*	Maltodextrin and lactose, galactooligosaccharides and fructooligo-*saccharides*	Ready to feed infant formula designed for growth faltering or high calorie needs Contains prebiotics
Gerber Good Start Gentle Soy (Nestle)	0.67	Soy protein isolate	Palm olein, soy, coconut, high-oleic safflower or sunflower oils	Corn maltodextrin, sucrose	
Gerber Good Start Gentle/Gentle Pro (Nestle)	0.67	Hydrolyzed whey protein concentrate	Palm olein, soy, coconut and high-oleic safflower or sunflower oils	Lactose, corn maltodextrin	Routine formula for full-term infants Contains probiotics (*B. lactis*) 100% partially hydrolyzed whey protein
Kendamil Classic (Kendal Nutricare)	0.67	Whole cow milk, demineralized whey powder, skimmed milk powder	Sunflower oil, coconut oil, rapeseed oil Contains DHA	Lactose, galactooligosaccharides and fructooligosaccharides	Routine formula for full-term infants Contains prebiotics

Kendamil Goat (Kendal Nutricare)	0.67	Whole goat milk, mineralized goat whey powder	Sunflower oil, coconut oil, rapeseed oil Contains DHA	Lactose, galacto-oligosaccharides	Routine formula for full-term infants No cow's milk ingredients Contains prebiotics
Monogen (Nutricia)	0.73	Whey protein concentrate	Oil blend (including coconut, walnut)	Corn syrup solids	90% fat as MCT oil
Neocate Syneo Infant (Nutricia)	0.67	Free amino acids	High-oleic sunflower oil, canola oil, MCT from palm kernel and/or coconut oils	Corn syrup solids	Amino acid-based formula for severe milk protein allergy 33% MCT Contains pre and probiotics (*B breve*) Lactose free
Neocate Infant DHA and ARA (Nutricia)	0.67	Free amino acids	High-oleic sunflower oil, canola oil, MCT from palm kernel and/or coconut oils. added DHA and ARA	Corn syrup solids	Amino acid-based formula for severe milk protein allergy 33% MCT Lactose free
Nutramigen with Probiotic LGG (Mead Johnson)	0.67	Extensively hydrolyzed casein	Vegetable oil blend containing one or more of: palm olein oil, coconut oil, soy oil, high-oleic sunflower oil	Corn syrup solids modified corn starch	Hypoallergenic for infant CMPA Lactose free Contains probiotics (*Lactobacillus rhamnosus* GG)
Pepticate (Nutricia)	0.67	Partially hydrolyzed whey protein	Palm oil, coconut oil, canola oil, sunflower oil Contains DHA and ARA	Maltodextrin, galactooligosaccharides and fructooligosaccharides	Hypoallergenic for infant CMPA Contains prebiotics

(continued)

TABLE 16.5 ENTERAL PRODUCT REFERENCES: ENERGY, MACRONUTRIENT, AND OTHER CONTENTS FOR INFANTS (*continued*)

PRODUCT (MANUFACTURER)	KCAL/ML	PROTEIN	FAT	CARBOHYDRATE	GENERAL COMMENTS
PurAmino *formerly Nutramigen AA* (Mead Johnson)	0.67	Free amino acids	High-oleic sunflower oil, MCT oil, soy oil	Corn syrup solids	Amino acid-based formula for severe milk protein allergy 33% MCT Lactose free
Similac 360 Total Care (Abbott)	0.67	Nonfat cow milk and whey protein concentrate	High-oleic safflower oil, soy oil, coconut oil. Contains DHA	Lactose, human milk oligosaccharides	Routine formula for full-term infants Contains prebiotics
Similac 360 Total Care-Sensitive (Abbott)	0.67	Cow milk protein isolate	High-oleic safflower oil, soy oil, coconut oil Contains DHA	Maltodextrin, sucrose and human milk oligosaccharides	Routine formula for full-term infants Designed for lactose sensitivity Contains prebiotics
Similac Advance (Abbott)	0.67	Nonfat cow milk and whey protein concentrate	High-oleic safflower oil, soy oil, coconut oil Contains DHA	Lactose, galacto-oligosaccharides	Routine formula for full-term infants Contains prebiotics
Similac Alimentum (Abbott)	0.67	Extensively hydrolyzed casein and free amino acids	Safflower oil, MCT, soy oil Contains DHA	Sucrose and modified tapioca starch	Hypoallergenic for infant CMPA 33% MCT Lactose free

Similac NeoSure 22 cal/oz (Abbott)	0.74	Nonfat cow milk and whey protein concentrate	Soy oil, coconut oil, MCT Contains DHA and ARA	Corn syrup solids and lactose	Designed for former premature infants >2 kg or >40 wk corrected age Additional Ca, P, vit A, vit D, folate, Zn 25% MCT
Similac PM 60/40 (Abbott)	0.67	Whey protein concentrate	High-oleic safflower oil, soy oil, coconut oil	Lactose	For infants requiring lower mineral provisions, such as in renal care Lower in Ca, P, maintaining 2:1 ratio Lower in K Low iron
Similac Sensitive (Abbott)	0.67	Cow milk protein isolate	High-oleic safflower oil, soy oil, coconut oil	Corn syrup, sucrose	Routine formula for full-term infants Lactose reduced Low osmolality (200 mOsm/kg water)
Similac Soy Isomil (Abbott)	0.67	Soy protein isolate	High-oleic safflower oil, soy oil, coconut oil Contains DHA and ARA	Corn syrup, sucrose and fru-tooligosaccharides	Indicated for Galactosemia Contains prebiotics Lactose free
Similac Special Care 20, 24, 30 cal/oz (Abbott)	0.67 0.81 1.0	Nonfat milk and whey protein concentrate	Soy oil, coconut oil, MCT Contains DHA and ARA	Corn syrup solids and lactose	Designed for low birth weight and premature infants High in protein Additional Ca, P, vit A, vit D, folate, Zn Ca:P ratio of 1.8:1

(*continued*)

TABLE 16.5 ENTERAL PRODUCT REFERENCES: ENERGY, MACRONUTRIENT, AND OTHER CONTENTS FOR INFANTS (*continued*)

PRODUCT (MANUFACTURER)	KCAL/ML	PROTEIN	FAT	CARBOHYDRATE	GENERAL COMMENTS
Similac Special Care-High Protein 24 cal/oz (Abbott)	0.81	Nonfat milk and whey protein concentrate	Soy oil, coconut oil, MCT Contains DHA and ARA	Corn syrup solids and lactose	Designed for low birth weight and premature infants High in protein: 0.3 g more per 100 kcal than Similac Special Care Additional Ca, P, vit A, vit D, folate, Zn Ca:P ratio of 1.8:1
Similac Total Comfort (Abbott)	0.67	Partially hydrolyzed whey	High-oleic safflower oil, soy oil, coconut oil Contains DHA and ARA	Corn maltodextrin, sucrose and fru-tooligosaccharides	Partially hydrolyzed proteins Contains prebiotics Lactose free

ARA, arachidonic acid; CMPA, cow's milk protein allergy; DHA, docosahexaenoic acid; MCT, medium-chain triglycerides.

TABLE 16.6 ENTERAL PRODUCT REFERENCES: ENERGY, MACRONUTRIENT, AND OTHER CONTENTS FOR OLDER CHILDREN (NON-INFANTS)

PRODUCT (MANUFACTURER)	KCAL/ML	PROTEIN	FAT	CARBOHYDRATE	GENERAL COMMENTS
Alfamino Jr (Nestle)	1.0	Free amino acids	MCT, soybean oil	Corn syrup solids, potato starch, maltodextrin	Amino acid based Unflavored or vanilla flavor
Boost (Nestle)	1.01	Cow milk protein concentrate Soy protein isolate	Canola oil	Glucose syrup, sugar	80% free water Gluten and lactose free, kosher
Boost Breeze (Nestle)	1.0	Whey protein isolate	None	Glucose syrup, sugar	82% free water Clear liquid, protein containing supplement, fat free, gluten free, lactose free, kosher
Boost Kid Essentials (Nestle)	1.0	Cow milk protein concentrate	Canola oil	Brown rice syrup, sugar	85% free water Multiple flavors Lactose and gluten free, kosher
Boost Kid Essentials 1.5 (Nestle)	1.5	Cow milk protein concentrate	Canola oil, soybean oil, MCT	Brown rice syrup, sugar	78% free water Lactose and gluten free, kosher Fiber-containing version available
Boost Plus (Nestle)	1.52	Cow milk protein concentrate Soy protein isolate	Canola oil	Glucose syrup, sugar	70% free water Gluten and lactose free, kosher
Compleat Pediatric original (Nestle)	1.0	Dehydrated chicken powder, cow milk protein concentrate, pea protein isolate	Canola oil MCT	Brown rice syrup, fruit and vegetable blend (tomato paste, peach puree, green bean powder, carrot powder, cranberry juice concentrate), pea powder, fructooligosaccharides, inulin	84% water Lactose and gluten free

(*continued*)

TABLE 16.6 ENTERAL PRODUCT REFERENCES: ENERGY, MACRONUTRIENT, AND OTHER CONTENTS FOR OLDER CHILDREN (NON-INFANTS) *(continued)*

PRODUCT (MANUFACTURER)	KCAL/ML	PROTEIN	FAT	CARBOHYDRATE	GENERAL COMMENTS
Compleat Pediatric Original Reduced calorie (Nestle)	0.6	Dehydrated chicken powder, cow milk protein concentrate, pea powder, pea protein isolate	Canola oil, MCT	Brown rice syrup, fruit and vegetable blend (green bean powder, tomato paste, peach puree, cranberry juice concentrate, carrot powder), pea fiber, fructooligosaccharides, inulin	90% water Lactose and gluten free
Compleat Pediatric Original Plant-based (Nestle)	1.5	Pea protein isolate, hydrolyzed pea protein isolate	High-oleic safflower oil/or sunflower oil, canola oil	Brown rice syrup, fruit and vegetable blend (apple puree, peach puree, cherry puree, banana puree, butternut squash puree, carrot powder)	Plant based Dairy free Lactose and gluten free
Compleat Pediatric Standard Plant-Based (Nestle)	1.0	Pea protein Isolate L-cystine	High-oleic sunflower oil, canola oil, MCT	Brown rice syrup, partially hydrolyzed guar gum, pea fiber	84% water Plant based, vegan, dairy free Available in 1.4 option Gluten, lactose free Kosher
Compleat Pediatric Organic Blends (Nestle)	1.2	Organic hydrolyzed pea protein, organic rice protein concentrate	Organic extra virgin olive oil, organic canola oil	Organic sweet potato puree, organic pear puree, organic brown rice flour, organic blueberry puree, organic kale puree	82% water blenderized whole food tube feeding formula Organic Lactose, gluten free, dairy free Two flavors chicken garden vegetable and plant based

EleCare Jr (Abbott)	1.0	Free L-amino acids	Soy oil, MCT, high-oleic safflower oil	Corn syrup solids	100% free amino 33% fat as MCT oil Unflavored and vanilla flavor Gluten, lactose, fructose, galactose, milk and soy protein free
Ensure (Abbott)	0.93	Cow milk protein concentrate, soy protein isolate, nonfat milk	Canola oil, corn oil	Corn maltodextrin, sugar	84% free water Gluten and lactose free Kosher High protein option
Ensure Plus (Abbott)	1.5	Cow milk protein concentrate, soy protein isolate	Canola oil, corn oil	Corn maltodextrin, sugar	76% free water Gluten and lactose free Kosher
Glucerna (Abbott)	0.93	Cow milk protein concentrate, soy protein isolate	Canola oil	Corn maltodextrin, fructose	85% free water Contains low glycemic carbohydrates 16 g fiber/L Gluten and lactose free Kosher Comes in 1.2 and 1.5 cal/mL
IsoSource HN (Nestle)	1.2	Soy protein isolate, sodium caseinate, calcium caseinate	Canola oil, MCT oil	Glucose syrup, maltodextrin	81% free water Higher calorie version available (1.5) Gluten and lactose free Kosher

(*continued*)

TABLE 16.6 ENTERAL PRODUCT REFERENCES: ENERGY, MACRONUTRIENT, AND OTHER CONTENTS FOR OLDER CHILDREN (NON-INFANTS) *(continued)*

PRODUCT (MANUFACTURER)	KCAL/ML	PROTEIN	FAT	CARBOHYDRATE	GENERAL COMMENTS
Jevity (Abbott)	1.05	Sodium caseinate, soy protein isolate, calcium caseinate	Canola oil, corn oil, MCT	Corn maltodextrin, corn syrup solids, soy fiber	84% free water 14.4 g fiber/L Higher calorie versions available (1.2, 1.5) Gluten and lactose free Kosher
Kate Farm Pediatric Standard (Kate Farms)	1.2	Organic pea protein	Organic MCT (from coconut), organic high linoleic sun-flower oil, organic flaxseed oil	Organic brown rice syrup solids, organic agave syrup, organic pea starch	75% water Plant-based protein Vanilla and chocolate flavor Kosher Lactose, gluten, and dairy free
Kate Farms Pediatric Peptide 1.0 (Kate Farms)	1.0	Organic hydrolyzed pea protein	Organic MCT (from coconut), organic high linoleic sun-flower oil, organic flaxseed oil	Organic brown rice syrup solids, organic agave syrup, organic pea starch	79% water Comes in 1.5 option Kosher Lactose-, gluten-, and dairy free
Neocate Junior (unflavored) (Nutricia)	1.0	Free amino acids	Refined vegetable oil, MCT, palm kernel and/or coconut oil, high-oleic sunflower oil, sunflower oil, canola oil	Corn syrup solids	Free amino acid formula Various flavors With or without prebiotics
Neocate Splash (Nutricia)	1.0	Free amino acids	High-oleic sunflower oil, MCT (modified palm kernel and/or coconut oil), canola oil	Maltodextrin, sugar	Flavors: orange-pineapple, grape, tropical fruit, vanilla, and unflavored Gluten free

Nepro (Abbott)	1.8	Caseinates (calcium, magnesium, sodium), milk protein isolate	High-oleic safflower oil, canola oil, soy lecithin	Corn syrup solids, sugar	73% water Gluten and lactose free Kosher Contains prebiotic
Nourish (Functional Formularies)	1.2	Organic garbanzo beans, organic pea protein	Organic Extra virgin olive oil, organic flax oil	Organic whole grain brown rice, organic sprouted quinoa, organic sweet potato	Plant based, gluten free, tree nut free (produced in a facility where tree nuts are used), dairy free, soy free, corn free, USDA Certified Organic, 7 g of naturally occurring dietary fiber in 12 oz
Nourish Peptide (Functional Formularies)	1.5	Organic garbanzo beans, organic hydrolyzed pea protein	Organic Extra virgin olive oil, organic coconut MCT oil, organic flax oil	Organic whole grain brown rice, organic sprouted quinoa, organic sweet potato	Plant-based peptide formula Free of tree nuts, gluten, dairy, soy, corn
Nutren Junior (Nestle)	1.0	Cow milk protein concentrate, whey protein concentrate	Soybean oil, canola oil, medium chain triglycerides	Maltodextrin, sugar	85% water Fiber-containing version available Gluten and lactose free kosher
Nutren 1.5 (Nestle)	1.5	Soy protein isolate Cow milk protein concentrate	Canola oil	Corn syrup, maltodextrin	76% water Gluten and lactose free
Nutren 2.0 (Nestle)	2.0	Sodium caseinate, soy protein isolate, calcium caseinate	MCT and canola oil	Corn syrup, maltodextrin	69% water Kosher, lactose and gluten free
Nutrihep (Nestle)	1.5	L-amino acids, whey protein concentrate	MCT (from coconut and/or palm kernel oil), canola oil, corn oil	Maltodextrin	76% water High in BCAA Kosher, lactose and gluten free

(continued)

TABLE 16.6 ENTERAL PRODUCT REFERENCES: ENERGY, MACRONUTRIENT, AND OTHER CONTENTS FOR OLDER CHILDREN (NON-INFANTS) *(continued)*

PRODUCT (MANUFACTURER)	KCAL/ML	PROTEIN	FAT	CARBOHYDRATE	GENERAL COMMENTS
Osmolite (Abbott)	1.2	Sodium and calcium caseinates	High-oleic safflower, canola, and MCT oils, soy lecithin	Corn maltodextrin	82% free water High calorie version available (1.5 cal/mL) Kosher, lactose and gluten free
PediaSure Enteral formula (Abbott)	1.0	Cow milk protein concentrate Soy protein isolate	High-oleic safflower, soy oil, MCT	Corn maltodextrin, sugar	84% free water Kosher, lactose and gluten free Also fiber-containing option
PediaSure 1.5 (Abbott)	1.5	Cow milk protein concentrate soy protein isolate	High-oleic safflower, soy oil, MCT	Corn, maltodextrin	78% water Lactose and gluten free, kosher Fiber-containing version
PediaSure Peptide	1.0	Whey protein hydrolysate, hydrolyzed sodium caseinate	Canola oil, MCT	Corn maltodextrin	85% free water 1.5 option available Lactose and gluten free, kosher
PediaSure Reduced Calorie (Abbott)	0.6	Milk protein concentrate, soy protein isolate, whey protein concentrate	Soy oil	Short-chain fructooligosaccharides, sugar	89% water Lactose free, gluten free, kosher Contains prebiotics
Peptamen (Nestle)	1.0	Hydrolyzed whey protein	MCT oil, soybean oil	Maltodextrin, corn starch	85% free water 70% fat from MCT Gluten free, lactose free, kosher Also in 1.5 cal/mL

Peptamen Junior (Nestle)	1.0	Hydrolyzed whey protein	MCT oil, canola oil, soybean oil	Maltodextrin, corn starch	85% free water, flavored version available 60% fat from MCT Gluten free, lactose free, kosher
Peptamen Junior 1.5 (Nestle)	1.5	Hydrolyzed whey protein	MCT oil, canola oil, soybean oil, refined fish oil (anchovy, sardine)	Maltodextrin, corn starch, partially hydrolyzed guar gum	77% free water 60% MCT Gluten free, lactose free, kosher
Peptamen 1.5 (Nestle)	1.5	Hydrolyzed whey protein	MCT oil, soybean oil	Maltodextrin, corn starch	77% free water, vanilla version available 70% fat from MCT Gluten free, lactose free, kosher
Promote (Abbott)	1.0	Sodium caseinate, soy protein isolate	Safflower oil, MCT oil, soy oil and soy lecithin	Corn maltodextrin, sugar	86% free water Kosher, lactose and gluten free Fiber option available
Pulmocare (Abbott)	1.5	Sodium and calcium caseinates	Canola oil, MCT oil, corn oil, high-oleic safflower oil	Sugar, corn maltodextrin	78% free water Low in glycemic index Kosher, lactose and gluten free
Puramino Jr (Mead Johnson)	1.0	Free amino acids	High-oleic sunflower oil, MCT, soy oil	Corn syrup solids, modified tapioca starch	Amino acid based Unflavored or vanilla flavor
Suplena with CARBSTEADY (Abbott)	1.8	Milk protein concentrate, sodium caseinate	High-oleic safflower oil, canola oil, soy lecithin	Corn maltodextrin, sugar, soluble corn fiber	73% water Low protein formula Lower in potassium and phosphorus Kosher, lactose and gluten free Contains sugar substitute

(*continued*)

TABLE 16.6 ENTERAL PRODUCT REFERENCES: ENERGY, MACRONUTRIENT, AND OTHER CONTENTS FOR OLDER CHILDREN (NON-INFANTS) *(continued)*

PRODUCT (MANUFACTURER)	KCAL/ML	PROTEIN	FAT	CARBOHYDRATE	GENERAL COMMENTS
Tolerex (Nestle)	1.0	Free amino acids	High linoleic safflower oil	Corn maltodextrin, modified corn starch	85% free water Free amino acid, high carbohydrate, low-fat formula (2%) Lactose and gluten free
TwoCal HN (Abbott)	2.0	Milk protein concentrate, sodium and calcium caseinates	Corn oil, canola oil,	Corn syrup solids, corn maltodextrin, sugar, fructose oligosaccharides	70% free water Kosher, lactose and gluten free Contains prebiotics
Vital HP (Abbott)	1.0	Whey protein hydrolysate, hydrolyzed sodium caseinate	MCT oil, marine oil, corn oil	Corn maltodextrin, sugar	84% water Peptide based High protein, low fat Gluten, lactose free
Vivonex Pediatric (Nestle)	0.8	Free amino acids	MCT oil, soybean oil	Corn syrup solids, potato starch	70% fat as MCT oil Suitable for gluten-free and lactose-free diet
Vivonex TEN (Nestle)	1.0	Free amino acids	Safflower oil	Maltodextrin, modified corn starch	83% free water Free amino acids High carbohydrate, Low-fat formula Lactose free, gluten free, kosher

BCAA, branched chain amino acids; MCT, medium-chain triglycerides

■ CONSIDERATIONS FOR EUROPEAN AND NON–FDA-REGULATED FORMULAS

Use of imported non–FDA-regulated formulas purchased from third-party online vendors is on the rise in the United States.[8,9] There may be several reasons why parents or caregivers choose these products, such as the belief these products contain higher quality ingredients, preference to avoid "corn syrup solids," or perceptions that European regulations are more stringent than in the United States.[9] There are no regulations for the transport and storage of non–FDA-regulated formulas.[8] Risks associated with using non–FDA-regulated formulas include inadequate or even excessive macro or micronutrient delivery, as these products do not have to meet the standards of the Infant Formula Act.[8] Different languages and different labeling regulations internationally can make identifying the type of formula and allergen ingredients difficult and increases risks associated with custom recipes.[8] There may be delays in notification of products that are recalled internationally.[8]

Following a large formula recall in the United States in 2022 and the supply chain constraints brought about by the COVID-19 pandemic, the FDA issued a guidance for enforcement discretion on a case-by-case basis to temporarily allow certain international infant formula products that were "safe and nutritionally adequate" to be sold in the United States.[10] In 2023, the FDA issued a pathway for these manufacturers to continue marketing and selling their products in the United States as they work toward meeting FDA requirements as a route for FDA approval.10 Clinicians should be aware of these products and potential nutritional and safety risks to discuss with the patient's caregivers.

■ CONCENTRATION AND MODULAR COMPONENTS

Formulas may be modified to enhance energy density by concentration of the formula base—adding less water or more concentrate—and/or by the addition of carbohydrate, protein, or fat modular components (Table 16.7). The standard dilution for infant formulas is 20 kcal/oz, and for pediatric formulas is 30 kcal/oz.

Children with increased energy requirements and/or volume restriction may benefit from a concentrated formula. Concentration of a base infant formula is generally recommended up to 24 to 26 cal/oz. Concentration of a base pediatric formula is generally recommended up to 45 cal/oz. When higher energy densities are required, use of modular components should be considered depending on clinical situation for further caloric enhancement. The addition of a modular allows increased calorie provision from formula without additional micronutrient contributions (which would alternately be present if one added more formula powder to achieve higher kcal/oz concentration). Modulars typically contain one to two macronutrients to contribute extra calories, which may be chosen for a different clinical implication (e.g., adding extra protein to meet dietary reference intakes, adding carbohydrates due to hypoglycemia, and so forth). Table 16.8 lists the suggested calorie distribution of feedings that should be considered when formulating recipes containing modular components. Table 16.9 lists situations in which particular types of macronutrient modulation may be indicated.

Excessively concentrated formula may have a high renal solute load, which may require additional fluids to meet estimated fluid needs which will increase potential

TABLE 16.7 ENTERAL FORMULA TYPES: MODULARS

- **Carbohydrate based**
  - Glycose polymers (example Polycose)
  - Hydrolyzed cornstarch
  - Partially hydrolyzed guar gum (e.g., Benefiber)
- **Fat based**
  - Vegetable-based oils
  - MCT oil
- **Protein based**
  - Calcium caseinate
  - Hydrolyzed collagen
  - Liquid protein fortifier
  - Whey protein isolates (e.g., Beneprotein)
- **Mixed sources**
  - Duocal (cornstarch + refined vegetable oils)
  - Benecalorie (calcium caseniate + refined vegetable oil + mono/diglycerides)
  - Human Milk Fortifiers (for use in preterm infants)

Adapted from EN modulator products. American Society for Parenteral and Enteral Nutrition. https://nutritioncare.org/clinical-resources/enteral-nutrition/

renal solute load (PRSL). When infants are fed a concentrated formula, urine solute concentration should be monitored and maintained less than 400 mOsm/kg of water. Practicing proper mixing of infant formulas is important to review with patient families to avoid accidental increase in renal solute load. Providing formulas that have high PRSL could provide more rapid dehydration than a low PRSL formula. The PRSL can be calculated by the following equation: PRSL (mOsm/L) = Na + Cl+ K + P + (protein/175), where the electrolyte units are mmol/L and the protein is expressed as mg/L.[11]

The osmolality of the final formula feeding must also be considered. Isotonic formulations have an osmolality of approximately 300 mOsm/L, similar to blood and other bodily fluids. Although diarrhea during enteral feeding is not uncommon and often multi-factorial, hyperosmolar formulas may be more difficult for children and infants to tolerate, and may contribute to looser stool output.[12]

TABLE 16.8 RECOMMENDED CALORIE DISTRIBUTION

	CARBOHYDRATE	PROTEIN	FAT
1-3 y of age	45%-65%	5%-20%	30%-40%
4-18 y of age	45%-65%	10%-30%	25%-35%
Over 18 y of age	45%-65%	10%-35%	20%-35%

From Institute of Medicine, Food and Nutrition Board. *Dietary Reference Intakes for Energy, Carbohydrate, Fiber, Fat, Fatty Acids, Cholesterol, Protein and Amino Acids.* National Academy Press; 2002.

TABLE 16.9 INDICATIONS FOR CALORIE ENHANCEMENT BY COMMONLY USED MODULARS

CARBOHYDRATE	LONG-CHAIN FATS	MEDIUM CHAIN TRIGLYCERIDES
Congenital heart disease	Bronchopulmonary dysplasia	Chylothorax
Delayed gastric emptying	Carbohydrate malabsorption	Fat malabsorption
Failure to thrive	Diarrhea	Lymphangiectasia
Gastroesophageal reflux	Failure to thrive	Prematurity
Glycogen storage disease	Hypermetabolic states	Thoracic duct trauma
Hypermetabolic states		

When selecting a modular, consider macronutrient profile for recommended calorie distribution and assessment of clinical needs.
Reproduced with permission from Davis A, Baker S. The use of modular nutrients in pediatrics. *JPEN J Parenter Enteral Nutr*. 1996;20:228–236.

■ RECOMMENDATIONS FOR CONCENTRATION OF FORMULAS

A step-by-step method to calculate formula recipes for concentrated formula can be found in Table 16.10. Energy density typically starts at the standard formula dilution and should be advanced by 2 to 4 cal/oz every 12 to 24 hours. Children receiving enhanced energy formulas should be closely monitored for signs of intolerance as well as adequacy of fluid and nutrient intake. Nutrition assessment, growth, and laboratory monitoring should occur periodically, particularly with changes in clinical status.[13]

It is important to be mindful of a formula regimen's contributions to renal solute load. Many manufacturers will not advise fortification of infant formula past 28 kcal/oz for this reason, due to the accumulation of protein, vitamins, and minerals. For children with fluid restrictions who require very high–calorie formulas, monitoring glomerular filtration rate (GFR) and hydration status is often indicated. Utilizing nutrition software can be helpful to calculate full micronutrient and protein contributions and compare them to upper limit (UL) values for age to assess appropriateness.

The osmolality of the final formula feeding must also be considered. It is not uncommon for fortified formulas of higher calorie concentration to cause diarrhea. Isotonic formulations have an osmolality of approximately 300 mOsm/L, similar to blood and other bodily fluids. Hyperosmolar formulas may not be well tolerated by some infants and children.[12]

■ INITIATION AND ADVANCEMENT OF FEEDINGS

Enteral feedings should be given in a manner appropriate to the child's clinical comorbidities and quality of life. Supplemental gastric feedings can be given at night to allow oral intake during daytime hours gastric enteral nutrition may be provided as a combination of bolus and/or continuous drip feedings. Bolus feedings can allow gravity to dictate the rate of infusion or a pump can be used to deliver formula at a constant rate.[14] Continuous feedings are given over 8 to 24 hour periods at a slower rate and require a pump for delivery. Postpyloric or jejunal feeds are required to be delivered as continuous. Table 16.11 outlines the advantages and disadvantages of each feeding method.

Progression of feedings as a bolus or continuous regimen is dictated by tolerance to the previous step in advancement. The final goal is a predetermined formula volume based on the child's estimated nutritional requirements. Rates of infusion and caloric concentration should not be increased simultaneously. Adjustments to the goal volume may be required when a child "outgrows" the calories provided by the formula volume or with changes in clinical condition. Recommendations for initiating tube feedings and attaining the desired goals are outlined in Table 16.12.

TABLE 16.10 FORMULA RECIPES

CREATING FORMULA RECIPES

- Note that using "water up" methods is less accurate than determining precise values for ingredients and mL of water needed—as outlined below.
- **We recommend using the formula product's medical provider website and product guides to obtain the most accurate and up to date information on calories per gram, grams per scoop, displacement, and other measurements from the manufacturer when calculating recipes.**

1. **Determine calories to be provided from formula.**

Example 1: 110 kcal/kg of routine infant formula (24 kcal/oz)

Example 2: 1750 kcal/d utilizing powdered elemental pediatric formula (30 kcal/oz) and carbohydrate/fat modular (5 kcal/oz)

2. **If applicable, determine daily total calories for infant by multiplying kcal/kg by current weight.**

Example 1: For an infant weighing 5.6 kg, a prescription of 110 kcal/kg would equal 616 kcal/d.

3. **Divide by the caloric density of the component**

Example 1: 616 kcal/d goal / 24 kcal/oz dilution = 25.6 oz (770 mL) needed per day to supply 616 kcal.

Example 2: Goal to provide 1750 kcal/d utilizing custom formula (35 kcal/oz), 30 kcal/oz from powdered elemental pediatric formula, 5 kcal/oz from modular powder

- 1750 kcal/d/35 kcal/oz formula = 50 oz/d (1500 mL) needed
- Calculate what nutrition each ingredient provides per oz
    - 30 kcal/oz × 50 oz = 1500 kcal from formula
    - 5 kcal/oz × 50 oz = 250 kcal from modular

4. **Using information from the manufacturer*, determine how many calories per gram (or mL) are provided by each ingredient, and how many mL each gram displaces in finished recipe.**

Example 1: Routine infant formula contains 5.12 kcal/g of powder. Each gram displaces 0.77 mL in final recipe.

Example 2:

- Elemental pediatric formula contains 4.72 kcal/g of powder. Each gram displaces 0.70 mL in final recipe.
- Carb and fat modular contain 4.92 kcal/g of powder. Each gram displaces 0.77 mL in final recipe.

TABLE 16.10 FORMULA RECIPES (*continued*)

5. **Using the following equation, determine how many grams of powder or mL of liquid ingredients are required for each recipe.**
   X = (Kcal/oz of ingredient) × (# of oz needed)/kcal per gram (or mL) of ingredient

Example 1:

X = (24) × (25.6/5.12)

X = 120 g Infant formula powder

Example 2:

X = (30) × (50/4.72)

X = 318 g Pediatric elemental formula powder

Y = (5) × (50/4.92)

Y = 51 g Carb/fat modular powder

6. Using information for displacement, calculate total displacement for each ingredient depending on amount above.

Example 1: 120 g powder × 0.77 mL/g displacement = 92 mL displaced by infant formula powder

Example 2:

X: 318 g powder × 0.70 mL/g displacement = 223 mL displaced by elemental formula powder

Y: 51 g modular powder × 0.77 mL/g displacement = 39 mL displaced by modular powder

$X + Y$ = 262 mL total displacement of ingredients

7. Determine the amount of water needed to make total final volume

W = Volume needed of formula – Displacement of (X) – Displacement of (Y)

Example 1:

W = 770 mL Infant formula – 92 mL displaced by powder

W = 678 mL

Example 2: W = 1500 mL Custom elemental formula (35 kcal/oz) – 223 mL displaced by elemental powder – 39 mL displaced by modular powder

W = 1228 mL

8. Combine all ingredients and water to make final recipe

Example 1: 120 g of powder + 678 mL of water = 770 mL formula at 24 kcal/oz dilution

Example 2: 318 g formula powder + 51 g of modular powder + 1228 mL water = 1500 mL formula at 35 kcal/oz dilution

For children transitioning to enteral nutrition from parenteral nutrition (PN), adequacy of fluid and nutrient intake must be closely monitored. Young infants are at greatest risk due to their proportionately higher nutrient needs. Most infants and children can successfully make the transition from to standard enteral formula once gut function has returned and enteral access is obtained. Patients with chronic gastrointestinal disease may require slower transitions, special formulas, and closer monitoring. Table 16.13 lists the steps in transitioning children from PN to EN, and Table 16.14 gives an example of transitional feeding.

For children who advance to goal enteral rates via continuous feeds, the ultimate goal should be transition to bolus or intermittent feeding regimen as it mimics typical

TABLE 16.11 ADMINISTRATION OF ENTERAL FEEDING

	ADVANTAGES	DISADVANTAGES
Bolus	Can mimic or supplement meals May not require a pump Freedom of movement between feedings	Increased risk of aspiration Not recommended for children with conditions associated with poor volume tolerance (e.g., gastroesophageal reflux, delayed gastric emptying)
Continuous	Preferred method for small bowel feedings Slow infusion may improve tolerance Can be given nocturnally to avoid disruption of daytime schedule and oral intake	Requires pump Child is attached to equipment for duration of feeding. Overnight feedings may result in morning fullness

TABLE 16.12 GUIDELINES FOR INITIATION AND ADVANCEMENT OF CONTINUOUS AND INTERMITTENT TUBE FEEDINGS

AGE	INITIAL INFUSION	ADVANCES	SUGGESTED TOLERATED RATE (JEJUNAL) OR GOAL (GASTRIC)
Jejunal Feeds			
Preterm	0.5-2 mL/kg/h	0.2-1 mL/kg/d q8h	4-8 mL/kg/h
0-12 mo	1-2 mL/kg/h	1-2 mL/kg q 2-8 h	5-6 mL/kg/h
1-6 y	1 mL/kg/h	1 mL/kg q 2-8 h	1-5 mL/kg/h
>7 y	25 mL/h	25 mL q 2-8 h	100-150 mL/h
Continuous Gastric Feeds			
Preterm	1-2 mL/kg/h	10-20 mL/kg/d	120-175 mL/kg/d
0-12 mo	1 mL/kg/h	1 mL/kg q 2-8 h	1-5 mL/kg/h
1-6 y	1-2 mL/kg/h	1-2 mL/kg/q 2-8 h	6 mL/kg/h
>7 y	25 mL/h	25 mL q 2-8 h	100-150 mL/h
Bolus/Intermittent Gastric Feeds			
Preterm (>1,200 g)	2-4 mL/kg/feed	2-4 mL/feed	120-175 mL/kg/d
0-12 mo	10-15 mL/kg q 2-3 h	10-30 mL/feed	20-30 mL/kg q 4-5 h
1-6 y	5-10 mL/kg q 2-3 h	30-45 mL/feed	15-20 mL/kg q 4-5 h
>7 y	90-120 mL q 3-4 h	60-90 mL/feed	330-480 mL q 4-5 h

Modified from Broekaert IJ, Falconer J, Bronsky J, et al. The use of jejunal tube feeding in children: a position paper by the gastroenterology and nutrition committees of the European Society for Paediatric Gastroenterology, Hepatology, and Nutrition 2019. *J Pediatr Gastroenterol Nutr*. 2019;69(2):239-258; Data from Davis A. Transitional and combination feeds. In: Baker SB, Baker RD, Davis A, eds. *Pediatric Enteral Nutrition*. Chapman and Hall; 1994.

TABLE 16.13 RECOMMENDATIONS FOR TRANSITIONING FROM PARENTERAL TO ENTERAL NUTRITION

1. Match PN caloric density with desired EN caloric density when feasible.
2. Once initial EN rate is tolerated, decrease PN rate milliliter for milliliter with further increases in EN (see initiation and advancement guidelines, Table 16.15).
3. For fluid restricted patients: continue lipid infusion until goal EN rate is tolerated, then concentrate formula as required to meet caloric requirements prior to discontinuing lipids. Calorie requirements of enterally fed patients are generally 10% higher than parenterally fed patients.

EN, enteral nutrition; PN, parenteral nutrition.

meal physiology[2] and allows for time to detach from the pump, allowing for participation in developmentally appropriate activities. See Table 16.15 for steps in transitioning from continuous to bolus enteral feedings and Table 16.16 for an example of transitional feeding to combined nighttime and bolus feedings.

HOME TUBE FEEDING

Home tube feeding can offer psychological benefits for the child and family and be markedly less expensive than hospitalization. Home tube feeding is indicated if the patient is medically stable and ready to be discharged from the hospital, and the child is tolerating tube feedings, and is expected to require them for longer than 1 week. It is important that caregivers and the patient (if old enough) be willing, able, and capable to administer tube feedings at home. Caregivers should be taught how to prepare, administer, and monitor the feedings, and be able to demonstrate their skills.

It should also be confirmed that caregivers have the necessary resources for administering tube feeds, such as running water, refrigeration, and storage space (Table 16.17).

TABLE 16.14 EXAMPLE OF TRANSITIONAL FEEDING FROM PARENTERAL TO ENTERAL NUTRITION

	PARENTERAL NUTRITION	20% LIPIDS	ENTERAL NUTRITION	TOTAL KCAL
Day 0	15 mL/h	2 mL/h	-	88 kcal/kg/d
Step 1	11 mL/h	2 mL/h	4 mL/h	90 kcal/kg/d
Step 2	7 mL/h	2 mL/h	8 mL/h	91 kcal/kg/d
Step 3	3 mL/h	2 mL/h	12 mL/h	93 kcal/kg/d
Step 4	Discontinue PN	2 mL/h	16 mL/h	98 kcal/kg/d
Step 5		1 mL/h	Increase to 24 kcal/oz	98 kcal/kg/d
Step 6		Discontinue lipids	18 mL/h	96 kcal/kg/d

For a 3.6 kg infant on PN with 15% dextrose and 2.5% amino acids.
Enteral nutrition = 20 cal/oz breastmilk; fluid limited to 120 mL/kg/d.

TABLE 16.15 RECOMMENDATIONS FOR TRANSITIONING TO BOLUS ENTERAL FEEDINGS

Attain goal feeding volume over 24 h.

Stop feedings for approximately 2 h then increase rate by 1-2 mL/kg or 25 mL/h (see Table 16.15) every 4-12 h, as tolerated, with a corresponding decrease in the number of hours of feedings per day. The total volume of feedings per 24 h should be constant.

When planning supplemental night tube feedings, consider running feeds only during planned feeding hours. Increase rate over these hours to the total volume desired.

Transition from continuous to bolus feedings:

- Consider combination bolus and nighttime continuous feedings for exclusively tube-fed patients.
- Cycle to desired rate of overnight feed, then decrease number of hours and provide remaining volume as bolus feedings; start bolus volume at 1-2 times the hourly rate.

Large volume bolus feedings may not be well tolerated in patients with delayed gastric emptying; many patients will require a pump to allow volume of bolus feed to run over 1/2 to 1 h.

TABLE 16.16 EXAMPLE OF TRANSITIONAL FEEDING TO COMBINATION NIGHTTIME AND BOLUS FEEDINGS

FEEDING	REGIMEN	SCHEDULE
Day 0	80 mL/h	Continuous
Day 1	100 mL/h for 19 h	4 PM-11 AM
Day 2	115 mL/h for 16 h + 150 mL bolus	5 PM-9 AM, bolus at 1 PM
Day 3	115 mL/h for 12 h + 250 mL bolus × 2	7 PM-7 AM, bolus at 11 AM and 3 PM
Day 4	115 mL/h for 10 h + 250 mL bolus × 3	8 PM-6 AM, bolus at 9:30 AM, 1 PM, and 4:30 PM

For a 9-year-old, 30 kg child on continuous intact protein nasogastric feedings of 30 kcal/oz formula

TABLE 16.17 REQUIRED INSTRUCTIONS FOR HOME TUBE FEEDING

Preparation

How to use sanitary techniques—e.g., proper handwashing, cleaning equipment before starting, avoiding contamination of formula, proper hang-time of formula

How to place and check the feeding tube, if using a nasogastric tube

How to prepare enteral feeding bags, program the feeding pump, and troubleshoot alarms

Monitoring

How to distinguish signs and symptoms of intolerance—e.g., vomiting, abdominal distention, and diarrhea. Excessive coughing, breathing difficulties, or skin color changes may indicate improper tube placement. The tube should be removed and replaced by either the caregiver if a G-tube, or hospital personnel in the case of J-tubes.

Support

Names and important phone numbers to be provided: physician, nutrition support nurse, dietitian, and 24-h hotline from infusion company for technical support.

A plan for insurance coverage of the cost of the formula and tube feeding equipment should be established prior to discharge. Outpatient medical and nutrition follow-up should be in place. It is imperative to establish the medical team responsible for enteral tube management (NG or gastrostomy tube), which often requires a pediatric gastroenterologist and trained GI nurse. Nutrition follow-up will involve continued assessment of the patient's nutritional needs and adjustments to feeding regimen as needed. A visiting nurse or social worker can provide support between clinic visits. Support groups in the area may also be available for the family.

MONITORING AND EVALUATION OF TUBE FEEDING

In the early stages of tube feeding, monitoring is focused on assessing the patient's tolerance to the feeding plan. Once a feeding regimen has been established, monitoring involves ensuring that the goals of nutritional therapy are being met and that tube feeding support is still required. Monitoring and evaluation of tube feedings include weight, height, biochemical and hematologic indices, monitoring for nutritional deficiencies/excesses, tube integrity, and any tube related complications. Table 16.18 lists some common complications of tube feeding and their solutions.

TABLE 16.18 COMPLICATIONS ENCOUNTERED IN TUBE FEEDING

COMPLICATION AND POSSIBLE CAUSES	INTERVENTION
Gastrointestinal	
Constipation	
Low fiber intake	Use fiber-containing formula or add fiber module.
	Watch for clogging of the tube if fiber used.
Diarrhea	
Formula delivered too rapidly	Decrease delivery rate.
Hypertonic formula	Change to isotonic formula and gradually increase concentration as tolerated.
	Alter carbohydrate and electrolyte content.
Medications that change the gut flora or have cathartic effects	If possible, change the type of medication or time it is given. Note sorbitol content in drugs.
Bacterial contamination of formula	Use aseptic preparation techniques and limit the feeding time to 4-8 h. Do not add new formula to bag containing old formula.
Cold formula	Allow formula to reach room temperature before feeding.
Mucosal atrophy and malnutrition	Use isotonic or diluted formula. Start at low rate and advance rate slowly.
Malabsorption	Use elemental or semi-elemental formula, MCT oil.

(continued)

TABLE 16.18 COMPLICATIONS ENCOUNTERED IN TUBE FEEDING (*continued*)

COMPLICATION AND POSSIBLE CAUSES	INTERVENTION
Hypoalbuminemia	Alter the protein and fat content. Dipeptide-based, low-fat formula may be beneficial.
Feeding intolerance	
Delayed gastric emptying of medications and other fluids being added to stomach	Consider prokinetic agent, patient positioning (place in right lateral oblique position), transpyloric feeds, continuous infusion, isotonic formula).
Vomiting, nausea, bloating	
Ileus/obstruction	Stop feedings. May require parenteral nutrition if ileus is prolonged
Complication and possible causes	**Intervention**
Improper tube placement	Check tube placement.
Infusion rate too rapid	Reduce rate and increase gradually as tolerated.
Delayed gastric emptying	Consider prokinetic agent, patient positioning, transpyloric feeds, continuous infusion, isotonic formula.
Hyperosmolar formula	Dilute formula to isotonicity then increase concentration gradually.
Hypertonic medications	Change timing or type of medication. Check for sorbitol content in drugs.
High fat formula	Change to lower fat formula.
Unpleasant odor of formula	Use flavor packets. Use different formula.
Formula too hot or too cold	Use formula at room temperature.
Patient positioning	Elevate head of bed 30°-45°.
Swallowing excess air	Stop feeding pump once feeding is complete.
Inadequate fluid intake	Monitor fluid balance closely. Increase fluid intake by changing formula concentration or rate or via fluid boluses.
Inactivity	Avoid prolonged bed rest.
Fecal impaction	Enemas or stool softeners, digital disimpaction, increase fiber and/or fluid intake.
Mechanical	
Aspiration	
Gastric hypomotility	Infuse formula past pylorus. Consider continuous infusion. Elevate head of bed 30°-45°.
GER	
Neurologic damage	

TABLE 16.18 COMPLICATIONS ENCOUNTERED IN TUBE FEEDING (*continued*)

COMPLICATION AND POSSIBLE CAUSES	INTERVENTION
Clogging of tube	
Improper or infrequent irrigation of the tube	Flush tubing with water every 4-8 h and after all medicines.
Administration of medications via a feeding tube	Crush medications well or use liquid form. Assess drug/formula interactions. Avoid mixing formulas with liquid medications with a pH <5.0 Use warm water to flush or a commercially prepared formula. Replace feeding tube.
Improper size or placement of tube	Change tube size. Check placement.
Nasopharyngeal discomfort, nasal or esophageal erosions	Wet the mucous membranes or use a smaller tube.
Pressure on the nares or esophagus	Alternate nares weekly
Gastrointestinal perforation	
Secondary to malpositioning of tube, excessive manipulation, use of guide wires	Can be avoided by radiologic confirmation of tube placement, minimizing manipulation, fluoroscopic guidance of nasoenteric tube placement, choice of proper size tube
Metabolic	
Azotemia recommended dietary allowances are met.	Decrease protein content while ensuring protein.
High protein intake, renal immaturity or dysfunction, liver disease, metabolic dysfunction	
Congestive heart failure	Reduce fluid and/or sodium content. Provide diuretics.
Dehydration	
Inadequate fluid intake	Increase fluid intake.
Hyperosmolar or high protein formula	Decrease formula concentration. Change to isotonic or lower protein formula.
Essential fatty acid deficiency	Change formula, add 5 mL of safflower oil, add modular fat.
Hyperglycemia	
Diabetes, insulin deficiency, severe malnutrition, trauma, sepsis or excessive carbohydrate intake	Monitor blood sugar. Initiate or adjust insulin. Reduce carbohydrate content.
Hyperkalemia	
High-potassium formula or IV potassium, renal insufficiency, acidosis	Monitor laboratory values. Change formula. Stop or decrease IV potassium. Give Kayexalate, insulin, glucose.
Hypokalemia	

(*continued*)

TABLE 16.18 COMPLICATIONS ENCOUNTERED IN TUBE FEEDING (*continued*)

COMPLICATION AND POSSIBLE CAUSES	INTERVENTION
Protein-calorie malnutrition, refeeding syndrome, diarrhea, insulin administration	IV/PO potassium. Evaluate potassium intake from formula for adequacy.
Hyponatremia	
Overhydration	Restrict water. Evaluate sodium intake from formula for adequacy.
Sodium depletion	Add sodium chloride.
Hyperphosphatemia	Change formula. Use phosphate binder or calcium supplement.
Hypophosphatemia	IV/PO phosphorus. Evaluate phosphorus intake from formula for adequacy.
Severe malnutrition (refeeding syndrome), insulin administration	
Liver function, abnormal	May need to stop or change formula
Overhydration	
Infusion rate too rapid	Decrease rate.
High sodium intake	Decrease sodium content.
Severe protein-calorie malnutrition	Monitor input and output.
Weight	
Rapid or excessive gain: excessive calories and/or fluid	Decrease concentration or amount of formula; evaluate electrolyte status.
Slow or no weight gain: inadequate caloric intake	Evaluate macro- and micronutrient intake. Evaluate input and output.
Psychomotor development	
Child kept on tube feeding for long period of time and missed important developmental steps for learning feeding skills	Nonnutritive sucking, taking very small amounts of food from a spoon, or taking liquid from a cup to desensitize the oral area, develop an association between oral activity and satiety and learn eating and feeding skills. Consult an occupational therapist or speech pathologist.

GER, gastroesophageal reflux; IV, intravenous; MCT, medium chain triglycerides; NG, nasogastric.

TRANSITION FROM ENTERAL TO ORAL NUTRITION

The transition to oral feedings is a process rather than a single event, but should be considered when a child no longer meets the indication for tube feeding support and is medically stable.[15] The process typically requires a multidisciplinary team, including experts in nutrition, pediatric gastroenterology, psychology, and speech and language pathology, as well as close partnership with the patient's caregiver. Common problems encountered in the transition to oral feeding include gagging, retching, and

TABLE 16.19 GUIDELINES FOR TRANSITION FROM ENTERAL TO ORAL FEEDINGS

ASSESSMENT

1. Assess the child's nutritional and medical status.
2. Assess the child's oral motor and swallowing skills.

If the child has a history of swallowing difficulties, have the child seen by a speech and language pathologist for a swallowing evaluation. Assess for aspiration of oral feeds.

3. Assess the caregiver's readiness to begin transition.

Caregivers will require education on process and reassurance that transition may be gradual.

TRANSITION TO ORAL FEEDS

1. Gradual transition to bolus feeding

   Increase the rate of feedings and lengthen the time between feedings.

2. Adjust bolus feeding to oral feeding schedule.

   Three meals and 2-3 snacks per day

3. Offer oral feeds first then bolus feed and/or nighttime feeds to make up caloric deficit.
4. Reduce tube feeding gradually.

Tube feeding can be reduced by 25% initially to promote hunger. Continue to gradually reduce by increments of 25%, based on improvements in oral intake, feeding problems, and growth. Once the child is consuming >75% from oral feeds, tube feeding can be stopped. Patient may need additional pedialyte or water when tube feeding is decreasing to meet fluid needs.

5. Other considerations

Consult a behavioral psychologist and/or speech therapist if feeding difficulties. Use behavior modification techniques—e.g. positive reinforcement and oral stimulation exercises. Offer variety in food texture, color, taste, temperature, and smell, without overwhelming the child. Do not force feed. Allow the child to play with different foods; tube feed during family mealtime to create an association between feeding and hunger.

vomiting when orally stimulated, and an absence of the hunger-satiety cycle.[16,17] To reduce the risk of oral hypersensitivities and feeding difficulties, early assessment and implementation of an oromotor stimulation program by a speech pathologist is recommended[2,18] (Table 16.19).

ACKNOWLEDGMENT:

Chapter was based on previous contributions by Ms. Amina Grunko, Ms. Erin Keenan, and Ms. Jenny Kinne.

REFERENCES

1. Irving SY, Rempel G, Lyman B, et al. Pediatric nasogastric tube placement and verification: best practice recommendations from the NOVEL Project. *Nutr Clin Pract*. 2018;33(6):921-927.
2. Braegger C, Decsi T, Dias JA, et al. Practical approach to paediatric enteral nutrition: a comment by the ESPGHAN committee on nutrition. *J Pediatr Gastroenterol Nutr*. 2010;51(1):110-122.

3. Broekaert IJ, Falconer J, Bronsky J, et al. The use of jejunal tube feeding in children: a position paper by the gastroenterology and nutrition committees of the European Society for Paediatric Gastroenterology, Hepatology, and Nutrition 2019. *J Pediatr Gastroenterol Nutr*. 2019;69(2):239-258.
4. Guha S, Herman A, Antonino M, Silverstein JS, Venkataraman-Rao P, Myers MR. Synthesis of research on ENFit gastrostomy tubes with potential implications for US patients using these devices. *Nutr Clin Pract*. 2022;37(4):752-761.
5. Guenter P, Lyman B. ENFit enteral nutrition connectors: benefits and challenges. *Nutr Clin Pract*. 2016;31(6):769-772.
6. Klepper CM, Moore J, Gabel ME, Fleet SE, Kassel R. Pediatric formulas: categories, composition, and considerations. *Nutr Clin Pract*. 2023;38(2):302-317.
7. Du N, DiMaggio DM, Porto AF. Nutrition content of young child formulas. *J Pediatr Gastroenterol Nutr*. 2023;76(4):512-516.
8. DiMaggio DM, Du N, Scherer C, et al. Comparison of imported European and US infant formulas: labeling, nutrient and safety concerns. *J Pediatr Gastroenterol Nutr*. 2019;69(4):480-486.
9. Du N, DiMaggio DM, Williams JK, et al. Non-FDA-reviewed imported European formula use among parents in urban pediatric private practice. *Clin Pediatr (Phila)*. 2020;59(6):566-572.
10. Human Foods Program. Enforcement discretion to manufacturers to increase infant formula supplies. U.S. Food and Drug Administration. Accessed November 1, 2021. https://www.fda.gov/food/infant-formula-guidance-documents-regulatory-information/enforcement-discretion-manufacturers-increase-infant-formula-supplies
11. Fomon SJ, Ziegler EE. Renal solute load and potential renal solute load in infancy. *J Pediatr*. 1999;134(1):11-14.
12. Tume, L.N., Valla, F.V. A review of feeding intolerance in critically ill children. *Eur J Pediatr*. 2018;177:1675–1683.
13. Davis A, Baker S. The use of modular nutrients in pediatrics. *JPEN J Parenter Enteral Nutr*. 1996;20(3):228-236.
14. Davis A. Transitional and combination feeds. In: Baker SB, Baker RD, Davis A, ed. *Pediatric Enteral Nutrition*. Chapman and Hall; 1994, 147-148
15. Clouzeau H, Dipasquale V, Rivard L, et al. Weaning children from prolonged enteral nutrition: a position paper. *Eur J Clin Nutr*. 2022;76(4):505-515.
16. Blackman JA, Nelson CLA. Reinstituting oral feedings in children fed by gastrostomy tube. *Clin Pediatr*. 1985;24:434–4388.
17. Blackman JA, Nelson CLA. Rapid introduction of oral feedings to tube-fed patients. *Dev Behav Pediatr*. 1987;8:63–66.
18. Clawson E, Kuchinski K, Bach R. Use of behavioral interventions and parent education to address feeding difficulties in young children with spastic diplegic cerebral palsy. *Neurorehabilitation* 2007;22:397-406.

INTERNET RESOURCES

1. American Society for Enteral and Parenteral Nutrition
2. Boston Children's Hospital Center for Nutrition
3. United States Department of Agriculture Children's Nutrition Research Center
4. Kennedy Krieger Institute

CHAPTER 17

Parenteral Nutrition

Coral Rudie, Margaret Murphy, Kathleen M. Gura, Jennifer McClelland, and Lissette Jimenez

The discovery and implementation of parenteral nutrition (PN) in the 1960s was a landmark in the history of nutrition, profoundly affecting the management of patients with gastrointestinal failure.[1] The application of PN in pediatric and adult patients with nongastrointestinal diseases such as malignancies, critical care, and other conditions soon followed.

■ INDICATIONS

Although enteral nutrition (EN) is the preferred route of nutrition support, there are several clinical conditions for which EN is not feasible or insufficient and PN is indicated (Table 17.1).[2,3] The initiation of PN is a clinical decision where the benefits of PN need to be weighed against both its risks as well as those of using intravenous fluids alone. An interdisciplinary nutrition support team reduces the inappropriate initiation and use of PN[4] (see Chapter 15).

Pediatric patients have increased metabolic requirements and limited fuel storage in the forms of fat and protein and are thus more susceptible to the effects of starvation than adults. An estimate of 3 to 5 days is often used as the length of time for which the provision of 10% dextrose is a reasonable alternative for nutrition support (Figure 17.1). If the period of time of minimal to no EN is anticipated to be longer than 5 days, most infants and young children would benefit from PN. In cases of malnutrition, low birth weight, hypermetabolism, or select other conditions, PN may be started even if the duration of inadequate enteral intake is anticipated to be fewer than 5 days. If the period of minimal to no EN is anticipated to be longer than 7 days (10-14 days in well-nourished adolescents), full PN with central venous access is usually indicated. Peripheral access and the infusion of a more dilute solution may be adequate for periods of less than 7 days, although the limitation of solution osmolarity can make it difficult to meet the patient's energy needs.

■ VENOUS ACCESS

A central catheter tip location allows for instantaneous dilution of hypertonic PN solution (>900 mOsm/L) into the blood stream and reduces the risk of thrombus and vascular intimal damage. Documentation of catheter tip location by radiographic confirmation is required for PN administration, since mispositioned catheters can have serious and even fatal consequences. In children, the superior vena cava, the junction of the superior vena cava (SVC) and the right atrium, and the inferior vena cava

TABLE 17.1 COMMON INDICATIONS FOR PARENTERAL NUTRITION

MECHANISM/INDICATION FOR PARENTERAL NUTRITION	EXAMPLE
Impaired absorption or loss of nutrients	Short bowel syndrome, extensive intestinal mucosal disease, chronic or secretory diarrhea (i.e., microvillus inclusion disease, tufting enteropathy), severe inflammatory bowel disease
Discontinuity of gastrointestinal tract	Intestinal atresia, esophageal atresia
Blockage of intestinal lumen	Mechanical bowel obstruction
Recurrent vomiting	
Need to restrict oral or enteral intake: bowel rest	Necrotizing enterocolitis, gastroschisis, volvulus, meconium ileus, prolonged postop ileus, peritonitis, gastrointestinal fistula, active gastrointestinal bleeding, pseudomembranous colitis
Motility disorders	Prolonged ileus, pseudo-obstruction
Circulatory	Congenital heart disease with decreased left-sided outflow, patent ductus arteriosus with left to right shunt or requiring medical/surgical treatment for closure
Critical illness	Hemodynamic instability, extracorporeal membrane oxygenation (ECMO), severe respiratory failure associated with hypoxia and acidosis
Failure of oral or enteral nutrition	Inability to achieve or maintain enteral access, contraindications to enteral access
Limited protein and energy stores and high metabolic demands	Preterm infants (<32 wk gestational age and/or birth weight <1.5 kg)

Table derived from Berlana D. *Parenteral nutrition overview. Nutrients.* 2022;**14**(21):4480; Worthington P, Balint J, Bechtold M, et al. *When is parenteral nutrition appropriate? JPEN J Parenter Enteral Nutr.* 2017;**41**(3):324-377.

(IVC) above the bifurcation of the iliac veins are all considered central locations for the catheter tip placement and offer the largest caliber lumen and high blood flows.[5] For umbilical venous catheters (UVC), commonly used in the first few weeks after birth, the ideal catheter tip location is between the junction between the IVC and the right atrium.[6] Appropriate UVC tip placement is crucially important as there is a risk of the line going into the liver, given how the umbilical vein connects with the IVC. The visual marker of the line tip being above the diaphragm is a reliable way to ensure appropriate UVC tip placement in the absence of congenital defects involving the diaphragm. Efforts to reduce technical and infectious complications of venous catheter placement and use are important in the safe delivery of the PN solution.

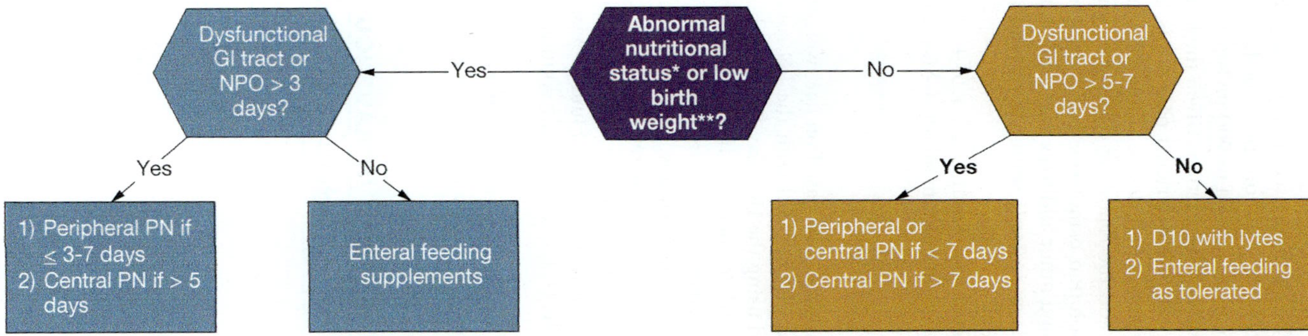

*BMI or weight for length z-score < -2
**< 2500 g

Figure 17.1 Decision tree used for the selection of method of nutrition support. BMI, body mass index; GI, gastrointestinal; NPO, nothing by mouth; PN, parenteral nutrition.

PERIPHERAL PARENTERAL NUTRITION

Peripheral parenteral nutrition (PPN) is often used in situations where central venous access is unavailable. Peripheral catheter locations preclude hyperosmolar solutions, and, therefore, PPN solutions should be limited to 900 mOsm/L or lower to help reduce the risk of phlebitis, infiltration, and infection. Given the limits on the solution concentration, PPN is unsuitable for fluid-restricted patients as large fluid volumes are typically necessary to deliver adequate calories. Table 17.2 lists the osmolarity of several common IV solutions, and the following equations can be used to calculate a rough estimate of the PN solution osmolarity, but it does not account for the impact vitamins, trace elements, and other additives may contribute. Intravenous fat emulsions (10% and 20%) provide an isotonic source of calories and can be infused through either a peripheral or a central vein.

PN solution osmolarity approximation = (Dextrose g/L × 5) + (Amino acids g/L × 10) + [(Sodium mEq/L + Potassium mEq/L + Calcium mEq/L + Magnesium mEq/L) × 2)]

FLUIDS AND ELECTROLYTES

Fluid requirements for the patient should be based on age, weight, and clinical condition. Typically, maintenance fluid is provided with the PN solution. Maintenance fluid requirements can be assessed using the Holliday-Segar method (see Chapter 5). Fluid requirements can be higher when there are increased insensible losses (fever or tachypnea) or sensible losses (diarrhea, vomiting, nasogastric output, ostomy, or excess urinary losses). In certain clinical situations, such as liver, cardiac, or kidney dysfunction, fluids may need to be restricted. Therefore, routine clinical monitoring of hydration status, including physical examination, serum electrolytes, and intakes and outputs, is essential in the patient receiving PN. Fluid provision from the PN solution and injectable lipid emulsions (ILEs) are typically counted toward meeting the patient's fluid requirements.

Basal electrolyte requirements for children and adults are shown in Table 17.3.[7] Clinical needs may vary if exogenous losses are high (e.g., diarrheal disease, diuretic

TABLE 17.2 OSMOLARITY OF SELECT INTRAVENOUS SOLUTIONS

SOLUTION	APPROXIMATE OSMOLARITY (MOSM/L)
5% dextrose	252
10% dextrose	505
20% dextrose	1010
10% dextrose + 2% amino acids	700
20% dextrose + 2% amino acids	1200
25% dextrose + 3% amino acids	1550
30% dextrose + 3% amino acids	1800
10% Omegaven	273
20% SMOFLipid	270
20% IntraLipid	260

TABLE 17.3 ASPEN RECOMMENDATIONS FOR BASAL ELECTROLYTE REQUIREMENTS FOR INFANTS AND CHILDREN

- Sodium: 2-5 mEq/kg recommended for preterm neonates, 2-5 mEq/kg recommended for infants/children, and 1-2 mEq/kg recommended for adolescents and children >50 kg
- Potassium: 2-4 mEq/kg recommended for preterm neonates, 2-4 mEq/kg recommended for infants/children, and 1-2 mEq/kg recommended for adolescents and children >50 kg
- Calcium: 2–4 mEq/kg recommended for preterm neonates, 0.5-4 mEq/kg recommended for infants/children, and 10-20 mEq/day recommended for adolescents and children >50 kg
- Magnesium: 0.3-0.5 mEq/kg recommended for preterm neonates, 0.3-0.5 mEq/kg recommended for infants/children, 10-30 mEq/day recommended for adolescents and children >50 kg
- Phosphorus: 1–2 mMol/kg recommended for preterm neonates, 1-2 mMol/kg recommended for infants/children, and 10-40 mMol/day recommended for adolescents and children >50 kg
- Chloride, Acetate as needed to maintain acid base-balance

Data from Appropriate Dosing for Parenteral Nutrition: ASPEN Recommendations 2019. https://nutritotal.com.br/pro/wp-content/uploads/2019/04/PN-DosingASPEN.pdf

use) or renal function is altered. Table 17.4 lists the estimated electrolyte losses and typical replacement fluids used in various gastrointestinal losses[8]; however, precise quantification is possible by sending a specimen to the chemistry lab for measurement of electrolyte concentrations.

COMPONENTS OF PARENTERAL NUTRITION

In pediatric PN solutions, dextrose, amino acids, electrolytes, and micronutrients are typically provided in a single solution (2:1 solution). Due to stability limitations of PN solution, ILE are usually infused separately from the dextrose-protein solution. In most adult and some pediatric facilities, however, total nutrient admixtures (TNA), in which the lipid are mixed directly with the PN solution, are used (3:1 solution).

Carbohydrate (Dextrose)

Of the macronutrients, dextrose provides the primary source of energy of the PN solution. In the intravenous form, dextrose monohydrate has an energy density of 3.4 kcal/g. This is slightly less than the 4 kcal/g caloric density attributed to all other carbohydrate (CHO) sources. Dextrose provision and advancement are typically thought of in terms of the glucose infusion rate (GIR), mg CHO/kg/min.

$$\text{GIR (mg/kg/min)} = \text{Dextrose (g/L)} \times \text{Volume (L)} \times 1000\ \text{(mg/g)} \div 24\ \text{hours} \div 60\ \text{(min/h)} \div \text{Weight (kg)}$$

Or more simply, $\text{GIR (mg/kg/min)} = \text{Dextrose (g/L)} \times \text{Volume (L)} \div 1.44 \div \text{Weight (kg)}$

A minimum GIR of 4 to 6 mg/kg/min should be provided for infants to meet obligatory needs. The increase in GIR will vary depending on the age, size, and tolerance to the dextrose infusion, although in most cases, dextrose advancement is performed in daily increments of 1 to 2.5 mg/kg/min (see Table 17.5).[9] The final GIR will be

TABLE 17.4 GASTROINTESTINAL ELECTROLYTE LOSSES AND SUGGESTED REPLACEMENT REGIMEN

SOURCE OF BODY FLUID LOSS	SODIUM (MEQ/L)	POTASSIUM (MEQ/L)	CHLORIDE (MEQ/L)	BICARBONATE (MEQ/L)	TYPICAL REPLACEMENT FLUID
Gastric	20-80	5-20	100-150	–	½ NS (normal saline) with 10 mEq/L of potassium[a]: mL replacement for mL losses as tolerated by patient hydration status
Ileostomy	45-135	3-15	20-115	50-70	½ to ¾ NS: mL replacement for mL losses as tolerated by patient hydration status If CO_2 is low could use Lactated Ringer's solution or may need 50% of sodium as NaCl and 50% of sodium as Na Acetate salts
Colostomy	50-120	30-40	90-95	20-30	½ to ¾ NS with 20mEq/L of potassium[a]: mL replacement for mL losses as tolerated by patient fluid status

[a]Any replacement solution with potassium needs to be infused over several hours depending on the total amount of potassium and total volume of replacement fluid required.

From Aune G. *Fluids and electrolytes*. In: *The Harriet Lane Handbook*. Elsevier Mosby; 2009.

TABLE 17.5 PARENTERAL NUTRITION AND INJECTABLE LIPID EMULSION ADVANCEMENT

		PREMATURE INFANT (≤1.5 KG)	TERM INFANT OR >1.5 KG	PEDIATRICS (1-10 Y)	ADOLESCENT (11-18 Y)
Dextrose *(Glucose Infusion Rate (GIR) mg/kg/min)*					
Initiate		4-6	4-7	3-6	2.5-3
		OR BASED ON CURRENT GIR, SERUM GLUCOSE AND OVERALL NUTRITION ASSESSMENT			
Advance GIR daily by (as tolerated)		1-2	2-2.5	1-2	1-2
Suggested maintenance GIR		10-14	10-14	8-10	5-6
Protein *(gm/kg/d)*					
Initiate		2	2	1	1
Advance by		2	0.5-1	0.5-1	0.5
Estimated protein requirements		3.5-4	2.5-3	1.5-2	1-1.5
Intravenous lipid emulsions *(gm/kg/d)*					
Initiate		1	1	1	1
Advance by (as tolerated)		0.5-1	0.5-1	0.5-1	0.5-1
Suggested maintenance dose	IntraLipid	1-3	1-3	1-2.5	1-1.5
	SMOFLipid	3	2.5-3	2.5-3	2-2.5
	Omegaven	1 (up to 1.5 g/kg/d has been used off label)			

Adapted from Boston Children's Hospital Center for Nutrition, PN ordering guidelines; Cober MP, Gura KM, Mirtallo JM, et al. *ASPEN lipid injectable emulsion safety recommendations part 2: neonate and pediatric considerations. Nutr Clin Pract.* 2021;*36*(6):1106-1125.

determined by calories needed to achieve the child's overall energy goal once targets for protein and fat are reached. The GIR should generally not exceed 18 mg/kg/min, the maximum glucose oxidation rate[10]; higher dextrose intake may contribute to the development of steatosis, cholestasis, hyperglycemia, or glucosuria. Tolerance to dextrose infusion is monitored by monitoring serum or urine glucose concentrations. If hyperglycemia or glucosuria occurs, the GIR may need to be reduced, even if temporarily. Tight glycemic control for critically ill children has not been proven to improve outcomes[11]; in some cases, however, low-dose insulin outside of the PN and titrated as needed is indicated.

Protein (Amino Acids)

Crystalline amino acids provide the protein source in PN solutions. Amino acid solutions commonly used in the United States in the pediatric population are listed in Table 17.6.[12-18] The solutions, designed for infants, have markedly different amino acid compositions than those used for older children and adults, with higher amounts of aspartic and glutamic acid and taurine and lower quantities of methionine, glycine, and phenylalanine. In extremely fluid-restricted children, the use of an adult 20% solution (e.g., Prosol [Baxter]) can be justified, but caution should be taken in neonates due to its high glycine content. Neonates should be switched back to an age-appropriate amino acid product as soon as fluids allow. Cysteine is commonly added to PN solution for premature infants to improve nitrogen balance. Additionally, cysteine reduces the pH of the PN solution, thus improving calcium and phosphorus solubility (see Chapter 35).

Protein provision is initiated at 1 to 2 g protein/kg/d and advanced to the goal the following day (Table 17.5). Protein provision is often reduced in chronic renal failure before dialysis is initiated or in severe liver failure; otherwise, provision of protein according to standard Dietary Reference Intakes (DRI) is typical practice.

Injectable Lipid Emulsions

ILE provide a rich source of energy, essential fatty acids, and a balance of macronutrients. ILEs commonly used for pediatric patients in United States are listed in Table 17.7.[9] IntraLipid and SMOFLipid are both 20% ILE (providing 10 kcal/g and 2 kcal/mL), while Omegaven is a 10% ILE (11 kcal/g and 1.1 kcal/mL). ILEs provide more calories than typically attributed to 1 g of fat as the phospholipid emulsifiers and glycerol provide additional calories. All solutions are oil based in water emulsions with egg yolk phospholipid emulsifiers and glycerin. ILEs are contraindicated in patients with known hypersensitivities to soy, egg, peanut, fish (for SMOFLipid and Omegaven), or to any of the active ingredients or excipients. At Boston Children's Hospital, Intralipid is the default ILE, and clinical indications for use of SMOFLipid and Omegaven are highlighted in Table 17.8.

ILE infusions are generally started at 1 g fat/kg/d and advanced by 1 g/kg/d to goal dose, which will vary by type of ILE (Table 17.5). Energy intake from fat should generally not exceed 40% of the total energy intake since higher percentages may cause ketosis. Tolerance to intravenous fats is performed by monitoring serum triglyceride (TG) concentrations following initiation and advancement, then weekly. Ideally, the fasting TG concentration should remain less than 250 mg/dL in children 1 year of age or younger and less than 400 mg/dL in children older than 1 year. Although

TABLE 17.6 BRAND-SPECIFIC COMPOSITION OF COMMON PEDIATRIC PARENTERAL AMINO ACID SOLUTIONS

	SOLUTIONS DESIGNED FOR INFANTS	STANDARD SOLUTIONS SUITABLE FOR AGES 1 Y AND ABOVE				
Product (Manufacturer)	TrophAmine 10% (B.Braun) & Premasol 10% (Baxter)	Aminosyn PF 10% Sulfite-Free (ICU medical)	Aminosyn PF 7% Sulfite-Free (ICU Medical)	Clinisol 15% (Baxter)	Travasol 10% (Baxter)	Prosol 20% (Baxter)
Total Nitrogen (g/L)	15.5	15.2	10.69	23.7	16.5	32.1
Essential Amino Acids (mg/100 mL)						
Isoleucine	820	760	534	749	600	1080
Leucine	1400	1200	831	1040	730	1080
Lysine	820	677	475	1180	580	1350
Methionine	340	180	125	749	400	760
Phenylalanine	480	427	300	1040	560	1000
Threonine	420	512	360	749	420	980
Tryptophan	200	180	125	250	180	320
Valine	780	673	452	960	580	1440
Nonessential Amino Acids (mg/100 mL)						
Alanine	540	698	490	2170	2070	2760
Arginine	1200	1227	861	1470	1150	1960
Histidine	480	312	220	894	480	1180
Proline	680	812	570	894	680	1340

TABLE 17.6 BRAND-SPECIFIC COMPOSITION OF COMMON PEDIATRIC PARENTERAL AMINO ACID SOLUTIONS

	SOLUTIONS DESIGNED FOR INFANTS	STANDARD SOLUTIONS SUITABLE FOR AGES 1 Y AND ABOVE				
Serine	380	495	347	592	500	1020
Taurine	25	70	50	0	0	0
Tyrosine	240	44	44	39	40	50
Glycine	360	385	270	1040	1030	2060
Glutamic acid	500	820	576	749	0	1020
Aspartic acid	320	527	370	434	0	600
Cysteine	<16	0	0	0	0	0

Data derived from 20% ProSol—sulfite-free (amino acid) injection. *Package insert*. Baxter Healthcare Corporation; 2014. https://baxterpi.com/pi-pdf/Prosol_PI.pdf; TRAVASOL (amino acids) injection. *Package insert*. Baxter Healthcare Corporation; 2020. https://baxterpi.com/pi-pdf/Travasol_PI.pdf; 15% CLINISOL—sulfite-free (amino acid) injection. *Package insert*. Baxter Healthcare Corporation; 2018. https://www.baxterpi.com/pi-pdf/Clinisol_PI.pdf; PREMASOL 10%—sulfite-free (amino acids) injection. *Package insert*. Baxter Healthcare Corporation; 2021. https://baxterpi.com/pi-pdf/PI%20PREMASOL10%2007-19-00-3923%20Nov2021.pdf; Aminosyn®-PF 10% sulfite-free (amino acid injection). *Package insert*. ICU Medical, Inc; 2018. https://www.icumed.com/media/h1rdh3jx/qen-4678-final.pdf; TrophAmine (10% amino acid injection). *Package insert*. 2023; Aminosyn®-PF 7% sulfite-free (amino acid injection). *Package insert*. ICU Medical, Inc; 2018. https://www.icumed.com/media/zf1ns4iu/qen-4682-final.pdf

TABLE 17.7 INJECTABLE LIPID EMULSION PRODUCT COMPARISON

	INTRALIPID (BAXTER)	SMOFLIPID (FRESENIUS KABI)	OMEGAVEN (FRESENIUS KABI)
% Fat emulsion	20%	20%	10%
Energy (kcal/mL)	2	2	1.1
Energy (kcal/g)	10	10	11
Source oil			
Soy oil	100%	30%	–
Fish oil	–	15%	100%
MCT oil	–	30%	–
Olive oil	–	25%	–
Additives			
Glycerol	2.25%	2.5%	2.5%
Egg phospholipid	1.2%	1.2%	1.2%
Phytosterols (mg/L)	422.4 ± 130.5	142.2 ± 15.3	0
Vitamin E (mg/100 mL)	0	16.3-22.5	15-30
Essential fatty acid %			
Linoleic	44-62	14-25	1.5 (mean)
α-Linolenic	4-11	1.5-3.5	1.1 (mean)
EPA	0	1-3.5	13-26
DHA	0	1-3.5	14-27
Arachidonic acid	0	Not reported	0.2-2

DHA, docosahexaenoic acid; EPA, eicosapentaenoic acid; MCT, medium-chain triglyceride.
Modified from Cober MP, Gura KM, Mirtallo JM, et al. *ASPEN lipid injectable emulsion safety recommendations part 2: neonate and pediatric considerations. Nutr Clin Pract.* 2021;*36*(6):1106-1125.

some cases of hypertriglyceridemia are attributable solely to excessive amounts of ILE, many patients receiving PN will have other reasons to have high TG levels, including acute phase stress response, sepsis, or hepatic and/or renal dysfunction. Multiple medications are also associated with hypertriglyceridemia, see Table 17.9. If persistent hypertriglyceridemia is noted, options include reducing the infusion time to 20 or fewer hours (and monitoring TG concentrations after a 4-hour "fast"), reducing dose, or infusing lipids on alternating days during the week.

The pathogenesis of intestinal failure associated liver disease (IFALD) is multifactorial but differential exposures to phytosterols (natural occurring compounds in plant-based lipids) and α-tocopherol have been hypothesized.[9] Table 17.7 reviews these components across the three main lipid products. Restricting the dose of Intralipid to 1 g/kg has become a mainstay therapy for IFALD prevention. From the perspective of the phytosterols load, 3 g/kg of SMOFLipid is roughly comparable to 1 g/kg of IntraLipid and allows a higher percentage of calories to be provided from fat and

TABLE 17.8 SMOFLIPID AND OMEGAVEN INDICATIONS FOR USE

SMOFLipid (Fresenius Kabi)	• Anticipated parenteral nutrition (PN) use for longer than 21 d and the presence of one of the following:
	  • Intestinal failure patients *without* hyperbilirubinemia (serum direct bilirubin <2 mg/dL) due to PN (short bowel syndrome, chronic intestinal pseudo-obstruction, congenital diarrhea).
	  • PN glucose infusion rate >20 mg/kg/min and/or challenge with cycling to 12 h after age 1 due to elevated glucose infusion rate.
	• Poor growth on lipid restriction, with need for additional caloric provision from lipids due to inability to advance dextrose, solution stability, or liver protection

Omegaven (Fresenius Kabi)	• FDA-approved indications include intestinal failure patients (i.e., diagnosis of short bowel syndrome, gastroschisis, chronic intestinal pseudo-obstruction, congenital diarrhea, and others) with hyperbilirubinemia (serum direct bilirubin or conjugated bilirubin >2 mg/dL) due to chronic PN use.
	• Special consideration for use in patient without intestinal failure
	  • Infants and children >14 d old with hyperbilirubinemia (serum direct or conjugated bilirubin >2 mg/dL) and who are not likely to advance to full oral or enteral nutrition within 21 d.
	    • Particularly if there is a history of hypertriglyceridemia and/or physical or biochemical findings of essential fatty acid deficiency (EFAD).
	  • Hypertriglyceridemia: fasting triglycerides >250 mg/dL (≤1 y old) and >400 mg/dL (>1 y old)
	  • EFAD: Triene:tetraene ratio of >0.2 and mead acid >30 nanomole/L
	  • The etiology of hyperbilirubinemia may be multifactorial but related in part to chronic PN use and not attributed solely to a primary liver disorder (including right heart failure or veno-occlusive disease), infection, or medication side effects.
	• Soy Allergy

Adopted from Boston Children's Hospital Clinical Guidelines for use of SMOFLipid and Omegaven.

limits the need for high GIRs to make up for lost calories when IntraLipid is restricted. It also includes a higher amount of α-tocopherol. The literature has been mixed on the effectiveness of low-dose Intralipid or full dose of SMOFLipid in preventing IFALD. Omegaven, which contains minimal phytosterols and has a high α-tocopherol content, has been evaluated only for the treatment of IFALD and is not currently indicated for IFALD prevention.[9]

Fat restriction or inappropriate dosing of ILEs potentially increases the risks of essential fatty acid deficiency (EFAD), inadequate energy intake for growth, or excessive carbohydrate intake. The total daily caloric intake needed from dietary linoleic acid (LA) and alpha-linolenic acid (ALA) are 1% to 3% and 0.2% to 1%,[19] respectively, or at least 3% to 10% of total calories coming from fat.[20,21] While the LA and ALA content of Omegaven is limited, it contains sufficient amounts of their downstream metabolites, eicosatetraenoic acid (EPA), docosahexaenoic acid (DHA), and arachidonic acid (AA) to prevent EFAD.[9] Patients on restricted doses of ILE for prolonged periods should be monitored for EFAD with a total fatty acid profile regularly (see Table 17.20). The biochemical hallmark of EFAD is an elevated ratio (> 0.2) of triene to tetraene fatty acids as well as an elevated mead acid concentration (>30 nanomole/L).[22] However,

TABLE 17.9 MEDICATIONS ASSOCIATED WITH HYPERTRIGLYCERIDEMIA

ABACAVIR	DIDANOSINE	NAFARELIN
Acitretin	Efavirenz	Olanzapine
Adalimumab	Eplerenone	Olmesartan
Amiodarone	Eprosartan	Paclitaxel
Amprenavir	Estrogen	Propofol
Aripiprazole	Estropipate	Raloxifene
Atevirdine	Febuxostat	Retinoids/vitamin A
Bazedoxifene	Fluconazole	Risperidone
β-Blockers	Fluoxetine	Ritonavir
Calcitriol	Fomepizole	Sertraline
Candesartan	Glucocorticoids	Sirolimus
Capecitabine	Indinavir	Somatropin
Cholestyramine	Interferons	Tacrolimus
Carvedilol	Isotretinoin	Tamoxifen
Clomiphene	Itraconazole	Thiazide diuretics
Clozapine	Ketoconazole	Thyrotropin
Cyclosporine	L-Asparaginase	Tipranavir
Darunavir	Leflunomide	Vitamin E
Delavirdine	Mirtazapine	
Dexrazoxane	Mitotane	

Derived from from Henkin J, Como JA, Oberman A. Secondary dyslipidemia: inadvertent effects of drugs in clinical practice. *JAMA.* 1992;267:961-968 and the Online Formulary, Boston Children's Hospital.

as more mixed oil lipids are being used, the triene to tetraene ratio should be assessed in the context of all components of the essential fatty acid profile.[22] Conversely, a "fat overload" syndrome has been described with excessive administration of lipids, characterized by focal seizures, fever, hepatosplenomegaly, and thrombocytopenia. This typically occurs when infusion rates exceed 0.15 g/kg/h.

MICRONUTRIENTS IN PN

Micronutrients should be added to all pediatric PN solutions as early as possible and not withheld for more than a few days at most.[23] The importance of vitamins in patients receiving PN has been underscored in the United States by several widespread shortages of parenteral multivitamins and reports of symptomatic thiamine deficiency.[24] Fatal vitamin deficiencies have been reported in patients receiving PN without vitamins in as short a time as a few weeks. Table 17.10 lists the current parenteral vitamin products available in the United States.[25,26] The pediatric version of multivitamins is notable for higher amounts of vitamins K and D and lower amounts of the B vitamins,

TABLE 17.10. COMPARISON OF PARENTERAL MULTIVITAMIN PREPARATIONS

PRODUCT	A	B_1 (MG)	B_2 (MG)	B_6 (MG)	B_{12} (μG)	BIOTIN (μG)	C (MG)	FOLIC ACID (μG)	D	E	K (μG)	NIACINAMIDE (MG)	DEXPANTHENOL (MG)
Pediatric (<11 y of age)													
Infuvite Pediatric (Baxter) *per 5 mL*	2300 IU (0.7mg)	1.2	1.4	1	1	20	80	140	400 IU (10 μg)	7 IU (7 mg)	200	17	5
Adolescents and Adults (≥11 y of age)													
Infuvite Adult (Baxter) *per 10 mL*	3300 IU (1 mg)	6	3.6	6	5	60	200	600	200 IU (5 μg)	10 IU (10 mg)	150	40	15

Data derived from Infuvite Adult (multiple vitamins injection). Prescribing information. Baxter Healthcare Corporation; 2016. https://www.accessdata.fda.gov/drugsatfda_docs/label/2004/21163s011lbl.pdf; Infuvite Pediatric (multiple vitamins injection). Prescribing information. Baxter Healthcare Corporation; 2016. https://www.accessdata.fda.gov/drugsatfda_docs/label/2008/021265s015lbl.pdf

as compared to the adult formulation. The adult formulation also includes propylene glycol, which may be toxic to neonates in large doses. There is currently no parenteral vitamin preparation designed especially for premature infants. Recommendations for parenteral vitamin doses for preterm infants, term infants, children, and adolescents are shown in Table 17.11.[28] Certain conditions may require adjustments to parenteral vitamin intake; hemodialysis, high ostomy losses, and other conditions may well alter vitamin requirements. The American Society for Parenteral and Enteral Nutrition (ASPEN) provides detailed recommendations for management in times of adult and pediatric IV multivitamin shortages.[28]

Trace elements commonly added to PN solutions include zinc, selenium, copper, manganese, and chromium. Table 17.12 lists recommendations for maintenance dosing of trace elements in PN.[7,27,29] Due to biliary excretion of copper and manganese, careful dosing is needed in patients with cholestasis. Serum copper and ceruloplasmin levels should be monitored to determine proper dosage in individuals on long-term PN. Hypocupremia can result in anemia, thrombocytopenia, osteopenia, and neutropenia.[30] Manganese and chromium are contaminants in PN solutions, and so additional supplementation via a multi-ingredient trace element product is controversial. If manganese toxicity is suspected, erythrocyte manganese levels and a 24-hour urine manganese level should be requested, and any additional manganese should be removed from PN solution. There are reports of abnormal cranial MRI findings consistent with manganese deposition, a concern for pediatric patients on long-term PN who may be

TABLE 17.11 RECOMMENDED DOSES FOR PARENTERAL SUPPLY OF FAT-SOLUBLE AND WATER-SOLUBLE VITAMINS FOR PRETERM INFANTS, INFANTS, AND CHILDREN

Vitamins	Preterm infant <37 wk' gestation	Infant >12 mo old	Children/adolescent 1-16 y old
Vitamin A	700-1500 IU/kg/d	500-1000 IU/kg/d	500 IU/d
Thiamin B_1	0.35-0.5 mg/kg/d	0.35-0.5 mg/kg/d	1.2 mg/d
Riboflavin	0.15-0.2 mg/kg/d	0.15-0.2 mg/kg/d	1.4 mg/d
Pyridoxine	0.15-0.2 mg/kg/d	0.15-0.2 mg/kg/d	1.0 mg/kg/d
Niacin	4-6.8 mg/kg/d	4-6.8 mg/kg/d	17 mg/d
Vitamin B_{12}	0.3 μg/kg/d	0.3 μg/kg/d	1 μg/d
Pantothenic acid	2.5 mg/kg/d	2.5 mg/kg/d	5 mg/d
Biotin	5-8 μg/kg/d	5-8 mg/kg/d	20 μg/d
Folic acid	56 μg/kg/d	56 μg/kg/d	140 μg/d
Vitamin C	15-25 mg/kg/d	15-25 mg/kg/d	80 mg/d
Vitamin D	200-1000 IU/d or 80-400 IU/kg/d	400 IU/d or 40-150 IU/kg/d	400-600 IU/d
Vitamin E	2.8-3.5 mg/kg/d	2.8-3.5 mg/kg/d	11 mg/d
Vitamin K	10 μg/kg/d	10 μg/kg/d	200 μg/d

Reproduced from Table 1 from Hardy G, Wong T, Morrissey H, et al. Parenteral provision of micronutrients to pediatric patients: an international expert consensus paper. *J Parenter Enteral Nutr.* 2020;44:S5-S23.

TABLE 17.12 MAINTENANCE REQUIREMENTS OF TRACE ELEMENTS IN PEDIATRIC PARENTERALNUTRITION (μG/KG)

	PRETERM INFANTS <3 KG	TERM INFANTS 3-10 KG	CHILDREN >10 KG	COMMENTS
Zinc (μg/kg)	400	250	50 (max 5000 μg/d)	Increase dose with increased intestinal losses
Copper (μg/kg)	20	20	20 (max 500 μg/d)	May need to decrease in cholestasis.
Selenium (μg/kg)	2	2	2 (max 100 μg/d)	May need to decrease for renal dysfunction; may have increased needs with increased intestinal losses.
Chromium (μg/kg)	0.05-0.3	0.2	0.2 (max 5 μg/d)	May need to decrease for renal dysfunction.
Manganese (μg/kg)	1	1	1 (max 55 μg/d)	Decrease/remove in cholestasis.
Iodine (μg/kg)	1-10	1	1	No product available in the United States

Data derived from Domellöf M, Szitanyi P, Simchowitz V, Franz A, Mimouni F. ESPGHAN/ESPEN/ESPR/CSPEN guidelines on pediatric parenteral nutrition: iron and trace minerals. *Clin Nutr*. 2018;*37*(6 pt B):2354-2359; American Society for Parenteral and Enteral Nutrition. *Appropriate dosing for parenteral nutrition: ASPEN recommendations*. 2020. Accessed November 26, 2024. https://nutritotal.com.br/pro/wp-content/uploads/2019/04/PN-DosingASPEN.pdf; Hardy G, Wong T, Morrissey H, et al. *Parenteral provision of micronutrients to pediatric patients: an international expert consensus paper*. *JPEN J Parenter Enteral Nutr*. 2020;**44**(suppl 2):S5-S23.

at risk of neurocognitive dysfunction due to prematurity and other medical problems already.[31] Chromium toxicity can result in decreased glomerular filtration rate (GFR) and renal tubular damage. Parenteral intake of selenium and chromium may need to be reduced or held in cases of renal dysfunction. For patients with intestinal failure who have greater zinc and selenium losses due to diarrhea/ostomy losses, it is common practice to add additional zinc to help replace those losses. If a multi-ingredient trace element product is used, practitioners should take the amount provided by the product into consideration when determining the added amount to supplement. For children receiving long-term PN, we commonly omit multi-ingredient products and individually dose zinc, selenium, and copper.

Intravenous iron is not routinely provided in pediatric PN but is recommended in patients with iron deficiency anemia if the enteral route is ineffective or contraindicated. The use of parenteral iron dextran to treat iron deficiency anemia has been controversial due to the risk of anaphylaxis. New formulations, including ferric gluconate and iron sucrose, are safer with less concern with anaphylaxis but still need monitoring for adverse reactions. Patients who receive blood transfusions may not require repletion doses of iron since blood transfusions provide a moderate amount of iron. The total amount of parenteral iron (as iron dextran) needed for repletion to normalize hemoglobin level can be estimated according to the following formula[32]:

$$\text{Dose (mL)} = 0.0442\,(Hb_n - Hb_o) \times LBW + (0.26 \times LBW).$$

LBW = lean body weight in kg.

Males: LBW (kg) = 50 + [2.3 × (Height in inches − 60)]

Females: LBW (kg) = 45.5 + [2.3 × (Height in inches − 60)]

Note: For patients weighing 5 to 15 kg, use actual body weight.

Hb_n = Desired hemoglobin (g/dL) = 12 g/dL if body weight $\leq$15 kg or 14.8 g/dL if >15 kg.

Hb_o = measured hemoglobin (g/dL).

An initial test dose of iron dextran should be given prior to the therapeutic dose to monitor for an anaphylactic response; subsequent doses can be administered in the home setting if no reaction is noted. Long-term, maintenance doses from 0.5 to 1 mg/kg/weekly may be indicated in some patients and added directly to lipid-free PN solutions. Currently, iron dextran is the only form of parenteral iron that can be added to PN solutions. Separate infusions of iron sucrose or ferric gluconate have been used, although the optimal dosing in the parenterally fed pediatric patient has yet to be established. Monitoring complete blood count (CBC), reticulocyte count, serum iron, TIBC, and ferritin initially and monthly are helpful to determine adequate repletion and maintenance dosing of intravenous iron.

Iodine is a required trace element for the synthesis of thyroid hormones. While added in other parts of the world, iodine is not routinely added to PN solutions in the United States as there is no IV iodine product currently available. Fully PN–dependent infants and children are likely to be at risk of iodine deficiency as supported by reports in the literature.[33] The European Society for Parenteral and Enteral Nutrition (ESPEN) and European Society for Pediatric Gastroenterology Hepatology and Nutrition (ESPGHAN) suggest that parenteral iodine supplementation of at least 1 μg/kg/d occur in infants and children receiving PN.[29]

■ CALCIUM, PHOSPHORUS, MAGNESIUM, SODIUM, POTASSIUM, CHLORIDE, AND ACETATE

Electrolyte disturbances may be corrected by increasing or decreasing the amount of component(s) in the volume of PN infused in the daily prescription. However, acute changes in serum electrolytes should not be treated with abrupt changes in PN infusion rate as changes in PN infusion rate will adversely affect macronutrient metabolism (e.g., increase blood glucose and potential excess protein intake) as well as alter the delivery of any medications added to PN.

Calcium, phosphorus, and magnesium balance are interrelated. Inadequate intakes of each may result in rickets, fractures, failure of appropriate bone mineralization, and reduced linear growth. In the PN-dependent growing child, high amounts of calcium and phosphorus are needed, but the provision of these nutrients in PN is challenging due to the physicochemical limitations of current PN additives. When compounding a solution with high amounts of calcium and phosphorus, it is imperative that the pH is low enough to optimize solubility and that the additions of these salts are done in the correct order. According to the U.S. Food and Drug Administration (FDA), calcium should always be the last ingredient added to the PN solution.[34] Phosphorus salts should be one of the first additives in order to be well diluted prior to the addition of calcium. Calcium gluconate is the preferred salt for use in PN solutions since it dissociates less than chloride salts and thereby remains in solution more readily. Other factors favoring the formation of calcium-phosphorus precipitates include low amino acid content, low dextrose content, high temperature, and high pH. Since pH is determined primarily by amino acid concentration, increasing amino acid intake, the use of more acidic brands of amino acid solutions, and/or the addition of cysteine hydrochloride are common strategies used to lower pH and help prevent precipitation. It is also recommended that if a PN solution contains less than 1 percent amino acids, then either calcium or phosphorus (not both) be added. Clinicians should refer to amino acid manufacturers' curves when evaluating calcium and phosphorus solubility in a PN solution. Additionally, TNA stability is affected by the total amount of divalent cations (i.e., calcium and magnesium).[35] Although not as well described as calcium-phosphorus incompatibility, PN solutions high in magnesium and phosphorus are also prone to precipitation.

Sodium and potassium are typically included in amounts to meet standard electrolyte requirements. Premature infants will have increased sodium needs due to their inability to conserve sodium. Similarly, in patients with chronic diarrhea or other gastrointestinal diseases, sodium requirements are greater due to intestinal losses via nasogastric or gastrostomy tube drainage and/or high ostomy output. Potassium requirements could also be greater in these situations of higher losses. The total amount of chloride and acetate varies depending on the amino acid brand and concentration as well as total sodium and potassium content. Acetate salt concentrations may need to be higher in cases of high ostomy losses. Due to the risk of metabolic alkalosis, the use of chloride-free PN solutions should be avoided.

MEDICATION AND PN

Patients requiring PN are often on multiple medications, and questions frequently arise concerning whether these medications can be safely coadministrated with PN. Because of the risks of precipitation and/or infection, coadministration of medications and PN should be avoided whenever possible. Moreover, medications should not be added directly to the PN bag itself except by pharmacy staff, although in home PN patients, it may be necessary to do so immediately prior to administration due to stability issues. Medications not directly added to PN should be coinfused via a "y" connection with the intravenous setup proximal to a filter. Whenever the PN formula changes, coadministered medications and potential compatibility problems should be reviewed, even whenever there are changes in the brands of amino acids or lipid emulsions.

Tables 17.13 list medications generally considered compatible or incompatible for coadministration with PN. Tables 17.14 list medications that are considered compatible or incompatible with 100% soybean ILE. Table 17.15 lists medications known to be compatible with SMOFLipid or Omegaven ILEs.[36] In all cases, consultation with a PN pharmacist is recommended. In the event that no information is available, the medication should be considerable incompatible with both PN and lipid emulsion.

In PN patients with limited venous access, it may be a challenge to administer parenteral medications if the medication is incompatible with PN. If possible, switching to a compatible medication should be considered. If that is not an option, the PN infusion will need to be interrupted to infuse the incompatible medication. Prior to infusing the medication, the PN infusion must be stopped, the line should be flushed with a neutral fluid compatible with the medication (i.e., saline or dextrose), the medication then infused, followed by another flush with a compatible fluid before the PN infusion is resumed. Children receiving PN with high dextrose concentrations may need to have the PN rate gradually reduced prior to the start of the drug infusion. In cases where the child cannot have their PN infusion interrupted because of an inability to maintain adequate blood glucose levels, the medication should be infused in a carrier fluid with a similar dextrose concentration as the PN. If a lipid infusion needs to be interrupted for the administration of an incompatible medication, no rate reduction before lipid discontinuation is necessary.

OTHER COMPOUNDING CONSIDERATIONS

In addition to the calcium-phosphorus compatibility, other factors have received attention regarding the prevention of PN-related complications: minimizing aluminum (Al) exposure, protecting the solutions from light, and avoidance of Di(2-ethylhexyl) phthalate (DEHP) materials. As children with intestinal failure and other conditions receive prolonged courses of PN, more long-term studies are needed to assess these complications.

Aluminum

Al exposure is a risk in patients receiving prolonged PN courses. Al is found in raw materials, incorporated into products during the manufacturing process, and leached from glass containers during autoclaving for sterilization.[37] When Al is administered parenterally, it bypasses the protective barrier of the gastrointestinal tract. Specific

TABLE 17.13 MEDICATION COMPATIBILITY WITH PARENTERAL NUTRITION SOLUTIONS

COMPATIBLE WITH PARENTERAL NUTRITION SOLUTIONS			INCOMPATIBLE WITH PARENTERAL NUTRITION SOLUTIONS	
Acetaminophen	Enalaprilat	Morphine	Acetazolamide	Furosemide
Albumin[a]	Epinephrine[b]	Nafcillin	Acyclovir	Ganciclovir
Amikacin[c]	Erythromycin	Ondansetron	Amphotericin	Imipenem
Atropine	Famotidine	Oxacillin	Amphotericin b lipid complex	Indomethacin
Aztreonam	Fentanyl	Penicillin G+ (aqueous)	Ampicillin	Mannitol
Bumetanide	Fluconazole	Phytonadione	Ampicillin/sulbactam	Methotrexate
Cefepime	Gentamicin[c]	Piperacillin/tazobactam	Calcium salts	Metoclopramide
Cefotaxime	Granisetron	Promethazine	Cefazolin	Metronidazole
Cefoxitin	Heparin	Pyridoxine	Ciprofloxacin	Midazolam
Ceftazidime	Hydrocortisone	Ranitidine	Cisplatin	Nitroglycerin
Cefuroxime	Hydromorphone	Tacrolimus	Cyclosporine	Nitroprusside
Chloramphenicol	Insulin (U-100 regular)	Ticarcillin	Cytarabine	Octreotide
Chlorpromazine	Iron dextran	Tobramycin[c]	Diazepam	Phenytoin
Cimetidine	Isoproterenol	Vancomycin[c]	Doxorubicin	Phosphate salts
Clindamycin	Leucovorin	Vecuronium	Filgrastim	Piperacillin
Dexamethasone	Levocarnitine	Zidovudine	Foscarnet	Promethazine
Digoxin	Lorazepam		Fluorouracil	Trimethoprim/sulfamethoxazole
Diphenhydramine	Meperidine			Tromethamine
Dobutamine[c]	Mesna			
Doxycycline				

[a]Will clog filter if albumin concentration >25 g/L.
[b]Incompatible with iron containing PN.
[c]Incompatible with heparin containing PN solutions.
Adapted from the 2025 Online Formulary, Boston Children's Hospital.

TABLE 17.14 MEDICATION COMPATIBILITY WITH 100% SOYBEAN INJECTABLE LIPID EMULSION

COMPATIBLE WITH 100% SOYBEAN INJECTABLE LIPID EMULSION		INCOMPATIBLE WITH 100% SOYBEAN INJECTABLE LIPID EMULSION	
Aldesleukin	Erythromycin	Acetazolamide	Furosemide
Bumetanide	Famotidine	Acyclovir	Ganciclovir
Ceftazidime	Hydrocortisone	Amikacin	Heparin
Ceftriaxone	Hydromorphone	Aminophylline	Imipenem
Chloramphenicol	Insulin, regular	Amphotericin	Indomethacin
Cimetidine	Isoproterenol	Amphotericin b lipid complex	Iron dextran
Clindamycin	Lidocaine	Ampicillin	Magnesium salts
Cyclosporine	Norepinephrine	Ampicillin/sulbactam	Metronidazole
Digoxin	Oxacillin	Calcium salts	Midazolam
Diphenhydramine	Ranitidine	Ciprofloxacin	Morphine
Dobutamine	Ticarcillin	Diazepam	Nitroglycerin
Dopamine	Tobramycin	Doxorubicin	Nitroprusside
		Filgrastim	Penicillin
		Fluorouracil	Phenytoin
		Foscarnet	Trimethoprim/ sulfamethoxazole
			Tromethamine

Adapted from the 2025 Online Formulary, Boston Children's Hospital.

TABLE 17.15 MEDICATIONS COMPATIBLE WITH SMOFLIPID AND OMEGAVEN INJECTABLE LIPID EMULSION

COMPATIBLE WITH SMOFLIPID INJECTABLE LIPID EMULSION	COMPATIBLE WITH OMEGAVEN INJECTABLE LIPID EMULSION
Ampicillin 10 mg/mL	Ampicillin 10 mg/mL
Dexmedetomidine 4 μg/mL	Cisatracurium besylate 0.1 mg/mL
Dopamine 1600 μg/mL	Dexmedetomidine 4 μg/mL
Fluconazole 2 mg/mL	Fluconazole 2 mg/mL
Norepinephrine 16 μg/mL	Gentamicin 2 mg/mL
	Norepinephrine 16 μg/mL

Medication compatibility tested with lipid emulsion as part of TNA via simulated Y-Site.
Adapted from Fresenius Kabi. *Y-site drug compatibility reference guide*. 2024. https://www.freseniuskabinutrition.com/wp-content/uploads/2024/03/4555-SMOFlipid-Compatibility-Tool-Brochure-2024.pdf

findings of this toxicity include encephalopathy, impaired neurodevelopment, bone pain with development of osteopenia or osteomalacia, microcytic anemia, and cholestasis. The amount of Al provided by PN should be less than 5 μg/kg/d, the threshold deemed "safe" by the US FDA. Since calcium gluconate salts are a large source of Al contamination, infants and children are at risk for developing toxicity due to their high calcium requirements coupled with renal immaturity.

Ambient Light

Intravenous components of PN admixtures and ILEs are susceptible to degradation and oxidation, when exposed to light in the presence of oxygen.[38] Vitamins and polyunsaturated fatty acids from ILE appear to be most sensitive to this photo-oxidation. The consequences of oxidative stress affect infants, especially preterm infants, more than children or adults and may contribute to associated morbidities, including bronchopulmonary dysplasia, retinopathy of prematurity, necrotizing enterocolitis, and IFALD.[38] Total photoprotection of PN admixtures and ILEs reduces indicators of oxidative stress in preterm infants.[38] Current ASPEN recommendations are for complete light protection of PN and ILE for infants beginning as soon as possible during the compounding process and continuing through the end of infusion. However, there is limited availability of materials necessary for complete photoprotection, such as amber-colored tubing. Each health care organization should assess and implement those steps for photoprotection that can be achieved.[38]

DEHP Toxicity

DEHP is an industrial additive plasticizer found in polyvinylchloride (PVC). PN infusion systems have been shown to be the most important source of DEHP load. Although DEHP has a rapid turnover (half-life less than 24 hours), this phthalate and its metabolites are consistently detected in human body fluids such as plasma, urine, amniotic fluid, or breast milk. In preterm neonates and infants who receive intensive care, DEHP has been shown to increase oxidative stress and toxicity.[39] PN infusion sets and containers containing DEHP have been implicated as contributing to this risk. Retrospective data showed that by changing to polyvinylchloride(PVC)-free infusion systems, a reduction in the incidence of cholestatic liver disease was noted.[40] Moreover, the use of PVC-containing infusion sets correlated strongly with the development of IFALD ($P = .0004$). DEHP-free containers and infusion sets should be used whenever possible so as to minimize this risk.

Supply Issues

In recent years, many of the ingredients used to formulate PN solutions have been in short supply. A variety of reasons have been cited, including discontinuation by a manufacturer, shortages of raw materials, and failure to meet FDA standards. Organizations such as ASPEN (Nutritioncare.org) have developed guidelines to help practitioners during these periods of supply shortages. In addition to reminding practitioners not to stockpile materials, these guidelines include recommendations for using alternative products or different dosing strategies until a stable supply stream is reestablished. In almost all instances, the need for PN should be reassessed and the provision of nutrition and/or supplements via the oral or enteral route considered. Due to their unique needs, special guidelines for neonates are typically included. All recommendations suggest compounding PN in a single, central location (either in a centralized pharmacy or as an outsourced preparation) in order to reduce inventory waste. Processes for regular communication among key stakeholders (e.g., prescribers, pharmacy and nutrition departments, central supply) should be implemented. Practitioners are also advised to consider supply outreach to other facilities within the same geographic area. Information about severe drug product shortages should be reported to the FDA Drug Shortage Program (DSP). Any patient-related issues concerning shortages should be reported to Institute for Safe Medication Practices (ISMP) Medications Errors Reporting Program (MERP). During shortages, laboratory monitoring schedules may need to be altered to ensure that alternative therapies meet the requirements and do not lead to potentially life-threatening deficiencies or toxicities.

CYCLING PARENTERAL NUTRITION INFUSIONS

The provision of one day's worth of PN over fewer than 24 hours has been termed "cycling." Figure 17.2 illustrates cycled PN with a ramp up over 30 minutes to max peak infusion rate, then ramps down over two 30 minutes rate changes. There are various mathematical approaches to cycling PN with potential risk for underdelivery of fluid/caloric provision with cycling. Figure 17.2 is based on 97% of total PN volume delivered during peak infusion of cycle with ramping (50%, 25%) based on peak infusion rate. Advantages of cycling include allowing the patient to be disconnected from intravenous tubing and pumps, avoiding chronic hyperinsulinemia, and, perhaps, an improved visceral protein status,[41] and a lower risk of developing IFALD. Suitable candidates for cyclic PN are those patients for whom long-term (>1 month) PN is anticipated and whose endocrine, renal, and cardiac function can tolerate shifts in dextrose and fluid delivery. Two to three days of metabolic stability on the solution

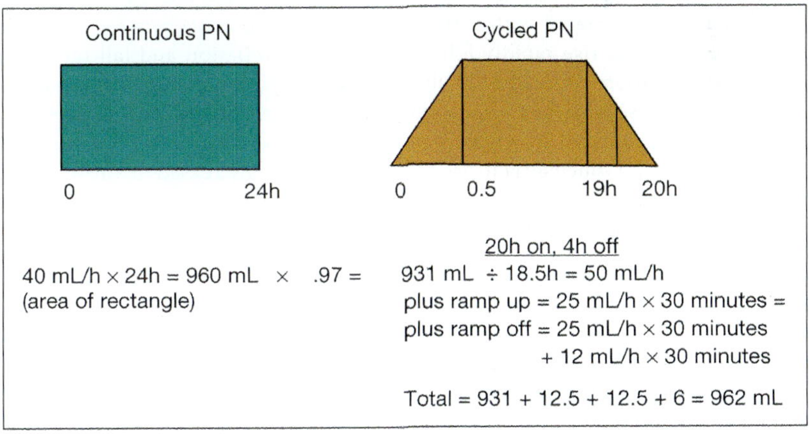

Figure 17.2 Cyclic administration of parenteral nutrition (PN).

TABLE 17.16 FACTORS TO CONSIDER WHEN DECIDING IF A PATIENT IS GOOD CANDIDATE FOR CYCLIC PARENTERAL NUTRITION

PATIENTS WHO MAY BENEFIT FROM CYCLIC PARENTERAL NUTRITION	PATIENTS WHERE ADDITIONAL MONITORING MAY BE NECESSARY OR CYCLING PARENTERAL NUTRITION IS CONTRAINDICATED
• Ambulatory patients whose mobility is impacted by infusion pump. • Home parenteral nutrition patients expected to be on long-term therapy. • Lifestyle benefits from breaks in infusion • Metabolic stability • Time of day (patients with frequent nocturnal urination may prefer daytime infusions)	• Fluid-sensitive patients • Long-acting insulin use • Low glycogen stores • Malnourished patients • Metabolic instability • Neonates

Adapted from Stout S, Cober M. *Cyclic parenteral nutrition infusion: considerations for the clinician. Pract Gastroenterol.* 2011;(97):11-24.

providing the desired amount of fluid and energy are also required before cycling can begin. Table 17.16 summarizes factors to consider when deciding if a patient is a good candidate for cyclic PN.[42]

Whereas cyclic PN infusion offers practical advantages over continuous infusion for patients receiving PN long term or at home, the potential metabolic changes that may result from this delivery technique must be considered. Unlike continuous PN infusion, patients receiving cyclic PN must be able to adapt to shifts in nutrients secondary to the starting and stopping of infusions. Furthermore, cyclic infusions utilize higher nutrient infusion rates to supply a comparable daily nutrient load over a shorter period of time but also result in a postinfusion period where no nutrients are infused. Some patients may not be able to withstand these altered delivery rates. Infusion of PN is associated with a rise in blood glucose concentrations. Similarly, insulin concentrations rise rapidly following infusion initiation and fall rapidly following discontinuation.[43] Conversely, abrupt discontinuation of PN infusion in children, especially those less than 2 to 3 years old, has been linked with elevated rates of hypoglycemia compared to when the infusion is tapered over 1 hour. Generally, urine is monitored for glucosuria to ascertain tolerance to increased dextrose infusion over shorter periods of time. Also, dextrose sticks are checked while off PN infusion to monitor for rebound hypoglycemia and for appropriate gluconeogenesis. Typically, blood sugar checks occur 30 minutes after the PN infusion ends and the halfway point of the total duration of time off PN.

MONITORING AND POTENTIAL COMPLICATIONS OF PARENTERAL NUTRITION

Table 17.17 lists multiple metabolic conditions commonly seen among patients receiving PN, as well as suggested therapeutic steps. Biochemical monitoring helps ensure tolerance to the individual components of PN and helps avoid the myriad metabolic

TABLE 17.17 COMMON METABOLIC CONDITIONS SEEN IN PATIENTS RECEIVING PARENTERAL NUTRITION

COMPLICATION	POSSIBLE CAUSES	CLINICAL FINDINGS	PREVENTION/MONITORING	TREATMENT
Macronutrient Substrate Complications				
Hyperglycemia	Diabetes mellitus Excessive dextrose infusion Metabolic stress/sepsis Medications (i.e., corticosteroids, thiazide diuretics, β-blockers) Peritoneal dialysis or CAVH-D Obesity Chromium deficiency Growth spurts	Elevated blood glucose (>200 mg/dL) Glucosuria > 2%	Limit dextrose infusion to approximately 10-15% Limit increments in dextrose to 2.5-5 mg glucose/kg/min Monitor serum glucose. Monitor urine glucose.	Decrease dextrose intake. Add regular insulin to PN or give IV insulin (starting dose 0.01 units/kg/h). Address underlying cause.
Hyperglycemic hyperosmolar state (HHS)	Sustained, uncontrolled hyperglycemia Infections Pancreatitis Trauma	Very high blood glucose levels Elevated serum osmolarity Osmotic diuresis Metabolic acidosis Lethargy and confusion Coma Dehydration	Goal ≤200 mg/dL Monitor: • Blood and urine glucose closely • Serum Osm • Fluid status	Immediate discontinuation of PN IV hydration, insulin Correction of metabolic acidosis

(continued)

TABLE 17.17 COMMON METABOLIC CONDITIONS SEEN IN PATIENTS RECEIVING PARENTERAL NUTRITION (*continued*)

COMPLICATION	POSSIBLE CAUSES	CLINICAL FINDINGS	PREVENTION/MONITORING	TREATMENT
Hypoglycemia	Sudden discontinuation of PN Exogenous insulin administration Sepsis	Blood glucose <50 mg/dL Diaphoresis Lethargy or palpitations Agitation/irritability Faintness Confusion Coma	Avoid abrupt cessation of PN. Check blood glucose one hour after PN discontinued in cycled patients.	IV dextrose bolus
Hypercapnia (elevated pCO_2)	Excessive dextrose or total caloric intake in patients with chronic lung disease Respiratory failure	Increased pCO_2 Respiratory distress	Avoid excessive caloric or dextrose infusion. Obtain indirect calorimetry measurement; adjust PN regimen to meet needs.	Decrease total caloric intake and/or increase calories as fat.
Azotemia	Dehydration Renal insufficiency Excessive amino acid infusion Lean tissue catabolism Immature liver Liver disease Inborn errors of protein metabolism	Elevated BUN Lethargy Coma	Adequate hydration prior to PN initiation Avoid excessive amino acid infusion. Provide adequate nutrition to minimize lean tissue catabolism. Monitor BUN and NH_3.	Free water administration Decrease amino acid infusion.

Abnormal amino acid profile	Inborn error of metabolism Liver disease Composition of PN solution	Serum amino acid profile out of normal range	Monitor serum amino acid levels. Avoid excess protein intake in liver disease.	Consider use of special amino acid solution.
Hypertriglyceridemia	Excessive lipid infusion Decreased clearance (stress/sepsis, liver failure) Sustained hyperglycemia Congenital hyperlipidemia Excessive caloric intake, especially glucose Medications (see Table 17.9)	Lipemia Serum TG >250 mg/dL	Avoid excessive lipid infusion. Monitor serum triglycerides weekly. Infuse lipids over 18-20 h (<0.15 g/kg/h).	Decrease lipid infusion. If sustained, provide only enough lipid to prevent essential fatty acid deficiency (EFAD) (0.5-1.0 g/kg/d).
Fluid and Electrolyte Disturbances				
Fluid overload	Excessive fluid administration Renal dysfunction Congestive heart failure Liver disease Trauma	Rapid weight gain Fluid intake> output Increased blood pressure Decreased serum sodium and hematocrit Edema	Avoid excessive fluid administration. Close monitoring of: • Weights • Intake/output • Physical exam • Electrolytes	Concentrate PN solution. Fluid restriction Sodium restriction and/or diuretics, if appropriate

(*continued*)

TABLE 17.17 COMMON METABOLIC CONDITIONS SEEN IN PATIENTS RECEIVING PARENTERAL NUTRITION (*continued*)

COMPLICATION	POSSIBLE CAUSES	CLINICAL FINDINGS	PREVENTION/MONITORING	TREATMENT
Dehydration	Inadequate fluid intake Excessive diuresis Increased GI losses Vomiting Diarrhea Fever	Decreased urine output Orthostasis Increased serum sodium, BUN, hematocrit Poor skin turgor Thirst Rapid weight loss	Provide adequate fluid. Replace insensible and GI losses. Monitor fluid status.	Fluid replacement with separate IV from PN
Hypokalemia	Inadequate potassium supplementation during anabolism/refeeding Increased GI losses (*vomiting, diarrhea,* furosemide) Medications (furosemide, amphotericin B, cisplatin, etc.)	Metabolic alkalosis Cardiac arrhythmias Muscle weakness Ileus	Adequate potassium in PN Adequate chloride in PN Measure and replace losses. Monitor serum levels daily until stable; biweekly thereafter.	Increase potassium in PN if mildly to moderately depleted. May need to increase chloride, decrease acetate in PN. Additional IV supplementation if severely depleted
Hyperkalemia	Renal insufficiency Excessive potassium administration Medications (e.g., spironolactone) Catabolism	Weakness Paresthesias Hyporeflexia Cardiac arrhythmias	Avoid excessive potassium administration. Monitor serum levels daily until stable; biweekly thereafter. Monitor serum potassium daily in patients with renal insufficiency/restrict as appropriate.	Decrease potassium in PN.

Hyponatremia	Fluid overload SIADH Excessive losses (urinary, GI, or through skin)	Irritability Confusion Lethargy Seizures	Adequate sodium in PN Avoid excessive fluid administration. Monitor serum sodium daily until stable; biweekly thereafter.	Fluid restriction Increase sodium in PN if sodium depleted. Replace with separate IV if increased losses.
Hypernatremia	Dehydration Excessive sodium administration Osmotic diuresis secondary to hyperglycemia Pituitary tumors Diabetes insipidus	Thirst Restlessness Muscle tremor and rigidity Hyperactive reflexes Coma Convulsions	Provide adequate fluid. Avoid excessive sodium administration. Monitor intake/output, urine sodium, osmolarity.	Fluid replacement if dehydrated Decrease sodium in PN if appropriate.
Metabolic acidosis	Increased intestinal losses of bicarbonate (diarrhea, fistulas) Renal bicarbonate losses Ketoacidosis (diabetes, starvation) Lactic acidosis (shock, cardiac arrest) Chronic renal failure or renal tubular acidosis Excessive chloride in PN (rare)	Headache Nausea/vomiting Diarrhea Convulsions	Measure and replace intestinal losses. Avoid excessive chloride in PN.	Increase acetate and decrease chloride in PN.
Metabolic alkalosis	Gastric acid losses (increased NG output) Excess base administration	Nausea/vomiting Diarrhea Sensory changes Tremoring Convulsions	Measure and replace NG output.	Treat underlying cause. Increase chloride and decrease acetate in PN. If severe, may need IV hydrochloric acid.

(continued)

TABLE 17.17 COMMON METABOLIC CONDITIONS SEEN IN PATIENTS RECEIVING PARENTERAL NUTRITION (*continued*)

COMPLICATION	POSSIBLE CAUSES	CLINICAL FINDINGS	PREVENTION/MONITORING	TREATMENT
Mineral Imbalances				
Hypocalcemia	Hypoalbuminemia Hypomagnesemia Hyperphosphatemia Hypoparathyroidism Malabsorption Inadequate calcium in PN	Muscular/abdominal cramping Irritability Confusion Tetany Seizures Prolonged QT interval	Adequate calcium in PN Monitor serum calcium biweekly: check ionized calcium if total calcium decreased. Check serum albumin and correct calcium level to determine if true deficiency Corrected calcium (mg/dL) = Measured total calcium (mg/dL) + 0.8 (4.0 − serum albumin [g/dL]). Monitor PTH and vitamin D levels.	Correct magnesium deficiency. Increase calcium in PN if ionized calcium low
Hypercalcemia	Neoplasm Renal insufficiency Excessive vitamin D administration Bone resorption caused by prolonged immobilization/stress	Confusion Lethargy Dehydration Muscle weakness Abdominal pain Nausea and vomiting Constipation Arrhythmias Extraskeletal calcification	Monitor serum levels daily until stable; biweekly thereafter. Restrict as appropriate.	Decrease calcium in PN. Hydrate with isotonic saline May need to remove vitamin D from PN.

Hypomagnesemia	Increased GI losses (vomiting, diarrhea, fistula) Increased urinary losses secondary to drugs (e.g., cisplatin, amphotericin B, aminoglycoside) Inadequate magnesium supplementation during anabolism/refeeding	Weakness Muscle tremors Ataxia Tetany Paresthesias Dizziness Disorientation/ irritability Seizures Cardiac arrhythmias	Adequate magnesium in PN Monitor serum levels daily until stable; biweekly thereafter. Check serum albumin and correct if true deficiency corrected magnesium = serum magnesium + 0.005 × (40 − albumin level).	Increase magnesium in PN if mildly to moderately depleted. Additional IV supplementation if severely depleted
Hypermagnesemia	Renal insufficiency Excessive magnesium administration	Nausea/vomiting Lethargy/weakness Cardiac arrhythmias Hypotension Respiratory depression	Monitor serum levels daily until stable; biweekly thereafter. Monitor serum levels daily in patients with renal insufficiency; restrict as appropriate. Avoid excessive magnesium administration.	Decrease magnesium in PN.
Hypophosphatemia	Inadequate phosphorous supplementation during anabolism/refeeding Exogenous insulin administration Chronic use of phosphate-binding antacids Alcoholism Diabetic ketoacidosis	Serum level <2 mg/dL Paresthesias Confusion Altered speech Lethargy Respiratory failure Decreased red blood cell function Coma	Supplement in PN above standard amounts in patients at risk (diabetes, alcoholism, protein-energy malnutrition) Monitor serum levels daily until stable; biweekly thereafter.	Increase phosphorous in PN if mildly to moderately depleted. Additional IV supplementation if severely depleted

(continued)

TABLE 17.17 COMMON METABOLIC CONDITIONS SEEN IN PATIENTS RECEIVING PARENTERAL NUTRITION (*continued*)

COMPLICATION	POSSIBLE CAUSES	CLINICAL FINDINGS	PREVENTION/MONITORING	TREATMENT
Hyperphosphatemia	Renal insufficiency Excessive phosphorus administration PTH deficiency	Prolonged elevations may lead to tissue calcification	Monitor serum levels daily until stable; biweekly thereafter. Monitor serum levels daily in patients with renal insufficiency/restrict as appropriate. Avoid excessive phosphorus administration.	Decrease phosphorus in PN.
Other				
Refeeding syndrome	Rapid or excessive dextrose infusion (especially in malnourished patients)	Hyperglycemia Hypophosphatemia Hypokalemia Hypomagnesemia Edema Pulmonary edema/CHF Anion gap metabolic acidosis	Identification of patients at risk (chronically malnourished, nutritionally depleted patients) Replete serum electrolyte deficiencies prior to PN initiation. Limit initial caloric intake to basal requirements. Supplement phosphorus in PN. Advance PN cautiously. Monitor serum glucose, electrolytes, phosphorus, and magnesium daily until stable; biweekly thereafter.	Decrease infusion rate. Replete serum electrolyte, *phosphorus*, magnesium. thiamine deficiencies; monitor closely. Limit fluid in presence of edema.
EFAD	Prolonged insufficient lipid infusion	Dry, scaly skin Hair loss Thrombocytopenia Elevated triene: tetraene ratio	Provide at least 0.5-1.0 g fat/kg/d as pure soybean oil (can be given 2-3×/wk). Higher doses of fat needed if mixed oil lipid emulsion used	Daily lipid infusion Cutaneous application of linoleic acid rich oils if IV lipid contraindicated

Hepatic dysfunction	Cholestasis	Elevated LFTs and direct bilirubin	Avoid excess energy intake. Avoid excess protein intake. Minimize soybean oil intake. Rule out infectious, metabolic, or anatomic causes of cholestasis.	Reduce copper and manganese intake. Reduce soybean oil dose. Reduce energy and protein to meet requirements. Cycle PN Advance enteral nutrition
Trace mineral deficiencies	Inadequate supplementation during long-term PN Excessive losses via GI tract (diarrhea, fistula output)	Varies depending on specific deficiency	Adequate supplementation	Supplement deficient nutrient
Trace Nutrient Deficiencies				
Iron (Fe)	Long-term NPO status without Fe supplementation Increased blood loss	Decreased ferritin Decreased transferrin saturation Decreased hemoglobin Tachypnea/tachycardia Poor weight gain Poor feeding	Monitor serum Fe levels.	Maintenance dose 1 mg/d as elemental iron in PN Do not give Fe if being transfused. Watch for anaphylaxis with initial infusion.
Zinc (Zn)	Increased GI losses Acrodermatitis enteropathica	Growth failure Perineal and perioral lesions Impaired wound healing Low serum alkaline phosphatase levels	Increase Zn if chronic GI losses Monitor serum Zn, serum alkaline phosphatase. Monitor growth Wound healing.	Increase Zn in PN if increased GI losses

(*continued*)

TABLE 17.17 COMMON METABOLIC CONDITIONS SEEN IN PATIENTS RECEIVING PARENTERAL NUTRITION (*continued*)

COMPLICATION	POSSIBLE CAUSES	CLINICAL FINDINGS	PREVENTION/MONITORING	TREATMENT
Selenium (Se)	Increased GI losses Inadequate supplementation Long-term NPO status without supplementation	Cardiomyopathy Muscle weakness Reduced glutathione peroxidase activity Hypopigmentation of hair and nails Hemolytic anemia	Provide Se supplementation with long-term NPO status. Monitor serum Se levels. Monitor serum or RBC glutathione peroxidase levels.	Supplement as necessary.
Carnitine	Long-term NPO status without supplementation	Liver dysfunction Steatosis Progressive myopathy Growth failure Hypertriglyceridemia Hypoglycemia	Monitor serum carnitine levels.	Supplement for long-term NPO, if low serum levels.
Metabolic bone disease	Etiology unclear/possibly multifactorial Possible etiologies include: • Altered vitamin D metabolism • Aluminum toxicity • Protein-induced calcium loss • Drug therapy (e.g., diuretics) • Inactivity • Inadequate Ca or PO_4 or Vit D	Demineralization Hypercalciuria Pathologic fractures Back pain Bone pain	Moderate nutrient provision Monitor minerals and other PN solutions for presence of aluminum.	Adequate Ca, PO_4, Vit D Weight bearing exercise Change diuretic therapy, if feasible.

BUN, blood urea nitrogen; CAVH-D, Continuous arteriovenous hemofiltration with dialysis; GI, gastrointestinal; IV, intravenous; LFT, liver function test; NG, nasogastric; PN, parenteral nutrition; PTH, parathyroid hormone; RBC, red blood cell; SIADH, syndrome of inappropriate antidiuretic hormone secretion; TG, triglyceride.

TABLE 17.18 GUIDELINES FOR THE INFUSION OF POTASSIUM

TOTAL IV POTASSIUM INTAKE (PER HOUR)	TOTAL POTASSIUM (IV AND ENTERAL PER DAY)	REQUIRED MONITORING
≤0.25 mEq/kg/h (max 10 mEq/h)	≤ 6 mEq/kg/d (or 180 mEq/d)	Plasma potassium Vital sign monitoring every 4 h
0.26-0.5 mEq/kg/h (min 10.1-max 20 mEq/h)	6.1-12 mEq/kg/d (min 180-max 360 mEq/d)	Plasma potassium every 12-24 h Continuous ECG monitoring Vital sign monitoring every 2 h
>0.5 mEq/kg/h (Not to exceed 20 mEq/h)	>12.1 mEq/kg/d (Not to exceed 360 mEq/day)	Frequent plasma potassium Continuous ECG monitoring Vital sign monitoring every 1 hour

ECG, electrocardiogram; IV, intravenous.
Adapted from Boston Children's Hospital Patient Care Manual: Administration of Supplemental Potassium, 2024.

complications of PN. Perhaps the most dangerous complication of PN is hyperkalemia, due to errors in PN ordering, transcription, and/or compounding. In order to reduce the risk of symptoms due to excessive potassium administration, our current institution policy is to limit parenteral potassium infusion rates to <0.25 mEq/kg/h and to institute continuous electrocardiogram (ECG) monitoring and increased vital signs monitoring if this amount is exceeded and (see Table 17.18). Phosphorus infusions should also be monitored for risk of hypocalcemia and hypotension; in our institution, we limit the phosphorus infusion rate to <0.1 mmol/kg/h (see Table 17.19). In addition, all PN orders at the administration and compounding levels should be double-checked to reduce the risk of error. Recommended monitoring parameters for inpatients are listed in Table 17.20. In the pediatric patient, an especially important parameter with which to assess the effectiveness of PN is growth (see Chapter 2).

TABLE 17.19 GUIDELINES FOR THE INFUSION OF PHOSPHORUS: INFUSION RATE, ADMINISTRATION, AND REQUIRED MONITORING

TOTAL INTRAVENOUS PHOSPHORUS INTAKE (PER HOUR)	REQUIRED MONITORING
0.1 mmol/kg/h Higher rates with additional monitoring have been used in the critical care setting (e.g., up to 0.12 mmol/kg/h).	Cardiac/apnea monitor Phosphorus level MUST be checked prior to infusion and then a minimum of 30 min following infusion. (plasma potassium if K Phos used). Vital signs every 30 min for first hour of infusion and hourly for the remainder of the infusion Rapid administration may also cause hypotension.

Adapted from Boston Children's Hospital Formulary 2025.

TABLE 17.20 SUGGESTED MONITORING SCHEDULE FOR PATIENTS RECEIVING PARENTERAL NUTRITION

	INPATIENT			OUTPATIENT (HPN)[a]
Parameter	Daily	Weekly[a]	Monthly[a]	
Weight	X			Per clinic schedule
Fluid balance	X			Per clinic schedule
Vital signs	X			Per clinic schedule
Catheter site/function	X			Daily
Laboratory test:				
Sodium		X		Q1-2 mo
Potassium		X		Q1-2 mo
Chloride		X		Q1-2 mo
CO_2		X		Q1-2 mo
Glucose		X		Q1-2 mo
Urine glucose/Ketones		As clinically indicated		
Blood urea nitrogen (BUN)		X		Q1-2 mo
Creatinine		X		Q1-2 mo
Triglycerides		X		Q1-2 mo
Calcium		X		Q1-2 mo
Magnesium		X		Q1-2 mo
Phosphorus		X		Q1-2 mo
Prealbumin		X		Q1-2 mo
Albumin		X		Q1-2 mo
Alanine aminotransferase (ALT)		X		Q1-2 mo
Aspartate aminotransferase (AST)		X		Q1-2 mo
Alkaline phosphatase		X		Q1-2 mo
Bilirubin (total and direct)		X		Q1-2 mo
Gamma-glutamyl transferase (GGTP)		X		Q1-2 mo

TABLE 17.20 SUGGESTED MONITORING SCHEDULE FOR PATIENTS RECEIVING PARENTERAL NUTRITION (*continued*)

	INPATIENT			OUTPATIENT (HPN)[a]
Parameter	Daily	Weekly[a]	Monthly[a]	
Selenium			X	Every 6 mo
Copper			X	Every 6 mo
Zinc			X	Every 6 mo
Iron			X	Q1-2 mo
Carnitine			X	Annually
C-reactive protein[b]			X	PRN
Vitamin D (25-OH vitamin D)			X	Q4-6 mo
Vitamin A + Retinol Binding Protein			X	Annually
Vitamin E			X	Annually
INR			X	Q4-6 mo
Aluminum				Annually
Iron studies (serum iron, ferritin total iron binding capacity, transferrin saturation, and reticulocyte count)			X	Q1-2 mo
Essential fatty acid profile			X	Q4-6 mo

HPN, home parenteral nutrition; INR, international normalized ratio.
[a]Stable PN schedule, more often as necessitated by clinical indication course.
[b]With micronutrient labs.

NURSING CARE IN PARENTERAL NUTRITION ADMINISTRATION

Meticulous nursing care is essential to successful PN administration in order to avoid potentially life-threatening complications. Several important nursing procedures are listed in Table 17.21.[44]

CATHETER-RELATED COMPLICATIONS

Table 17.22 lists common technical or catheter-related complications and recommended approaches for prevention and treatment.[45] Obstruction of the intravenous infusion system is one of the most common complications of PN use. Initial management consists of repositioning the patient, changing the needleless connector using

TABLE 17.21 NURSING CARES IN PARENTERAL NUTRITION ADMINISTRATION

I. PN ADMINISTRATION

ACTION	RATIONALE
Change PN administration sets every 24 h), using strict aseptic technique. Solution is to be changed every 24 h. Administration sets should be changed if not used for greater than 4 h.	Administration sets, solutions, or filters may be a source of contamination.
Any connections in the PN system must be Luer locked.	Luer lock connectors reduce the incidence of accidental uncoupling of joints.
Scrub every connector and entry site with alcohol.	Alcohol is a disinfectant and will also remove any traces of solution that might accumulate on connectors during setup.
Stopcocks are not to be used; avoid the use of added extension tubing or T-connectors.	Extra tubing may be a source of contamination.
Keep a smooth-edged clamp or Kelly clamps at the bedside.	If the PN system should become disconnected or break, immediate clamping of the catheter above the break will prevent air embolism or blood loss.
A volumetric infusion pump must be used.	A volumetric pump will accurately deliver desired volume as well as signal air and/or obstruction in the system.
Cover solution with UV-resistant light sensitive bag.	Decrease potential risk of nutrient oxidation.
Independent double-check should be performed to ensure appropriate pump settings/right tubing-right pump.	

II. PREVENTION OF INFECTION

ACTION	RATIONALE
A single lumen CVC placed for nutrition is not intended to serve any other purpose (i.e., to measure central venous pressures, administer blood products, "piggyback" medications or obtain blood samples).	Frequent manipulation of the PN system increases the risk of infectious and mechanical complications.
Cover the CVC exit site with a sterile dressing, and change at least every 7 d or as needed.	
THE FOLLOWING PRECAUTIONS MUST BE TAKEN BEFORE ENTERING THE LINE:	
All entry points are to be scrubbed with alcohol for at least 15 s.	Alcohol is a disinfectant.
No medications may be added to the PN solution outside the pharmacy.	Medication may precipitate in PN solution. The addition of a medication is also a potential source of contamination.

TABLE 17.21 NURSING CARES IN PARENTERAL NUTRITION ADMINISTRATION (*continued*)

If blood must be withdrawn from any catheter, it must be done by a physician or nurse specifically trained in this procedure.	If done improperly, blood withdrawal may cause clotting or infectious complications.
III. LIPID ADMINISTRATION	
ACTION	**RATIONALE**
Lipid may be administered with PN solution, provided:	
A separate pump is used.	Use of a pump ensures accurate infusion and prevents backflow of PN into the lipid circuit.
A 1.2-μm filter is used in the system, closest to the patient.	
Lipid volumes <60 mL are administered through a syringe pump.	Lipid must be administered at a steady rate to prevent fat overload.
Change tubing every 24 h. Solution is to be changed every 12 h.	Administration sets, solutions, or filters may be a source of contamination.
Coordinate lipid administration setup change with the change in solution to minimize manipulation of the line.	This decreases the risk of infection.
IV. CYCLIC PN	
ACTION	**RATIONALE**
A neutral pressure cap is placed on the CVC and changed twice weekly or at the same time as the catheter dressing is changed or after lab draws.	A Luer lock cap closes off the infusion system and prevents disconnection of the cap. It also provides a site for heparin instillation.
After PN administration complete, disconnect PN and ILE line.	For prevention of infection
Scrub CVC with alcohol for 15 s and flush with 3-10 mL normal saline.	
Scrub connection site with alcohol and flush CVC with 3 mL heparin 10 units/mL.	Heparin will prevent blood from clotting.
Place alcohol-impregnated cap on needleless connector.	For prevention of infection

CVC, central venous catheter; ILE, injectable lipid emulsion; PN, parenteral nutrition.
From Canada T, Crill C, Guenter P. *Home parenteral nutrition*. In: *ASPEN Parenteral Nutrition Handbook*. American Society for Parenteral and Enteral Nutrition; 2009:253-278.

aseptic technique, and ensuring that there are no clamps or kinks present (mechanical obstruction). The inline filter should never be removed unless it is replaced with a new one. Using aseptic technique, a 3-10 mL flush with normal saline should be attempted. If occlusion is sudden, consideration for infusate composition and intracatheter precipitate should be considered. Depending on the nature of an intracatheter precipitate, Table 17.23 lists commonly used agents and doses for treatment.[46]

TABLE 17.22 COMMON MECHANICAL AND CENTRAL LINE–RELATED COMPLICATIONS IN PATIENTS RECEIVING PARENTERAL NUTRITION

COMPLICATION	CLINICAL SIGNS AND SYMPTOMS	MANAGEMENT	PREVENTIVE MEASURE
Obstruction in the infusion system	PN does not flow to gravity. Occlusion alarm sounds	• Check that all clamps in the system are open. • Check the IV tubing and catheter for kinks. • If the catheter has clotted, one may attempt to dislodge the clot by careful flushing with 1 mL of normal saline directly attached to catheter hub, using sterile technique. If unsuccessful, a fibrinolytic agent may be necessary (see Table 17.23).	• Use a pump that detects obstruction immediately. • Careful taping of catheter and dressing to prevent kinking of tubing
Dislodgment of the catheter with subcutaneous collection of PN solution	Swelling at the insertion site of the catheter	• Removal of the catheter	• Careful handling of catheter • Securing line with tape
Venous thrombosis	Venous distention or edema of the part of the body drained by that vein	• Instillation of a fibrinolytic agent may dissolve a small thrombus. • Attempt to aspirate blood to verify if catheter is patent and intact. • Evaluate need for removal.	• Use a pump that detects obstructions.
Breakage of silastic catheter	Leakage of PN fluid or blood Ballooning of catheter during flushing/infusion	• Clamp catheter immediately. • Obtain proper size repair kit. • Repair the catheter.	• Careful handling of the catheter • Clamping only where indicated on CVC • Avoid forceful flushing. • Keep entirety of catheter under dressing. • Consider use of protective vests/clothing.

Accidental uncoupling of joints in the infusion system	• Leakage of PN solution or spontaneous blood return • May cause hypoglycemic reaction or infection.	• Clamp off system • Clean joints with alcohol before reconnecting	• Use of Luer lock connectors • If concern for contamination, consider new bag/infusion set.
Air embolus	Sudden onset of respiratory distress Cyanosis	• Immediately clamp catheter. • Place patient in Trendelenburg position with right side up.	• Use a pump that detects air in the system. • Use air eliminating filters in setup. • Clamping catheter when system is opened
Transient arrhythmias	Irregular heartbeat usually occurring during insertion	May require repositioning of catheter.	• Careful monitoring of heartbeat immediately after insertion
Skin sloughing due to infiltration of PN solution	Swelling at peripheral IV site with discoloration of surrounding skin	• Immediately remove IV. • Elevate limb to reduce edema. • Cover skin slough with sterile dressing. • Apply warm compresses. • Consider aspirating fluid from extravasated area. • Consider use of hyaluronidase 15 u/mL inject 0.5 mL × 5 doses SQ around site or apply nitroglycerin ointment 2% 4 mM per Kg q 8 h.	• Hourly observation of IV site for infiltration • Changing peripheral IV sites as needed • Using clear tape or dressings to allow for visual inspection of the infusion site

CVC, central venous catheter; IV, intravenous; PN, parenteral nutrition; SQ, subcutaneous.

TABLE 17.23 TREATMENT OF CENTRAL VENOUS CATHETER OCCLUSION

PRECIPITATE SUSPECTED	CLINICAL SCENARIO	PHARMACOLOGIC AGENT	DOSE
Particulate (e.g., Ca-P) with drugs that are soluble in acidic solution.	PN, Calcium and/or Phosphorus; use of etoposide or Aminoglycosides + heparin	50 mg/mL Cysteine hydrochloride	1-2 mL or catheter volume in 30-60 min dwell time
Particulate with drugs that are soluble in basic solutions.	Phenytoin, imipenem, oxacillin, ticarcillin	1 mEq/mL Sodium bicarbonate	1-2 mL or catheter volume in 30-60 min dwell time
Lipids	PN/ILE propofol	Ethanol 70% in water	1-2 mL or catheter volume in 30-60 min dwell time
None (i.e., thrombus suspected)	No precipitate suspected, line sluggish, difficulty drawing blood from catheter	Alteplase 1 mg/mL	2 mg for >30 kg child Use CVC prime volume if <30 kg child. 120 min dwell time-May repeat 1 time if unsuccessful.

CVC, central venous catheter; ILE, injectable lipid emulsion; PN, parenteral nutrition.
Adapted from Boston Children's Hospital CVC occlusion algorithm 2022; van Miert C, Hill R, Jones L. *Interventions for restoring patency of occluded central venous catheter lumens. Cochrane Database Syst Rev.* 2012;*2012*(4):CD007119.

Persistent obstructions are often treated with thrombolytic agents. Diagnostic imaging (ultrasound, x-ray, MR angiography, or venogram) can be helpful in distinguishing between malpositioned catheters, a fibrin sheath at the central venous catheter (CVC) tip, or mural thrombi. Complete occlusions, however, cannot be evaluated by contrast studies. Figure 17.3 describes the algorithm used at Boston Children's Hospital for the evaluation and treatment of CVC occlusions. For catheter occlusions refractory to tPA (Alteplase), refer to Table 17.23 for suspected precipitate troubleshooting.[46]

■ CATHETER INFECTION PROPHYLAXIS

At Boston Children's Hospital, we have instituted the use of 70% ethanol locks for patients who are at risk for frequent CVC-associated blood stream infections.[47] Ethanol is both bactericidal and fungicidal, and there is no known microbial resistance to ethanol. Our criteria for the use of 70% ethanol lock therapy include silicone (not polyurethane) vascular access device, weight greater than or equal to 5 kg, age 6 months or greater, a history of a confirmed CVC-related blood stream infection, and PN cycled at least 4 hours each day. The priming volume of the catheter is measured by a competent clinician to decrease risk for ethanol exposure. A test dose is administered, and the patient is observed for adverse reactions to the therapy.

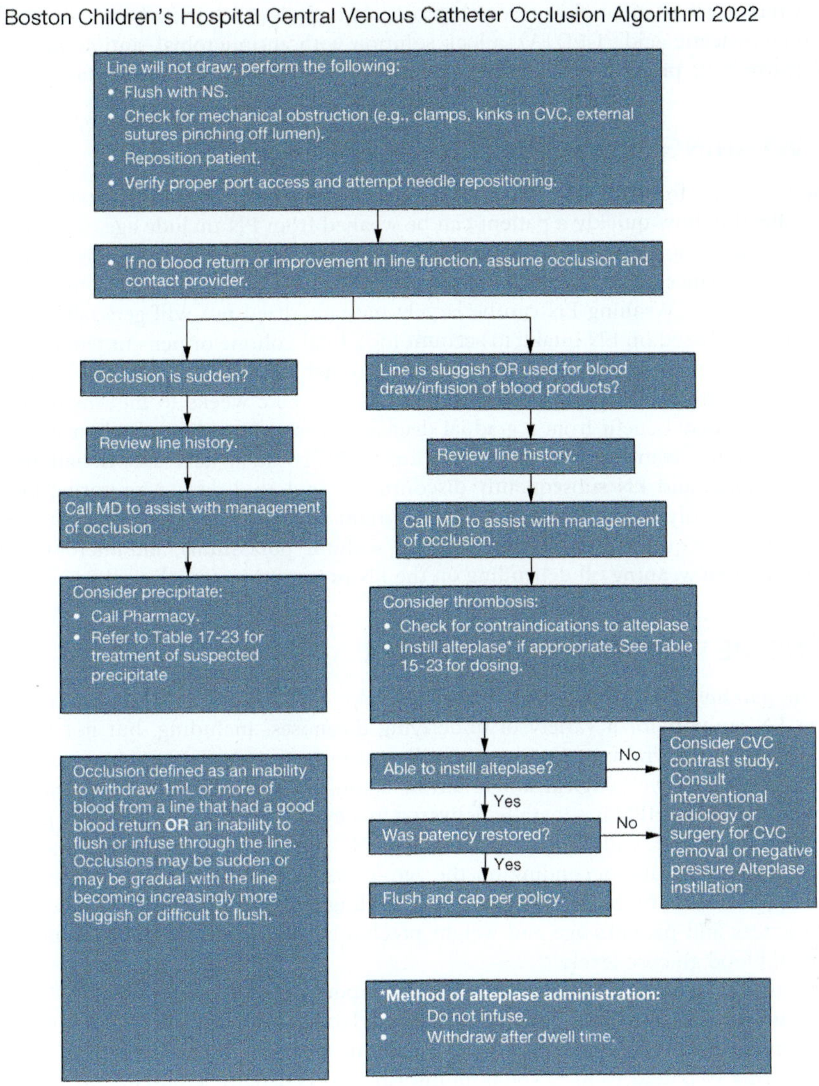

Figure 17.3 Central venous catheter occlusion algorithm. CVC, central venous catheter; MD, medical doctor; NS, normal saline.

During use, ethanol is instilled into the catheter and allowed to dwell for at least 2 hours and up to 14 hours. The catheter is flushed with normal saline prior to use; blood alcohol levels are negligible when ethanol lock is injected.[48] Ethanol locks are generally used from 3 to 7 days per week. Ethanol and heparin are incompatible and will cause a precipitate in the catheter. Because of this, heparin is not used in the catheter the days the patient is receiving ethanol locks. Over time, prolonged use of ethanol locks may increase mechanical complications, including fibrin formation, catheter occlusion, and catheter fracture.[49]

Alternatives to ethanol in research protocols include 4% tetrasodium ethylenediaminetetraacetic acid (T-EDTA), a lock solution with antimicrobial, antibiofilm, and antithrombotic properties[50] as well as sodium bicarbonate and citrate solutions.

WEANING FROM PARENTERAL NUTRITION

The transition from PN to enteral autonomy (EN, PO) can be highly variable. Factors affecting how quickly a patient can be weaned from PN include age, underlying disease, indication for PN, tolerance to enteral advancement, psychological factors (e.g., compliance), and previous medical interventions (e.g., prolonged intubation, enteral access). Weaning PN can be largely individualized but will generally aim at titrating PN based on EN intake to account for a total volume or percent reduction of PN support. Younger patients, those with questionable tolerance to enteral feedings, and those with a history of feeding difficulties may take weeks to months to wean off PN and may benefit from a gradual decrease in rate. For older children who are anticipated to advance EN rapidly, the volume of PN could be decreased in half, lipids discontinued, and PN subsequently discontinued in 1 to 2 days. Monitoring blood glucose, electrolytes, and fluid status is important during the weaning process. Some patients may require enteral electrolyte (e.g., sodium, potassium), and micronutrient support when weaning off depending on the PN prescription and clinical needs.

HOME PARENTERAL NUTRITION

Home parenteral nutrition (HPN) may be an option for children who require long-term PN support for a variety of underlying diagnoses, including, but not limited to, short bowel syndrome, primary motility disorders, and congenital enteropathy. Medical, social, psychological, and financial factors must all be considered in the decision to use HPN. HPN is generally delivered in a cyclic schedule allowing the patient to perform normal, daily functions while off PN. The duration of infusion may vary from 10 to 20 hours, depending on the age, nutritional requirements, medications, and enteral intake of the patient. Barriers to cycling HPN include fluid and electrolyte imbalances and patient's age and weight precluding the patient's ability to maintain normal blood glucose levels.

Continual primary care giver education is important for the duration of HPN therapy with the goal to reduce complications related to HPN such as infusion errors, central venous catheter complications, and infections that can be life threatening.[22] HPN monitoring is similar to in-hospital monitoring but is usually less frequent. We generally recommend the following parameters to be monitored every 4 to 8 weeks: (1) height or length, weight, head circumference (if applicable), and triceps skinfold measurements; (2) a record of enteral and oral intake should be reviewed; (3) assessment of catheter function and care; and (4) biochemical monitoring (see Table 17.20). Periodic monitoring includes fat-soluble vitamins and trace elements.[51] Long-term HPN patients are at risk for metabolic bone disease secondary to composition limitations (e.g., calcium, phosphorus, vitamin D) of PN solutions. Bone mineral density correlates well with future fracture risk; thus, evaluation by DXA scan should start at age 5 years and be repeated as clinically indicated.[52] Long-term PN support also places patients at risk for liver and kidney disease with routine screening (e.g., laboratory trends, ultrasound, transient elastography) required for ongoing risk assessment and management. Assessing growth and enteral intake, in addition to biochemical parameters, helps determine necessary changes in the amount and composition of the solution.

The length of therapy for HPN depends on the underlying medical reason for initiating nutrition support and can be as short as a few months to as long as several years. Because of the high rate of infectious and noninfectious complications of prolonged PN in pediatric patients, it is imperative that every effort be made to wean patients from prolonged PN dependence. Tolerance to EN in this setting must be managed through a transition that is carefully monitored by all caretakers.

■ CONCLUSION

Since its introduction in 1968, PN has become a life-sustaining therapy in the management of children unable to meet their nutritional needs exclusively by the enteral route. Although numerous advancements have been made to provide more balanced solutions, PN continues to be an artificial high-risk therapy. By working collaboratively with an interdisciplinary team utilizing nutrition and catheter guidelines, and care giver education, these risks may be lowered. Given the inherent risks of PN therapy, continued advocacy for innovation and research is needed to improve outcomes.

■ REFERENCES

1. Dudrick SJ, Wilmore DW, Vars HM, Rhoads JE. Long-term total parenteral nutrition with growth, development, and positive nitrogen balance. *Surgery*. 1968;64(1):134-142.
2. Berlana D. Parenteral nutrition overview. *Nutrients*. 2022;14(21):4480.
3. Worthington P, Balint J, Bechtold M, et al. When is parenteral nutrition appropriate? *JPEN J Parenter Enteral Nutr*. 2017;41(3):324-377.
4. Mistiaen P, Van den Heede K. Nutrition Support Teams: a systematic review. *JPEN J Parenter Enteral Nutr*. 2020;44(6):1004-1020.
5. Bahoush G, Salajegheh P, Anari AM, Eshghi A, Aski BH. A review of peripherally inserted central catheters and various types of vascular access in very small children and pediatric patients and their potential complications. *J Med Life*. 2021;14(3):298-309.
6. D'Andrea V, Prontera G, Rubortone SA, et al. Umbilical venous catheter update: a narrative review including ultrasound and training. *Front Pediatr*. 2021;9:774705.
7. American Society for Parenteral and Enteral Nutrition. Appropriate dosing for parenteral nutrition: ASPEN recommendations. 2020. Accessed November 26, 2024. https://nutritioncare.org/wp-content/themes/aspen/validate-protected-media.php?file=2025/08/Appropriate-Dosing-for-PN.pdf
8. Aune G. Fluids and electrolytes. In: *The Harriet Lane Handbook*. Elsevier Mosby; 2009.
9. Cober MP, Gura KM, Mirtallo JM, et al. ASPEN lipid injectable emulsion safety recommendations part 2: neonate and pediatric considerations. *Nutr Clin Pract*. 2021;36(6):1106-1125.
10. Bresson JL, Narcy P, Putet G, Ricour C, Sachs C, Rey J. Energy substrate utilization in infants receiving total parenteral nutrition with different glucose to fat ratios. *Pediatr Res*. 1989;25(6):645-648.
11. Agus MS, Wypij D, Hirshberg EL, et al. Tight glycemic control in critically ill children. *N Engl J Med*. 2017;376(8):729-741.
12. 20% ProSol—sulfite-free (amino acid) injection. Package insert. Baxter Healthcare Corporation; 2014. https://baxterpi.com/pi-pdf/Prosol_PI.pdf
13. TRAVASOL (amino acids) injection. Package insert. Baxter Healthcare Corporation; 2020. https://baxterpi.com/pi-pdf/Travasol_PI.pdf
14. 15% CLINISOL—sulfite-free (amino acid) injection. Package insert. Baxter Healthcare Corporation; 2018. https://www.baxterpi.com/pi-pdf/Clinisol_PI.pdf
15. PREMASOL 10%—sulfite-free (amino acids) injection. Package insert. Baxter Healthcare Corporation; 2021. https://baxterpi.com/pi-pdf/PI%20PREMASOL10%2007-19-00-3923%20Nov2021.pdf
16. Aminosyn® -PF 10% sulfite-free (amino acid injection). Package insert. ICU Medical, Inc; 2018. https://www.icumed.com/media/h1rdh3jx/qen-4678-final.pdf

17. TrophAmine (10% amino acid injection). Package insert. 2023.
18. Aminosyn® -PF 7% sulfite-free (amino acid injection). Package insert. ICU Medical, Inc; 2018. https://www.icumed.com/media/zf1ns4iu/qen-4682-final.pdf
19. Anez-Bustillos L, Dao DT, Fell GL, et al. Redefining essential fatty acids in the era of novel intravenous lipid emulsions. *Clin Nutr*. 2018;37(3):784-789.
20. Barr LH, Dunn GD, Brennan MF. Essential fatty acid deficiency during total parenteral nutrition. *Ann Surg*. 1981;193(3):304-311.
21. Mogensen KM. Essential fatty acid deficiency. *Pract Gastroenterol*. 2017;41(6):37-44.
22. Wolff J, Cober MP, Huff KA. Essential fatty acid deficiency in parenteral nutrition: historical perspective and modern solutions, a narrative review. *Nutr Clin Pract*. 2025;40(2):350-367.
23. Zemrani B, McCallum Z, Bines JE. Trace element provision in parenteral nutrition in children: one size does not fit all. *Nutrients*. 2018;10(11):1819.
24. Hahn JS, Berquist W, Alcorn DM, Chamberlain L, Bass D. Wernicke encephalopathy and beriberi during total parenteral nutrition attributable to multivitamin infusion shortage. *Pediatrics*. 1998;101(1):E10.
25. Infuvite Adult (multiple vitamins injection). Prescribing information. Baxter Healthcare Corporation; 2016. https://www.accessdata.fda.gov/drugsatfda_docs/label/2004/21163s011lbl.pdf
26. Infuvite Pediatric (multiple vitamins injection). Prescribing information. Baxter Healthcare Corporation; 2016. https://www.accessdata.fda.gov/drugsatfda_docs/label/2008/021265s015lbl.pdf
27. Hardy G, Wong T, Morrissey H, et al. Parenteral provision of micronutrients to pediatric patients: an international expert consensus paper. *JPEN J Parenter Enteral Nutr*. 2020;44(suppl 2):S5-S23.
28. Directors APNCaBo. 2024 Parenteral nutrition product shortage recommendations: intravenous multivitamins 2024. Published October 09, 2024. Accessed November 19, 2024. https://nutritioncare.org/wp-content/uploads/2024/12/Intravenous-Multivitamin-Shortage-Recommendations.pdf
29. Domellöf M, Szitanyi P, Simchowitz V, Franz A, Mimouni F. ESPGHAN/ESPEN/ESPR/CSPEN guidelines on pediatric parenteral nutrition: iron and trace minerals. *Clin Nutr*. 2018;37(6 pt B):2354-2359.
30. Hurwitz M, Garcia MG, Poole RL, Kerner JA. Copper deficiency during parenteral nutrition: a report of four pediatric cases. *Nutr Clin Pract*. 2004;19(3):305-308.
31. Takagi Y, Okada A, Sando K, Wasa M, Yoshida H, Hirabuki N. Evaluation of indexes of in vivo manganese status and the optimal intravenous dose for adult patients undergoing home parenteral nutrition. *Am J Clin Nutr*. 2002;75(1):112-118.
32. INFeD® (iron dextran injection). Ppackage insert. Allergan; 2021. Accessed June 25, 2025. https://www.accessdata.fda.gov/drugsatfda_docs/label/2021/017441s179lbl.pdf
33. Ikomi C, Cole CR, Vale E, Golekoh M, Khoury JC, Jones NY. Hypothyroidism and iodine deficiency in children on chronic parenteral nutrition. *Pediatrics*. 2018;141(4):e20173046.
34. McKinnon BT. FDA safety alert: hazards of precipitation associated with parenteral nutrition. *Nutr Clin Pract*. 1996;11(2):59-65.
35. Boullata JI, Mirtallo JM, Sacks GS, et al. Parenteral nutrition compatibility and stability: a comprehensive review. *JPEN J Parenter Enteral Nutr*. 2022;46(2):273-299.
36. Fresenius Kabi. Y-site drug compatibility reference guide. 2024. https://www.freseniuskabinutrition.com/wp-content/uploads/2024/03/4555-SMOFlipid-Compatibility-Tool-Brochure-2024.pdf
37. Bohrer D, do Nascimento PC, Binotto R, Becker E, Pomblum S. Contribution of the raw material to the aluminum contamination in parenterals. *JPEN J Parenter Enteral Nutr*. 2002;26(6):382-388.
38. Robinson DT, Ayers P, Fleming B, et al. Recommendations for photoprotection of parenteral nutrition for premature infants: An ASPEN position paper. *Nutr Clin Pract*. 2021;36(5):927-941.
39. Calafat AM, Needham LL, Silva MJ, Lambert G. Exposure to di-(2-ethylhexyl) phthalate among premature neonates in a neonatal intensive care unit. *Pediatrics*. 2004;113(5):e429-e434.
40. von Rettberg H, Hannman T, Subotic U, et al. Use of di(2-ethylhexyl)phthalate-containing infusion systems increases the risk for cholestasis. *Pediatrics*. 2009;124(2):710-716.
41. Morimoto T, Tsujinaka T, Ogawa A, et al. Effects of cyclic and continuous parenteral nutrition on albumin gene transcription in rat liver. *Am J Clin Nutr*. 1997;65(4):994-999.
42. Stout S, Cober M. Cyclic Parenteral Nutrition Infusion: Considerations for the Clinician. *Pract Gastroenterol*. 2011;(97):11-24.
43. Lienhardt A, Rakotoambinina B, Colomb V, et al. Insulin secretion and sensitivity in children on cyclic total parenteral nutrition. *JPEN J Parenter Enteral Nutr*. 1998;22(6):382-386.
44. Canada T, Crill C, Guenter P. Home parenteral nutrition. In: ASPEN Parenteral Nutrition Handbook. American Society for Parenteral and Enteral Nutrition; 2009:253-278.
45. Knöfler R, Dinger J, Kabus M, et al. Thrombolytic therapy in children—clinical experiences with recombinant tissue-plasminogen activator. *Semin Thromb Hemost*. 2001;27(2):169-174.

46. van Miert C, Hill R, Jones L. Interventions for restoring patency of occluded central venous catheter lumens. *Cochrane Database Syst Rev*. 2012;2012(4):CD007119.
47. Oliveira C, Nasr A, Brindle M, Wales PW. Ethanol locks to prevent catheter-related bloodstream infections in parenteral nutrition: a meta-analysis. *Pediatrics*. 2012;129(2):318-329.
48. Cober MP, Kovacevich DS, Teitelbaum DH. Ethanol-lock therapy for the prevention of central venous access device infections in pediatric patients with intestinal failure. *JPEN J Parenter Enteral Nutr*. 2011;35(1):67-73.
49. Fligor SC, Hirsch TI, Tsikis ST, et al. Ethanol lock therapy increases mechanical catheter complications in a pediatric intestinal failure population: a retrospective cohort study. *JPEN J Parenter Enteral Nutr*. 2023;47(5):662-669.
50. Hirsch TI, Fligor SC, Tsikis ST, et al. Administration of 4% tetrasodium EDTA lock solution and central venous catheter complications in high-risk pediatric patients with intestinal failure: a retrospective cohort study. *JPEN J Parenter Enteral Nutr*. 2024;48(5):624-632.
51. Vanek VW, Borum P, Buchman A, et al. A.S.P.E.N. position paper: recommendations for changes in commercially available parenteral multivitamin and multi-trace element products. *Nutr Clin Pract*. 2012;27(4):440-491.
52. Pastore S, Londero M, Barbieri F, Di Leo G, Paparazzo R, Ventura A. Treatment with pamidronate for osteoporosis complicating long-term intestinal failure. *J Pediatr Gastroenterol Nutr*. 2012;55(5):615-618.

PART III

Nutrition and Specific Disease States

CHAPTER 18

Sepsis, Trauma, and Critical Care

Melanie V. Connolly and Nilesh Mehta

Trauma and injury continue to be the leading cause of death for children in the United States.[1] Many of these critically ill patients, often with multi-organ involvement, are admitted to the pediatric intensive care unit (PICU), and provision of optimal nutrition support remains a key component of the care of these children. Malnutrition, both undernutrition and overweight/obesity, is prevalent in children with severe injury or other critical illnesses admitted to the PICU. A child with underweight or obesity in the PICU presents with unique challenges in determining nutrition goals and may have an increased risk of hospital-acquired complications.[2] Furthermore, being underweight in the PICU is associated with a significantly higher risk of 60-day mortality and fewer ventilator-free days.[2]

In addition to changes in metabolism reviewed in the following section, a variety of barriers impede the delivery of nutrients in the PICU population.[3] These factors may lead to deterioration of nutritional status, subsequently affecting the ability to recover, and increasing the risk of morbidity and mortality.[2] In this chapter, we will describe some of the unique nutritional challenges facing children in the PICU.

■ METABOLISM

The metabolic stress response that follows a variety of injuries, such as sepsis, surgery, trauma, and burns, is characterized by protein catabolism and increased metabolic demands. Muscle atrophy is common in children admitted to the PICU.[4] To prevent accelerated loss of lean body mass during this catabolic phase, it is crucial to provide adequate macronutrients and micronutrients. Detailed knowledge of the metabolic stress response following injury is essential, to allow appropriate, individualized energy prescriptions.

The body's response to injury, stress, surgery, or inflammation is difficult to predict and is characterized by dynamic metabolic alterations during the hospital course of illness.[5] Both a period of hypermetabolism and hypometabolism are thought to occur during the hospital course; however, the transition and exact timing of these metabolic states remain unclear. In some cases, the hypermetabolism associated with the body's stress response may be offset by therapies such as mechanical ventilation and sedative/muscle relaxant medications, which reduce energy expenditure, leading to challenges in accurately predicting energy expenditure of children in the PICU. Children have significantly less metabolic stores compared to adults, specifically protein and fat stores.[6] Following critical illness, children are at a much greater risk of deleterious effects, such as acute malnutrition with loss of lean body mass, if nutrition support is not initiated following adequate fluid resuscitation.

NUTRITION REQUIREMENTS

Energy

The primary goal of nutrition therapy is to meet energy, macronutrient, and micronutrient requirements, as well as to preserve lean body mass during the catabolic stress response following injury and critical illness. Failure to accurately estimate energy and protein needs and barriers to delivering the prescribed macronutrients could result in overfeeding or underfeeding, precipitating nutritional deterioration during illness.[6] Difficulties with wound healing, loss of lean body mass, and a depressed immune system can result from underfeeding.[7] On the other hand, overfeeding can precipitate hyperglycemia and hypertriglyceridemia, as well as increase ventilator load with carbon dioxide production, which may be poorly tolerated by patients with an existing respiratory insufficiency.[5,7]

The most accurate clinical measure of resting energy expenditure is obtained through indirect calorimetry (IC). In the absence of IC, consensus guidelines recommend goal energy intake of calculated REE/BEE using the Schofield or FAO/WHO/UNU equations, without the use of a stress factor.[5] This includes children on extracorporeal membrane oxygenation support (ECMO).[8] Sole reliance on equations for estimating energy requirements can result in cumulative energy imbalance during critical illness, although they continue to be routinely used. The use of IC to guide energy prescriptions during critical illness is recommended whenever possible.[5] See Chapter 14 for details of IC.

Once goal energy needs are established, ongoing reassessment is crucial due to the dynamic medical course of children in the PICU, including changes in sedative, paralytic, and vasopressor medication, respiratory status, and surgical interventions. It is important to be aware of the macronutrient composition being provided, either enterally or parenterally, as substrate utilization may be altered during critical illness.

Protein

Critical illness is characterized by increased protein turnover, with ongoing protein degradation and synthesis.[6] This adaptive response allows for amino acids to be available in the free amino acid pool, which are then redistributed away from skeletal muscle for tissue repair, wound healing, and participation in a variety of inflammatory response pathways. This contribution to the amino acid pool, as well as overall protein breakdown during critical illness, tends to exceed actual dietary protein intake, creating a net negative nitrogen balance. A minimum of 1.5 g/kg of protein intake may be necessary to maintain a positive balance during critical illness,[5] with higher amounts in infants and malnourished children. For obese children in the PICU, protein should be prescribed at 1.5 g/kg using ideal body weight.[5] Consensus guidelines for children on ECMO recommend 3 g/kg protein for neonates and at least 1.5 g/kg for children.[8] Current protein recommendations for injured children with the aim to achieve protein balance are based on limited data and consensus, which supports the need for further research.[5]

Studies have shown that actual protein delivery in the PICU is often far lower than recommended.[9,10] Ongoing protein turnover that is not matched by simultaneous adequate protein intake can result in loss of lean body mass.[7] Muscle atrophy in critically ill children can lead to reduced diaphragm thickness with difficulty weaning from mechanical ventilation, prolonged intensive care unit (ICU) admission, worse functional outcomes,[4] and in one large observational study, higher 60-day mortality.[10] To this end, clinicians should work to identify and eliminate barriers in the provision of goal protein and energy intakes in the PICU.

It should be noted that adequate protein intake alone may be insufficient to prevent muscle atrophy in PICU patients. A recent systematic review identified risk factors for muscle atrophy in PICU: length of PICU stay, length of hospital stay, length of mechanical ventilation, corticosteroid use, neuromuscular blockade use, and elevated C-reactive protein.[11] Using techniques such as ultrasound measurement of quadriceps muscle changes, ongoing research focuses on strategies to attenuate muscle loss—for example, safe mechanical muscle stimulation (mobilization and rehabilitation) for PICU patients, as well as functional impacts of muscle atrophy after a PICU stay.

Carbohydrates

The metabolism of carbohydrates during critical illness is characterized by an increase in glucose production and insulin resistance. Gluconeogenesis ensures a steady energy source for glucose-dependent organs, such as the brain, erythrocytes, and renal medulla. Owing to an association between high serum glucose levels and poor outcomes during critical illness,[6,7] studies have examined the role of tight glucose control, using insulin, in the intensive care unit. A large multicenter trial noted severe hypoglycemia and increased hospital-associated infections when tight glucose control (80-110 mg/dL, compared to a higher range of 150-180 mg/dL) was achieved in children admitted to the PICU[12]; therefore, using insulin to achieve target blood sugar levels in the 80-100 mg/dL range is not currently recommended. Current management of hyperglycemia in the PICU includes the avoidance of overfeeding[5,7,13] and the use of insulin to treat persistent hyperglycemia (defined as two serial blood glucose measurements >180 mg/dL).[14] Optimal target glucose levels and glycemic control strategies in critically ill children continue to be investigated.

Lipids

Like protein and carbohydrates, lipids have increased turnover rates during critical illness, with free fatty acids acting as the primary source of energy for patients under physiologic stress.[6] It is important to ensure adequate delivery of essential fatty acids during critical illness to prevent deficiency. This is usually achieved by providing 30% to 40% of the total calories from fat, which is the recommended upper limit to maintain a mixed fuel system of macronutrients, while preventing associated complications, such as hypertriglyceridemia. Lower intake levels of intravenous fat, 0.5 to 1 g/kg/d of soybean oil-based preparations, are usually enough to prevent essential fatty acid deficiency. Currently, there is insufficient evidence to support the use of omega-3 fatty acids as an anti-inflammatory agent in critically ill children.

Electrolytes, Vitamins, and Minerals

Routine monitoring of electrolytes in critically ill patients is recommended to detect alterations, particularly for children deemed at risk of refeeding syndrome. Chapter 14 discusses the electrolyte alterations commonly seen with refeeding syndrome.

The body relies on a complex system of enzymes, cofactors (copper, zinc, iron, selenium, and manganese), and vitamins (C and E) to act as a defense system against oxidant stress that exists in the acute phase of injury or illness. Vitamins and minerals are redistributed from central circulation to tissues, and fluid losses from wounds and third spacing may alter micronutrient balance and result in possible deficiencies during the early phase of illness.[15] The association of low micronutrient levels in serum with poor outcomes has fueled the desire to provide micronutrient supplements in this population. However, the inflammatory state of critically ill patients, including those with sepsis, reduces the serum levels of micronutrients in the absence of true deficiency.[15,16] These abnormal levels may take weeks to return to normal. Thus, the role of micronutrient supplementation in critically ill children continues to be researched, including the use of glutamine, arginine, zinc, and antioxidants to attenuate inflammation or modulate immune response. There is currently insufficient evidence to support either the use of specific vitamin or mineral supplements in critically ill children, or the use of "immune enhancing" formulas.

ROUTE, TIMING, AND BARRIERS TO NUTRITION SUPPORT

Once the individualized nutrition prescription is determined for the critically ill child, the next decision is to select the appropriate route to deliver the nutrients. The enteral route is preferred in patients with a functional gastrointestinal tract, due to its established benefits, such as preservation of intestinal mucosa integrity, enhanced mucosal immunity, safety, and cost-effectiveness, compared to parenteral nutrition (PN).[5,6] It is recommended that low-volume enteral nutrition (EN) be initiated within 24 to 48 hours of PICU admission, unless contraindicated.[5,13]

PN may be used either alone or as a supplement to EN in patients with EN contraindications or intolerance, such as those with increased risk of bowel ischemia. The optimal timing of PN initiation has been studied in adult and pediatric trials.[17,18] The use of early PN (initiated within 24 hours of PICU admission) was associated with poorer outcomes compared to late initiation (day 8 of PICU admission), including longer hospital stay, longer ICU stay, increased new infections, longer duration of mechanical ventilation (adult), and longer duration of renal replacement therapy (adult).[17,18] In an adult trial, individual optimization of nutrition with supplemental PN starting on day 4 after ICU admission was associated with lower rates of nosocomial infection.[19] In a recent international, multicenter prospective observational study, achievement of 60% of the prescribed energy and protein goal between days 3 and 7 of PICU admission, from EN alone or EN + PN, was associated with lower mortality compared with achievement of these nutrition goals after day 7 of PICU admission.[20]

Current consensus guidelines recommend delaying initiation of PN until 1 week after PICU admission in adults and children,[5,13] although clinical judgment should be used to identify those patients who may benefit from earlier PN initiation, for example a child with an anticipated lengthy NPO course. Additionally, PN may have a role as a supplement to EN, particularly in malnourished children who are unable to be initiated on or advanced past low-volume EN within the first week of PICU admission.[5,20] A pragmatic approach of individualized timing of PN initiation, with strict aseptic delivery and avoiding overfeeding, may be appropriate in critically ill patients. We refer the reader to Chapter 17 for the indications for initiation of PN.

Many barriers exist when attempting to provide adequate nutrition via EN in the PICU, such as delays in initiating EN and frequent interruptions to feeds (due to procedures or subjective opinions related to enteral feeding intolerance).[3] Many of these barriers are avoidable and can be reassessed by a uniform, evidence-based approach to enteral nutrition in the PICU, including a consistent definition of "feeding intolerance". The use of feeding protocols in PICUs facilitates early initiation of EN, prevents unnecessary interruptions, increases the likelihood of reaching nutrition goals, and increases the overall use and success of EN.[5,13]

Chapters 16 and 17 provide additional details on these modes of nutrition support.

SPECIAL CONSIDERATIONS IN TRAUMA, SEPSIS, AND MULTISYSTEM INFLAMMATORY SYNDROME IN CHILDREN

Research examining nutritional support in pediatric traumatic brain injury (TBI) is limited. Consensus guidelines regarding care of children with severe TBI recommend nutrition support consistent with current PICU nutrition guidelines,[5] including initiation of early EN (within 72 hours of injury) to reduce mortality and improve outcomes.[21] In a number of studies in recent years, the anticipated increase in energy expenditure during the acute illness phase of critical illness has not been uniformly observed. Furthermore, in the modern ICU, the use of sedative and muscle relaxant medications, synchronized mechanical ventilation, temperature and humidity control, and advanced surgical and anesthetic techniques, might contribute to a lower energy expenditure in patients. The use of old equations based on healthy subjects to estimate energy requirements may result in overestimation of energy goals and therefore overfeeding. The use of IC to guide energy prescription in this population is highly recommended.[22]

Current nutritional approaches for children with severe sepsis focus on the above PICU nutrition support principles to attenuate the normal metabolic stress response and to prevent a decline in nutritional status. Recent point-prevalence data revealed a high incidence (67%) of malnutrition in a large international PICU sample with severe sepsis.[23] Severe undernutrition (body mass index z score (BMIZ) <-3) was associated with higher all-cause mortality, and severe overnutrition (BMIZ $>+3$) was associated with increased ICU length of stay in this population,[23] highlighting the need for accurate anthropometric measurements to identify those septic patients at highest nutritional risk. Early attention to micronutrients in formulas or PN might help avoid severe deficiencies. The addition of supraphysiologic doses of micronutrients in patients with sepsis or other forms of inflammation has not been adequately proven and continues to be studied.

Multisystem inflammatory syndrome (MIS) has been reported in children (MIS-C) and adults (MIS-A) after infection with the SARS-CoV-2 virus that was responsible for the COVID-19 pandemic. The condition was more common and severe in children, although all age groups were affected. Patients with MIS manifested with fever and inflammation of several organs. There was considerable interest in the role of nutrition in MIS, both as a preventative and therapeutic intervention.

Nutritional assessment and intervention for critically ill children infected with COVID-19 do not differ from the general PICU nutrition guidelines discussed in this chapter.[24] The potential for boosting immunity and therefore preventing or alleviating symptoms of MIS with optimal nutrition was explored in the absence of any specific therapies available for this illness. A variety of diets (e.g., plant-based, Mediterranean diet, healthy eating index) and micronutrient deficiencies have been studied for their role in this inflammatory condition[25,26]; however, there are no evidence-based specific therapeutic relationships proven between specific individual or groups of nutrients and MIS. The nutrition and COVID-19 relationship might be seen in the broader context of the benefits of adaptable choices such as optimal and balanced nutrition, exercise, and healthy lifestyle on boosting immune health.[27] The socioeconomic impact of a global pandemic, particularly reduced access to adequate and optimal nutrient intake, may put certain groups at a higher risk of immune dysregulation and therefore at a higher risk of severe disease.

CONCLUSION

Nutrition therapy is an essential component in the treatment and recovery of critically ill children. Due to the dynamic metabolic response to stress and barriers to nutrient delivery, critically ill children are at risk of nutritional deterioration during their illness course. Hence, close monitoring of the nutritional status, individualized nutritional prescription, careful attention to maintaining nutritional intake, and continued reassessment of nutritional needs are crucial. A multidisciplinary, evidence-based approach to optimize the provision of energy, macronutrients and micronutrients during critical illness should improve clinical outcomes in critically ill children.

REFERENCES

1. Curtin SC, Tejada-Vera B, Bastian BA. *National Vital Statistics Report: Deaths: Leading Causes for 2021*. National Center for Health Statistics; 2024. Accessed April 8, 2025. https://www.cdc.gov/nchs/data/nvsr/nvsr73/nvsr73-04.pdf
2. Bechard LJ, Duggan CP, Touger-Decker R, et al. Nutritional status based on Body Mass Index is associated with morbidity and mortality in mechanically ventilated critically ill children in the PICU. *Crit Care Med*. 2016;44(8):1530-1537.
3. Mehta NM, McAleer D, Hamilton S, et al. Challenges to optimal enteral nutrition in a multidisciplinary pediatric intensive care unit. *JPEN J Parenter Enteral Nutr*. 2010;34(1):38-45.
4. Johnson RW, Ng KWP, Dietz AR, et al. Muscle atrophy in mechanically-ventilated critically ill children. *PLoS One*. 2018;13(12):e0207720.
5. Mehta NM, Skillman HE, Irving SY, et al. Guidelines for the provision and assessment of nutrition support therapy in the pediatric critically ill patient: Society of Critical Care Medicine and American Society for Parenteral and Enteral Nutrition. *JPEN J Parenter Enteral Nutr*. 2017;41(5):706-742.
6. Sparks EA, Fisher JG, Khan FA, et al. The critically ill child. In: Duggan C, Watkins JB, Koletzko B, Walker WA, eds. *Nutrition in Pediatrics*. 5th ed. PMPH; 2016:957-969.
7. Hulst JM, Joosten KF, Tibboel D, et al. Causes and consequences of inadequate substrate supply to pediatric ICU patients. *Curr Opin Clin Nutr Metab Care*. 2006;9(3):297-303.
8. Lee AE, Munoz E, Al Dabbous T, et al. Extracorporeal Life Support Organization guidelines for the provision and assessment of nutritional support in the neonatal and pediatric ECMO patient. *ASAIO J*. 2022;68(7):875-880.
9. Tume LN, Latten LL, Compton V, Valla FV. Association between protein intake and muscle wasting in critically ill children: a prospective cohort study. *JPEN J Parenter Enteral Nutr*. 2024;48(5):615-623.
10. Mehta NM, Bechard LJ, Zurakowski D, et al. Adequate enteral protein intake is inversely associated with 60-d mortality in critically ill children: a multicenter, prospective, cohort study. *AJCN*. 2015;102(1):199-206.
11. Stacey LJ, Valla FV, Huang C, et al. The relationship between muscle mass changes and protein or energy intake in critically ill children: a systematic review and meta-analysis. *JPEN J Parenter Enteral Nutr*. 2025;49:152-164.

12. Agus MSD, Wypij D, Hirshberg EL, et al. Tight glycemic control in critically ill children. *N Engl J Med.* 2017;376(8):729-741.
13. Tume LN, Valla FV, Joosten K, et al. Nutritional support for children during critical illness: European Society of Pediatric and Neonatal Intensive Care (ESPNIC) metabolism, endocrine and nutrition section position statement and clinical recommendations. *Intensive Care Med.* 2020;46(3):411-425.
14. Honarmand K, Sirimaturos M, Hirshberg E, et al. Society of Critical Care Medicine guidelines on glycemic control for critically ill children and adults 2024. *Crit Care Med.* 2024;52(4): e161-e181.
15. Dresen E, Pimiento JM, Patel JJ, et al. Overview of oxidative stress and the role of micronutrients in critical illness. *JPEN J Parenter Enteral Nutr.* 2023;47:S38-S49.
16. Singer P, Blaser AR, Berger MM, et al. ESPEN practical and partially revised guideline: clinical nutrition in the intensive care unit. *Clin Nutr.* 2023;42(9):1671-1689.
17. Casaer MP, Mesotten D, Hermans G, et al. Early versus late parenteral nutrition in critically ill adults. *N Engl J Med.* 2011;365(6):506-517.
18. Fivez T, Kerklaan D, Mesotten D, et al. Early versus late parenteral nutrition in critically ill children. *N Eng J Med.* 2016;374(12):1111-1122.
19. Heidegger CP, Berger MM, Graf S, et al. Optimisation of energy provision with supplemental parenteral nutrition in critically ill patients: a randomised controlled clinical trial. *Lancet.* 2013;381(9864):385-393.
20. Bechard LJ, Staffa S, Zurakowski D, Mehta NM. Time to achieve delivery of nutrition targets is associated with clinical outcomes in critically ill children. *Am J Clin Nutr.* 2021;114:1859-1867.
21. Kochanek PM, Tasker RC, Carney N, et al. Guidelines for the management of pediatric severe traumatic brain injury, third edition: update of the Brain Trauma Foundation guidelines, executive summary. *Pediatr Crit Care Med.* 2019;20(3):280-289.
22. Wallinga MM, Newkirk MM, Gardner MT, Ziegler J. Variation in metabolic demand following severe pediatric traumatic brain injury: a case review. *Nutr Clin Pract.* 2024;39(1):246-253.
23. Irving SY, Daly B, Verger J, et al. The association of nutrition status expressed as Body Mass Index z score with outcomes in children with severe sepsis: a secondary analysis from the Sepsis Prevalence, Outcomes, and Therapies (SPROUT) study. *Crit Care Med.* 2018;46(11):e1029-e1039.
24. Marino LV, Valla FV, Tume LN, et al. Considerations for nutrition support in critically ill children with COVID-19 and paediatric inflammatory multisystem syndrome temporally associated with COVID-19. *Clin Nutr.* 2021;40(3):895-900.
25. Moludi J, Qaisar SA, Alizadeh M, et al. The relationship between Dietary Inflammatory Index and disease severity and inflammatory status: a case-control study of COVID-19 patients. *Br J Nutr.* 2022; 127(5):773-781.
26. Ponzo V, Pellegrini M, D'Eusebio C, et al. Mediterranean diet and SARS-COV-2 infection: is there any association? A proof-of-concept study. *Nutrients.* 2021;13(5):1721.
27. Messina G, Polito R, Monda V, et al. Functional role of dietary intervention to improve the outcome of COVID-19: a hypothesis of work. *Int J Mol Sci.* 2020;21(9):3104.

CHAPTER 19

Cardiac Disease

Emily Finnan, Tina Sun, and Kimberly I. Mills

Congenital heart disease (CHD) is the most common birth defect in the United States, affecting 1 in 100 newborns. The substantial improvement in survivorship over the past four decades has led to an increasing burden of noncardiac morbidities among children with CHD. Malnutrition is present in 15% to 41% of children with CHD.[1] As one of the most prevalent morbidities in CHD, nutrition-related challenges are a significant source of stress for families.

Issues related to growth and nutrition in this patient population are multifactorial. Contributing factors are noted in Figure 19.1. CHD lesions can also be classified based on the presence or absence of cyanosis, which may help determine a patient's expected nutrient needs and growth patterns (Table 19.1). Malnutrition is associated with important clinical outcomes such as (1) ICU and total hospital length of stay, (2) duration of mechanical ventilation, (3) wound healing, and (4) mortality.[2] Viewing malnutrition as a modifiable risk factor in children with CHD underscores the importance and potential impact of nutritional management.

NUTRITIONAL ASSESSMENT

Many components can be considered for a thorough assessment of patients with CHD, including, but not limited to, anthropometrics and biomarkers.

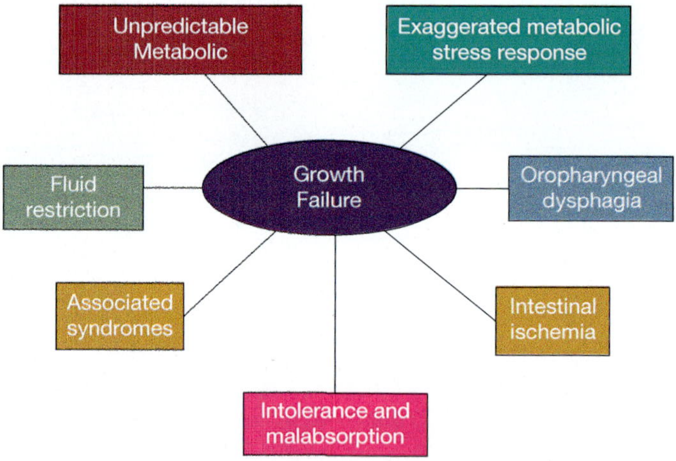

Figure 19.1 Factors contributing to malnutrition in congenital heart disease.

TABLE 19.1 ACYANOTIC VERSUS CYANOTIC CONGENITAL HEART LESIONS

ACYANOTIC (LEFT-TO-RIGHT SHUNT; HIGH/NORMAL $Q_P:Q_S$)	CYANOTIC (RIGHT-TO-LEFT SHUNT; LOW/NORMAL $Q_P:Q_S$)
Atrial septal defect (ASD)	Pulmonary atresia/stenosis
Ventricular septal defect (VSD)	Transposition of the great arteries (TGA)
Patent ductus arteriosus (PDA)	Hypoplastic left heart syndrome (HLHS)
Common atrioventricular canal (CAVC)	Single ventricle
Aortic stenosis	Tetralogy of Fallot (TOF)
Cardiomyopathy	Truncus arteriosus
Coarctation of the aorta	Tricuspid atresia
	Total anomalous pulmonary venous return (TAPVR)
	Ebstein anomaly

Anthropometrics

Several factors make accurate anthropometric assessment uniquely challenging in the CHD population. Preoperative measures ideally are obtained when the patient is euvolemic and free of medical devices. However, subsequent serial measures of weights can fluctuate depending on a patient's volume status. Fluctuations are more often indicative of response to diuretics versus somatic growth. Moreover, it may not be conceivable to safely obtain weights for several days post cardiac surgery or during an acute illness due to clinical instability. Therefore, alternative anthropometric measures may become useful for this population.

Arm anthropometrics such as mid-upper arm circumference (MUAC), triceps skinfold (TSF), and subscapular skinfold thickness (SST) can be used to track growth, changes in body composition, and assess for malnutrition. Arm anthropometrics have the advantage of being easier to obtain during periods of prolonged clinical instability, although positioning of the child and freedom from lines and tubes is required (see Chapter 2).

Biomarkers

Biomarkers of nutritional status can be difficult to interpret in children in the early postoperative stages of treatment for CHD since cardiopulmonary bypass and acute illnesses are often characterized by an inflammatory state. Classic markers, such as prealbumin, retinol and transferrin, are acute-phase proteins and can be falsely depressed when acutely ill[3] (see Chapter 4).

■ NUTRITION SUPPORT CONSIDERATIONS

An individualized and dynamic assessment is required when considering the enteral and parenteral needs for children in the inpatient stages of treatment of children with CHD. Daily nutrition prescriptions are based on several factors to include patient's age, baseline nutritional status, phase of illness, presence of ductal-dependent circulation, fluid restriction, tolerance of enteral feeds, and oral feeding abilities.

Enteral Nutrition

The safety of preoperative enteral nutrition (EN) in neonates with CHD is often determined by the patient's clinical status and presence of a ductal-dependent lesion (i.e., a lesion wherein systemic or pulmonary blood flow depends on a patent ductus arteriosus). The primary concern for initiating preoperative EN in neonates with CHD is mesenteric ischemia—due to reduced diastolic blood flow and resultant intestinal hypoperfusion.[4] (This is often referred to as "necrotizing enterocolitis (NEC)" in the literature and at the bedside but differs from the condition that plagues premature infants in many ways. The term "cardiac-NEC" may be more appropriate.) Similarly, neonates with hemodynamic instability are often supported with vasoactive infusions, which increase the risk for mesenteric ischemia. There are known advantages of EN in the support of critically ill children, including preoperative neonates with ductal-dependent CHD. The administration of exclusive unfortified human milk has been associated with a decrease in the risk of preoperative NEC for neonates with CHD.[5] In addition, the initiation of preoperative feeds (either by mouth or via nasoenteral tube) has been associated with reduced hospital length of stay and utilization of feeding tubes at the time of discharge.[6] Therefore, although the practice varies widely, the trend across institutions is to allow for preoperative EN in hemodynamically stable neonates with ductal-dependent CHD.[7]

Early provision of EN following congenital cardiac surgery is generally safe and recommended. To minimize intestinal atrophy that may lead to impaired absorption and increased mucosal permeability, the initiation of trophic feeds (10-20 mL/kg/d) within 4 to 6 hours of surgery has been shown to reduce the duration of mechanical ventilation and ICU length of stay while not increasing gastrointestinal complications in children with CHD.[8] However, infants with single ventricle physiology undergoing Stage 1 palliation often remain *nil per os* (NPO) for a prolonged period of time given hemodynamic instability and vasoactive requirements to minimize the risk of cardiac-NEC. The development and adherence to an institutional enteral feeding protocol reduces practice variation, utilization of parenteral nutrition and the incidence of NEC, even in infants with single ventricle physiology.[9]

Parenteral Nutrition

Parenteral nutrition (PN) is often required for hospitalized children with CHD. There are no specific guidelines for PN provision in children with CHD; therefore, clinicians apply the American Society for Parenteral and Enteral Nutrition (ASPEN) and European Society of Paediatric and Neonatal Intensive Care (ESPNIC) guidelines for critically ill children and neonates, respectively, when considering timing of PN initiation.[10,11] While a late PN strategy (defined as withholding PN for 7 days from ICU admission) has been associated with better outcomes in critically ill children, PN provision before that time is frequently utilized in children with CHD due to prolonged perioperative NPO periods, imposed fluid restriction limiting provision of adequate nutrition, enteral feeding intolerance, and frequent interruptions to EN.[12] Common scenarios in which "early" PN is considered include patients with single ventricle physiology undergoing Stage 1 palliation, ductal-dependent CHD, associated gastrointestinal anomalies preventing initiation of timely EN, open sternum, and mechanical support (extracorporeal membrane oxygenator and ventricular assist device). PN is generally delivered via central venous catheters in infants and young children with CHD since peripheral PN requires a volume of fluid not aligned with imposed fluid restrictions to meet minimum energy and protein goals.

Oral Feeding

Children with CHD experience delays in oral feeding progression due to potential vocal cord injury, developmental delay of the suck-swallow-breathe sequence, and associated upper airway/gastrointestinal anomalies. Vocal fold immobility is a known postoperative complication of congenital cardiac surgery. The recurrent laryngeal nerve is proximal to the aortic arch and ligamentum arteriosus and can often be injured during cardiac surgery. Vocal fold immobility can lead to aspiration and is associated with increased hospital length of stay, costs, and feeding tube utilization.[13] Vocal fold immobility often improves with time but is most likely to require a modified diet (i.e., thickened feeds). Close partnership with a feeding therapist, otolaryngology and gastroenterology can aid in safely providing EN and progressing toward full oral intake for children with CHD.

■ MACRO AND MICRONUTRIENT CONSIDERATION

Energy

Infants with unrepaired CHD may have increased energy requirements when compared to age-matched peers without CHD. Infants with unrepaired CHD have been reported to have a 35% higher total daily energy expenditure compared with healthy controls.[14] Following surgical correction, energy expenditure slowly returns to normal although patients may continue to require additional caloric provision to promote catch-up growth.

Indirect calorimetry (IC) is the gold standard to estimate energy expenditure in acutely ill children. No "stress factor" is added initially while the patients are muscle relaxed, therapeutically cooled, and/or inflamed. As the patient recovers, a modest "stress factor" may be added to estimate needs for surgical recovery and catch-up growth. Serial measurement with IC can help tailor dynamic energy goals. If IC is unavailable or not feasible, predictive equations (e.g., Schofield) are employed to estimate energy requirements (see Chapters 5 and 14).

Protein

Protein requirements are likely higher in patients with postoperative CHD due to higher protein turnover after cardiopulmonary bypass (CPB). Furthermore, patients with CHD experience high protein loss conditions secondary to losses from wounds, chylous effusions, or protein-losing enteropathy. Current guidelines from ASPEN and Society for Critical Care Medicine (SCCM) for the critically ill pediatric patient recommend a minimum protein intake of 1.5 g/kg/d with higher needs in the neonatal and specific populations to prevent a cumulative negative nitrogen balance.[10] For neonates with CHD, the goal protein intake is 3 g/kg/d, and for infants and children, it is 1.5 to 2 g/kg/d. Zhang et al. randomized infants after CPB to receive 1.3, 2.5, or 4 g/kg/d protein via enteral formula.[15] Infants in the highest protein group obtained

TABLE 19.2 DETERMINATION OF ESTIMATED MACRONUTRIENT NEEDS FOR THE PEDIATRIC PATIENT WITH CONGENITAL HEART DISEASE

	CRITICAL CARE	STEP-DOWN/ACUTE CARE
Energy Requirements	Determine by indirect calorimetry (if available). Acutely (72 h post CPB) aim for no stress factor. Stress factor may gradually increase to 1.1-1.3 pending recovery.	Catch-up Growth Stress factors will vary widely depending on preoperative status. Stress factors as high as 2 may be needed, particularly in the preoperative state.
Protein[a]	3+ g/kg/d (infant) 1.5+ g/kg/d (pediatric)	RDA as a minimum
Carbohydrate	May require lower GIR acutely postop if hyperglycemia present. Minimum GIR 4 mg/kg/min for infants	45%-65% of kcal, as needed for growth
Fat[b]	Minimum 1 g/kg/d when given intravenously	40%-55% of kcal for infants 25%-40% of kcal for children

CPB, cardiopulmonary bypass; GIR, glucose infusion rate; PLE, protein-losing enteropathy; RDA, recommended dietary allowance.
[a]Special consideration for conditions with increased losses (i.e., chylothorax, PLE, wound healing, renal replacement therapy).
[b]Special consideration for chylothorax minimum intake of essential fats 2% to 4% of total calories.

faster positive nitrogen balance than the other groups, as well as greater increases in serum prealbumin levels, MUAC, and triceps skinfold without an increase in feeding intolerance. Table 19.2 explores macronutrient needs for hospitalized children with CHD.

Micronutrients

Micronutrient status may be impacted in patients with CHD, due to the presence of malnutrition, medications, and various CHD-related morbidities.

Fat-Soluble Vitamins

As discussed below, fat-soluble vitamins A, D, E, and K may be affected if there are alterations in fat metabolism. Vitamin K is a nutrient of interest in patients with CHD, as vitamin K antagonists are a commonly prescribed anticoagulant. Acute changes in dietary intake of vitamin K may impact a patient's therapeutic ranges of international normalized ratio (INR). Patients on these medications are counseled to consume a consistent vitamin K diet. Assessment of vitamin K status using prothrombin time or INR levels is not appropriate for patients on vitamin K antagonists, as these levels more accurately reflect the therapeutic response of the medication than vitamin K status. Table 19.3 explores drug-nutrient interactions of common medications used in the CHD population.

TABLE 19.3 COMMON MEDICATIONS USED IN CONGENITAL HEART DISEASE WITH DRUG-NUTRIENT INTERACTIONS

MEDICATION	*DRUG-NUTRIENT INTERACTION*
Captopril	• Anorexia • Increased potassium • Decreased sodium
Coumadin (Warfarin)	• Vitamin K decreases efficacy.
Digoxin	• Nausea, vomiting, diarrhea • Decrease in magnesium • Increase/decrease in potassium
Epinephrine	• Nausea • Hyperglycemia
Flecainide	• Calcium may decrease efficacy. Do not take with breast milk/formula if possible.
Loop diuretics (Bumetanide [Bumex], Furosemide [Lasix])	• Decrease levels of sodium, potassium, magnesium, calcium, and thiamine • Increase water loss
Propranolol	• Nausea, vomiting • Hypoglycemia
Spironolactone (Aldactone)	• Retention of potassium and magnesium • Increase losses of sodium and water
Thiazide diuretics (Hydrochlorothiazide, Diuril)	• Decrease levels of sodium, potassium and magnesium • Increase water loss

Water-Soluble Vitamins

Two water-soluble vitamins of potential concern in CHD patients are vitamin C and thiamine. Serum vitamin C concentrations are low following CPB likely secondary to the significant inflammatory state.[16] The impact of this hypovitaminosis on outcomes is unclear and, therefore, high dose IV vitamin C is generally not indicated.

CHD patients on loop diuretics are at risk of thiamine deficiency, given increased renal losses. Thiamine deficiency can exacerbate heart failure and ventricular dysfunction. The classic deficiency, known as wet beriberi, leads to cellular dysfunction of myocardial cells as well as increased venous return, leading to volume overload and heart failure. Trials of IV thiamine in adult heart failure patients have not demonstrated improvements in symptoms.[17] Currently, routine surveillance of thiamine deficiency in the CHD population is not recommend although suspected deficiency, particularly where refeeding syndrome is concerned, should be treated.

Minerals and Electrolytes

The status of sodium, potassium, chloride, magnesium, and calcium can all be affected by medication effects and changes in volume status in children with CHD. Patients are typically instructed to limit sodium intake while on chronic diuretic therapy to help alleviate volume overload. However, administration of diuretics can result in the increased loss of sodium in the urine leading to hyponatremia and hypochloremia. Total body depletion of sodium can impact a patient's growth, particularly in infants.

However, in the CHD patient sodium supplementation beyond what is needed to normalize severe hyponatremia is generally not recommended, given the concern for worsening volume overload. Additionally, a urine sodium level, which is used to assess total body sodium depletion, is not a useful measure in patients taking diuretics, as urinary excretion of sodium will remain high despite a total body depletion.

Calcium loss in the urine is a known side effect of loop diuretics that can lead to a compensatory hyperparathyroidism and bone resorption leading to metabolic bone disease. Thiazide diuretics, particularly in infants, are often a preferred choice due to less impact on calcium excretion. Chronic use of diuretics, poor dietary intake of calcium, vitamin D deficiency, hyperparathyroidism, and immobility all impact a patient's risk and severity of metabolic bone disease. Metabolic bone disease is a complex morbidity that benefits from a multidisciplinary approach for treatment. Safe handling, physical therapy, assessment and correction of parathyroid and calcitriol alterations as well as improvement in intake of calcium and correction for inadequate vitamin D stores may improve patient's risk of fractures.

Iron

Iron deficiency is prevalent in those with CHD and heart failure—impacting up to 50% patients and can be associated with higher risks of hospitalization, worse echocardiographic features, heart transplant, and death.[18] In patients with cyanotic heart disease, iron deficiency can be more difficult to diagnosis since hemoglobin and mean corpuscular volume levels may not decline due to hypoxemia leading to polycythemia. A full iron panel consisting of ferritin, total iron binding capacity, transferrin, transferrin saturation, and plasma iron is needed for complete assessment of iron status in a patient with CHD. IV iron may be more effective than oral iron for repletion in heart failure patients.[19]

CHYLOUS EFFUSION MANAGEMENT

Chylothorax, accumulation of lymphatic fluid in the pleural space, can develop after congenital cardiac surgery due to damage of the thoracic duct or collateral lymphatics, elevated central venous pressure, right ventricular dysfunction, or congenital malformations of the lymphatic duct. The overall incidence of chylothorax following surgery ranges between 2.8% and 3.8%.[20] There is a higher incidence of postoperative chylothorax in neonates, single ventricle physiology, chromosomal/genetic anomalies, and major noncardiac anomalies. Chyle is composed of 5 to 30 g/L of fat, 20 to 30 g/L of protein, fat-soluble vitamins, lymphocytes, and electrolytes. Continued chylous drainage can cause electrolyte disturbances, increase risk of infection, and contribute to nutrient losses in the postoperative phase, thus worsening a patient's nutritional state.[20] Chylothorax is diagnosed by pleural fluid analysis, with either a lymphocyte count greater than 80%, a triglyceride concentration greater than 110 mg/dL or the presence of chylomicrons.[20] The absence of a milky fluid appearance does not exclude the diagnosis of chylothorax, especially in fasting patients.

The treatment goal for chylothorax is to cease thoracic lymph flow and allow the lymphatic vessels time to heal.[20] Nutritional interventions to encourage treatment of chylothorax include NPO and PN support or enteral feeding with a fat-modified diet (high medium-chain triglyceride (MCT) formula, skimmed human milk, or a low-fat oral diet). Complete removal of fat is not recommended, as fat is crucial in providing adequate calories for supporting growth and brain development, especially in infants who have a diet high in long-chain triglycerides (LCT).[21] MCTs can reduce lymphatic flow along the thoracic duct, thus decreasing chyle output, as MCTs are absorbed by intestinal cells and directly transported into the portal system without chylomicron formation.[20] Skimmed human milk is a safe and effective option for reducing chylous drainage.[21] Fat is removed from human milk through centrifugation, commercial cream separation, or natural separation techniques, with the refrigerated centrifuge method being the most effective method for fat removal. Once fat is removed, human milk is only 10 to 12 kcal/oz on average, so fortification is needed from MCT-based formulas, sometimes with additional modulars high in MCTs, to provide human milk at an age-appropriate energy density.

A multisite algorithm has been developed to manage chylothorax following CHD surgery to decrease variability in clinical practice and improve clinical outcomes.[22] Recent recommendations are to start treatment with an age-appropriate fat-modified diet for 24 to 72 hours. If unable to feed, NPO status with parental nutrition support is recommended. Intravenous lipid emulsions can also bypass the lymphatic system and enter the bloodstream directly, allowing for adequate fat and calorie intake. After a 24- to 72-hour trial of a fat-modified diet, it is recommended to determine if the chest tube output is high volume (>20 mL/kg/d) or low-volume (≤20 mL/kg/d). If it is high volume, NPO status with PN support is recommended, with considerations for refractory management (surgical or lymphatic evaluation) if chest tube output is still high volume (≥10 mL/kg/d) after 7 days of NPO status. While a 6-week fat-modified diet is the most common one reported in the literature, recent consensus recommendations have noted that chylothorax can resolve in less time. New proposed recommendations are to be on a fat-modified diet 2 to 4 weeks, starting from when enteral feeding or an oral diet has commenced.

Being on a fat-modified diet that provides less than 10% calories from LCTs increases the risk for developing essential fatty acid deficiency.[21] Screening for essential fatty acid deficiency is recommended for patients receiving a fat-modified diet for more than 3 weeks. Lab evidence of fatty acid deficiency occurs earlier than clinical signs and symptoms, which include dry scaly skin, skin lesions, dry dull hair, brittle nails, hair loss, poor wound healing, and poor growth. Essential fatty acid deficiency can be prevented with intakes of 2% to 4% of total calories from linoleic acid and 0.2% to 1% of calories from α-linolenic acid. Oral intake of fat sources rich in linoleic acid and α-linolenic acid, such as sunflower, safflower, corn, soybean, flaxseed, canola, walnut, and fish oils, or intravenous lipid emulsions can prevent the development of essential fatty acid deficiency.[21]

Lab monitoring of other vitamins and minerals is recommended while on a fat-modified diet.[21] Due to concerns for macronutrient and micronutrient losses with large-volume chylous output, some monitoring labs are recommended early on in the fat-modified diet course including albumin, immunoglobulins, and protein-bound minerals (i.e., zinc, copper, and selenium). Being on a fat-modified diet can also increase the risk of fat-soluble vitamin deficiencies, necessitating regular monitoring as well.

■ PROTEIN-LOSING ENTEROPATHY MANAGEMENT

Patients who undergo Fontan palliative cardiac surgery are at risk for developing protein-losing enteropathy (PLE), a syndrome of excessive protein loss into the gastrointestinal tract.[23] The incidence of PLE in the Fontan population is around 4%. While the etiology of PLE post-Fontan is not completely understood, it is felt to be due to a combination of chronic low cardiac output and systemic venous hypertension. Low cardiac output increases mesenteric vascular resistance and leads to decreased intestinal perfusion, compromising gut mucosal integrity. Elevated systemic venous pressures increase lymphatic hydrostatic pressure, thereby increasing lymph production. In patients with PLE, this increased lymphatic pressure is associated with chyle leak into the intestinal lumen, which leads to low serum protein concentration and associated edema, as well as metabolic disturbances and nutritional deficiencies.

Typical clinical manifestations of PLE include chronic diarrhea, abdominal pain, ascites, effusions, and peripheral edema. Symptoms can start from a few weeks to years following the Fontan palliation. Secondary clinical manifestations come from the loss of enteric proteins in the gastrointestinal tract, such as hypocalcemia, sepsis, and growth failure. PLE can be confirmed with detection of an increased α-1-antitrypsin protein level in a spot stool sample or 24-hour collection of stool.

The primary goal of nutrition management for PLE is to decrease the loss of nutritionally rich lymphatic fluid into the intestinal lumen. Reducing intake of dietary LCTs can reduce chyle production and subsequent chyle flow into the intestine. The initial recommendation is for a fat-modified diet in which LCT intake is limited to approximately 10% to 15% of total calories. LCT intake may be increased back slowly as clinical symptoms and nutrition derangements improve. It can be especially difficult to manage PLE in a Fontan patient with malnutrition, as the fat restriction is a barrier to consuming a high calorie diet to support weight gain. To address the reduced energy intake from restricting LCT intake, diets can be supplemented with MCTs. Protein intake is the secondary focus of nutrition management. To address the increased protein losses in the gastrointestinal tract, higher protein intake is recommended (2-3.5 g/kg in infants and children and 1.5-3 g/kg in adolescents).

PLE increases the risk for fat-soluble vitamin deficiencies due to decreased enteral intake, decreased absorption efficiency, and enteric lymphatic loss. Also, when on a LCT restricted diet, patients often need higher doses of fat-soluble vitamin supplementation to overcome inefficient absorption. Vitamin B_{12} concentrations should also be monitored when on a low LCT diet, due to decreased intake of higher fat foods that are rich in vitamin B_{12}, as well as gastrointestinal (GI) malabsorption. Lymphatic losses from PLE also increase the risk of trace mineral deficiencies, such as of iron, zinc and copper, as many of these minerals are bound to albumin. Electrolytes (such as sodium, potassium, chloride, calcium, and phosphate) should also be monitored and supplemented appropriately, due to lymphatic losses and excessive stool losses from PLE. Labs including fat-soluble vitamins, B_{12}, lipid profile, essential fatty acid profile, albumin, trace elements, and iron studies should be evaluated at the time of PLE diagnosis and every 3 to 6 months while treating nutrient deficiencies.

■ TRANSPLANTATION

Heart transplantation is an option for those patients who reach end-stage heart failure. The most common underlying diagnosis in infants younger than 1 year of age is CHD, while in older patients, cardiomyopathy is the predominant diagnosis. Malnutrition is common among pediatric patients at time of heart transplantation.[24] Poor growth pretransplantation has been found to be a risk factor for posttransplantation mortality, as well as decreased time to first rejection, decreased graft survival, and increased graft vasculopathy.[24] Ventricular assist device support has been suggested to be a helpful tool for nutritional rehabilitation pretransplantation, as it can reduce heart failure symptoms and improve hemodynamics, allowing for an increase in dietary intake with a reduction in metabolic demand and nutrient losses. One study found that ventricular assist device (VAD) therapy was associated with a reduced need for enteral feeding support and lower risk for developing a feeding disorder after heart transplant.[25]

There can be rapid increases in weight-for-age z-scores after heart transplantation, especially in the first year. However, stunting can persist, in both patients with single ventricle CHD as well as cardiomyopathy posttransplant.[24] Other identified nutrition complications posttransplantation include hypertension, hyperglycemia, and hyperlipidemia, due to common side effects of posttransplant medications and immunosuppression (Table 19.4). Osteoporosis is common, due to both the suboptimal nutrition status prior to transplant and the decreased calcium absorption and bone formation that result from the use of immunosuppression medications and steroids. It is recommended to draw lipid profiles and hemoglobin A1C values at least once a year to monitor for some of these nutrition complications, as well as trending vitamin D levels at least every 6 to 12 months. Lifestyle intervention, which includes exercise sessions and regular nutrition education, delivered via telehealth has been shown to significantly improve cardiac, vascular, nutritional and functional health in pediatric heart transplant recipients. As with transplant recipients of other organs,

TABLE 19.4 NUTRITION-RELATED SIDE EFFECTS OF COMMON IMMUNOSUPPRESSIVE MEDICATIONS USED IN ORGAN TRANSPLANTATION (ADAPTED FROM BCH PEDIATRIC TRANSPLANT CENTER)

MEDICATION NAME	BRAND NAME	USE	NUTRITION-RELATED SIDE EFFECTS
Prednisone		To prevent onset of early rejection	Moon face, increased appetite, salt/fluid retention, high blood pressure, slowed height growth, osteoporosis
Tacrolimus	Prograf	Immunosuppression	High blood pressure, kidney dysfunction, diabetes, anemia, diarrhea
Mycophenolate mofetil	CellCept, Myfortic	Immunosuppression	Nausea, vomiting, diarrhea, or anemia
Azathioprine	Imuran, Azasan	Immunosuppression	Nausea, vomiting, diarrhea, infection, bruising, or anemia
Sirolimus	Rapamune	Immunosuppression	Increased cholesterol levels, high blood pressure
Cyclosporine	Gengraf, Neoral	Immunosuppression	High blood pressure, kidney dysfunction, diabetes, anemia, mild diarrhea
Bactrim		Antibiotic (for first 6-12 mo)	Nausea

immunosuppressive medications increase the risk of developing foodborne illnesses, so proper education on food safety practices is also important.

SUMMARY

Nutritional provision in children with CHD is complex and requires situational considerations. Growth and nutrition-related issues are highly prevalent and impactful to children with CHD. Assessment of baseline and ongoing nutritional state is important but challenging. EN provision should be prioritized when possible; however, PN in the acute postoperative period is often required to ensure adequate energy and protein intake. Vitamin and micronutrient deficiencies are common in children with CHD and require regular monitoring. The presence of chylous effusions and PLE are disease-specific conditions associated with CHD and not only greatly impact the nutritional state of children with CHD but also are managed by alterations to patient's nutrition prescription. Finally, the diagnosis of malnutrition and nutritional management of pediatric patients with heart failure and following cardiac transplant is of paramount importance. Although great strides have been made to better evaluate and manage growth and nutrition in children with CHD, research and quality improvement efforts are needed to move the field forward.

REFERENCES

1. Diao J, Chen L, Wei J, et al. Prevalence of malnutrition in children with congenital heart disease: a systematic review and meta-analysis. *J Pediatr*. 2022;242:39-47.e4.
2. Anderson JB, Kalkwarf HJ, Kehl JE, Eghtesady P, Marino BS. Low weight-for-age z-score and infection risk after the Fontan procedure. *Ann Thorac Surg*. 2011;91(5):1460-1466.
3. Paparella D, Yau TM, Young E. Cardiopulmonary bypass induced inflammation: pathophysiology and treatment. An update. *Eur J Cardiothorac Surg*. 2002;21(2):232-244.
4. Becker KC, Hornik CP, Cotten CM, et al. Necrotizing enterocolitis in infants with ductal-dependent congenital heart disease. *Am J Perinatol*. 2015;32(7):633-638.
5. Cognata A, Kataria-Hale J, Griffiths P, et al. Human milk use in the preoperative period is associated with a lower risk for necrotizing enterocolitis in neonates with complex congenital heart disease. *J Pediatr*. 2019;215:11-16.e12.
6. Sagiv E, Tjoeng YL, Davis M, et al. Assessing the association between pre-operative feeding and the development of oral feeding skills in infants with single ventricle heart disease: an analysis of the NPC-QIC dataset. *Pediatr Cardiol*. 2022;43(5):1141-1155.
7. Alten JA, Rhodes LA, Tabbutt S, et al. Perioperative feeding management of neonates with CHD: analysis of the Pediatric Cardiac Critical Care Consortium (PC4) registry. *Cardiol Young*. 2015;25(8):1593-1601.
8. Kalra R, Vohra R, Negi M, et al. Feasibility of initiating early enteral nutrition after congenital heart surgery in neonates and infants. *Clin Nutr ESPEN*. 2018;25:100-102.
9. Simsic JM, Carpenito KR, Kirchner K, et al. Reducing variation in feeding newborns with congenital heart disease. *Congenit Heart Dis*. 2017;12(3):275-281.
10. Mehta NM, Skillman HE, Irving SY, et al. Guidelines for the provision and assessment of nutrition support therapy in the pediatric critically ill patient: Society of Critical Care Medicine and American Society for Parenteral and Enteral Nutrition. *JPEN J Parenter Enteral Nutr*. 2017;41(5):706-742.
11. Tume LN, Valla FV, Joosten K, et al. Nutritional support for children during critical illness: European Society of Pediatric and Neonatal Intensive Care (ESPNIC) metabolism, endocrine and nutrition section position statement and clinical recommendations. *Intensive Care Med*. 2020;46(3):411-425.
12. Fivez T, Kerklaan D, Mesotten D, et al. Early versus late parenteral nutrition in critically ill children. *N Engl J Med*. 2016;374(12):1111-1122.
13. Ambrose SE, Ongkasuwan J, Dedhia K, et al. Analysis of vocal fold motion impairment in neonates undergoing congenital heart surgery. *JAMA Otolaryngol Head Neck Surg*. 2018;144(5):406-412.
14. van der Kuip M, Hoos MB, Forget PP, et al. Energy expenditure in infants with congenital heart disease, including a meta-analysis. *Acta Paediatr*. 2003;92(8):921-927.

15. Zhang J, Cui YQ, Luo Y, et al. Assessment of energy and protein requirements in relation to nitrogen kinetics, nutrition, and clinical outcomes in infants receiving early enteral nutrition following cardiopulmonary bypass. *JPEN J Parenter Enteral Nutr*. 2021;45(3):553-566.
16. Al-Subu AM, Long MT, Nelson KL, et al. Risk of hypovitaminosis and vitamin C deficiency in pediatric patients undergoing cardiopulmonary bypass. *Pediatr Cardiol* 2023;44(7):1487-1494.
17. Smithline HA. Thiamine for the treatment of acute decompensated heart failure. *Am J Emerg Med*. 2007;25(1):124-126.
18. Higgins D, Otero J, Jefferis Kirk C, et al. Iron laboratory studies in pediatric patients with heart failure from dilated cardiomyopathy. *Am J Cardiol*. 2017;120(11):2049-2055.
19. Puri K, Spinner JA, Powers JM, et al. Poor efficacy of oral iron replacement therapy in pediatric patients with heart failure. *Cardiol Young*. 2022;32(8):1302-1309.
20. Samanidis G, Kourelis G, Bounta S, et al. Postoperative chylothorax in neonates and infants after congenital heart disease surgery-current aspects in diagnosis and treatment. *Nutrients*. 2022;14(9):1803.
21. Fogg KL, Trauth A, Horsley M, et al. Nutritional management of postoperative chylothorax in children with CHD. *Cardiol Young*. 2023;33(9):1663-1671.
22. Lion RP, Winder MM, Amirnovin R, et al. Development of consensus recommendations for the management of post-operative chylothorax in paediatric CHD. *Cardiol Young*. 2022;32(8):1202-1209.
23. Al Balushi A, Mackie AS. Protein-losing enteropathy following Fontan palliation. *Can J Cardiol*. 2019; 35(12):1857-1860.
24. Rossano JW, Grenier MA, Dreyer WJ, et al. Effect of body mass index on outcome in pediatric heart transplant patients. *J Heart Lung Transplant*. 2007;26(7):718-723.
25. Zook N, Schultz L, Rizzuto S, et al. Supplemental nutrition, feeding disorders, and renourishment in pediatric heart failure through transplantation. *Pediatr Transplant*. 2023;27(8):e14601.

CHAPTER 20

Cystic Fibrosis

Jessica Leonard and Sabina Sabharwal

OVERVIEW AND EPIDEMIOLOGY

Overview

Cystic fibrosis (CF) is an autosomal recessive genetic disorder caused by mutations in the gene that encodes for the CF transmembrane conductance regulator protein (CFTR). The CFTR protein is responsible for chloride ion exchange across cells; a defect in this protein results in the production of abnormally thick secretions from epithelial cells throughout the body. These secretions can clog tubules and airways (e.g., bronchioles and pancreatic ducts) as well as act as a medium for bacterial growth leading to infection and inflammation, primarily in the respiratory tract.

Major clinical manifestations of CF include:

- Chronic pulmonary infections resulting in progressive lung failure
- Malnutrition
- Exocrine pancreatic insufficiency
- CF-related diabetes mellitus (CFRD)
- Constipation
- Distal intestinal obstruction syndrome (DIOS)
- CF hepatobiliary involvement (CFHBI)
- CF-related sinus disease

Epidemiology

In the United States the incidence of CF is approximately 1 in every 4000 live births. CF affects people of all races and ethnic groups but remains most common among White. With the introduction of highly effective modulator therapy (HEMT) over the last decade, patients with CF are living longer. Based on 2023 CF Registry data, the median age of survival for people with CF who were born between 2019 and 2023 is predicted to be 61 years. HEMT and the associated improvement in pulmonary outcomes in CF has brought more attention to gastrointestinal manifestations of CF and to nutritional outcomes such as overweight/obesity, which increase cardiometabolic risk in adulthood.[1] There are now 4 times as many CF patients with a body mass index (BMI) classification of overweight/obese compared to underweight.[2] While improved weight status does not guarantee improvement in lung function, the correlation is strong enough that nutrition is a core discipline of the interdisciplinary CF team. When patients with CF are experiencing a respiratory illnesses, referred to as a CF exacerbation, energy needs increase, which can greatly impact nutritional status.[3]

■ NUTRITIONAL ASSESSMENT AND MONITORING

Nutritional assessment of the patient with CF involves a thorough review of medical history, nutrient intake, medications, laboratory values, and psychosocial and behavioral factors (Table 20.1). Maintaining optimal BMI or weight-for-length status plays an active role in extending CF life expectancy and reducing disease severity. Early diagnosis, coupled with aggressive nutritional interventions, can enhance long-term nutritional status.[4]

Pediatric feeding disorder (PFD) is common in children with CF, with most patients studied qualifying for a diagnosis of PFD based on nutritional factors.[5] The need for enteral nutrition support is a primary influence on this domain's dysfunction. Caregivers of children and adolescents with CF report more disruptive child feeding behaviors, and inappropriate parental responses to these behaviors, than non-CF controls.[6] Behavioral interventions paired with nutrition education are needed to optimize BMI status in children with CF (see Chapter 24).

TABLE 20.1 NUTRITIONAL ASSESSMENT IN CYSTIC FIBROSIS

Medical History

- Pulmonary
  - Number of pulmonary exacerbations
  - Change in pulmonary function tests
- Gastrointestinal
  - History of gastrointestinal disease, meconium ileus, DIOS, intussusception, or gastrointestinal surgery
  - Symptoms of malabsorption (e.g., gas and bloating, frequent, bulky, loose stools, floating, fatty, foul smelling, and frothy stools)
  - Abdominal pain, vomiting, and gastroesophageal reflux
- Endocrine
  - Polyuria, polydipsia, unexplained weight loss, poor growth, steroid use, history of abnormal blood sugars
- Liver disease
  - History of biliary cirrhosis, ascites, or esophageal varices

Growth and Development

- Biological parental height—note on growth chart (Determine mid-parental height [see Chapter 2])
- Measure every 3 mo for children <2 y of age then annually
  - Weight, height/length, and head circumference
- Measure annually
  - Tanner stage; in collaboration with team members

Diet History and Analysis

- Intake history, including total calorie and protein intake, meal patterns, and eating environment
- Percent of total calories from fat and grams of fat per meal
- Food allergies or intolerances
- Baseline appetite and variations during illness
- Use of oral nutritional supplements or tube feeding
- Grams of carbohydrate at meals and snacks if on insulin
- Types and amounts of vitamin supplements
- Use of complementary/alternative medicines
- Food insecurity

(continued)

TABLE 20.1 NUTRITIONAL ASSESSMENT IN CYSTIC FIBROSIS (*continued*)

Medications
Enzymes
Timing and method of pancreatic enzyme administration
Number of enzymes with meals, snacks, and tube feeding
Units of lipase/kg of body weight per day, or units/gram of fat
CFTR modulators
Timing and method of administration
Duration of use; cumulative and per type
Other medications
Antibiotics, acid blockers (H2 antagonists), steroids, and alternative/ complimentary medicines
Biochemical Values (at least annually regardless of exocrine pancreatic function)
Vitamin A (retinol)
• If low, check retinol-binding protein
Vitamin D (25 (OH) D)
Vitamin E (α-tocopherol)
Vitamin K (PIVKA-II, if available, or PT and INR)
Psychosocial
Socioeconomic status, medical insurance, employment, history of depression, anxiety, substance misuse, and social supports
Behavioral
Behaviors around eating/mealtime, positive/negative reinforcement to behavior, stage or readiness for change, history of eating disorder, or disordered eating patterns.

CFTR, cystic fibrosis transmembrane conductance regulator; DIOS, distal intestinal obstruction syndrome; INR, international normalized ratio; PIVKA, proteins induced by vitamin K; PT, prothrombin time.
Borowitz D, Baker RD, Stallings V. Consensus report on nutrition for pediatric patients with cystic fibrosis. *J Pediatr Gastroenterol Nutr.* 2002;35(3):246-259.

In addition, due to CF's intensive focus on diet, nutrition, and growth from an early age, the condition may be a precursor to disordered eating, mental and physical health disturbances, and can progress to an eating disorder. When adolescents and young adults with CF were screened, 10% of participants screened positive for an eating disorder on the Eating Disorder Examination Questionnaire (EDE-Q)[7] (see Chapter 23).

■ MALNUTRITION

Nutritional goals for pediatric patients with CF are to promote normal growth and development through the provision of adequate nutrients. The Cystic Fibrosis Foundation (CFF) recommends using weight-for-length or BMI percentile to assess nutritional status in CF. Weight, supine length or standing height, and head circumference (in patients <2 years corrected age) should be measured regularly and plotted on the pediatric growth chart "according to the regular practice in the country or (CF) center."[8] Increased monitoring is needed when poor growth trajectory or growth faltering occur. To maintain optimal health, the CFF recommends a goal of a weight-for-length greater than or equal to 50th percentile for children less than 2 years and BMI greater than or equal to 50th percentile for children aged 2 to 18 years. In patients over

18 years old, the goal BMI is 22 kg/m^2 for females and 23 kg/m^2 for males.[8] These goals were established based on their correlation with improved lung function at these anthropometric classifications. Obtaining mid-upper arm circumference and triceps' skinfold thickness can help classify nutritional status by categorizing the body composition of patients with CF (see Chapter 2).

Patients with CF can experience poor appetite from pulmonary exacerbations, symptoms of malabsorption, constipation, DIOS, zinc deficiency, hyponatremia, depression, eating disorders, CFRD, sinusitis/nasal polyps, delayed gastric emptying, and gastroesophageal reflux disease. When these causes have been ruled out and/or treated, appetite stimulants may be used to improve nutritional status. Cyproheptadine hydrochloride is commonly used as an appetite stimulant, although some individuals have reported fatigue and irritability. This medication is commonly used cycled (e.g., 3 weeks on and 1 week off) to prevent tachyphylaxis and is normally well tolerated.[9]

PANCREATIC INSUFFICIENCY

Diagnosis

According to the 2023 CF patient registry, 81.1% of the CF population receives pancreatic enzyme replacement therapy.[10] A 72-hour fecal fat balance test, while laborious, is the gold standard for determining the degree of fat malabsorption. It is defined as follows:

$$\text{CFA (\%)} = 100 \times ([\text{grams fat intake} - \text{grams fat excretion}]/\text{grams fat intake})$$

The fecal elastase-1 test is a highly sensitive and specific way to indirectly measure severe exocrine pancreatic insufficiency (EPI). The amount of pancreatic elastase in stool is representative of the pancreas producing enzymes. Patients with a fecal elastase greater than 200 μg/g of stool classify as normal, 100 to 200 μg/g classify as having moderate EPI, and less than 100 μg/g classify as having severe EPI.[11] In mild EPI, fecal elastase testing may not be as useful, and results should be interpreted with this consideration.

Fat Intake and Metabolism

Observational studies from the 1960s support the importance of avoiding dietary fat restriction and instead offering a high-fat diet. Current recommendations are requiring re-alignment as the patient population experiences widespread use of HEMT, and patients with CF are now represented along the full spectrum of BMI classifications. The CF Foundation Patient Registry Report showed an increase in average BMI percentile for age 2 to 19 from 49.4% in 2008 to 61.2% in 2023, and an increase in the frequency of BMI equal to, or above, the 95th percentile from 3.3% in 2008 to 8.1% in 2023.[10]

Medium-chain triglycerides (MCT) require less lipase than long-chain fats for absorption and are found in infant and enteral formulas as well as in individual supplements. They are not a source of essential fatty acids and can be expensive and unpalatable.

Essential Fatty Acid Deficiency

Low plasma levels of essential fatty acids are seen in patients with CF, although symptoms of essential fatty acid deficiency (EFAD) are rare. It has been proposed that

EFAD is due to impaired fatty acid metabolism in CF rather than malabsorption of fat caused by EPI; however, the root cause of EFAD observed in CF remains unclear.[12] The Consensus Report on Nutrition for Pediatric Patients with CF suggests the use of linolenic acid-rich foods and supplements as a source of energy, in addition to the promotion of human milk, which is rich in docosahexaenoic acid (DHA). Although some studies have suggested that omega-3 fatty acid supplements offer theoretical anti-inflammatory advantages, not enough research exists to make recommendations for supplementation in CF.[8] If patients are taking omega-3 or fish oil supplements, it is important to increase the dosage of pancreatic enzymes to compensate for the fat content of these supplements.[13]

Pancreatitis

People with CF who develop pancreatitis are generally pancreatic sufficient, and 20% of these patients will develop acute pancreatitis (AP).[14] Management revolves around early intravenous fluid resuscitation. Early enteral refeeding by oral or nasogastric access is recommended (over parenteral nutrition) in both children and adults with pancreatitis and may reduce the risk of infectious complications. There remains little to no evidence that a low-fat diet compared to a general well-balanced and healthy diet is helpful in patients with pancreatitis. Further, interpretation of a low-fat diet differs by dietitians, and a lower fat dietary intake during mild AP attacks does not improve pain scores or length of hospitalization.[15] Children with acute recurrent and chronic pancreatitis need ongoing assessment for growth and nutritional deficiencies, including exocrine and endocrine insufficiencies.

■ PANCREATIC ENZYME REPLACEMENT THERAPY

Dosing and Administration

Malabsorption in CF can be in the range of 5% to 20% of gross energy intake, even in the presence of pancreatic enzyme replacement therapy (compared to <5% among healthy children). Individuals with pancreatic insufficiency take oral pancreatic enzymes to aid in absorption and digestion. These gelatin capsules contain mini-microspheres of lipase, amylase, and protease that are usually porcine derived[16] (see Table 20.2).

Enzyme dosages are prescribed in units of lipase per kilogram of body weight per meal or snack, or can be prescribed based on units of lipase per gram of fat consumed (Figure 20.1).[16,17] Dosage is titrated based on symptoms of steatorrhea and/or coefficient of fat absorption, though the latter is not often utilized. Enzymes available in the United States are listed in Table 20.2. The CF Foundation does not recommend the use of generic enzymes that may not be equivalent to brand enzymes.

High dosages of pancreatic enzymes have historically been associated with fibrosing colonopathy, an inflammatory condition of the large intestine of unclear etiology. Recommended maximum pancreatic enzyme dosing is 2500 units of lipase/kg/meal and 10,000 units of lipase/kg/d although some CF patients require higher dosages to adequately treat signs and symptoms of malabsorption and promote weight gain.[18] See Figure 20.1 for more info.

TABLE 20.2 ENTERIC-COATED PANCREATIC ENZYMES

ENZYME	COMPANY	BEAD SIZE (MM)	OPTIMAL DISSOLUTION PH	LIPASE USP UNITS	PROTEASE USP UNITS	AMYLASE USP UNITS
Creon 3	Abbott	<1.7	<5.5	3000	9500	15,000
Creon 6	Abbott	<1.7	<5.5	6000	19,000	30,000
Creon 12	Abbott	<1.7	<5.5	12,000	38,000	60,000
Creon 24	Abbott	<1.7	<5.5	24,000	76,000	120,000
Pancreaze MT4	Janssen Pharmaceuticals, Inc.	<3	<5.5	4200	10,000	17,500
Pancreaze MT10	Janssen Pharmaceuticals, Inc.	<3	<5.5	10,500	25,000	43,750
Pancreaze MT16	Janssen Pharmaceuticals, Inc.	<3	<5.5	16,800	40,000	70,000
Pancreaze MT 21	Janssen Pharmaceuticals, Inc.	<3	<5.5	21,000	37,000	61,000
Zenpep (3)	Aptalis	1.8-1.9	<5.5	3000	10,000	16,000
Zenpep (5)	Aptalis	1.8-1.9	<5.5	5000	17,000	27,000
Zenpep (10)	Aptalis	2.2-2.5	<5.5	10,000	34,000	55,000
Zenpep (15)	Aptalis	2.2-2.5	<5.5	15,000	51,000	82,000
Zenpep (20)	Aptalis	2.2-2.5	<5.5	20,000	68,000	109,000
Zenpep (25)	Aptalis	2.2-2.5	<5.5	25,000	85,000	136,000
Ultresa 13,800	Aptalis	2-2.4	<5.5	13,800	27,600	27,600
Ultresa 20,700	Aptalis	2-2.4	<5.5	20,700	41,400	41,400

(*continued*)

TABLE 20.2 GLUTEN-FREE DIET GUIDELINES (*continued*)

ENZYME	COMPANY	BEAD SIZE (MM)	OPTIMAL DISSOLUTION PH	LIPASE USP UNITS	PROTEASE USP UNITS	AMYLASE USP UNITS
Ultresa 23,000	Aptalis	2-2.4	<5.5	23,000	46,000	46,000
Viokace 10,440	Aptalis	Tablet	<5.5	10,440	39,150	39,150
Viokace 22,880	Aptalis	Tablet	<5.5	22,880	78,300	78,300
Pertzye 8000[a]	Digestive Care, Inc.	0.8-2.2	<5.5	8000	28,750	30,250
Pertzye 16,000[a]	Digestive Care, Inc.	0.8-2.2	<5.5	16,000	57,500	60,500

[a]**Bicarbonate**-buffered enteric-coated microspheres.

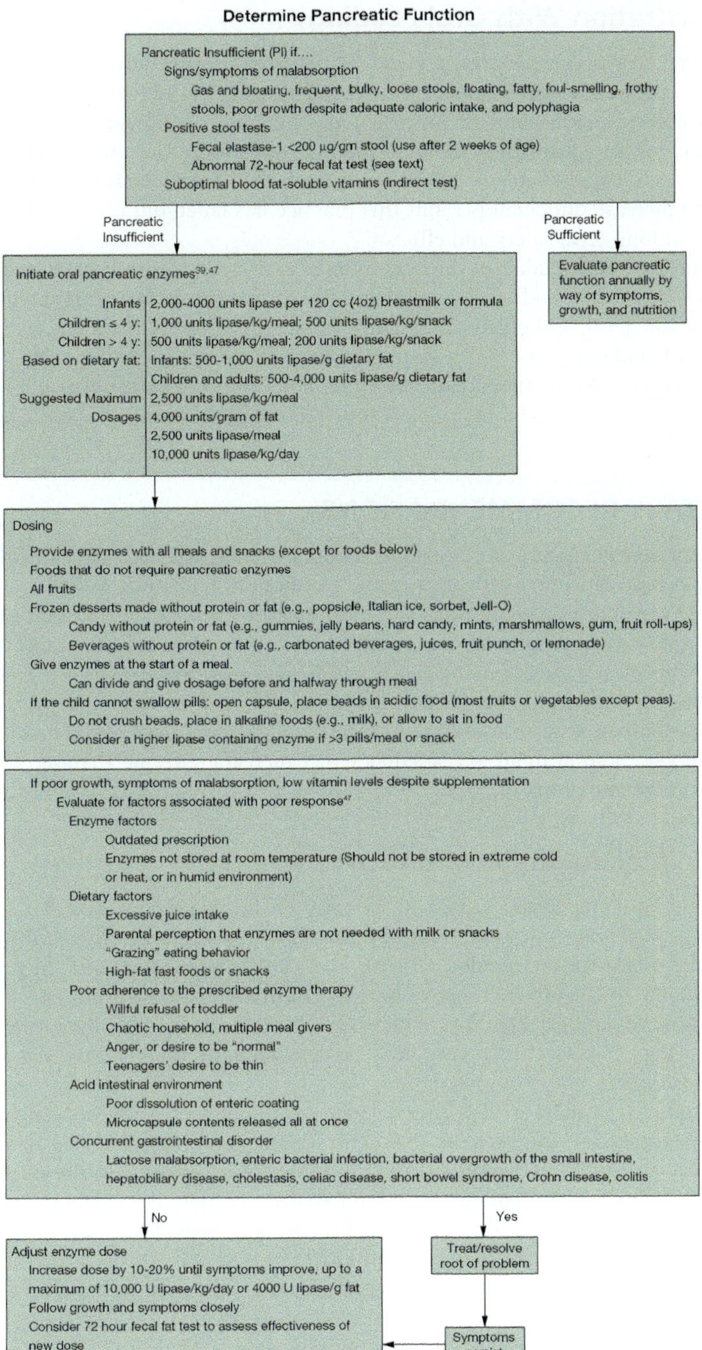

Figure 20.1 Dosing and adjusting pancreatic enzyme treatment in CF. (Data from van der Haak N, King SJ, Crowder T, et al. Highlights from the nutrition guidelines for cystic fibrosis in Australia and New Zealand. *J Cyst Fibros*. 2020;19[1]:16-25; Borowitz DS, Grand RJ, Durie PR. Use of pancreatic enzyme supplements for patients with cystic fibrosis in the context of fibrosing colonopathy. Consensus Committee. *J Pediatr*. 1995;127[5]:681-684.)

Administration With Oral Feedings

The enteric coating on pancreatic enzymes prevents inactivation of enzymes in the acidic environment of the stomach. Once in the higher pH of the upper small intestine, the enteric coating breaks down and the enzymes are released. Poor bicarbonate production in CF leads to an abnormally acidic pH in the duodenum, reducing enzyme effectiveness. Acid blocking medications had therefore been routinely prescribed to increase duodenal pH, but this practice has fallen out of favor due to concerns about long-term safety and efficacy.[19]

Enzymes should be taken at the beginning of each oral meal and snack. Infants and children who cannot swallow capsules should take the beads coated in applesauce or another acidic food, and given orally with a spoon.[20] It is important to sweep the infant's mouth and chin for enzyme beads, as they can cause skin and mouth irritation. Foods that do not require pancreatic enzymes include popsicles, fruit snacks, and fruit juice; however, these foods are typically low in energy and nutritional value.

DIETARY RECOMMENDATIONS

Nutritional management and counseling are an essential aspect of CF care, given the correlation between nutritional status and pulmonary outcomes as well as the impact that gastrointestinal symptoms can have on patients with CF. The 2024 updated CFF CF care model recommends a reduced frequency of in-person clinic visits for patients who are not experiencing severe pulmonary exacerbations or CF comorbidities, while recommending that all patients should be seen at least once per year by a registered dietitian who can analyze accurate anthropometric measurements, assess dietary intake, help evaluate the adequacy of pancreatic enzyme therapy, and make dietary recommendations.[21]

Energy Intake and Expenditure

Resting energy expenditure (REE) in CF may be influenced by pancreatic insufficiency, type of genetic mutation, stage of pulmonary infection, severity of lung disease, degree of malabsorption, gender, CFHBI, and CFRD. Studies on REE in CF found levels from 4% to 20% above those of healthy controls or predicted values.[22,23] In presymptomatic CF, energy expenditure may be closer to normal, while hypermetabolism is seen during CF exacerbations and may be dependent on the severity lung disease[24] (see Table 20.3).

Traditionally patients with CF have been recommended to follow a high energy, high protein, high fat, and high salt diet, with weight gain prioritized over diet quality. CF physiology continues to support the need for diet monitoring in these areas, and the diet recommended for patients on HEMT has been updated to reflect the goal of an age-appropriate healthy diet that promotes healthy outcomes. This shift is the result of patients on HEMT who have experienced a reduction in the energy intake needed to achieve their growth goals, a decrease in gut inflammation, and decrease in fat malabsorption defined as changes in coefficient of fat absorption (CFA%).[25] A personalized nutritional approach is the new standard that recognizes the needs of each individual patient, their growth stage, and if they are ineligible for HEMT and may require higher energy intake.

TABLE 20.3 DIAGNOSTIC CRITERIA FOR CYSTIC FIBROSIS-RELATED DIABETES

Tests Used to Diagnose Cystic Fibrosis-Related Diabetes (CFRD)

TEST		RESULTS	DIAGNOSIS	NEXT STEPS
Oral glucose tolerance test (OGTT)	Done in the morning after an 8-h fast	2-h glucose ≥200 mg/dL (≥11.1 mmol/L)	CFRD	You will be followed by your CF and endocrinology team and may be treated with insulin.
		2-h glucose 140-199 mg/dL (7.8-11.0 mmol/L)	*Impaired glucose tolerance (IGT)*	You are at higher risk for developing diabetes; you will be closely monitored by your CF team. Repeat OGTT annually or earlier if symptoms occur.
		Mid-OGTT glucose ≥200 mg/dL (≥11.1 mmol/L). OGTT otherwise normal	*Indeterminate glycemia (INDET)*	You are at higher risk for developing diabetes; you will be closely monitored by your CF team. Repeat OGTT annually or earlier if symptoms occur.
		2-h glucose <140 mg/dL (<7.8 mmol/L)	Normal	Repeat OGTT annually.
Fasting blood glucose	Done first thing in the morning after an 8-h fast	<100 mg/dL (<5.6 mmol/L)	Normal	Starting at age 10, or earlier if symptoms occur, do OGTT annually.
		100-125 mg/dL (5.6-6.9 mmol/L)	*Impaired fasting glucose (IFG)*	You are more likely to develop diabetes; you will be closely monitored by your CF team. Repeat OGTT annually or earlier if symptoms occur.
		≥126 mg/dL (≥7.0 mmol/L)	CFRD	You will be followed by your CF and endocrinology team and may be treated with insulin.
Casual (random) blood glucose	Done at any time regardless of time of last meal or snack	<200 mg/dL (11.1 mmol/L)	*Nondiagnostic*	Starting at age 10, or earlier if symptoms occur, do OGTT annually.
		≥200 mg/dL (≥11.1 mmol/L)	High risk of CFRD	If symptoms are present, do a fasting blood glucose test; otherwise, do OGTT.
Hemoglobin A1c (HbA1c)	Done at any time regardless of time of the meal or snack. Typically done at 3 mo intervals once diabetes is diagnosed	>6.5%	CFRD	This test should not be solely used for screening since a normal test could miss cases of CFRD. However, if the level is above 6.5%, then this is diagnostic.

Benge T, Brunzell C, Elshaar N, Moran A, Sandouk Z. *Managing Cystic Fibrosis-Related Diabetes (CFRD): An Instruction Guide for Parents and Families.* Cystic Fibrosis Foundation; 2023.

Carbohydrates and Cystic Fibrosis-Related Diabetes

Increased CF life expectancy, as well as the aging patient population, has made CFRD the most common complications in patients with CF with an overall prevalence of 19%.[10] CFRD manifests with characteristics of both type 1 (insulin insufficiency) and type 2 (insulin resistant) diabetes. Insulin resistance can worsen during illness and steroid treatment.[26] CFRD may present similarly to type I or type II diabetes (polydipsia, polyuria, weight loss/poor growth, fatigue, unexplained decline in lung function, increased pulmonary exacerbations or infections), but ketoacidosis is rare.

The CF Foundation regularly updates and publishes *Managing Cystic Fibrosis-Related Diabetes (CFRD) An Instruction Guide for Patients and Families,* which outlines the current recommendations on the testing, treatment, monitoring, and education needs of patients with CFRD. These care guidelines recommend screening for CFRD beginning at age 10 with an oral glucose tolerance test (OGTT) and regularly monitoring hemoglobin A1c (HbA1c) trends. Diagnostic criteria for CFRD can be found in Table 20.3.

The American Diabetes Association and the CF Foundation recommend the use of insulin to treat CFRD.[18] Patients should meet with a dietitian at the time of diagnosis and thereafter to obtain education on carbohydrate counting and the effect of oral intake on blood sugars. The diet recommendations for CFRD are based on the personalized nutritional goals of the patient. Carbohydrates, proteins, and fats should all be in the diet and the amounts are largely based on the patient's weight goals. Sugar-sweetened beverages and simple sugars should be limited in the diet, and foods high in carbohydrates are best ingested along with fat and protein-containing foods to provide a mixed meal profile.

Complications of diabetes such as retinopathy, microalbuminuria, chronic renal insufficiency, peripheral neuropathy, and severe hypoglycemia are uncommon (see Chapter 22).

Protein

Due to nitrogen losses in the presence of pancreatic insufficiency, children with CF have been estimated to need at least 1.5 to 2 times the Dietary Reference Intake (DRI) for protein for age, which is usually met if energy goals are being met.[27]

Human Milk and Infant Formulas

Human milk, with appropriate enzyme replacement therapy, is optimal for infants with CF.[28] Routine CF infant care does not require the use of specialized formulas (semi-elemental, elemental, or high MCT) though other clinical factors may indicate their use.[29] Human milk and formula can be made at higher calorie concentrations, either by the use of formula or high-calorie additives, with the goal of promoting age-appropriate weight gain. All formulas, including protein hydrolysates, require pancreatic enzymes. The amount of pancreatic enzymes to administer will vary with the fat profile of the formula and the patient's volume of intake.

Oral Nutrition Supplements

A variety of commercially available oral nutrition supplements may be utilized to help patients with CF meet their calorie needs. Patients with CF using oral supplements should be monitored to make sure that the supplements complement intake of regular food, rather than replacing it.[12] Pancreatic enzymes are required for oral nutrition supplements (see Chapter 16).

Enteral Nutrition Therapy

When oral intake fails to achieve weight gain goals, enteral tube feedings should be considered as a tool to promote weight gain.[30] It is important to begin discussions about enteral nutrition therapy before moderate or severe malnutrition is diagnosed.

The 2016 CF Foundation evidence-informed guideline on enteral tube feeds for individuals with CF states, "The CF Foundation recommends enteral tube feeding as a means to improve age-dependent anthropometrics in individuals with CF that are unable to consume adequate calories and protein to meet growth/weight maintenance goals, despite appropriate evaluation and intervention by the multidisciplinary team."[30] The type of enteral access varies based on the patient's needs, degree of pulmonary disease, and gastrointestinal history and complications. Overnight tube feedings are recommended to promote maintenance of oral intake during the day and should provide 30% to 50% of the patient's estimated energy needs[12] (refer to Chapter 16).

PANCREATIC ENZYME REPLACEMENT THERAPY ADMINISTRATION WITH ENTERAL FEEDINGS

Pancreatic enzymes are required for all formulas. Amino acid-based and protein hydrolysate formulas (which may contain medium chain fats) may require a lower dose of pancreatic enzymes than formulas with higher amounts of long-chain fats. The general recommendation is to give a meal dose of enzymes at the beginning of the feed and a meal dose at the end of the feed. It is preferable to take enzymes by mouth with tube feedings. Most methods for administering enzymes with tube feedings when a patient is unable to take the capsules orally have not been well studied.

One method for patients with a gastrostomy tube (GT) is to open the enzyme capsules, crushing the beads with a pill crusher, and mixing them directly into the formula. The formula must sit for 30 to 45 minutes, occasionally agitating the mixture before infusing. For jejunostomy tube (JT) feeds, the crushed enzymes can be dissolved in a small volume of sodium bicarbonate, to mimic the intestinal environment, and either flushed via the JT or added to the formula bag and mixed before infusing.[27] Avoid mucus membrane exposure to crushed enzyme powders. The enteral feeding bag containing the enzymes mixed with the formula may only hang for 4 hours.

Immobilized Lipase Cartridge

Patients can also use the Relizorb immobilized lipase cartridge if their formula regimen is compatible. This in-line cartridge is attached to the enteral feeding bag tubing and when the formula flows through the cartridge the fat is hydrolyzed by the lipase beads in the cartridge. Manufacturer guidelines dictate the compatibility of formulas and feeding regimens.[31] One advantage for overnight or continuous feeds is that increasing fat hydrolysis can contribute to a reduction in feelings of fullness and discomfort with enteral tube feeding for patients with EPI.[32] Of note, only the fat in the formula is hydrolyzed when the Relizorb immobilized lipase cartridge is used as stand-alone treatment. If enzymes have been added to the feed bag the mixture can not be infused through the cartridge.

NUTRITIONAL SUPPLEMENTS

Vitamin and Mineral Supplementation

Supplementation of fat-soluble vitamins is recommended for all patients with CF who have pancreatic insufficiency. CF-formulated vitamins provide water-miscible forms of the fat-soluble vitamins A, D, E, and K. Serum vitamins A, E, and 25-hydroxyvitamin D should be measured at diagnosis and annually[12] (see Table 20.4).

If serum concentrations indicate deficiency, compliance and financial ability to obtain vitamins should be reviewed before initiating additional supplementation. If additional supplementation is initiated, serum levels should be repeated 1 to 2 months later.

Vitamin toxicity can occur with high dose supplement use. Vitamin A toxicity is more likely to occur with increasing plasma levels of retinyl esters, and laboratory measurements of these esters are the most direct way to assess overdosage of retinol supplements. Excess free retinol may also be diagnosed by measuring the molar ratio of retinol-to-retinol binding protein. A serum vitamin A level should not be measured if the patient has evidence of inflammation, as vitamin A is a negative acute phase reactant.[12]

Since serum vitamin K levels do not reflect vitamin K stores, Vitamin K is traditionally evaluated indirectly via plasma prothrombin concentrations (PT). If PT is prolonged, then supplementation would be recommended. The PIVKA-II (Proteins Induced by vitamin K Absence or Antagonist-II) is a more sensitive indicator of vitamin K status and is considered the gold standard for assessing vitamin K status but is not universally available for clinical use.[12] Additional vitamin K may be required with CFHBI and/or prolonged antibiotic use.[1,27]

Serum 25-hydroxyvitamin D (25(OH)D) remains the optimal lab value to assess vitamin D status. If deficiency is identified, additional supplementation may be required. The CF Foundation recommends cholecalciferol for treatment of vitamin D deficiency in CF. It is recommended to measure 25(OH)D annually during the winter months, and re-checking 25(OH)D after 3 months of increased dosage.[33] The recommendations for vitamin D supplementation and stepwise treatment of low vitamin D status are summarized in Table 20.5.

Salt Homeostasis

Given the relatively low amount of sodium in human milk, infant formulas, and some baby foods, infants with CF should receive table salt added to formula or to the applesauce used to give enzymes. From birth to 6 months of age, ¼ teaspoon (13 mEq) of salt should be given daily, and from 6 months to 1-year ¼ teaspoon (26 mEq) of salt should be given daily. For growth failure, patients can be adjusted to receive 2 to 4 mEq/kg of sodium per day.[12]

TABLE 20.4 NUTRITIONAL MANAGEMENT IN CYSTIC FIBROSIS

DIET		HIGH CALORIE, HIGHER FAT
Calories		1.2-2 × DRI for age
Protein		1.5-2 × DRI for age
Fat		35%-40% total calories
Essential fatty acids		3%-5% of total calories
Vitamin A		
	0–12 mo:	1500 IU/d
	1-3 y:	5000 IU/d
	4-8 y:	5000-10,000 IU/d
	>8 y:	10,000 IU/d
Vitamin D—Cholecalciferol		
	0-12 mo:	10 μg/d
	1-3 y:	10-20 μg/d
	4-8 y:	20-50 μg/d
	>8 y:	20-50 μg/d
Vitamin E		
	0-12 mo:	40-50 IU/d
	1-3 y:	80-150 IU/d
	4-8 y:	100-200 IU/d
	>8 y:	200-400 IU/d
Vitamin K		At least 0.3-0.5 mg/d
Calcium		DRI
	0-6 mo:	200 mg[a]
	7-12 mo:	260 mg[a]
	1-3 y:	700 mg
	4-8 y:	1000 mg
	9-13 y:	1300 mg
	14-18 y:	1300 mg
Iron		DRI unless deficient
Sodium		Increased needs at times of sweating and during hot weather.
	0-6 mo:	13 mEq/d (1/8 teaspoon salt)
	7-12 mo:	26 mEq/d (1/4 teaspoon salt)
	Children/adolescents:	At least the DRI
Water-soluble vitamins		At least the DRI
Zinc		DRI unless deficient Consider 6 mo trial of zinc supplementation if poor growth or stunting

DRI, Dietary Reference Intakes (see Chapter 10).
[a]Adequate intake rather than Recommended Dietary Allowance.
Borowitz D, Baker RD, Stallings V. Consensus report on nutrition for pediatric patients with cystic fibrosis. *J Pediatr Gastroenterol Nutr*. 2002;35(3):246-259.

TABLE 20.5 STEPWISE THERAPY FOR VITAMIN D DEFICIENCY

AGE	ROUTINE DOSING OF CF-SPECIFIC VITAMINS	STEP 1: IF 25(OH)D <30 NG/ML[A]	STEP 2: IF STILL <30 NG/ML[A]	STEP 3: IF STILL <30 NG/ML
Birth-12 mo	10-12.5 µg/d	20-25 µg/d	Not >50 µg/d	Refer to Endocrinologist
> 12 mo-10 years	20-25 µg/d	40-75 µg/d	Not >100 µg/d	Refer to Endocrinologist
> 10-18 y	20-50 µg/d	400-150 µg/d	Not >250 µg/d	Refer to Endocrinologist

[a]Recheck 3 months after dose increase.
From Tangpricha V, Kelly A, Stephenson A, et al. An update on the screening, diagnosis, management, and treatment of vitamin D deficiency in individuals with cystic fibrosis: evidence-based by permission of Oxford University recommendations from the Cystic Fibrosis Foundation. *J Clin Endocrinol Metab.* 2012;97(4):1082-1093.

When patients are over 1 year, transition to a liberal salt diet is recommended. Use of HEMT modulators has produced normalization of sweat chloride for some patients and therefore they require a personalized recommendation based on assessment of their sodium balance.

■ BONE DISEASE

Low bone mineral density (BMD) may begin in childhood with osteopenia defined as BMD that falls one standard deviation below normal, and osteoporosis defined as bone mineral density that falls greater than or equal to 2 standard deviations below normal. Osteopenia is found in 28%, and osteoporosis is found in 10% to 34% of children with CF.[34] Low BMD occurs in 50% to 70% of adults with CF[2] and is also common after lung transplantation.[35]

CF-bone disease (CFBD) is multifactorial and may be due to a range of issues, including altered sex hormone production, inflammation, physical inactivity, glucocorticoid therapy, malnutrition, low calcium intake, and malabsorption of vitamin D. Dual energy x-ray absorptiometry (DXA) is the gold standard for assessment of CFBD. Recommendations for management of CFBD include increased weight-bearing exercise, and supplementation with calcium, vitamin D, and vitamin K. Bisphosphonate therapy should be considered in pediatric CF patients who have osteoporosis and have failed conservative therapy[36] (see Table 20.6).

■ CYSTIC FIBROSIS HEPATOBILIARY INVOLVEMENT

Cystic fibrosis hepatobiliary involvement (CFHBI) covers a spectrum of liver involvement in CF, including elevated liver enzymes, neonatal cholestasis, and gallbladder, and biliary tract disorders. The incidence of severe CF liver disease in the pediatric population is 5% to 10% and is marked by biliary cirrhosis and portal hypertension.[37]

Patients with a severe phenotype of liver disease are at risk for malnutrition, including micro- and macronutrient deficiencies.[38] Gastrointestinal issues related

TABLE 20.6 NUTRITIONAL RECOMMENDATIONS FOR PREVENTION AND TREATMENT OF BONE DISEASE IN CYSTIC FIBROSIS

- Screen children >8 y old with risk factors and adults for bone disease by DXA. If bone mineral density (BMD) is normal, re-screen every 5 y or sooner if change in risk factors: IBW <90% or BMI <25th percentile, FEV1 <50%, glucocorticoids >5 mg/d for >90 d out of the year, delayed puberty, or a history of fractures.

  Normal – Children: z-score = 0 ± 1 SD
  Adults: T-score = 0 ± 1 SD
  Moderate Demineralization= T-score or z-score between −1.0 and −2.0; Repeat DXA every 2-4 y.
  Severe Demineralization = T-score or z-score <−2.0; repeat DXA yearly

- *Weight*: Maintain at ≥90% IBW or 25th percentile BMI
- *Calcium*: At least the Dietary Reference Intake (DRI)/age
- *Vitamin D*: Monitor annually in all age groups (at the end of the Winter months). Supplement to achieve a serum 25(OH)D >30 ng/mL.
- *Vitamin K*: 0.3-0.5 mg vitamin K per day
- *Other minerals*: At least the DRI for magnesium, zinc and copper
- *Exercise*: Foster weight-bearing exercise
- *Medications*: pamidronate, and IV bisphosphonate under study in adults with CF. No data in children.

BMI, body mass index; DXA, dual energy x-ray absorptiometry; IBW, ideal body weight.
Use of z-scores is recommended in children aged 18 and under. Data from Sermet-Gaudelus I, Castanet M, Retsch-Bogart G, Aris RM. Update on cystic fibrosis-related bone disease: a special focus on children. *Paediatr Respir Rev.* 2009;10(3):134-142.

to this include increased energy expenditure, malabsorption, and decreased oral intake in the setting or early satiety and delayed gastric emptying from abdominal distension (hepatosplenomegaly, ascites).[39] A multidisciplinary team (including gastroenterologists and experienced dietitians) is key to the management of severe liver disease in CF. Guidelines include a need for higher daily calories up to 130% to 150% of the estimated requirement for age, preferably by increasing the proportion of dietary fat to 40% to 50%, with supplementation in MCT and polyunsaturated fatty acids.[18] It is important to ensure adequate daily protein intake, pancreatic enzymes to optimize fat absorption, and fat-soluble vitamins and zinc, to prevent deficiency. Frequent monitoring is important to prevent vitamin toxicity. Although salt supplementation is common in CF patients, it should be avoided for those with cirrhosis and portal hypertension due to the risk of developing or worsening ascites.

NUTRITION FOR CYSTIC FIBROSIS TRANSMEMBRANE CONDUCTANCE REGULATOR MODULATOR THERAPY

HEMT is a class of oral medications that improve the function of the CFTR protein. HEMT is associated with weight gain in CF.[40] This weight gain is multifactorial: HEMT may improve appetite, improve respiratory function with decreased energy expenditure, and result in thinned mucous secretions, which may improve nutrient absorption. In younger CF patients, HEMT is associated with reversal of EPI and improved absorption of nutrients.[41] As previously noted, CF adults are at higher risk of overweight/obesity than in the past. This has resulted in a shift in nutritional management of CF patients which has broadly supported a high-calorie and high-fat diet, resulting in diets of low nutrient quality and the presence of obesity comorbidities in adults with CF, including hypertension and insulin resistance.

CONCLUSION

The relationship between nutrition and CF is well defined. Individuals with CF benefit from early and aggressive nutritional intervention to prevent malnutrition and to ensure longer and healthier lives. However, in this new age of HEMT, with longer patient survival and attention to issues such as overweight/obesity, it is also important to consider the quality of high-calorie foods with attention to nutrient density, in order to prevent adverse cardiometabolic complications long-term. This requires a more individualized weight-neutral approach to patient nutrition, with a greater focus on body composition and health outcomes versus actual body weight.

REFERENCES

1. Leonard A, Bailey J, Bruce A, et al. Nutritional considerations for a new era: a CF foundation position paper. *J Cyst Fibros*. 2023;22(5):788-795.
2. McDonald CM, Alvarez JA, Bailey J, et al. Academy of Nutrition and Dietetics: 2020 cystic fibrosis evidence analysis center evidence-based nutrition practice guideline. *J Acad Nutr Diet*. 2021;121(8): 1591-1636.e3.
3. Zemel BS, Kawchak DA, Cnaan A, Zhao H, Scanlin TF, Stallings VA. Prospective evaluation of resting energy expenditure, nutritional status, pulmonary function, and genotype in children with cystic fibrosis. *Pediatr Res*. 1996;40(4):578-586.
4. Farrell PM, Kosorok MR; Wisconsin Cystic Fibrosis Neonatal Screening Study Group, et al. Nutritional benefits of neonatal screening for cystic fibrosis. *N Engl J Med*. 1997;337(14):963-969.
5. Bashir A, Antos N, Miller T, et al. A cross-sectional study of pediatric feeding disorder in children with cystic fibrosis. *J Pediatr Gastroenterol Nutr*. 2023;77(6):819-823.
6. Duff AJ, Wolfe SP, Dickson C, Conway SP, Brownlee KG. Feeding behavior problems in children with cystic fibrosis in the UK: prevalence and comparison with healthy controls. *J Pediatr Gastroenterol Nutr*. 2003;36(4):443-447.
7. Kass AP, Berbert L, Dahlberg S, et al. Eating disorders in adolescents and young adults with cystic fibrosis. *Pediatr Pulmonol*. 2022;57(11):2791-2797.
8. Wilschanski M, Munck A, Carrion E, et al. ESPEN-ESPGHAN-ECFS guideline on nutrition care for cystic fibrosis. *Clin Nutr*. 2024;43(2):413-445.
9. Nasr SZ, Drury D. Appetite stimulants use in cystic fibrosis. *Pediatr Pulmonol*. 2008;43(3):209-219.
10. Cystic Fibrosis Foundation. *Cystic Fibrosis Foundation Patient Registry Report. 2023 Annual Data Report*. Cystic Fibrosis Foundation; 2023.
11. Labs MC. Pancreatic elastase, feces. Mayo Clinic Labs. 2021. https://www.mayocliniclabs.com/test-catalog/overview/609492
12. Borowitz D, Baker RD, Stallings V. Consensus report on nutrition for pediatric patients with cystic fibrosis. *J Pediatr Gastroenterol Nutr*. 2002;35(3):246-259.
13. Shamseer L, Adams D, Brown N, Johnson JA, Vohra S. Antioxidant micronutrients for lung disease in cystic fibrosis. *Cochrane Database Syst Rev*. 2010;(12):CD007020.
14. Abu-El-Haija M, Kumar S, Quiros JA, et al. Management of acute pancreatitis in the pediatric population: a clinical report from the North American Society for Pediatric Gastroenterology, Hepatology and Nutrition Pancreas Committee. *J Pediatr Gastroenterol Nutr*. 2018;66(1):159-176.
15. Abu-El-Haija M, Uc A, Werlin SL, et al. Nutritional considerations in pediatric pancreatitis: a position paper from the NASPGHAN Pancreas Committee and ESPGHAN Cystic Fibrosis/Pancreas Working Group. *J Pediatr Gastroenterol Nutr*. 2018;67(1):131-143.
16. van der Haak N, King SJ, Crowder T, et al. Highlights from the nutrition guidelines for cystic fibrosis in Australia and New Zealand. *J Cyst Fibros*. 2020;19(1):16-25.

17. Borowitz DS, Grand RJ, Durie PR. Use of pancreatic enzyme supplements for patients with cystic fibrosis in the context of fibrosing colonopathy. Consensus Committee. *J Pediatr*. 1995;127(5):681-684.
18. Padula L, Kofsky R, Mascarenhas M. Pulmonary disorders. In: Corkins MR, ed. *ASPEN Pediatric Nutrition Support Core Curriculum*. 3rd ed. American Society of Parenteral and Enteral Nutrition; 2024:533-552.
19. Phillips AE, Brownell JN, Tindall A, et al. Proton-pump inhibitors and fat absorption in cystic fibrosis and pancreatic insufficiency: a randomized crossover pilot trial. *Dig Dis Sci*. 2025;70(3):968-977.
20. Van de Vijver E, Desager K, Mulberg AE, et al. Treatment of infants and toddlers with cystic fibrosis-related pancreatic insufficiency and fat malabsorption with pancrelipase MT. *J Pediatr Gastroenterol Nutr*. 2011;53(1):61-64.
21. Goetz DM, Brown RF, Filigno SS, et al. Cystic fibrosis foundation position paper: redefining the CF care model. *J Cyst Fibros*. 2024;23(6):1055-1065.
22. Allen JR, McCauley JC, Selby AM, et al. Differences in resting energy expenditure between male and female children with cystic fibrosis. *J Pediatr*. 2003;142(1):15-19.
23. Tomezsko JL, Stallings VA, Kawchak DA, Goin JE, Diamond G, Scanlin TF. Energy expenditure and genotype of children with cystic fibrosis. *Pediatr Res*. 1994;35(4 pt 1):451-460.
24. Marin VB, Velandia S, Hunter B, et al. Energy expenditure, nutrition status, and body composition in children with cystic fibrosis. *Nutrition*. 2004;20(2):181-186.
25. Stallings VA, Sainath N, Oberle M, Bertolaso C, Schall JI. Energy balance and mechanisms of weight gain with ivacaftor treatment of cystic fibrosis gating mutations. *J Pediatr*. 2018;201:229-237.e4.
26. Benge T, Brunzell C, Elshaar N, Moran A, Sandouk Z. *Managing Cystic Fibrosis-Related Diabetes (CFRD): An Instruction Guide for Parents and Families*. Cystic Fibrosis Foundation; 2023.
27. Leonard A, Schindler T, Padula L, et al. *Cystic Fibrosis Nutrition 101: Getting Started*. Cystic Fibrosis Foundation; 2022.
28. Holliday KE, Allen JR, Waters DL, Gruca MA, Thompson SM, Gaskin KJ. Growth of human milk-fed and formula-fed infants with cystic fibrosis. *J Pediatr*. 1991;118(1):77-79.
29. Ellis L, Kalnins D, Corey M, Brennan J, Pencharz P, Durie P. Do infants with cystic fibrosis need a protein hydrolysate formula? A prospective, randomized, comparative study. *J Pediatr*. 1998;132(2):270-276.
30. Schwarzenberg SJ, Hempstead SE, McDonald CM, et al. Enteral tube feeding for individuals with cystic fibrosis: Cystic Fibrosis Foundation evidence-informed guidelines. *J Cyst Fibros*. 2016;15(6):724-735.
31. RELiZORB Immobilized Lipase Cartridge. Patient guide. 2025. https://www.relizorbhcp.com/pdf/RELiZORB-Patient-Guide.pdf
32. Stevens J, Wyatt C, Brown P, Patel D, Grujic D, Freedman SD. Absorption and safety with sustained use of RELiZORB evaluation (ASSURE) study in patients with cystic fibrosis receiving enteral feeding. *J Pediatr Gastroenterol Nutr*. 2018;67(4):527-532.
33. Tangpricha V, Kelly A, Stephenson A, et al. An update on the screening, diagnosis, management, and treatment of vitamin D deficiency in individuals with cystic fibrosis: evidence-based recommendations from the Cystic Fibrosis Foundation. *J Clin Endocrinol Metab*. 2012;97(4):1082-1093.
34. Sermet-Gaudelus I, Castanet M, Retsch-Bogart G, Aris RM. Update on cystic fibrosis-related bone disease: a special focus on children. *Paediatr Respir Rev*. 2009;10(3):134-142.
35. Yankaskas JR, Marshall BC, Sufian B, Simon RH, Rodman D. Cystic fibrosis adult care: consensus conference report. *Chest*. 2004;125(1 suppl):1S–39S.
36. Ullal J, Kutney K, Williams KM, Weber DR. Treatment of cystic fibrosis related bone disease. *J Clin Transl Endocrinol*. 2022;27:100291.
37. Debray D, Kelly D, Houwen R, Strandvik B, Colombo C. Best practice guidance for the diagnosis and management of cystic fibrosis-associated liver disease. *J Cyst Fibros*. 2011;(10 suppl 2):S29-S36.
38. Singh H, Coffey MJ, Ooi CY. Cystic fibrosis-related liver disease is associated with increased disease burden and endocrine comorbidities. *J Pediatr Gastroenterol Nutr*. 2020;70(6):796-800.
39. Mouzaki M, Bronsky J, Gupte G, et al. Nutrition support of children with chronic liver diseases: a joint position paper of the North American Society for Pediatric Gastroenterology, Hepatology, and Nutrition and the European Society for Pediatric Gastroenterology, Hepatology, and Nutrition. *J Pediatr Gastroenterol Nutr*. 2019;69(4):498-511.
40. Bailey J, Rozga M, McDonald CM, et al. Effect of CFTR modulators on anthropometric parameters in individuals with cystic fibrosis: an evidence analysis center systematic review. *J Acad Nutr Diet*. 2021;121(7):1364-1378.e2.
41. Nichols AL, Davies JC, Jones D, Carr SB. Restoration of exocrine pancreatic function in older children with cystic fibrosis on ivacaftor. *Paediatr Respir Rev*. 2020;35:99-102.

CHAPTER 21

Developmental Disabilities

Heidi Quinn and Sharon Weston

Developmental disabilities (DD) are conditions characterized by physical, cognitive, psychological, sensory, adaptive, and/or communication impairments that manifest during development.[1] Children with chronic diseases and/or developmental disorders, also referred to as children with special health care needs (CSHCN), require adequate nutrition for growth and development, but have more frequent nutritional risk factors, which may pose additional challenges (Table 21.1). Oral-motor and feeding difficulties are common in children with DD and are discussed in Chapter 24.[1] Other common nutrition concerns include constipation and reduced bone density, especially in children who are nonambulatory.[1]

SPECIAL ASPECTS OF NUTRITIONAL ASSESSMENT AND MANAGEMENT

In children with DD, a thorough review of birth, medical, and feeding history is needed to determine the potential effects of long-term hospitalizations, surgeries, and medical procedures (e.g., intubation, supplemental tube feedings) on overall development, as well as on oral feeding and feeding skill development. Early medical and feeding history can provide insight into feeding problems, such as oral aversion.

Obtaining accurate measurements of weight, length/height, and head circumference, along with serial tracking over time, is critical in assessing adequacy of growth. Growth should be plotted on The Centers for Disease Control and Prevention (CDC) and/or World Health Organization (WHO) growth charts, as well as specialized syndrome-specific growth charts if available. Specialized growth charts are currently available for achondroplasia, cerebral palsy (quadriplegia), Down syndrome, Marfan syndrome, myelomeningocele, Noonan syndrome, Turner syndrome, Prader-Willi syndrome, Williams syndrome, and sickle cell disease (see Appendix 3).[1] Specialized charts have limitations because they are based on a small sample size, so should be used alongside the CDC/WHO growth charts. In children with DD, measuring linear growth may be complicated by the presence of contractures, scoliosis, kyphosis, or the inability to stand. Alternative methods of linear measurement, such as crown-rump length, sitting height, arm span, tibial length, or segmented body length, can be used but may also be compromised by contractures and/or scoliosis.[1]

Children with DD may be small for their age, with growth parameters below the fifth percentile on standard growth charts.[1] Assessment of weight-for-length/height is especially important in this population, as it indicates individual proportionality, which is often a more appropriate way to evaluate adequacy of growth in children with DD. It is also important to note that alterations in head circumference (micro/macrocephaly) and body composition (lean mass vs. body fat) seen in some children with DD can skew the weight-for-age and weight-for-length parameters. Triceps

TABLE 21.1 NUTRITIONAL RISK FACTORS FOR CHILDREN WITH DEVELOPMENTAL DISABILITIES

- Altered Growth
  - Obesity (Prader-Willi, Laurence-Moon-Biedl, Carpenter, and Down syndromes)
  - Failure to thrive (Rett syndrome, athetoid cerebral palsy)
  - Short stature (Down, Hurler, Russell Silver, and Cornelia de Lange syndromes)
- Gastrointestinal Symptoms
  - Diarrhea
  - Constipation
  - Vomiting/gastroesophageal reflux
- Oral-Motor Difficulties
  - Discoordination of suck/swallow
  - Structural abnormalities (cleft lip/palate; dentition)
  - Poor oral containment (food/fluid loss)
  - Tone abnormalities (hypo/hypertonic)
  - Altered oral sensory response (hypo/hyper responsive)
  - Delayed oral-motor skill development
  - Aspiration
- Altered Nutrient Needs/Nutrient Deficiencies
  - Drug-nutrient interactions (anticonvulsants, diuretics, laxatives, tranquilizers)
  - Restricted intake (metabolic disease, food allergies, food texture aversion)
  - Inadequate intake (poor appetite, poor oral-motor control, malabsorption)
  - Increased calorie requirement (athetoid crebral palsy, spasticity)
  - Inadequate fluid intake
- Behavior
  - Oral aversion
  - Pica
  - Rumination
  - Hyperactivity
  - Distractibility
  - Perseverative behaviors
  - Binge eating /overeating
- Positioning for Feeding
  - Adaptive seating devices
- Feeding Skill Development
  - Self-feeder vs. dependent feeder
  - Adaptive feeding equipment

skinfold and subscapular skinfold measurements can be useful for assessing body composition and resting energy expenditure.[2]

Children with DD may experience a range of alterations in activity level and movement, which has important implications for nutrition assessment (e.g., weight goals) and overall health. For nonambulatory children, weight-for-length in the 10th to 25th percentile is generally an acceptable goal, as additional weight is often accumulated as increased fat stores rather than as muscle mass. Excessive weight can compromise care in terms of cardiorespiratory health, as well as ease of transfers (bed, bath, wheelchair) and progression with gross motor skills. While physical activity may be limited, children should be encouraged to be as physically active as possible within their abilities. Engaging in physical activity can help promote healthy growth and development, and has also been shown to encourage social interaction, build motor skills, and support cognitive development.[3]

Given the complexity of assessing adequacy of growth in children with DD, a visual clinical assessment, in conjunction with growth history is essential. Utilizing Nutrition Focused Physical Exam (NFPE) techniques can provide additional information that can be used as part of the nutrition assessment.[4]

Nutrient Requirements

Energy

Calorie requirements can be assessed in several ways, including[1]:

1. Calories per centimeter of body height/length (Table 21.2)
2. Catch-up growth equations using height age instead of weight age (Table 21.3)
3. Standardized equations (see Chapter 5)

These methods produce estimates, and individual calorie needs should be assessed based on changes in weight over time and/or through measurement of basal metabolic rate (e.g., indirect calorimetry). Regular weight monitoring is an essential component in managing children with DD, particularly in children with syndromes that may impact linear growth. Calorie requirements may be as low as 5 kcal/cm of height in children with severe central nervous system impairment.[1]

Protein

Protein requirements are estimated using Recommended Dietary Allowance (RDA) for chronological age or height age if growth parameters are significantly below chronological age (Table 21.3).[1]

TABLE 21.2 GUIDELINES FOR ESTIMATING CALORIC REQUIREMENTS IN CHILDREN WITH DEVELOPMENTAL DISABILITIES

CONDITION	CALORIC RECOMMENDATION
Ambulatory, ages 5-12 y	13.9 kcal/cm height
Nonambulatory, ages 5-12 y	11.1 kcal/cm height
Cerebral palsy with severely restricted activity	10 kcal/cm height
Cerebral palsy with mild to moderate activity	15 kcal/cm height
Athetoid cerebral palsy, adolescence	Up to 6000 kcal/d
Down syndrome, boys ages 5-12 y	16.1 kcal/cm height
Down syndrome, girls ages 5-12 y	14.3 kcal/cm height
Myelomenigocele	Approximately 50% of Recommended Dietary Allowance for age after infancy; may need as little as 7 kcal/cm height
Prader-Willi syndrome	10-11 kcal/cm height for weight maintenance; 8-9 kcal/cm height for weight loss

TABLE 21.3 CATCH-UP GROWTH EQUATIONS USING HEIGHT AGE

$$\text{kcal/kg} = \frac{\text{IBW for height} \times \text{RDA kcal/kkg height age}^{a}}{\text{actual weight}}$$

$$\text{g protein/kg} = \frac{\text{IBW for height} \times \text{RDA g protein/kg height age}^{a}}{\text{actual weight}}$$

IBW, ideal body weight; RDA, Recommended Dietary Allowance.
[a]Height age is the age at which a child's current height would place them at the 50th percentile on a standardized growth chart for their sex. It is determined by comparing the child's measured height to the growth chart and identifying the age at which that height corresponds to the 50th percentile.

Vitamins/Minerals

The most common nutrient deficiencies seen in children with DD are vitamins: A, C, D, and folate, as well as iron, zinc, and calcium.[1]

Fluid

Fluid requirements may be higher in some children with DD due to constipation, increased fluid losses (e.g., drooling, excessive sweating), and/or medications. Standard guidelines for fluids based on body weight should be followed, with adjustment for these special considerations.

Drug-Nutrient Interactions

Some children with DD are on multiple medications that can interfere with nutrient absorption, appetite, elimination patterns, and level of alertness for feeding. For example, children on some seizure medications (e.g., phenytoin [Dilantin]) may require increased vitamin D and folic acid intake.[1] Certain medications can contribute to constipation, which often inhibits appetite. Due to potential concerns with drug-nutrient interactions, especially in the context of concerns of inadequate dietary intake and/or decreased mobility or weight-bearing activities, laboratory values reflecting iron, protein, vitamin D, calcium, and phosphorus status should be monitored regularly (see Appendix 2).[1]

Developmental Disabilities With Nutrition and Feeding Concerns

Several DD, such as Down syndrome, cerebral palsy, attention-deficit/hyperactivity disorder, autism, spina bifida, and Prader-Willi syndrome, have distinct nutrition and feeding concerns.

Down Syndrome

Down syndrome (DS) is a chromosomal anomaly resulting from trisomy of chromosome 21 and is associated with several medical concerns (Table 21.4) that can affect their nutritional status and overall development (Table 21.5).[1] Approximately 40% to 50% of children with DS are born with congenital heart defects, 8% to 12% are

TABLE 21.4 MEDICAL DIAGNOSES ASSOCIATED WITH DOWN SYNDROME

Cardiac anomalies
Intestinal malformations (e.g., duodenal atresia, Hirschsprung disease)
Celiac disease
Increased incidence of infections (ear, respiratory)
Endocrine (diabetes, hypothyroidism)
Orthopedic (atlanto-axial instability, hip dislocation)
Dental (delayed/missing dentition)
Increased risk of leukemia
Hearing loss

born with gastrointestinal malformations, and 31% to 80% have feeding difficulties.[5] The incidence is reported to be 1 in 640 live births, with increasing incidence with increased maternal age.[5]

DS-specific growth charts (Appendix 3), along with the CDC growth charts, should be used to monitor growth. Although DS-specific weight-for-length and body mass index (BMI) charts are available, the optimal weight-for-length and BMI levels for individuals with DS are not yet established, so the CDC chart should be used to plot BMI. One study showed that the CDC BMI growth chart using the 85th percentile was more sensitive for excess adiposity than the new DS-specific BMI chart.[6] Given the short stature inherent to Down syndrome, calorie requirements for children with Down syndrome aged 5 to 12 years should be based on body height rather than on body weight to avoid overestimating calorie requirement (Table 21.2).[1] Approximately 25% of children with DS are affected by obesity.[1] Early promotion of healthy eating habits and avoiding use of food as a reward for good behavior is recommended.

Studies have not shown consistent evidence that nutritional supplementation improves the outcome in DS. If dietary variety is limited due to issues such as oral-motor difficulty, oral sensory issues, or constipation, a multivitamin with iron may be indicated. Supplementation with additional nutrients beyond a standard multivitamin is not currently recommended, and children who receive supplementation at levels well above the RDA should be monitored for signs of nutrient excess (Table 3.1). Extra fluid may be indicated for children with Down syndrome who have constipation.[1]

TABLE 21.5 NUTRITIONAL AND FEEDING RISK FACTORS ASSOCIATED WITH DOWN SYNDROME

Poor weight gain associated with cardiac anomalies, recurrent infections, hypothyroidism)
Short stature
Obesity
Constipation (related to hypotonia, hypothyroid, fluid loss)
Delayed oral-motor skill development: weak lip seal, difficulty with thin fluids, prolonged tongue thrust, delayed chewing
Delayed feeding skill development: delayed self-feeding skills
Selective intake: prolonged preference for pureed foods, difficulty with transition to textures
Reduced activity (associated with hypotonia, orthopedic concerns)
Behavior difficulties

Cerebral Palsy

Cerebral palsy (CP) is a group of chronic, nonprogressive disorders of the nervous system that produce abnormalities of posture, muscle tone, and motor coordination. It is classified according to the specific abnormality in muscle tone (hypertonia, hypotonia) and extrapyramidal signs (choreoathetosis, ataxia, and dystonia). The estimated prevalence ranges between 1 and 4 per 1000 live births, and is more common among children born preterm or at low birth weight.[7] Due to their motor involvement, children with CP may have many of the feeding problems listed in Table 21.1, including poor growth and oral-motor feeding difficulties due to poor oral-motor control. In addition, medications commonly used to help treat spasticity, seizures, constipation, and/or gastroesophageal reflux can impact nutrient intake and feeding skills as well as behavioral state (lethargy, distraction, drowsiness) at mealtime. Regular monitoring of growth, diet intake, and oral-motor feeding skills by a multidisciplinary team is essential to maximize growth, intake, oral-motor skills, and feeding skills. Feeding evaluations should also include assessment for adaptive seating and adaptive feeding utensils to facilitate intake.[1]

Attention-Deficit/Hyperactivity Disorder

Attention-deficit/hyperactivity disorder (ADHD) is one of the most common neurobehavioral problems exhibited in children today, affecting an estimated 3% to 10% of school-aged children.[8,9] Children with ADHD may present with increased levels of impulsiveness, hyperactivity, and/or inattentiveness. Diagnosis of ADHD often occurs in the early grade school years when rapid growth and development are still occurring. Treatment of ADHD involves medication, behavioral management, and modifying the environment at home and at school to optimize the child's potential for success.[1] Although alternative treatments such as nutritional supplementation, dietary modifications, and homeopathy have been proposed, there is no clear evidence that supports their effectiveness.[10] Some research suggests that certain artificial food colors and additives may exacerbate ADHD-like symptoms, so a balanced diet that includes a minimal intake of highly processed foods is encouraged.[11] Children who are treated with stimulant medications may exhibit decreased appetite and weight loss as a side effect. To ensure optimal nutritional intake, meals should be scheduled during times when hunger is typically highest. Nutritional supplements and a calorically dense diet may be helpful to address any nutritional gaps and support optimal growth and development.

Autism Spectrum Disorder

Autism spectrum disorder (ASD) is a neurodevelopmental disorder characterized by deficits in social/communication, restricted interests, and repetitive behaviors.[1] The etiology of ASD is unclear; it is extraordinarily complex and may be related to both genetic and environmental problems. Children with certain medical conditions, such as Fragile X syndrome, tuberous sclerosis, Tourette syndrome, and seizure disorders, have a higher-than-normal risk of having ASD.[8] Although the number of children diagnosed with ASD appears to be rising, it is unclear if this is due to better detection and screening, actual increases, or both.[8] In 2020, the estimated prevalence of ASD in the United States was found to be 27.6 per 1000 (1 in 36) children aged 8 years and was 3.8 times as prevalent among boys as among girls (1 in 43.0 vs. 11.4).[12]

TABLE 21.6 COMMON FEEDING CONCERNS FOR CHILDREN WITH AUTISM SPECTRUM DISORDER

Difficulty with texture transition
Heightened sensory responses
Restricted intake due to color/brand name/presentation style/shape or texture
Decreased selection of foods over time
Difficulty accepting new foods
Difficulty with administration of multivitamin/mineral supplement
Difficulty with changes in mealtime environment—may eat at school but not in the home
Disruptive mealtime behaviors

Many children with ASD have selective eating patterns, putting them at risk for suboptimal nutritional deficiencies (Table 21.6). Restrictive food acceptance may be due to sensory processing, ritualistic patterns of behaviors, or excessive resistance to change (e.g., insistence on same foods with extreme distress/anxiety at small changes) (Table 21.7). For some children, intake may be limited in variety to as few as two to three foods or beverages. Foods may be refused due to color, temperature, texture, smell, or simply because they are new.[13] Supplementation with a multivitamin with minerals in a form that the child will accept may be difficult, possibly requiring multiple trials with various forms (liquid, powder, and tablet). Despite selective intake,

TABLE 21.7 HELPFUL MEALTIME STRATEGIES FOR CHILDREN WITH AUTISM SPECTRUM DISORDER

PATTERNS OF LIKEABLE FOODS

- Identify patterns in texture, taste, temperature, and colors that the child prefers.
- Introduce new foods that are most similar to those they already like.
- Food chaining involves gradually adding new foods with similar characteristics to those the child tolerates.[13]

TOO MANY CHOICES

- Avoid overwhelming the child with too many foods options.
- Too many choices may lead to refusal of all foods.

NEW FOODS

- Use desensitization by placing a new food near the child's plate at mealtime without pressure.
- Over time, encourage them to lick, taste, and eventually swallow the food; this process may take several weeks.
- Pairing the new food item with a positive role model (e.g., a parent or sibling enjoying it) may also help with acceptance.

MEALTIME

- For children who struggle with sitting at the table:
  - Use a visual schedule with pictures or words for the day that defines meals and activities.
  - Plan physical activity before mealtime.
  - Set a timer for short, manageable times that the child should remain seated.
  - Allow quiet activities during meals.
  - Maintain a positive attitude and avoid force feeding.

TABLE 21.7 HELPFUL MEALTIME STRATEGIES FOR CHILDREN WITH AUTISM SPECTRUM DISORDER (*continued*)

BETWEEN MEALS

- Avoid offering preferred foods throughout the day.
- Do not allow grazing on foods and beverages between meals to encourage better intake during meals.

DIFFERENT FOODS

- Offer a mix of preferred foods and less-preferred foods.
- Use positive reinforcement to encourage the child to try less-preferred foods (e.g., "*First* try your favorite food, A, and try a bite of B. *Then* you can play with your train.").

TIME LIMIT

- Set a specific time limit for meals.
- If the child refuses to eat, calmly end the meal with "dinner is done" and clear the table.
- Do not offer any more food until the next planned mealtime.

EXPECTATIONS

- Set clear expectations using visual cues like a number board, which shows how many bites or chew required.
- Mark progress by crossing off numbers as the child eats, providing structure and clarity for the mealtime.

adequate growth is generally seen in children with ASD, with the exception of late infancy/early toddlerhood when there is sometimes poor growth as a result of the transition from baby foods to table foods.

Specific energy requirements for children with ASD have not been established, but the RDA for age is typically used, with modifications made based on activity level. Some children with ASD are quite sedentary, while others are constantly active, often with self-stimulatory behavior (e.g., spinning, hand flapping, rocking). Some medications used to treat behavioral and anxiety symptoms of ASD such as selective serotonin re-uptake inhibitors (SSRIs), and antipsychotics can cause weight gain. Children with ASD consuming a selective diet of mostly refined carbohydrates with limited intake of fruit and vegetables are at risk for obesity and other related consequences.[1] Nutritional needs for children with ASD should be assessed using a team approach, including a registered dietitian, an occupational therapist or speech therapist with training in feeding therapy, and a psychologist/psychiatrist specializing in behavioral medicine.[1,13]

Parents of children with ASD are often drawn to investigate alternative therapies, such as following a gluten-free/casein-free diet. There is no clear evidence that supports the effectiveness of this diet, in the absence of celiac disease/gluten sensitivities and/or lactose intolerance. In addition, restrictive diets can be harmful in young children, particularly those who already have a selective eating pattern.[1]

Spina Bifida

Spina bifida refers to a group of neural tube defects caused by incomplete closure of the spinal cord during early pregnancy (21-28 days after conception). When the neural tube fails to close, it leaves a sac or lesion along the midline of the spinal cord. The level and severity of the lesion determines the level of sensation and motor function in the individual.[14] About 1 in 2875 babies is born with spina bifida in the United States each year.[15] Folate plays a critical role in the closure of the neural tube during embryonic development. Mandatory fortification of grain products with folic acid began in the United States in 1998. Fortification has helped to reduce both the incidence and severity of spina bifida.[16]

Feeding difficulties are common in children with spina bifida due to Arnold Chiari malformation, hypotonia, and dysphagia. Due to neurogenic bowel, decreased fluid intake, and decreased mobility, other nutritional risk factors seen in children with spina bifida include constipation, urinary tract infections, obesity, and osteopenia. Monitoring nutrition and growth in this population requires special considerations due to mobility limitations and other medical challenges.[14]

Prader-Willi Syndrome

Prader-Willi syndrome (PWS) is the most common syndromic cause of obesity, with an incidence of 1 in 15,000 live births, affecting both males and females across all ethnic groups.[17] This neurodevelopmental genetic disorder is characterized by hypothalamic dysfunction leading to hyperphagia and obesity, as well as cognitive and behavioral problems (learning issues, anxiety, tantrums, compulsive behavior, skin picking).[17] Historically, PWS has been thought to present as two nutritional phases, initially presenting as hypotonia and poor feeding in infancy, and then transitioning to hyperphagia and weight gain during childhood. However, more recent classifications describe a gradual progression of five main nutritional phases, which may be altered by the use of growth hormone treatment (Table 21.8).[17]

In addition to hyperphagia, an unrelenting hunger drive, and a lack of satiety, children with PWS have lower energy expenditure and reduced exercise performance.[18]

TABLE 21.8 PROGRESSION OF NUTRITIONAL PHASES IN PRADER-WILLI SYNDROME

PHASE	AGE RANGE	DESCRIPTION
Phase 0	Prenatal	Decreased fetal movement and growth
Phase 1a	Birth to 9 mo	Poor feeding skills, hypotonia, may require nutrition support
Phase 1b	9-25 mo	Improved feeding and growth with normal growth velocity
Phase 2a	2.1-4.5 y	Weight gain occurs without a change in caloric intake.
Phase 2b	4.5-8 y	Increased interest in food, weight gain
Phase 3	8 y to adulthood	Hyperphagia, insatiable appetite, food seeking
Phase 4	Adulthood	Some adults may progress to this stage, able to feel full, insatiable appetite no longer present.

Butler MG, Miller JL, Forster JL. Prader-Willi Syndrome—clinical genetics, diagnosis and treatment approaches: an update. *Curr Pediatr Rev*. 2019;15(4):207-244.

Close supervision of food access may be necessary to prevent overeating episodes that could lead to serious complications, including gastric dilation and rupture, aspiration, food poisoning, and intestinal blockage.[17] To prevent excess weight gain, early dietary intervention is recommended, with a diet consisting of 8 to 11 kcal/cm height staring at approximately 2 years of age shown to help maintain weight in a healthy range.[19] A Mediterranean-style diet (~30% fat, 45% carbohydrates and 25% protein, and at least 20 g of fiber per day) combined with energy restriction, exercise, and environmental controls has been shown to be effective for weight management.[19] While many children with PWS dislike plain water, encouraging hydration with minimal sweeteners (natural or artificial) is recommended to reduce cravings and a dependence on sweet tastes.[19] Additionally, fostering a safe, low-stress food environment with structured meal and snack times, where the family eats together, can support success.[19]

Routine growth monitoring using PWS-specific growth charts (age 0-18, sex-specific; see Appendix 3) can be done in conjunction with the WHO and CDC growth charts to monitor growth, track trends, and guide nutrition interventions.[20]

REFERENCES

1. Academy of Nutrition and Dietetics. *Pocket Guide to Pediatric Nutrition Assessment*. 2nd ed. Academy of Nutrition and Dietetics; 2021.
2. Bellou TF. Skinfold measurements enhance nutrition assessments and care planning for children with developmental delays and disabilities. *ICAN Infant Child Adolesc Nutr*. 2011;3:158-170.
3. Howells K, Sivaratnam C, May T, Lindor E, Rinehart N. A Pilot Acceptability Study of an 'AllPlay Pre-Learn' day program to facilitate participation in organised physical activity for children with disabilities. *Int J Environ Res Public Health*. 2019;16(24):5058.
4. Chen ST, Ong SH, Lim PY, Chong KS. Nutrition-focused physical exam in assessing nutritional status of children with neurological impairment. *Hum Nutr Metab*. 2024;37:200279.
5. Bull MJ, Trotter T, Santoro SL, Christensen C, Grout RW. Health supervision for children and adolescents with Down syndrome. *Pediatrics*. 2022;149(5):1.
6. Hatch-Stein JA, Zemel BS, Prasad D, et al. Body composition and BMI growth charts in children with Down syndrome. *Pediatrics*. 2016;138(4):e20160541.
7. McIntyre S, Goldsmith S, Webb A, et al. Global prevalence of cerebral palsy: a systematic analysis. *Dev Med Child Neurol*. 2022;64:1494.
8. American Psychiatric Association. *Diagnostic and Statistical Manual of Mental Disorders: DSM-V-TR*. American Psychiatric Association; 2022.
9. Centers for Disease Control and Prevention. QuickStats: percentage* of children and adolescents aged 5-17 years who had ever received a diagnosis of attention-deficit/hyperactivity disorder,† by urbanization level§ and age group—National Health Interview Survey, United States, 2020-2022¶. *MMWR Morb Mortal Wkly Rep*. 2024;73:116.
10. Pellow J, Solomon EM, Barnard CN. Complementary and alternative medical therapies for children with attention-deficit/hyperactivity disorder (ADHD). *Altern Med Rev*. 2011;16(4):323-337.
11. McCann D, Barrett A, Cooper A, et al. Food additives and hyperactive behaviour in 3-year- old 8/9-year-old children in the community: a randomised, double-blinded, placebo-controlled trial. *Lancet*. 2007; 370:1560-1567.
12. Maenner MJ, Warren Z, Williams AR, et al. Prevalence and characteristics of autism spectrum disorder among children aged 8 years—autism and developmental disabilities monitoring network, 11 sites, United States, 2020. *MMWR Surveill Summ*. 2023;72(2):1-14.
13. Fraker C, Fishbein M, Walbert S, Cox S, Barker SC. *Food chaining: the proven 6-step plan to stop picky eating, solve feeding problems, and expand your child's diet*. Marlowe; 2007.
14. Wittenbrook, W. Best practices in nutrition for children with myelomeningocele. *ICAN Infant Child Adolesc Nutr*. 2010;2(4):237.
15. Stallings EB, Isenburg JL, Rutkowski RE, et al. National population-based estimates for major birth defects, 2016–2020. *Birth Defects Res*. 2024;116(1):e2301.
16. Williams J, Mai CT, Mulinare J, et al. Updated estimates of neural tube defects prevented by mandatory folic acid fortification—United States, 1995-2011. *MMWR Morb Mortal Wkly Rep*. 2015;64:1-5.

17. Butler MG, Miller JL, Forster JL. Prader-Willi syndrome—clinical genetics, diagnosis and treatment approaches: an update. *Curr Pediatr Rev*. 2019;15(4):207-244.
18. Alsaif M, Elliot SA, MacKenzie ML, Prado CM, Field CJ, Haqq AM. Energy metabolism profile in individuals with Prader-Willi syndrome and implications for clinical management: a systematic review. *Adv Nutr*. 2017;8(6):905-915.
19. Miller JL, Tan M. Dietary management for adolescents with Prader-Willi syndrome. *Adolesc Health Med Ther*. 2020;11:113-118.
20. Hoybye C, Tauber M. Approach to the patient with Prader-Willi syndrome. *J Clin Endocrinol Metab*. 2022;107(6):1698-1705.

CHAPTER 22

Diabetes Mellitus

Sarah Federoff, Heidi Quinn, and Katharine Garvey

Diabetes mellitus is a chronic condition characterized by high glucose levels, resulting from insulin deficiency or inadequate insulin response. Diabetes affects both children and adults, although, in youth, type 1 diabetes is more prevalent than type 2 diabetes and the prevalence of both is increasing. Diabetes is one of the most common chronic diseases in youth, and nutrition management is an essential aspect of therapy for all diabetes types. This chapter provides an overview of diabetes in youth, including a detailed approach to nutrition therapy.

BACKGROUND

Diabetes occurs when insulin is either absent or insufficient, or when the target tissues do not respond normally to insulin. When insulin is unavailable, glucose cannot enter the cells of insulin-sensitive tissues, causing glucose to accumulate in the blood. High levels of blood glucose can lead to both acute and chronic complications in the body, which are discussed further in this chapter.

Type 1 diabetes is an autoimmune disease that results in the destruction of the insulin secreting β cells of the pancreas, leading to absolute insulin deficiency. Symptoms do not typically present until late in the process of β cell destruction, when most of the β cells have been destroyed. Common symptoms at the time of diagnosis include polyuria, polydipsia, and weight loss. According to the SEARCH for Diabetes in Youth Study data, the estimated prevalence type 1 diabetes in youth aged 19 years or younger increased significantly from 1.48 per 1000 in 2001 to 1.93 per 1000 in 2009 to 2.15 per 1000 (or 1 in 465 youth) in 2017, a relative increase of about 45% over 16 years.[1] Type 1 diabetes typically manifests in childhood, with a peak incidence occurring around age 10 years.[2] Initial therapy involves medical management to correct hyperglycemia, glycosuria, and ketonuria, which are responsible for symptoms occurring at diagnosis. In type 1 diabetes, exogenous insulin is essential for survival and is provided via daily multiple insulin injections or insulin pump.

Type 2 diabetes results from insulin resistance and, in many cases, a relative inability to produce sufficient insulin. Data from the SEARCH for Diabetes in Youth Study show that the prevalence of type 2 diabetes in youth aged 19 years or younger increased significantly from 0.34 per 1000 in 2001 to 0.46 per 1000 in 2009 to 0.67 per 1000 (or 1 in 1492 youth), a 95% relative increase over 16 years.[2] Childhood obesity, which is strongly associated with the insulin resistance seen in type 2 diabetes, increased from 13.9% in 1999 to 2000 to 18.5% in 2015 to 2016.[3]

Most cases of type 2 diabetes in youth occur in older children and adolescents, typically after the onset of puberty. The peak age at diagnosis for youth-onset type 2 diabetes is around 16 years.[2] Type 2 diabetes is more common in children with a family history of the condition and disproportionately affects Hispanic, Black, Native

American, Asian American, and Pacific Islander youth in the United States compared to White youth. Insulin resistance in type 2 diabetes can often be improved through weight loss, improved nutrition, and exercise, in addition to oral medications (e.g., metformin). In some cases, intensification of therapy with glucagon-like peptide-1 (GLP-1) agonists or insulin may be necessary.

GLYCEMIC CONTROL

Prospective, randomized trials have shown that improved glycemic control decreases the risks of developing chronic microvascular complications such as retinopathy, nephropathy, and neuropathy.[4,5] Routine testing of glycated hemoglobin, also known as hemoglobin A1c (HbA1c), is the gold standard for assessing glycemic control. The American Diabetes Association recommends a target HbA1c of less than 7% (equivalent to an estimated average glucose <154 mg/dL) for youth with diabetes. This metric is typically monitored every 3 months at diabetes clinic visits. In addition, continuous glucose monitoring (CGM) technology allows for real-time glucose trend monitoring and provides aggregate glucose data to guide management.

CONTINUOUS GLUCOSE MONITORS

CGM technology captures glucose readings from interstitial fluids approximately every 5 minutes using a sensor wire placed under the skin. The sensor transmits glucose data to a receiver, insulin pump, or a compatible smart phone. The duration of wear varies with the brand used, but typically ranges from 7 to 14 days. CGM has become standard of care for individuals with type 1 diabetes, particularly in youth. From 2010 to 2019, the use of CGM in youth with type 1 diabetes with commercial insurance increased from 20% to 50%.[6] The American Diabetes Association's 2025 Standards of Care recommend offering CGM for diabetes management at diagnosis or as soon as possible in youth on insulin therapy.[7]

In addition to glucose values, CGM systems display directional arrows that indicate whether glucose is rising or falling and at what rate. The system can also alert the wearer if the glucose levels are too low or too high, with individualized targets established with guidance from the diabetes care team. Data from the CGM can also be shared with caregivers through a mobile app, enabling remote monitoring. Aggregate CGM data offer valuable insights into overall glycemic control for individuals with diabetes as well as caregivers and health care provider teams. International expert consensus recommends a goal of greater than or equal to 70% "time-in-range" (time between 70 and 180 mg/dL on CGM), which is approximately equivalent to an HbA1c less than or equal to 7%.[8]

INSULIN REPLACEMENT IN TYPE 1 DIABETES

As noted above, insulin replacement is central to type 1 diabetes therapy, ideally mimicking physiologic insulin production. While some individuals with type 2 diabetes require insulin treatment, this section focuses on typical insulin regimens used for complete replacement in type 1 diabetes. Multiple insulin regimens are available and can be injection-based or pump-based. It is important to choose an insulin regimen that best fits the needs of the patient and the family.

Insulin Injections

To allow increased dietary flexibility, contemporary insulin injection regimens often follow a "basal-bolus" approach. This includes two types of insulin: (1) a long-acting, basal insulin (e.g., insulin glargine or insulin degludec) administered once daily to provide steady coverage over approximately 24 to 36 hours, and (2) a rapid-acting insulin (e.g., insulin lispro or insulin aspart) given periodically throughout the day to cover carbohydrates consumed at meals and snacks and to correct high glucose levels. Insulin doses may need to be adjusted for physical activity, considering the type, intensity, and timing of activity in relation to meals and snacks.

Insulin Pumps and Automated Insulin Delivery

Insulin pumps are often used in place of multiple daily injections. Insulin pumps deliver rapid-acting insulin, providing a continuous basal rate of insulin and larger boluses for carbohydrate coverage and correction. Insulin pumps can be especially beneficial in children, who often require smaller, more precise doses. There are a variety of insulin pumps available with different features and form factors. Pump reservoirs typically hold up to 200 to 300 units of insulin, requiring infusion site changes every 2 to 3 days. The most advanced insulin pumps are integrated with CGM systems and are referred to as a hybrid closed-loop system. These pumps automatically adjust insulin delivery based on CGM glucose readings, though the user still needs to program bolus dosing for carbohydrate intake. Insulin pump therapy, when used appropriately, can improve glycemic control and quality of life.[9]

ACUTE AND CHRONIC COMPLICATIONS OF DIABETES

The major acute complications of diabetes in children are hypoglycemia (in insulin-treated patients) and diabetic ketoacidosis (DKA; predominantly in type 1 diabetes due to severe insulin deficiency). Common nutrition-related factors that may contribute to hypoglycemia in youth on intensive insulin therapy include delayed or missed meals and snacks, excessive insulin (from inaccurate carbohydrate estimation or insufficient carbohydrate intake), increased exercise without adjustment to food or insulin, or alcohol consumption without food. Hyperglycemia may occur due to inadequate insulin, excessive carbohydrate intake, inaccurate carbohydrate estimation, or reduced physical activity. DKA occurs when the body is unable to use glucose as fuel due to severe insulin deficiency, causing body to burn fat for fuel instead. Ketones, the byproducts of fat breakdown, can accumulate to toxic levels, leading to ketoacidosis.

Chronic complications of diabetes, which can affect all individuals with diabetes, whether insulin-treated or not, include microvascular disease (neuropathy, nephropathy, and retinopathy) and macrovascular disease (ischemic heart disease, cerebrovascular disease, peripheral vascular disease). These chronic complications can be prevented or delayed by maintaining glucose levels within the target range, managing dyslipidemia and hypertension, maintaining a healthy weight, and avoiding smoking.

NUTRITION ASSESSMENT FOR DIABETES

A comprehensive nutrition assessment in young people with diabetes should consider their unique developmental stages, growth patterns, activity levels, eating habits, and psychosocial factors to ensure tailored dietary recommendations that support optimal

TABLE 22.1 SPECIAL ASPECTS OF NUTRITIONAL ASSESSMENT FOR CHILDREN AND ADOLESCENTS WITH DIABETES

Client history	Past medical history (celiac disease, nephropathy, hyperlipidemia, eating disorder, high blood pressure, asthma, attention deficit disorder, hypothyroidism, and other autoimmune diseases), duration of disease, medication (insulin regimen, oral glucose-lowering medications), and supplement history, family history, and social history
Food/nutrition-related history	Food intake (composition, carbohydrate, adequacy, meal/snack patterns, environmental cues to eating, tolerance, current diets, or food modifications), nutrition health awareness and management (knowledge and beliefs about nutrition recommendations, self-monitoring/management practices, prior education), physical activity and exercise (functional status, activity patterns, sedentary time, exercise intensity, frequency, and duration), food availability (food planning, purchasing, preparation abilities and limitations, food safety, food program utilization, food insecurity)
Biochemical data/medical Tests	ADA guideline based on age and type of diabetes should be followed (8), including hemoglobin A1c, lipid profile, microalbuminuria, blood pressure, fasting/nonfasting blood glucose, screening for autoimmune diseases (thyroid, celiac disease), vitamin D levels if concern for deficiency
Anthropometric measurements	Height, weight, BMI, growth rate, rate of weight change
Nutrition-focused physical findings	General physical appearance, body language, polyuria, polydipsia, polyphagia, stool patterns, acanthosis nigricans

ADA, American Diabetes Association; BMI, body mass index.
From American Diabetes Association; Bantle JP, Wylie-Rosett J, et al. Nutrition recommendations and interventions for diabetes: a position statement of the American Diabetes Association. *Diabetes Care*. 2008;31(suppl 1):S61-S78.

glycemic control and overall health. Table 22.1 summarizes nutrition assessment using the Nutrition Care Process for pediatric patients with diabetes.

■ GOALS OF MEDICAL NUTRITION THERAPY FOR DIABETES

The American Diabetes Association established the following goals for all people with diabetes[10]:

1. Achieve and maintain:
   a. Blood glucose levels in the normal range or as close to normal as is safely possible
   b. Blood lipid and lipoprotein profile that reduces the risk for cardiovascular and peripheral vascular disease
   c. Blood pressure levels in the normal range or as close to normal as is safely possible
2. Prevent or slow the rate of development of the chronic complications by modifying nutrient intake and lifestyle factors, such as following a heart-healthy diet and incorporating regular physical activity.
3. Address individual nutrition needs, taking into account personal and cultural preferences and readiness to change.

4. Maintain the pleasure of eating by only limiting food choices when indicated by scientific evidence or dietary restrictions due to allergies.
5. Encourage regular physical activity to maintain a healthy weight range, promote healthy bone mass, and help manage glucose levels.

NUTRITION THERAPY GOALS FOR TYPE 2 DIABETES

The goal of managing type 2 diabetes is to achieve and maintain optimal blood glucose and lipid control, as well as a healthy weight, through nutrition and lifestyle changes. Recommendations may include a reduced-calorie, nutrient-dense diet and reduced intake of sugar-sweetened beverages, saturated fat, cholesterol, and sodium. Reducing the frequency of eating out, especially fast food, and increasing family meals at home can also help reach these goals. It is also important to emphasize regular physical activity. Youth with type 2 diabetes should engage in moderate to vigorous physical activity for 60 minutes daily and strength training at least 3 times per week. Sedentary activities such as watching television, playing video games, and computer/phone use should be limited to no more than 2 hours/d.[11]

Insulin sensitivity improves with even modest weight loss. Weight loss goals should aim for a 7% to 10% reduction in weight if linear growth has been completed and a target body mass index (BMI) less than or equal to 95th percentile for those who are still growing. Initially, weight maintenance may be a more achievable goal. Once weight maintenance has been achieved, further diet modification can focus on gradual weight loss to reach BMI of less than 85th percentile. A safe weight loss rate of 0.5 to 1 kg/mo for growing children is suggested. Adolescents who have completed puberty should have a target goal of 0.5 to 1 kg/wk. Behavior modification can be challenging for some patients to achieve safely,[11] so support from a mental health provider is recommended.

NUTRITION THERAPY IN TYPE 1 DIABETES

Individuals with type 1 diabetes can achieve optimal postprandial glycemic control with 40% to 50% of their energy from carbohydrates, provided insulin-to-carbohydrate ratios (ICR) and insulin delivery are appropriately matched.[12] Healthy sources of carbohydrates, including whole grain breads and cereals, legumes (peas, beans, and lentils), fruits, vegetables, and low-fat dairy products (full fat for children under 2 years), should be encouraged to help minimize glycemic excursions, meet nutrient needs, and provide a balanced diet intake. Protein intake should focus on high-quality protein sources such as lean meat, poultry, fish, eggs, milk, cheese, and soy. To help reduce the risk of cardiovascular disease, intake of saturated fat, and *trans*-fatty acids, and dietary cholesterol should be limited.

DIETARY INTAKE PLANNING IN TYPE 1 DIABETES

Dietary recommendations should be developed based on the child's usual intake, schedule, and food preferences, with a focus on providing adequate nutrition in age-appropriate portion sizes to promote growth. At diagnosis, many children experience weight loss due to dehydration and inadequate absorption of carbohydrates due to inadequate availability of insulin. Weight is typically regained quickly once rehydrated and exogenous insulin is available. Appetite is often significantly increased for the first few weeks after diagnosis, as the body compensates for previous inadequate nutrient absorption. It is important for families to understand this common response.

To meet nutrient and calorie needs, young children typically require three meals and two to three snacks daily, ideally spaced 2½ to 3 hours apart. Older children and adolescents may not have a morning snack built into their school schedule but often have an earlier lunch time. Their morning insulin regimen may need to be modified to accommodate this change.

LOW-CARBOHYDRATE DIETS IN TYPE 1 DIABETES

Low-carbohydrate (<26% energy from carbohydrates) and very low-carbohydrate (20-50 g/d) diets are becoming increasingly popular, including among people with type 1 diabetes.[12] While there is some evidence that following a low-carbohydrate (<26% energy from carbohydrate), higher protein, higher quality fat diet can be beneficial for adults with diabetes,[12] neither the American Diabetes Association nor International Society for Pediatric and Adolescent Diabetes endorse these diets for children with diabetes. The evidence supporting their benefits in pediatric populations is limited, although further research is underway.[13]

Strict adherence to very low-carbohydrate diets may result in ketosis, dyslipidemia, and disordered eating behaviors. Additionally, maintaining a low-carbohydrate diet for long term can be challenging due to the need to limit or eliminate a wide array of foods.[12] Families interested in adopting a low-carbohydrate diet should consult their health care team, including a registered dietitian, to ensure adequate nutrient intake, particularly for calcium, B vitamins, vitamin D, iron, and fiber, and to monitor the child's linear growth.

ESTIMATING CARBOHYDRATE INTAKE IN TYPE 1 DIABETES

Accurate estimation of carbohydrate intake is an important skill for calculating rapid-acting insulin doses to match food intake. Carbohydrates, found in starches, fruits, milk, yogurt, and other sugar-containing foods, have the greatest effect on blood glucose levels. Most children with type 1 diabetes use carbohydrate counting to help determine insulin dosing for meals and snacks. This method allows flexibility in food choices and is taught to parents and children, who learn to identify which foods contain carbohydrates, how to measure/weigh foods those foods, and how to read food labels to calculate grams of carbohydrates.

INSULIN COVERAGE WITH CARBOHYDRATE RATIOS IN TYPE 1 DIABETES

Carbohydrates eaten must be covered with rapid-acting insulin to prevent hyperglycemia. The insulin-to-carbohydrate ratio is individualized based on child's age and diabetes duration, and adjusted as needed based on glucose patterns. For example, for a child with a 1:10 insulin-to-carbohydrate ratio, 1 unit of insulin is needed for every 10 g of carbohydrates consumed; for a meal that contains 60 g of carbohydrates, an insulin dose of 6 units of rapid-acting insulin would be required. Tools such as insulin calculator apps are available to help assign dosing for carbohydrate content. Insulin pumps will calculate the meal/snack dose if carbohydrate grams are entered.

RESOURCES FOR CARBOHYDRATE ESTIMATION

Estimating carbohydrate content of foods without labels, restaurant meals, or school lunches can be challenging, but there are resources (e.g., apps, websites) available to help with estimating carbohydrate in these foods. Calorie King functions as a search engine and allows users to search specific foods, name brands, and chain restaurants and adjust for specific measurements (i.e., ounces, grams, cups) to help estimate the carbohydrate content of the food. The Figwee Calorie Counter provides a visual representation of a food, displayed on a plate, bowl, or cup, allowing the user to adjust the quantity of the food/beverage on the app to match the portion they plan to consume. Cronometer is an app and website where the user can input recipes of home-cooked meals to help determine single-serving carbohydrate counts.

MANAGING HIGH-FAT/HIGH-PROTEIN MEALS IN TYPE 1 DIABETES

While carbohydrates have the largest impact on glucose levels, fat and protein can also influence them. Fat and protein in meals can delay digestion, preventing a rapid rise in glucose after a meal, but may cause elevated glucose several hours after eating, depending on the amount consumed. Meals that are high in fat and/or protein may require additional insulin to prevent late postprandial hyperglycemia. It is important to monitor glucose trends after eating to determine if the insulin regimen is working well. If glucose rises several hours after a high-protein or high-fat meal or snack, additional insulin may be needed.[12] There is no formal consensus on adjusting insulin doses, but current considerations are as follows:

- If glucose levels drop less than 80 mg/dL 30 minutes after eating:
  - Split insulin dose: 70% before meal, 30% 1 to 2 hours after meal.
- If glucose levels rise greater than 150 mg/dL 3 to 6 hours after eating:
  - Increase insulin dose for carbohydrates, starting with 20% (multiply by 1.2).
- If the glucose level decreases within 30 minutes of eating, but rise 3 to 6 hours later:
  - Increase carbohydrates by 20% (multiply by 1.2).
  - Gradually increase carbohydrates in 10% increments (multiply by 1.1) up to a 50% increase (multiply by 1.5) based on glucose response.

FIBER

Dietary fiber is not completely digested and absorbed like other carbohydrates. Because fiber does not cause the blood glucose to rise in the same way as other carbohydrates, the American Diabetes Association recommends subtracting half of the fiber from the total grams of carbohydrate content for foods with more than 5 g of fiber per serving. Some families may find this rule difficult to remember, so may be instructed to cover the full amount of carbohydrates and monitor glucose trends to assess if modifications are needed.

GLYCEMIC INDEX

Foods with a lower glycemic index, such as whole grains and beans, result in a more moderate postprandial glucose rise compared to food with a higher glycemic index, such as white bread, white rice, and white pasta. Lower glycemic index foods also promote satiety as they tend to have more fiber. CGM reports can help educate families about the impact of low versus high glycemic index foods on glucose trends and the importance of choosing low glycemic index options. A balanced meal that includes protein and low–glycemic index carbohydrates can help achieve more stable glucose trends.

NONNUTRITIVE SWEETENERS

There are eight U.S. Food and Drug Administration (FDA)-approved nonnutritive sweeteners: Acesulfame Potassium, Aspartame, Neotame, Advantame, Saccharin, Sucralose, Luo Han Guo (monk fruit), and Rebaudioside A (stevia). According to the FDA, all can be safely used in moderation by people with diabetes. Additional research on the effects of nonnutritive sweeteners on the gut microbiome and overall health is ongoing.[14] Sugar alcohols, often found in low-sugar products, are incompletely absorbed and can cause gastric distress (e.g., gas, bloating) in some individuals and are not recommended for children. To estimate the amount of carbohydrate in a food product sweetened with a sugar alcohol, subtract half of the sugar alcohol grams from the total carbohydrate grams of the food item. For example, a sugar-free chocolate bar that contains 40 g of total carbohydrate, including 20 g of sugar alcohols, should be counted as containing 30 g of carbohydrate.

ALCOHOL AND SUBSTANCE USE

Alcohol inhibits gluconeogenesis and interferes with the counterregulatory response to insulin-induced hypoglycemia. Adolescents with diabetes should be educated about how alcohol affects blood sugar and the potential risks associated with its use. Abstinence from alcohol is recommended for those under 21 years of age. Adolescents who choose to drink should consume alcohol with food and should be instructed not to administer extra insulin for the carbohydrates in alcohol due to the hypoglycemic effect of alcohol and increased risk for hypoglycemia. The health implications of using cannabis and other substances (e.g., tobacco, vaping, illicit drugs) should also be discussed. Cannabis can alter appetite and eating behaviors and may contribute to inconsistent glucose monitoring and increased risk of missed insulin administration, which together can increase risk of hyperglycemia and complications such as DKA.[12]

SPECIAL CONSIDERATIONS

Illness

Infection, illness, and surgery can all complicate glycemic control due to multiple factors, including increased counterregulatory hormone levels and reduced appetite and food intake. In general, sick children should continue their usual insulin regimen, though they may need additional insulin as acute illness may cause insulin resistance with resultant hyperglycemia. Families should follow the guidance provided by their medical provider, but will typically be encouraged to check blood glucose every 3 to 4 hours (or utilize CGM to monitor trends) and to check urine or blood concentrations of ketones. If the child is able to eat their usual meal plan and/or blood glucose is greater than 200 mg/dL, they should be given 4 to 6 oz of sugar-free fluid each hour. If the child is not able to eat their usual meals and snacks and/or blood glucose is less than 200 mg/dL, sugar-free drinks should be alternated with sugar-containing drinks. The carbohydrate grams or servings allotted in the meal plan should be replaced with sugar-containing sodas, popsicles, juices, and gelatin.

Exercise

All types of exercise or physical activity can lower glucose levels both during and 6 to 24 hours after the activity. Blood glucose should be checked before and after the activity, with additional checks for prolonged activity (e.g., sports events, long bike rides, hiking trips). Exercise is not recommended if the glucose level is greater than 250 mg/dL with ketones or greater than 300 mg/dL without ketones. To prevent hypoglycemia during physical activity, insulin doses may be adjusted and/or additional carbohydrate (15 g of carbohydrate for every 30-60 minutes of physical activity) may be consumed. The benefits of regular physical activity should be emphasized for all patients with diabetes, but it is particularly important for improved glycemic control in patients with type 2 diabetes.

STAGES OF LIFE

Infants and Toddlers

Young children often have inconsistent appetites and unpredictable eating habits. In addition, they often cannot recognize and/or verbalize symptoms of hypoglycemia, making the management of glucose trends challenging. Consistent with the division of responsibility in feeding, parents are responsible for establishing regular meal and snack times and providing age-appropriate portions of healthy foods, including low–glycemic index carbohydrates paired with protein and fiber, which can help stabilize glucose trends.[15] In addition, this approach can help keep the child full for longer and reduce the desire to graze. Grazing throughout the day is discouraged, as it adds to glucose variability and reduced intake at meals.

Preschool and School Age

A structured meal and snack schedule should be established for preschool and school-aged children to help improve glycemic control. This schedule should align with the child's school routine and periods of physical activity. For children who eat school-provided meals, breakfast and lunch menus should be reviewed for carbohydrate content, while taking the child's preferences into account. Children can be encouraged to help with preparing meals and choosing snacks. Families should also receive education on how to navigate food choices at events like parties or sleepovers and when dining out.

Adolescents

Adolescence presents unique challenges in diabetes management, including increasing independence (e.g., more meals may be eaten away from home, less parental supervision) and periods of physiologic insulin resistance due to growth and puberty, often requiring significantly increased insulin in adolescents with type 1 diabetes.[16] Appetite, growth parameters, and activity levels should all be considered when determining carbohydrate recommendations for adolescents with type 1 diabetes and to help guide their food choices. Education should focus on managing meals away from home, adjusting insulin for physical activity, and accommodating busy schedule and activities. Basal-bolus insulin regimens or insulin pump therapy offer a distinct advantage in this age group as they provide greater flexibility. Ultrarapid insulins (e.g., Fiasp, Lyumjev) offer a slightly faster onset and shorter duration, which may help improve glucose control.[17]

REFERENCES

1. Lawrence JM, Divers J, Isom S, et al. Trends in prevalence of type 1 and type 2 diabetes in children and adolescents in the US, 2001-2017. *JAMA*. 2021;326(8):717-727.
2. Wagenknecht LE, Lawrence JM, Isom S, et al. Trends in incidence of youth-onset type 1 and type 2 diabetes in the USA, 2002-18: results from the population-based SEARCH for diabetes in Youth study. *Lancet Diabetes Endocrinol*. 2023;11(4):242-250.
3. Hales CM, Carroll MD, Fryar CD, Ogden CL. Prevalence of obesity among adults and youth: United States, 2015-2016. *NCHS Data Brief*. 2017;(288):1-8.
4. Diabetes Control and Complications Trial Research Group; Nathan DM, Genuth S, et al. The effect of intensive treatment of diabetes on the development and progression of long-term complications in insulin-dependent diabetes mellitus. *N Engl J Med*. 1993;329(14):977-986.
5. Holman RR, Paul SK, Bethel MA, Matthews DR, Neil HA. 10-year follow-up of intensive glucose control in type 2 diabetes. *N Engl J Med*. 2008;359(15):1577-1589.
6. Lacy ME, Lee KE, Atac O, et al. Patterns and trends in continuous glucose monitoring utilization among commercially insured individuals with type 1 diabetes: 2010-2013 to 2016-2019. *Clin Diabetes*. 2024;42(3):388-397.
7. American Diabetes Association Professional Practice Committee. 14. Children and adolescents: standards of care in diabetes-2025. *Diabetes Care*. 2025;48(suppl_1):S283-S305.
8. Battelino T, Danne T, Bergenstal RM, et al. Clinical targets for continuous glucose monitoring data interpretation: recommendations from the international consensus on time in range. *Diabetes Care*. 2019; 42(8):1593-1603.
9. Berget C, Messer LH, Forlenza GP. A clinical overview of insulin pump therapy for the management of diabetes: past, present, and future of intensive therapy. *Diabetes Spectr*. 2019;32(3):194-204.
10. American Diabetes Association; Bantle JP, Wylie-Rosett J, et al. Nutrition recommendations and interventions for diabetes: a position statement of the American Diabetes Association. *Diabetes Care*. 2008;31(suppl 1):S61-S78.
11. Shah AS, Zeitler PS, Wong J, et al. ISPAD clinical practice consensus guidelines 2022: type 2 diabetes in children and adolescents. *Pediatr Diabetes*. 2022;23(7):872-902.
12. Annan SF, Higgins LA, Jelleryd E, et al. ISPAD clinical practice consensus guidelines 2022: nutritional management in children and adolescents with diabetes. *Pediatr Diabetes*. 2022;23(8):1297-1321.
13. Lennerz BS, Barton A, Bernstein RK, et al. Management of type 1 diabetes with a very low-carbohydrate diet. *Pediatrics*. 2018;141(6):e20173349.
14. Conz A, Salmona M, Diomede L. Effect of non-nutritive sweeteners on the gut microbiota. *Nutrients*. 2023;15(8):1869.
15. Hatun Ş, Gökçe T, Can E, et al. Current management of type 1 diabetes in children: guideline-based expert opinions and recommendations. *J Clin Res Pediatr Endocrinol*. 2024;16(3):245-255.
16. Gregory JW, Cameron FJ, Joshi K, et al. ISPAD clinical practice consensus guidelines 2022: diabetes in adolescence. *Pediatr Diabetes*. 2022;23(7):857-871.
17. Wong EY, Kroon L. Ultra-rapid-acting insulins: how fast is really needed? *Clin Diabetes*. 2021;39(4):415-423.

PROFESSIONAL ORGANIZATIONS AND INTERNET RESOURCES

1. American Diabetes Association
   www.diabetes.org
2. Academy of Nutrition and Dietetics
   www.eatright.org
3. Beyond Type 1
4. Welcome to Beyond Type 1 and Type 2
5. Breakthrough T1D (formerly JDRF)
   https://www.breakthrought1d.org
6. Association of Diabetes Care and Education Specialists
   www.adces.org
7. National Institute of Diabetes and Digestive and Kidney Diseases
   www.niddk.nih.gov
8. CDC Diabetes
   www.cdc.gov/diabetes
9. Children with Diabetes
   www.childrenwithdiabetes.com
10. International Society of Pediatric and Adolescent Diabetes (ISPAD)
    www.ispad.org

CHAPTER 23

Eating Disorders

Katrina A.S. Smith, Annette Schille, and Tracy Richmond

Eating disorders (EDs) are common yet underrecognized biologically based mental illnesses.[1] Recent studies have estimated that by the age of 40, 1 in 5 females and 1 in 7 males will develop an ED.[2,3] These disorders typically emerge during adolescence, with a median onset of age 12 to 13[4] and occur along the continuum of weight, not only affecting those severely underweight, but also those with weights in the ranges considered healthy, overweight, and obese.

EDs are frequently underrecognized, resulting in an average delay of 30 months before treatment begins.[5] Even after diagnosis, the course of illness for EDs is often prolonged (averaging 6 years),[5] and marked by cycles of recovery and relapse. EDs carry the second highest mortality among all psychiatric illnesses, and at least one-third of survivors do not achieve full recovery in their lifetimes.[6] The burden of illness is substantial, both personally and societally.[7] Given the high burden of these illnesses, early recognition and comprehensive treatment strategies are needed.

The *Diagnostic and Statistical Manual of Mental Disorders (DSM)* outlines the diagnostic criteria for the various feeding and EDs[8] (see Table 23.1 for Diagnostic criteria).

MEDICAL AND NUTRITIONAL COMPLICATIONS

EDs are associated with numerous complications, including cardiac arrhythmias, electrolyte abnormalities, and skeletal fractures, and are often accompanied by psychiatric comorbidities such as depression and anxiety.[9] While complications are most common in patients with anorexia nervosa (AN) or bulimia nervosa (BN), they can occur in any type of ED. Table 23.2 outlines the most frequently observed complications in AN and BN. Among the most severe complications are sudden cardiac arrest and refeeding syndrome, which can result in death. Refeeding syndrome refers to severe extracellular hypophosphatemia as the body moves from using catabolized muscle and fat as the energy source to carbohydrate with refeeding. Ultimately, this may result in decreased adenosine triphosphate (ATP), which can lead to cardiac and respiratory failure. See Chapter 14 (Nutritional Assessment in Sick or Hospitalized Patients) for a discussion of refeeding syndrome. Nutrition-focused physical findings may include calluses on hands (from self-induced vomiting), lanugo, or swollen salivary glands. Depending on the type and severity of their ED, patients may be at risk for micronutrient deficiencies or macronutrient deficiencies (Table 23.3).[10-12]

TABLE 23.1 DIAGNOSTIC CRITERIA FOR EATING DISORDERS BASED ON THE DIAGNOSTIC AND STATISTICAL MANUAL OF MENTAL DISORDERS, FIFTH EDITION TEXT REVISION (DSM-5-TR)

ANOREXIA NERVOSA

- Restriction of food and drink leading to a body weight that is less than expected
- Fear of weight gain
- Inability to see the severity of the energy restriction

Subtypes:

- **Restricting Type:** lacks binge eating or purging
- **Binge-Eating/Purging Type:** restriction that includes binge eating and/or purging

BULIMIA NERVOSA

- Episodes of binge eating, characterized by a lack of control during the episode and consumption of a large amount of food, occurring approximately once per week for 3 months or more
- After each binge episode, inappropriate compensatory behaviors are used to prevent weight gain, such as self-induced vomiting, laxatives misuse, excessive exercise, or use of other medications

BINGE EATING DISORDER

- Episodes of binge eating, characterized by a lack of control during the episode and consumption of a large amount of food, occurring approximately once per week for 3 months or more
- No use of compensatory behaviors such as purging, restricting, or excessive exercise
- Feelings of distress related to the binge eating episodes, along with three or more of the following symptoms: unusually fast eating, continuing to eat past fullness, consuming excessive amounts without physical hunger, eating in private due to embarrassment, or experiencing strong negative emotions like guilt, shame, or sadness afterward

AVOIDANT/RESTRICTIVE FOOD INTAKE DISORDER

- Difficulty or unwillingness to eat an amount of energy and nutrients to maintain or sustain an appropriate weight; this may be due to decreased interest in food, sensory issues associated with the food, or concern of adverse effects (e.g., vomiting or choking) when eating or drinking
- May present as weight loss, slowed growth, and/or nutrient deficiencies, potentially requiring supplementation or enteral feeds
- Restriction is not driven by fear of weight gain or attempts at weight control.

OTHER SPECIFIED FEEDING AND EATING DISORDERS (OSFED)

Subtypes:

- **Atypical Anorexia Nervosa:** Restriction of energy without significant weight loss or a weight loss that falls into a "healthy" BMI category
- **Subthreshold Bulimia Nervosa:** Binge eating and purging (or other compensatory behaviors) occurring less frequently than the requirements for Bulimia Nervosa diagnosis
- **Subthreshold Binge Eating Disorder:** Binge eating that occurs less frequently than the requirements for the Binge Eating Disorder diagnosis
- **Night Eating Syndrome:** Eating exclusively upon waking at night, causing significant distress
- **Purging Disorder:** Recurrent purging behaviors (e.g., self-induced vomiting) for the purpose of weight loss, without the presence of binge eating

Data from American Psychiatric Association. Diagnostic and Statistical Manual of Mental Disorders, Fifth Edition, Text Revision. Arlington, Virginia: American Psychiatric Publishing; 2022.

TABLE 23.2 MEDICAL COMPLICATIONS OF EATING DISORDERS

CLINICAL SIGNS	ANOREXIA NERVOSA	BULIMIA NERVOSA
Labs	Low potassium, magnesium, or phosphorus related to refeeding	Low potassium, magnesium, and/or elevated CO_2 due to purging
Gastrointestinal	Bloating, constipation, delayed gastric emptying	Bloating, constipation, delayed gastric emptying, dysmotility, reflux, gastrointestinal bleeding
Cardiovascular	Hypotension, orthostasis, bradycardia	Cardiac arrhythmias, palpitations
Skeletal and dental	Osteopenia, osteoporosis	Dental caries and erosion
Weight	Underweight	Variable
Growth	Can delay growth	Growth typically not affected
Endocrine	Secondary amenorrhea/irregular menstrual cycles, sick euthyroid	Irregular menstrual cycles
Other	Fatigue, cold sensitivity	Fluid retention with edema, enlargement of parotid gland

TABLE 23.3 MICRONUTRIENT AND MACRONUTRIENT DEFICIENCIES

MICRONUTRIENT DEFICIENCIES

Iron

- Clinical Presentation: fatigue, anemia, pallor, hair loss
- Complications: impaired cognitive and immune function
- Populations at Risk: patients with restrictive eating patterns or limited food variety

Vitamin D

- Clinical Presentation: bone pain, muscle weakness, fatigue
- Complications: osteopenia, rickets in severe cases, or fractures
- Risk Factors: low sun exposure, low-fat diets, malabsorption syndromes

Calcium

- Clinical Presentation: muscle cramps, tingling in extremities
- Complications: osteoporosis, dental issues, and arrhythmias
- Contributing Factors: insufficient intake from dairy or fortified foods

B Vitamins (e.g., B_1, B_{12}, Folate)

- Clinical Presentation: neurologic symptoms (e.g., tingling or itching sensation, memory issues)
- Complications: anemia, nerve damage, cognitive dysfunction
- Common in: vegan diets or prolonged malnutrition

Zinc

- Clinical Presentation: poor wound healing, hair thinning
- Complications: growth delays in children, impaired taste/smell
- Risk Factors: ARFID, restrictive diets

TABLE 23.3 MICRONUTRIENT AND MACRONUTRIENT DEFICIENCIES (*continued*)

Potassium and Magnesium

- Clinical Presentation: fatigue, muscle weakness, cardiac arrhythmias
- Complications: cardiac and neuromuscular dysfunction
- Risk in: purging behaviors like vomiting or laxative misuse

MACRONUTRIENT DEFICIENCIES

Protein-Energy Malnutrition

- Clinical Presentation: muscle wasting, fatigue, edema (in severe cases)
- Complications: poor wound healing, compromised immunity
- Seen in: prolonged restriction or imbalance in dietary intake

Fat Deficiency

- Clinical Presentation: dry skin, hormonal imbalances
- Complications: impaired fat-soluble vitamin absorption (A, D, E, K)
- Causes: avoidance of fats

Carbohydrate Deficiency

- Clinical Presentation: fatigue, hypoglycemia, irritability
- Complications: ketoacidosis in extreme cases, impaired exercise tolerance
- Context: avoidance of carbohydrates, extreme low-carb dieting

Essential Fatty Acid (Omega-3, Omega-6) Deficiency

- Clinical Presentation: dry, scaly skin; cognitive issues
- Complications: growth delays in children, inflammatory issues
- Risk Factors: avoidance of fats or animal products

Dietary Fiber Deficiency

- Clinical Presentation: constipation, GI/gut-related issues
- Complications: increased risk for gastrointestinal issues and nutrient malabsorption

ARFID, avoidant/restrictive food intake disorder; GI, gastrointestinal.

NUTRITION ASSESSMENT

A comprehensive nutrition assessment is a critical component of evaluation and care of individuals with EDs, providing insight into the patient's nutritional status, growth patterns, dietary behaviors, and medical risks.[10] See Table 23.4 for an example of what components might be included in a nutrition assessment for individuals with EDs.

INTERDISCIPLINARY TREATMENT

Successful treatment of an ED begins with an interdisciplinary team evaluation, ideally including a medical provider, registered dietitian, mental health provider, and, in some cases, family therapist and/or psychiatrist.[14,15] Treatment planning, including recommendations for the level of care appropriate for an individual patient, is based on the severity of the patient's medical, psychological, and nutritional presentation symptoms. See Table 23.5 for descriptions of levels of care in ED treatment.

TABLE 23.4 COMPONENTS OF A COMPREHENSIVE NUTRITION ASSESSMENT

A. Clinical History

Dietary History:

- Typical daily intake: identify safe/unsafe foods, meal patterns, and portion sizes.
- Food preferences, aversions, and avoidance along with recent changes in dietary habits
- Episodes of bingeing, purging (vomiting, laxative use, diuretic use, or excessive exercise), or restrictive eating
- Fluid intake: over hydration or dehydration practices
- Use of supplements or meal replacements

Weight History:

- Weight trajectory over time (including highest/lowest weights and changes in either/both weight and BMI growth curve percentiles)
- Goal weight vs. perceived ideal weight
- History of weight changes, including intentional or unintentional weight loss

Activity Level:

- Exercise patterns, including excessive or compulsive behaviors

Medical History:

- Comorbid conditions (e.g., gastrointestinal issues, diabetes)
- Menstrual history in females (amenorrhea or irregular periods)

Psychosocial History:

- Psychological factors: anxiety, depression, trauma, body image concerns
- Social factors: family dynamics, peer influence, or cultural factors impacting eating

B. Anthropometric Measurements

Weight and Height:

- Monitor trends, growth charts, and percentiles for pediatric patients.
- Percent median body weight and BMI percentiles
- Assessment of stunted growth or delayed growth patterns in children

Body Composition:

- Optional use of tools like skinfold thickness
- Signs of muscle wasting or fat depletion

Mid-upper arm circumference (MUAC):

- Useful in cases of severe malnutrition or growth assessment

Growth Velocity:

- Critical for children and adolescents to assess stunted growth or catch-up

C. ***Biochemical Data***

Lab Markers to Evaluate:

- Vitamin and mineral levels (e.g., iron, folate, B vitamins, vitamin D, zinc)
- Markers of malnutrition (e.g., albumin, prealbumin)
- Hematological status (e.g., hemoglobin, ferritin, transferrin)
- Electrolyte imbalances (potassium, magnesium, sodium)
- Thyroid function tests (to assess metabolic function)
- Liver function tests (elevated transaminases in malnutrition)
- Bone health (serum calcium, phosphate, alkaline phosphatase, vitamin D)

TABLE 23.4 COMPONENTS OF A COMPREHENSIVE NUTRITION ASSESSMENT (*continued*)

D. Assessment

Methods:

- 24-h dietary recall or food frequency questionnaires
- Use of apps or journals to capture intake
- Observation during meals for ARFID or behavioral patterns

Evaluation:

- Energy adequacy compared to estimated energy requirements (EER)
- Macronutrient distribution (protein, carbohydrates, fats)
- Micronutrient sufficiency (e.g., calcium, vitamin D for bone health)
- Fiber insufficiency or excess, impacting gastrointestinal health

Assess Eating Behaviors:

- Ritualistic food preparation or eating habits (e.g., vegetarian or vegan)
- Use of compensatory mechanisms (e.g., cutting food into small pieces, hiding food)

Physical Assessment:

- Look for signs of malnutrition or eating disorder behaviors:
  - Hair: thin, brittle hair or hair loss
  - Skin: dry skin, lanugo, bruising
  - Nails: brittle or ridged nails
  - Oral health: dental erosion (from vomiting), swollen parotid glands
  - Musculoskeletal: muscle wasting, joint pain, or osteoporosis
  - Cardiovascular: bradycardia, orthostatic hypotension, arrhythmias
- Assess for signs of refeeding syndrome during nutritional rehabilitation.
- Impact of nutritional status on physical activity, school performance, and daily life

Monitor for:

- Delayed pubertal development
- Growth stunting or failure to meet genetic growth potential
- Catch-up growth following nutritional rehabilitation

Tailor the Assessment Based on:

- Specific eating disorder diagnosis (e.g., anorexia nervosa, bulimia nervosa, ARFID)
- Severity of medical and nutritional complications
- Patient and family's understanding of and willingness to address the disorder

Interdisciplinary Collaboration:

- Work with interdisciplinary team members (e.g., MD, psychologist, psychiatrist, social worker).

ARFID, avoidant/restrictive food intake disorder; BMI, body mass index.

Awareness of common psychological therapies can be helpful for the nutrition professional to facilitate their collaboration with the interdisciplinary team. Common approaches used in the treatment of EDs include:

- Cognitive Behavioral Therapy (CBT): A goal-oriented approach that focuses on identifying and changing disordered thoughts and behaviors
- Dialectical Behavioral Therapy (DBT): A skills-based approach that emphasizes emotional regulation, mindfulness, and distress tolerance

TABLE 23.5 LEVELS OF CARE[a] FOR THE TREATMENT OF PATIENTS WITH EATING DISORDERS

Inpatient Hospitalization

- Provides: 24/7 medical monitoring, nasogastric feeds when necessary
- Patient criteria: low body weight, acute food refusal even if not low weighted, low heart rate and/or blood pressure, abnormal electrolytes, unsuccessful with outpatient treatment and in need of supervision during and after meals and/or support of nasogastric feedings

Residential Treatment

- Provides: 24/7 monitoring, all meals and snacks supervised
- Patient criteria: does not require daily feeding tubes, labs, or IV fluids, support/supervision during and after meals needed

Partial Hospitalization Program (PHP, full-day outpatient care)

- Provides: several supervised meals and snacks, ability to sleep at home, group and individual therapy, nutrition counseling
- Patient criteria: generally >80% of target body weight, needs some structure around meal times to support recovery, medically stable enough to travel to and from program daily, support/supervision during and after some meals needed

Intensive Outpatient Program (IOP, often an evening program several days per week)

- Provides: one supervised meal and snack per session, group and individual therapy and nutrition counseling
- Patient criteria: generally >80% of target body weight, some support/supervision during and after meals needed

Outpatient

- Provides: weekly, biweekly, or monthly check-ins with therapist and/or dietitian depending on progress
- Patient criteria: generally >85% of target body weight, minimal support/supervision during and after meals needed

[a]Recommended levels of care may differ between institutions and will vary on a case-by-case basis.
Hackert AN, Kniskern MA, Beasley TM. Academy of Nutrition and Dietetics: revised 2020 standards of practice and standards of professional performance for registered dietitian nutritionists (competent, proficient, and expert) in eating disorders. *J Acad Nutr Diet*. 2020;120(11):1902-1919.e54; Ozier AD, Henry BW; American Dietetic Association. Position of the American Dietetic Association: nutrition intervention in the treatment of eating disorders. *J Am Diet Assoc*. 2011;111(8):1236-1241.

- Acceptance and Commitment Therapy (ACT): A behavioral therapy that encourages patients to accept their thoughts and emotions as valid, while acting in line with personal values
- Family-Based Treatment (FBT): A structured approach in which parents take control of food and refeeding, gradually returning autonomy to the child or adolescent; considered the first-line approach for the treatment of anorexia nervosa in younger patients and has been proven effective for treatment of bulimia nervosa

NUTRITION INTERVENTION

Outpatient nutrition counseling for individuals with EDs should be done by a registered dietitian with training and experience in treating complex disorders with psychological and medical complications. The primary goals of outpatient nutrition intervention are to reduce the use of disordered eating behaviors, restore weight (if medically necessary), and establish a consistent meal pattern, all in a setting that allows the patient to remain a participant in as much of their current life and preferred activities as possible.

The outpatient registered dietitian's (RD) role includes assessing energy and macronutrient needs, monitoring dietary intake and growth, and determining weight goals in collaboration with the treatment team. The RD should also identify and implement appropriate interventions to address nutrition-related concerns, disordered eating behaviors, and contributing environmental or psychosocial factors. Interventions may include setting nutrition goals, expanding food variety, increasing portion sizes, teaching hunger/fullness awareness, or providing a structured meal plan.

Many individuals with EDs may be ambivalent or resistant to nutritional changes recommended by the RD. Understanding the transtheoretical "stages of change" model—from precontemplation to contemplation, preparation, and action—can help guide individualized counseling approaches.[16] Partnering and collaborating with the young person, rather than simply educating or prescribing, can enhance engagement and improve the likelihood of sustained behavior change, even when motivation appears low.

In inpatient settings, nutrition interventions are typically more protocolized and closely monitored. See Tables 23.6 [17] and 23.7 [18,19] for examples of inpatient medical and nutrition protocols for restrictive EDs and avoidant/restrictive food intake disorder (ARFID).

TABLE 23.6 SUMMARY OF RESTRICTIVE EATING INPATIENT MEDICAL AND NUTRITION PROTOCOL

GOALS

- Stabilize heart rate, blood pressure, electrolytes, body weight, and body temperature via improving nutritional status and overall health, by providing prescribed meals and limiting physical activity.
- Demonstrate ability and improve self-efficacy around taking in adequate nutrition.
- Identify and address psychiatric comorbidities while supporting movement away from disordered eating behaviors.

Medical monitoring

- Vital signs (heart rate and blood pressure), temperature, labs (concern for refeeding syndrome), body weight, and urine-specific gravity
- Multivitamin with minerals and supplement providing K/Na/P (to prevent refeeding syndrome) given daily; amount of K/Na/P may be adjusted based on lab value

Nutrition therapy

- All meal plans start at 2000 calories unless otherwise determined by team.
- Meal plans are increased by 250 calories per day until goal.
- Standard meals are provided (i.e., patients do not choose their meal).
- Available menus: regular, vegetarian, nut free, gluten free, lactose free
- Each patient can identify five "dislikes."
- Other deviations from standard preselected menus require consultation.

Supplementation

- If a meal is not completed within 30 min, the supplement equivalent is offered.
- If a patient is unable to drink the supplements in the allotted amount of time, the use of a nasogastric tube may be considered.

(continued)

TABLE 23.6 SUMMARY OF RESTRICTIVE EATING INPATIENT MEDICAL AND NUTRITION PROTOCOL (*continued*)

Weight-gain expectations

- Inpatient weight gain is expected to be 0.2 kg/d.
- If weight gain expectation is not met, liquid supplement is added (additional 500 kcal first day, 750 kcal second day, 1000 kcal third, and subsequent days).
- If weight gain expectation not consistently met, meal plan may be increased or weight expectation may be reset.

Physical activity

- Two to three 10-min supervised walks on the inpatient unit once the patient is medically cleared.
- Patients are encouraged to be out of bed and in a chair to support blood pressure.

Family education

- Parents receive psychoeducation regarding the disorder and coaching around how best to support around meal times.

Discharge goals

- Resolutions of vital sign or lab abnormalities
- Achievement of weight goal necessary to move toward the next appropriate level of care

Boston Chidren's Hospital. *Restrictive eating —clinical pathways*. https://clinical.pathways.childrenshospital.org/pathways/63f42a869ebd7600129eed4d

TABLE 23.7 SUMMARY OF AVOIDANT RESTRICTIVE FOOD INTAKE INPATIENT MEDICAL AND NUTRITION PROTOCOL

GOALS

- Optimize nutritional intake, develop mealtime structure to optimize the patient's appetite and natural desire to eat, and support desired behaviors to allow for graduated sustainable achievements.
- Address underlying triggers and comorbidities associated with ARFID.
- Help family and patient with their feeding challenges and to improve their quality of life.

Medical monitoring

- Observe patient's eating behaviors and identify their risk of malnutrition and analyze the quality and quantity of macro and micronutrients.
- Correct micronutrient deficiencies with supplements.

Nutrition therapy

- Create structure for the patient and family around feeding to optimize appetite and awareness and importance of hunger and thirst sensation.
- Offer three to five meal exposures daily, up to three meals and two snacks.
- All 30 min for meals, 20 min for snacks, remove food/tray following exposure.
- Observe the patient eating their meal in an environment both with the caregiver and without the caregiver to better understand the patient's feeding behaviors.

Supplementation

- Individualized determination of oral vs. enteral supplemental nutrition needs (decision about need for supplemental enteral nutrition is based on degree of nutritional insufficiency and patient's motivation and ability to implement oral nutritional restoration).
- Supplementation may be used to promote weight gain in some patients, though there is no predetermined criteria for rate of weight gain.

TABLE 23.7 SUMMARY OF AVOIDANT RESTRICTIVE FOOD INTAKE INPATIENT MEDICAL AND NUTRITION PROTOCOL (*continued*)

Physical activity

- Physical activity may be limited due to the medical state of patient (e.g., weakness, dizziness).
- Bed rest or wheelchair use might be recommended.

Family education

- As the hospitalization continues, the multidisciplinary team works to empower the caregivers to implement the feeding plan to the best of their abilities through team member modeling and engagement in supportive nonaccommodative behaviors.
- Behavioral parent training, psychoeducation regarding ARFID, and nutrition education are provided.

Discharge goals

- Achievement of weight goal necessary to move toward the next appropriate level of care. Optimize discharge planning to allow for progressive recovery.
- Discharge planning is discussed in the framework of the patient's projected needs and the caregiver's competency with the intent of providing medical stabilization and positioning the family successfully to continue treatment via outpatient care.
- Options for discharge may include transition to residential or intensive outpatient programs to address the eating disorder, comorbidities such as anxiety or depression or follow-up in the multidisciplinary outpatient ARFID program.

ARFID, avoidant/restrictive food intake disorder.
Bern EM, Milliren CE, Tsang KK, et al. Variation in care for inpatients with avoidant restrictive food intake disorder leads to development of a novel inpatient clinical pathway to standardize care. *J Eat Disord*. 2024;12(1):66; Boston Chidren's Hospital. *Avoidant/restrictive food intake disorder (ARFID) —clinical pathways.* https://clinical.pathways.childrenshospital.org/pathways/63d9638f9ebd7600129ed97c

REFERENCES

1. Klump KL, Bulik C, Kaye W, Treasure J, Tyson E. Academy for Eating Disorders Position paper: eating disorders are serious mental illnesses. *Int J Eat Discord*. 2009;42(2):97-103.
2. Herpertz-Dahlmann B. Adolescent eating disorders: update on definitions, symptomatology, epidemiology, and comorbidity. *Child Adolesc Psychiatr Clin N Am*. 2015;24(1):177-196.
3. Ward ZJ, Rodriguez P, Wright DR, Austin SB, Long MW. Estimation of eating disorders prevalence by age and associations with mortality in a simulated Nationally Representative US Cohort. *JAMA Netw Open*. 2019;2(10):e1912925.
4. Swanson SA, Crow SJ, Le Grange D, Swendsen J, Merikangas KR. Prevalence and correlates of eating disorders in adolescents: results from the national comorbidity survey replication adolescent supplement. *Arch Gen Psychiatry*. 2011;68(7):714-723.
5. Austin A, Flynn M, Richards K, et al. Duration of untreated eating disorder and relationship to outcomes: a systematic review of the literature. *Eur Eat Disord Rev*. 2021;29(3):329-345.
6. Arcelus J, Mitchell AJ, Wales J, Nielsen S. Mortality rates in patients with anorexia nervosa and other eating disorders: a meta-analysis of 36 studies. *Arch Gen Psychiatry*. 2011;68(7):724-731.
7. Streatfeild J, Hickson J, Austin SB, et al. Social and economic cost of eating disorders in the United States: evidence to inform policy action. *Int J Eat Disord*. 2021;54(5):851-868.
8. American Psychiatric Association. *Diagnostic and Statistical Manual of Mental Disorders*. 5th ed. American Psychiatric Association; 2013.
9. Fichter MM, Quadflieg N. Six-year course and outcome of anorexia nervosa. *Int J Eat Disord*. 1999;26(4):359-385.

10. Ozier AD, Henry BW; American Dietetic Association. Position of the American Dietetic Association: nutrition intervention in the treatment of eating disorders. *J Am Diet Assoc*. 2011;111(8):1236-1241.
11. American Dietetic Association. Position of the American Dietetic Association: nutrition intervention in the treatment of anorexia nervosa, bulimia nervosa, and other eating disorders. *J Am Diet Assoc*. 2006; 106(12):2073-2082.
12. Setnick J. Micronutrient deficiencies and supplementation in Anorexia and Bulimia Nervosa: a review of literature. *Nutr Clin Pract*. 2010;25(2):137-142.
13. Hackert AN, Kniskern MA, Beasley TM. Academy of Nutrition and Dietetics: revised 2020 standards of practice and standards of professional performance for registered dietitian nutritionists (competent, proficient, and expert) in eating disorders. *J Acad Nutr Diet*. 2020;120(11):1902-1919.e54.
14. Ozier AD, Henry BW; American Dietetic Association. Position of the American Dietetic Association: nutrition intervention in the treatment of eating disorders. *J Am Diet Assoc*. 2011;111(8):1236-1241.
15. Hoetzel K, von Brachel R, Schlossmacher L, Vocks S. Assessing motivation to change in eating disorders: a systematic review. *J Eat Disord*. 2013;1:38.
16. Boston Chidren's Hospital. *Restrictive eating —clinical pathways*. https://clinical.pathways.childrenshospital.org/pathways/63f42a869ebd7600129eed4d
17. Boston Chidren's Hospital. *Avoidant/restrictive food intake disorder (ARFID) —clinical pathways*. https://clinical.pathways.childrenshospital.org/pathways/63d9638f9ebd7600129ed97c
18. Bern EM, Milliren CE, Tsang KK, et al. Variation in care for inpatients with avoidant restrictive food intake disorder leads to development of a novel inpatient clinical pathway to standardize care. *J Eat Disord*. 2024;12(1):66.

SUGGESTED RESOURCES

■ EATING DISORDER ORGANIZATIONS:

- Multi-service Eating Disorders Association, Inc. (MEDA)
  www.medainc.org
- National Eating Disorder Association (NEDA)
  www.nationaleatingdisorders.org

■ EATING DISORDER RESOURCES:

- GÜRZE Books: Eating Disorder Resource Catalogue
  www.gurzebooks.com
- Center for Young Women's Health
  www.youngwomenshealth.org

Note: Clinicians should be cautious when advising internet browsing, as pro eating disorder web sites are very easily accessible to this vulnerable population.

CHAPTER 24

Feeding and Swallowing Difficulties

Daniel R. Duncan, Kayla Hernandez, and Heather Stone

Feeding and swallowing difficulties are frequently diagnosed in children and require coordinated, multidisciplinary management involving specialists in nutrition, speech-language pathology, and gastroenterology.[1] Dysphagia, or difficulty swallowing, may result from abnormal oropharyngeal anatomy or dysfunction in any phase of swallowing.[2,3] More severe complications can result when there is incomplete laryngeal vestibule closure in the pharyngeal phase of the swallow, resulting in either laryngeal penetration (entry of foreign material into the laryngeal vestibule above the vocal folds) or aspiration (entry of foreign material below the level of the vocal folds into the airway).

Feeding and swallowing difficulties may also stem from altered oral-motor or oral-sensory development, common among children with broader developmental delays and/or medical comorbidities.[4]

The estimated prevalence of oropharyngeal dysphagia ranges from 25% to 45% in typically developing children and up to 80% in children with developmental disabilities.[1] An apparent increase in the prevalence of these conditions in pediatrics may be due to the higher rate of survival of preterm infants and children with medical complexity.

The diagnosis of pediatric feeding disorder (PFD) encompasses an even broader set of clinical conditions related to inadequate oral intake. PFD unifies the medical, nutritional, feeding skill, and/or psychosocial concerns associated with feeding disorders.[4] This diagnosis highlights the importance of a multidisciplinary approach to care.[5]

CAUSES

Feeding is a complex skill involving multiple organ systems, including coordination of the central nervous, gastrointestinal (GI), respiratory, and musculoskeletal systems, as well as behavioral and sensory regulation.[2] Causes of feeding and swallowing difficulties may be developmental, structural, GI, neurologic, iatrogenic, or cognitive/behavioral.[2,6] Dysphagia can occur in any of the phases of swallowing, each of which can be impacted by structural anomalies and difficulties related to peripheral or central nervous system function:

- **Preoral phase:** Involves hunger cues and readiness to eat. Negative feeding experiences (e.g., GI discomfort, forceful feeding) may lead to oral feeding aversion.
- **Oral phase:** Involves mechanical manipulation of food to prepare the bolus for swallowing. Children with orofacial anomalies such as cleft lip and palate often experience difficulties with oral feeding coordination and efficiency prior to surgical repair, often due to difficulty with suction and sealing on a bottle.

- **Pharyngeal phase:** Involuntary phase initiated as the bolus moves from the oral cavity to the hypopharynx. Poor coordination due to conditions such as laryngomalacia or structural aerodigestive anomalies (e.g., laryngeal cleft, tracheoesophageal fistula) may disrupt this phase, leading to aspiration.
- **Esophageal phase:** Begins as the bolus enters the upper esophageal sphincter and is propelled to the stomach via peristaltic contractions. Structural abnormalities of the esophagus, mucosal inflammation, or motility disorders can interfere with transit and increase aspiration risk.

In otherwise healthy infants and young children with oropharyngeal dysphagia, the majority will have developmental swallow dysfunction, which improves with growth and development.[3] GI conditions such as gastroesophageal reflux disease, eosinophilic esophagitis, and food allergy can also contribute to dysphagia or feeding difficulties and may mimic or overlap with signs of aspiration, especially in young children. Accurate diagnosis is essential, given the symptom overlap and differing treatment approaches.[7,8]

ASSESSMENT/EVALUATION

Clinical signs or symptoms suggestive of oropharyngeal dysphagia can include respiratory symptoms such as coughing, choking, congestion, or wet breath sounds associated with feeding. However, most aspiration in infants and young children is clinically silent, occurring without associated cough.[9,10]

When a dietitian identifies potential feeding or swallowing difficulties, referral to a speech-language pathologist specializing in pediatric feeding and swallowing disorders is warranted. Table 24.1 outlines "red flags" and common reasons for referral.

A clinical feeding evaluation completed by a speech-language pathologist is often the first evaluation for a child presenting with feeding and/or swallowing difficulties.[6] Refer to Table 24.2 for the components of a clinical feeding evaluation.

If there are concerns for swallowing difficulties or impaired airway protection with swallowing, an instrumental swallowing assessment, such as videofluoroscopic swallow study (VFSS) or flexible endoscopic evaluation of swallowing (FEES), may be indicated.[6] These assessments, described in Table 24.3, help characterize the physiology of the oral and pharyngeal swallow mechanism and may include a brief esophageal screen. Instrumental swallowing assessment findings often lead to further diagnostic testing and specialist referrals.

Timely diagnosis and treatment are essential to prevent long-term adverse effects of chronic aspiration, including severe pulmonary sequelae, bronchiectasis, intractable feeding difficulties, oral aversion, and/or malnutrition.[1,2] If available, a multidisciplinary feeding program and/or aerodigestive program, which may include a gastroenterologist, pulmonologist, otolaryngologist, registered dietitian, speech-language pathologist, occupational therapist, psychologist, developmental pediatrician, and/or social worker, can provide comprehensive and coordinated evaluation and care.

TREATMENT

Treatment plans should be informed by a thorough evaluation of a child's feeding and swallowing skills and developed in collaboration with families. The treatment plan should balance considerations related to safety, efficiency, and developmental appropriateness.

TABLE 24.1 RED FLAGS AND COMMON REASONS FOR REFERRAL

AGE GROUP	INDICATIONS FOR REFERRAL TO A FEEDING SPECIALIST
All ages	Coughing or choking
	Frequent gagging with swallowing
	Cyanosis or color change (red/blue around lips)
	Wet, congested breathing
	Unexplained fevers or respiratory symptoms
	Recurrent respiratory infections
	Excessive drooling
≤6 mo	Large amounts of liquid loss
(Breast and/or bottle feeding)	Difficulty latching to nipple
	Short sucking bursts
	Prolonged feeding times (>30 min)
	Failure to gain weight
	Consistently fussy or refusing feedings
	Only feeds while drowsy/asleep ("dream feeding")
	Arching, pulling away from nipple despite hunger cues
6-18 mo	Any of the above
	Excessive food loss while eating
	Consistently gags when trying a new food
	Consistently refuses categories of food (fruits, vegetables, meats, purees)
	Not interested in mouthing objects or food
	Difficulty transitioning to cup drinking by 12-18 mo
	Not engaging in self-feeding (finger feeding/utensil use) by 12-18 mo
>18 mo	Any of the above
	Inefficient with solid foods (i.e., swallowing food whole, taking a long time to swallow each bite, pocketing food in cheeks, overstuffing of food)
	Not consuming age-appropriate solid food textures
	Gags, chokes, or vomits when offered new or nonpreferred foods
	Refuses to try new foods
	Extremely sensitive/particular about tastes, textures, smells, brands, and presentation of food
	Stress and anxiety at mealtime
	Lack of interest in food/low appetite
	Lengthy mealtimes that might involve leaving the table repeatedly
	Maladaptive feeding behaviors

If nutrition and hydration needs cannot be met through oral feeding alone, nonoral methods of supplemental nutrition should be considered. Treatment approaches vary based on the underlying cause of a child's feeding difficulty.[2] Under the guidance of a speech-language pathologist with expertise in pediatric feeding and swallowing disorders, treatment approaches may include:

- **Changes in delivery method**: for example, slower flow nipples, alternative cups

TABLE 24.2 COMPONENTS OF A CLINICAL ASSESSMENT OF FEEDING AND SWALLOWING

Case history	• Medical, developmental, and early feeding history • Current diet and feeding and swallowing skills, including types of foods/liquids consumed, mealtime behaviors, feeding schedule, self-feeding skills, utensils and methods of delivery, feeding environment • Concerns regarding feeding and swallowing and goals of assessment
Physical examination	• Level of alertness, attention, self-regulation, communication • Oral mechanism evaluation, including structure and function of oral anatomy, oral reflexes, saliva management, and vocal quality • Oral-sensory observations
Feeding observation	• Assessment of typical feeding tasks • Observation of swallowing; identifying any adverse clinical signs suggestive of possible aspiration • Assess stability during feeding. • Trial feeding strategies, positional changes, different feeding equipment, and modifications to food/liquid consistency • Assess caregiver and child interactions during feeding.
Other considerations	• Developmental profile, underlying medical diagnosis, GI function, growth and nutritional status, family structure, cultural views on feeding, social determinants of health

TABLE 24.3 INSTRUMENTAL ASSESSMENT OF SWALLOWING

VIDEOFLUOROSCOPIC EVALUATION OF SWALLOWING (VFSS) OR MODIFIED BARIUM SWALLOW STUDY (MBS)	FLEXIBLE ENDOSCOPIC EVALUATION OF SWALLOWING (FEES)
Both assessments define the physiology of the swallowing mechanism and diagnose swallowing impairments/dysphagia. Findings should be integrated with the clinical assessment of feeding and swallowing, as well as information from the history and other diagnostic testing and factors. Compliance with both assessments can be challenging, particularly for toddlers and young children.	
Radiographic study performed jointly by a speech-language pathologist and radiologist	Nasal endoscopy performed by a speech-language pathologist ± an otolaryngologist. A flexible endoscope is passed transnasally to the hypopharynx, above the vocal cords.
Assesses the **oral, pharyngeal, and upper esophageal phase** of the swallow. May include an esophageal screening	Only assesses the **pharyngeal phase** of the swallow.
Child consumes barium contrast of different consistencies of liquids and textures of solids (as appropriate), while continuous fluoroscopic images are captured.	Child consumes food or liquid while the flexible endoscope is in place. Food coloring is sometimes added to improve visibility of food/liquid.
Directly visualizes moments of laryngeal penetration and/or aspiration during the swallow	Visualizes only before and after the swallow. "White out" occurs during the swallow when the view is obscured.
Involves radiation exposure	Can assess structural anomalies in the throat and secretion management
Cannot assess swallowing during breastfeeding	Can be used to assess swallowing during breastfeeding

- **Dietary modification:** for example, thickened liquid, food texture modification
- **Feeding techniques:** for example, positioning changes, pacing, swallowing maneuvers
- **Oral-motor/sensory therapy:** to improve bolus control, developmental feeding skills (e.g., chewing development, cup or straw drinking), or expand food repertoire[4,5]

For PFDs involving food aversion/avoidance and behavioral feeding difficulties, cotreatment with behavioral health providers may be necessary. Refer to Table 24.4 for additional treatment considerations.

Thickening liquids may be recommended for children who present with concerns for aspiration or to improve swallowing efficiency and coordination.[11,12] Commonly utilized thicknesses are described as slightly thick, mildly thick, and moderately thick. Factors influencing liquid thickness include[11,13]:

- **Liquid type** (e.g., expressed breastmilk, type and caloric density of formula, water, juice)
- **Thickening agent type** (e.g., starch-based, gum-based, food-based)
- **Mixing method** (e.g., amount of thickening agent, thickening time, temperature)

Table 24.5 outlines important considerations for thickening liquids. Dietitians must monitor for nutritional adequacy, as thickening agents can alter the caloric density and nutritional composition of breastmilk and formula. Food-based thickeners (e.g., food purees or yogurt) may affect micronutrient intake.

Semisolid foods that melt into a thin liquid in the mouth (e.g., ice, gelatin desserts, ice cream, and popsicles) must be avoided if thickening is required to avoid aspiration. Juicy fruits such as pineapple and watermelon should also be avoided.

TABLE 24.4 EXAMPLES OF FEEDING AND SWALLOWING TREATMENT OPTIONS

	Swallowing Difficulties
Modified fluids	• Adding thickener to liquids • Trialing naturally thicker liquids (i.e., smoothies, yogurt drinks) • Altering the sensory properties of liquids (i.e., temperature, carbonation)
Feeding equipment	• Changing the bottle type, nipple shape, or nipple flow rate for infants. • Using specialty feeding systems for children with anatomic differences (i.e., one-way valve system for cleft palate) • Trialing different cups based on oral-motor patterns and developmental skills (i.e., open cup, straw cup, spouted cup)
Feeding strategies	• Changing the feeding position for infants (i.e., side-lying or upright position to control the flow of fluids and improve coordination) • Trialing postural changes in older children (i.e., neutral head posture, slight head down/chin tuck to encourage airway protection, head turn for unilateral weakness) • Changing the volume (i.e., controlling sip size or bite size) • Changing the pace or rate of delivery (i.e., imposed breaks, single sips)

(continued)

TABLE 24.4 EXAMPLES OF FEEDING AND SWALLOWING TREATMENT OPTIONS (*continued*)

	Oral-Sensory and Oral-Motor Difficulties
Modified foods	• Modifying the sensory properties of food to increase sensory feedback and promote increased chewing (i.e., crunchy foods, stronger flavors) • Modifying the texture of foods for children with delayed or impaired chewing skills (i.e., pureed, mashed, minced, bite size)
Functional feeding goals	• Improving oral-motor skills to support a new developmental skill (i.e., advancement from bottle to cup drinking) • Improving oral-motor skills for chewing more advanced textures • Targeting oral-sensory responses to improve acceptance of new foods, textures, and flavors
	Behavioral Considerations
	• Set mealtimes and routines that include a 2-3 h spacing between meals and snacks to ensure appetite. • Avoid grazing between meals and snacks as this can interfere with appetite. This includes caloric beverages. Offer water only between meals and snacks. • Encourage family meals (socialization). • Verbal praise and attention for desired behaviors • Include children in meal preparation and cleanup. • Talk about the physical properties of food (i.e., color, shape, texture, taste, smell). • Do not have "battles" over food or force feed. Offer exposure without pressure to take a bite—*touch, smell, lick, kiss.* • Encourage mindful eating by removing distractions (i.e., screens, books, toys).

Thickened liquids may be contraindicated for some children, such as those with a history of prematurity with increased risk of necrotizing enterocolitis (NEC) and children with congenital heart disease with decreased GI perfusion.[12] These situations underscore the need for multidisciplinary management for children requiring modified diets, especially those with medical complexity.

Clinicians should use standardized terminology and recommend testing methods for food texture and liquid thickness provided by the International Dysphagia Diet Standardisation Initiative (IDDSI) when managing children with feeding and swallowing difficulties for which modified liquid or food diets are recommended.[14] The IDDSI Flow Test, a syringe-based gravity test, is a practical tool used to verify liquid thickness. Caregivers should be trained to perform this test, especially when changes are made to the type of thickener, type of formula/milk, or caloric concentration.[15] Refer to Figure 24.1 for an overview of the IDDSI framework.

■ CONCLUSION/SUMMARY

Feeding and swallowing difficulties are increasingly recognized in the pediatric population and may arise from a wide range of medical, developmental, and behavioral conditions. Effective treatment depends on accurate diagnosis and may involve a range of strategies tailored to the child's needs. Multidisciplinary assessment and collaborative management are essential for achieving optimal outcomes.

TABLE 24.5 THICKENER OPTIONS AND CONSIDERATIONS

THICKENER[a]	PRIMARY INGREDIENTS	CALORIES PER SERVING[b]	CAN BE USED TO THICKEN BREASTMILK	APPROVED AGE/WEIGHT[c]	LIMITATIONS/OTHER CONSIDERATIONS
Infant rice cereal	Rice flour	5 kcal per teaspoon	No	No restrictions	• Potential change in bowel movements (constipation) • Arsenic/heavy metal contamination concern • Fortified to provide additional micronutrients
Infant oatmeal cereal	Oat flour	4-5 kcal per teaspoon of cereal (varies by brand)	No	No restrictions	• Increased risk of clogging nipple • May be fortified to provide additional micronutrient intake • May contain wheat.
Other infant grain cereals	Varies by brand May contain combinations of wheat, oat, spelt, barley, corn	5 kcal per teaspoon of cereal	No	No restriction	• Nutritional considerations and consistencies vary depending on the grain(s). • May be fortified to provide additional micronutrient intake.
GelMix	Tapioca Maltodextrin, Carob bean gum	5 kcal per scoop[b]	Yes	Age: >42 wk postmenstrual age; Weight: >6 lbs[c]	• Lukewarm liquid required to achieve thickening • Stable in most liquids for up to 24 h • May cause gas and loose stools for the first 1-2 wk of use.
SimplyThick	Xanthan gum Soluble fiber	0 kcal per slightly thick packet[b] 5 kcal per mildly thick packet[b]	Yes	>12 mo depending on institutional policy[c] (Manufacturer warning: "Do not use in infants or children under 12 y of age without consulting a health care professional")	• Case reports of necrotizing enterocolitis (NEC) • Note that recipe includes soluble fiber

(continued)

TABLE 24.5 THICKENER OPTIONS AND CONSIDERATIONS (*continued*)

THICKENER[a]	PRIMARY INGREDIENTS	CALORIES PER SERVING[b]	CAN BE USED TO THICKEN BREASTMILK	APPROVED AGE/WEIGHT[c]	LIMITATIONS/OTHER CONSIDERATIONS
Thick-It	Corn starch	20 kcal per packet	No	>24 mo corrected age depending on institutional policy[c] (Manufacturer guideline: "Should only be used with children under the age of 12 in consultation with a physician")	• Thickens hot and cold liquids • Grainy texture reported • May further thicken over time (recommended to consume within 30 min).
Purathick	Tara gum Tapioca Maltodextrin	10 kcal per packet[b]	Yes	>12 mo corrected age[c]; not safe in galactosemia	• Thickens hot and cold liquids • Requires mixing thoroughly (blender bottle recommended) to fully incorporate the powder • Can prepare with most liquids up to 24 h in advance
ThickenUp Clear	Xanthan gum	5 kcal per packet or scoop[b]	Yes	>3 y[c]	• Does not further thicken over time • Thickens hot and cold liquids
Enfamil A.R. Infant Formula	Rice starch	Varies depending on concentration	No	No restrictions	• Thickness will vary depending on concentration of formula and use of powder vs. ready-to-feed. • May further thicken over time.
Food purees	Fruit, vegetable, yogurt, other pureed foods	Varies depending on foods used	Yes	Typically only after 6 mo corrected age for yogurt and after 4 mo of age for other purees	• Work with team, including registered dietitian and feeding specialist, to ensure appropriate nutrient content and liquid consistency. • Volume used is added to final volume of recipe. • Yogurt adds protein and can also be used to provide calcium and vitamin D.

[a]Thickening agent availability may vary based on country. These agents are approved and available at the time of publication.
[b]Note that calories from gel thickeners are not completely absorbed.
[c]Note that approved ages for commercial thickeners can vary by institution.

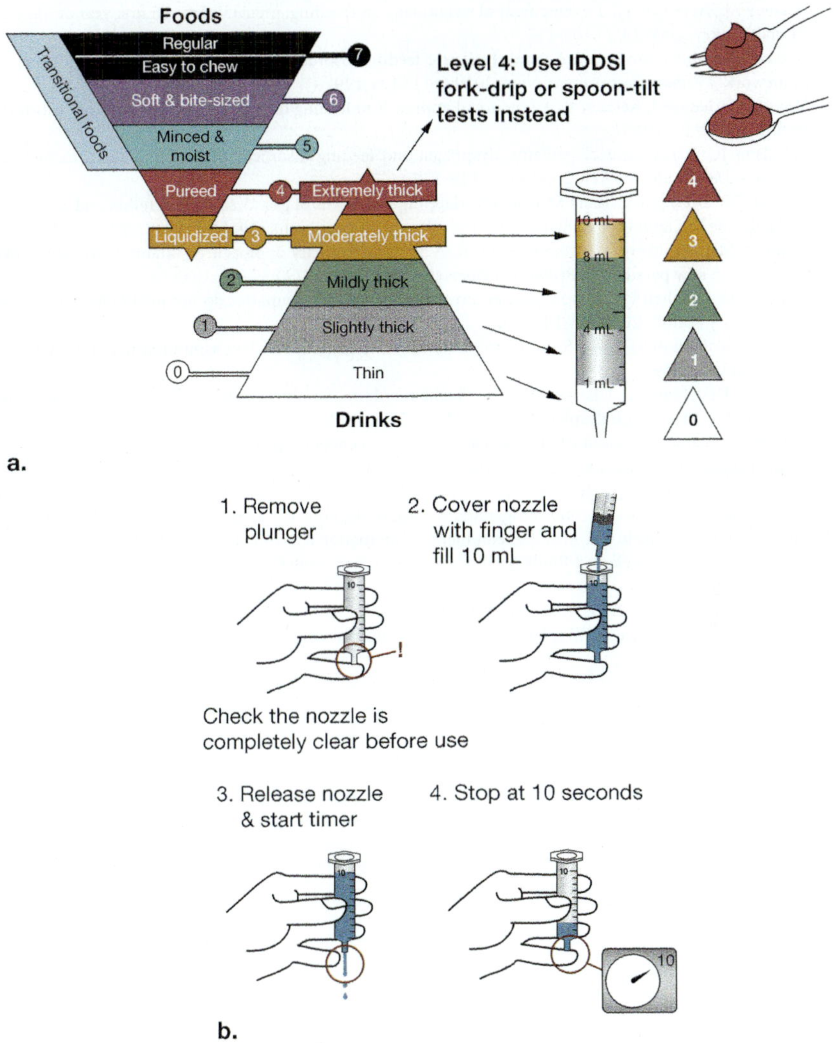

■ **Figure 24.1** IDDSI terminology and syringe flow test. A. The International Dysphagia Diet Standardisation Initiative (IDDSI) Framework shows standardized names for describing food texture and liquid thickness. B. The IDDSI Flow Test, a gravity flow test to determine liquid viscosity using a 10 mL syringe. Data from International Dysphagia Diet Standardisation Initiative. 2019. https://iddsi.org

■ REFERENCES

1. Lefton-Greif MA, Arvedson JC. Pediatric feeding and swallowing disorders: state of health, population trends, and application of the international classification of functioning, disability, and health. *Semin Speech Lang*. 2007;28(3):161-165.
2. Dodrill P, Gosa MM. Pediatric dysphagia: physiology, assessment, and management. *Ann Nutr Metab*. 2015;66(suppl 5):24-31.

3. Delaney AL, Arvedson JC. Development of swallowing and feeding: prenatal through first year of life. *Dev Disabil Res Rev*. 2008;14(2):105-117.
4. Goday PS, Huh SY, Silverman A, et al. Pediatric feeding disorder: consensus definition and conceptual framework. *J Pediatr Gastroenterol Nutr*. 2019;68(1):124-129.
5. Milano K, Chatoor I, Kerzner B. A functional approach to feeding difficulties in children. *Curr Gastroenterol Rep*. 2019;21(10):51.
6. Arvedson JC. Assessment of pediatric dysphagia and feeding disorders: clinical and instrumental approaches. *Dev Disabil Res Rev*. 2008;14(2):118-127.
7. Duncan DR, DiFilippo C, Kane M, et al. Overlapping symptoms of gastroesophageal reflux and aspiration highlight the limitations of validated questionnaires. *J Pediatr Gastroenterol Nutr*. 2021;72(3):372-377.
8. Fishbein MH, Kronberg J, Alvarado S, et al. A multidisciplinary approach to infants with GERD-like symptoms: a new paradigm. *J Pediatr Gastroenterol Nutr*. 2023;77(1):39-46.
9. Duncan DR, Mitchell PD, Larson K, et al. Presenting signs and symptoms do not predict aspiration risk in children. *J Pediatr*. 2018;201:141-146.
10. Weir KA, McMahon S, Taylor S, et al. Oropharyngeal aspiration and silent aspiration in children. *Chest*. 2011;140(3):589-597.
11. Brooks L, DiStefano CC, Clayton H, et al. Thickening human milk: the effect of time, temperature, and thickener for infants with dysphagia. *Eur J Pediatr*. 2024;183(4):1839-1848.
12. Duncan DR, Larson K, Rosen RL. Clinical aspects of thickeners for pediatric gastroesophageal reflux and oropharyngeal dysphagia. *Curr Gastroenterol Rep*. 2019;21(7):30.
13. McGrattan KE, Spoden A, Sterkowitz A, et al. Validity of anti-reflux formulas as a slightly thick liquid: effect of time, caloric density, and refrigerated storage on formula thickness. *Pediatr Med*. 2021;5:14.
14. Cichero JA, Lam P, Steele CM, et al. Development of international terminology and definitions for texture-modified foods and thickened fluids used in dysphagia management: the IDDSI framework. *Dysphagia*. 2017;32(2):293-314.
15. Duncan DR, Cohen A, Du M, et al. A prospective study of parental experience with thickening feeds for children with oropharyngeal dysphagia and gastroesophageal reflux. *J Pediatr*. 2023;260:113510.

CHAPTER 25

Food Allergies

Wendy Elverson and Erin P. Syverson

Food allergy refers to a reproducible adverse immunologic reaction to a food protein resulting in clinical symptoms. Food allergies can be classified as immunoglobulin E (IgE)-mediated, non-IgE-mediated, or mixed mechanism (involving both IgE and non-IgE pathways).

IgE-mediated food allergy has rapid symptom onset, caused by activation of the T helper 2 response, leading to IgE binding to effector T cells and resulting in histamine release. Non-IgE-mediated food allergies typically present with delayed symptoms and are mediated by other immune pathways. The terms "food intolerance" or "food sensitivity" are used to describe an undesired reaction to ingested food(s), although these terms lack specificity and do not necessarily indicate an immune-mediated process.

■ IGE-MEDIATED FOOD ALLERGY

The prevalence of IgE-mediated food allergy in children has increased significantly over the past 30 years, likely due to complex interactions between genetics and a number of environmental factors, with an estimated 8% of children affected by food allergies.[1,2] Although any food can cause an allergic reaction, nine major food allergens account for the majority of cases in the United States: cow's milk, egg, peanut, tree nut, soy, wheat, fish, shellfish, and sesame.[3]

IgE-mediated food allergy often begins in infancy and early childhood. Allergies to cow's milk, soy, egg, and wheat typically develop in infancy and frequently resolve during childhood, whereas tree nut, fish, and shellfish allergies develop slightly later and are more likely to persist into adulthood.[4] Clinical symptoms of food allergies can involve the gastrointestinal and respiratory tract, skin, and/or cardiovascular system (see Table 25.1).

When diagnosing IgE-mediated food allergy, a thorough history of symptoms associated with the ingestion of specific food(s) is necessary. While a double-blind, placebo-controlled food challenge remains the "gold standard" for diagnosing an IgE-mediated food allergy, it is resource-intensive and used primarily to confirm resolution or in research settings (see Table 25.2). During a food challenge, the food is given in gradually increasing amounts in a controlled environment so that the child can be observed closely and treated for adverse reactions if they occur. In a typical six-step food challenge, the patient consumes a total dose of a typical serving size for age, starting with 1% of the total dose for step 1, followed by 4%, 10%, 20%, 30%, and, finally, 35% of the total dose.

In clinical practice, most diagnoses rely on symptom history combined with diagnostic tests to diagnose IgE-mediated food allergies. Two commonly used tests are skin prick tests (SPT) and serum immunoassays, which quantify serum specific IgE antibodies to foods (sIgE) (see Table 25.3). Higher sIgE level and larger SPT wheal size

TABLE 25.1 FOOD ALLERGY SIGNS AND SYMPTOMS

IGE-MEDIATED	
Classic food allergy or anaphylaxis	Immediate and reproducible symptoms such as hives, vomiting, wheezing, chest tightness, throat itching/swelling, angioedema, hypotension, tachycardia after ingestion of a food allergen
NON-IGE-MEDIATED	
Food protein-induced enterocolitis (FPIES)	Acute presentation: profuse vomiting ± diarrhea, lethargy, pallor, vital sign instability beginning 1-4 h after ingestion Chronic presentation: intermittent progressive vomiting and/or diarrhea, growth faltering, ± electrolyte derangements, metabolic acidosis
Food protein-induced allergic proctocolitis (FPIAP)	Mucusy, blood-streaked stools, reflux, irritability, constipation

can suggest sensitization to a particular food, which may indicate a higher likelihood of having an allergic reaction. Because a "positive" test indicates only the possibility of an IgE-mediated allergy, SPT and sIgE testing is best performed and interpreted by an allergist in the context of the patient's specific clinical history to avoid unnecessary food avoidance and the associated nutritional risks. There is no role for SPT or sIgE testing for non-IgE-mediated food allergies.

TABLE 25.2 FOOD CHALLENGES

TYPE OF FOOD CHALLENGE	DESCRIPTION	EXAMPLE
Double-blind, placebo-controlled (DBPC)	• Most objective test • The patient, parent(s), and medical personnel administering the challenge are blinded to the food being challenged	• Dried egg white powder or milk powder mixed into a carrier (i.e., applesauce or fruit juice), placebos can be dextrose, cornstarch, baby food dry cereal, or others
Single-blind	• The patient and parent are unaware of the food being challenged • This type of challenge eliminates the bias of the patient and family	
Open challenge	• Unblinded food challenge • The patient and parent know what food will be consumed • An open challenge can help the individual to realize that a particular food is not responsible for the symptoms • An open challenge may be performed at the end of a DBPC or a single-blind challenge if the challenge is successful	• If an individual is challenged to a food such as milk, they could be provided with milk, yogurt, or cheese • If challenging an individual to food such as egg, they could be provided with scrambled or hard-boiled egg

TABLE 25.3 COMMON LABORATORY TESTS FOR IGE-MEDIATED FOOD ALLERGIES

LABORATORY TEST	PROCEDURE	UTILITY
Skin prick test (SPT)	• A small amount of the allergen is introduced to the skin; a wheal 3 mm or greater than the control is usually considered positive	• Rapid method to confirm sensitivity to an allergen but does not confirm diagnosis • A positive SPT may persist even when clinical symptoms are no longer present • 90% sensitive but only 50% specific. Wheal size does not correlate with reaction severity • Recent anaphylactic reaction, antihistamine use, and certain skin conditions can interfere with result interpretation
Serum food-specific IgE testing (sIgE)	• Blood test measuring level of food sIgE antibodies	• Helpful in evaluating IgE-mediated food allergies • May be substituted for SPT when recent anaphylaxis, skin conditions, or recent antihistamine use limits SPT use • Like SPT, high sensitivity but lower specificity • sIgE level does not correlate with reaction severity

Baked Milk and Baked Egg

Up to 70% of children with milk and/or egg allergies tolerate baked milk and/or egg.[5] Heat can alter the shape of conformational epitopes in proteins, including whey and ovalbumin, making them no longer recognizable to epitope specific IgE. Furthermore, the flour matrix of baked products may reduce the IgE binding capacity to milk and egg proteins. Tolerance to baked products often precedes tolerance to the less-heated form with the absence of a flour matrix.[6,7]

A medically supervised oral food challenge may be recommended for initial introduction of baked milk and/or egg due to the potential risk of anaphylaxis. Standard baked recipes (e.g., muffins) typically contain 1.33 g of milk protein and 2 g of egg with a minimum amount of 1 cup of flour and are baked at 350 °F for 30 minutes. The American Academy of Allergy Asthma and Immunology's *Muffins and More: A Baked Milk and Baked Egg Recipe and Guidebook* provides standardized recipes for use after successfully passing a baked milk or baked egg oral food challenge.[8]

Primary Prevention of IgE-Mediated Food Allergy

The American Academy of Pediatrics (AAP) recommends exclusive human milk feeding for 6 months and introduction of a wide variety of complementary foods, including common allergens, beginning at 6 months.[9] Multiple randomized control studies, including the Learning Early About Peanut (LEAP) Study and the Enquiring About Tolerance (EAT) Study, have led to recommendations for early allergen introduction.[10,11] The LEAP study randomized infants with moderate to severe eczema and/or egg allergy to early introduction and consistent intake of peanut (4-11 months of age) versus avoidance of peanut until age 5 years and found greater than 80% reduction in the incidence of peanut allergy at age 5 years in the peanut consuming group of children. The EAT Study randomized human milk–fed infants to early introduction of six foods (cow's milk, egg, sesame, fish, peanut, and wheat) between 3 and 6 months of age versus continued exclusive human milk feeding until 6 months. While the study failed to show the efficacy of early introduction in an intention-to-treat analysis, an analysis that included only those who adhered to the study protocol demonstrated significantly less prevalence of peanut and egg allergy in the early introduction group.

Although the benefits of early introduction likely extend to the general population, early introduction may be most important for infants with severe eczema as they are at the highest risk of developing food allergy, followed by infants with mild to moderate eczema, infants with a family history of atopy in either or both parents, and infants with one known food allergy.[12] Consensus guidelines published by the American Academy of Allergy, Asthma, and Immunology, American College of Allergy, Asthma, and Immunology, and the Canadian Society for Allergy and Clinical Immunology recommend introduction of peanut and cooked egg to all infants irrespective of their risk, starting around 6 months, although not before 4 months, and not to deliberately delay introduction of other potentially allergenic complementary foods once introduction of solids foods has started.[12] Additional randomized trials are needed to specify timing and dosing of allergen introduction beyond peanut and egg (see Table 25.4).

TABLE 25.4 PRACTICAL CONSIDERATION FOR EARLY ALLERGEN INTRODUCTION

ALLERGEN	DOSE RECOMMENDED[a]	FOOD IDEAS
Peanut	2 g peanut protein, 2-3 times per week	2 teaspoons of peanut butter, 2 teaspoons peanut butter powder, or 21 Bamba (for infants mixed into puree or thinned with water)
Egg	2 g egg protein, 2-3 times per week	1/3 medium boiled egg, 1/3 scrambled egg or omelet style egg
Wheat	–	Infant wheat cereals (iron-fortified for the breastfed infant); whole wheat toast, pasta, or crackers for older infants
Milk	–	Cow's milk-based formula, grated cheese, whole milk plain yogurt, cottage cheese, ricotta cheese
Soy	–	Tofu, soybean butter (thinned with water for younger infants)
Sesame	–	Tahini (sesame seed paste), hummus containing tahini
Fish	–	Cooked fish (low mercury options)
Tree nuts	–	Mixed nut butter (thinned with water for younger infants), tree nuts grated or finely ground mixed into cereal or other foods

[a]If no dose recommended, insufficient data available to know if early introduction is preventive for allergy development.

Schroer B, Groetch M, Mack DP, Venter C. Practical challenges and considerations for early introduction of potential food allergens for prevention of food allergy. *J Allergy Clin Immunol Pract*. 2021;9(1):44-56.e1.
Togias A, Cooper SF, Acebal ML, et al. Addendum guidelines for the prevention of peanut allergy in the United States. *JAAPA*. 2017;30(3):1-5.

Diet and Nutritional Management of Allergy

There is currently no cure for IgE-mediated food allergies. While oral immunotherapy (OIT) and medications like omalizumab may be options for some patients with IgE-mediated food allergies, the current standard of care for treatment of most IgE-mediated food allergies remains strict allergen avoidance. This requires reading ingredient labels of all foods, beverages, medications, and supplements. For young children who may ingest nonfood items, ingredients in craft materials and topical applications such as lotions, sunscreens, and soap should also be examined. Cross-contamination and changes in product formulations pose ongoing risks.

Under the Food Allergy Safety, Treatment, Education, and Research (FASTER) Act and Food Allergen Labeling and Consumer Protection Act (FALCPA) Act, US food labels must disclose the top nine allergens. This law also requires labels to indicate the presence of these allergens in spices, flavorings, additives, and colorings. Food manufacturers must label the allergen's common name either in the ingredient list or in a "contains" statement at the end of the ingredient list. Exceptions to the law include raw fruits and vegetables sold in their natural state, highly refined oils and ingredients derived from these, and foods regulated by the U.S. Department of Agriculture such as raw meat, raw poultry, and egg products. The FALCPA and FASTER Act do not recommend or regulate precautionary/advisory labeling statements such as "may contain" or "made in a factory with" or "made on shared equipment with." If an allergen is present, or cannot be ruled out, the product must be avoided.[13] Allergen-free substitution ideas are provided in Table 25.5.

TABLE 25.5 FOOD ALLERGY SUBSTITUTIONS FOR BAKING AND COOKING

WHEAT	COW'S MILK	EGG
Gluten-free all-purpose flour: ½ cup rice flour ¼ cup tapioca flour/starch ½ cup potato starch or cornstarch	**Milk substitute for baking:** Use any plant-based "milk"; for thinner varieties of plant-based "milk" (e.g., rice, almond), consider reducing volume by 10%	**For baking:** Replace each egg with: Option 1: 1 1/2 tbsp water + 1 1/2 tbsp oil + 1 tsp baking powder Option 2: 1 tsp baking powder + 1 tbsp liquid (water) + 1 tbsp vinegar Option 3: Mix 1 tbsp of ground flaxseed with 3 tbsp of water and let stand for 5 min
Gluten-free high-fiber flour: 1 cup sorghum or brown rice flour ½ cup light teff flour ½ cup Montina or millet flour 2/3 cup tapioca flour/starch 1/3 cup potato starch or corn starch	**Butter substitute for baking:** Use a plant-based, milk-free margarine	
Bread, pasta, crackers, cereal substitute: Corn, rice, millet, almond, and quinoa-based products	**Cheese substitute:** Try legumes, avocado, seed, or bean spreads or plant-based "cheese" (pea, coconut, oat, nut)	**For cooking:** Replace each egg with 2 tbsp pureed vegetable
Lunch and snack ideas: Soup with corn chips with quinoa or rice added, corn tacos with fillings, gluten-free pasta with vegetables and beans or chicken	**Yogurt substitute:** Soy, nut, or coconut yogurt	**For thickening cream dishes and sauces:** Add extra flour, cornstarch, or xanthan gum

For allergens not covered under current labeling laws, caregivers must be educated to identify ingredient synonyms (e.g., "spices" may contain mustard). Most children with soy allergy generally tolerate the highly refined soybean oil and soy lecithin included in foods, as residual levels of protein are very low.

NON-IGE-MEDIATED ALLERGIC CONDITIONS

Eosinophilic Gastrointestinal Disease

Eosinophilic gastrointestinal diseases (EGID) are immune-mediated allergic conditions characterized by eosinophilic infiltration of one or more portions of the gastrointestinal tract. See Chapter 26 for further discussion on EGIDs.

Food Protein-Induced Enterocolitis

Food protein-induced enterocolitis (FPIES) is a non-IgE-mediated gastrointestinal food hypersensitivity. FPIES typically initially presents in infants under 1 year of age with an incidence of about 0.5% of the population. Although much less common, FPIES can also present later in childhood and adulthood. FPIES presents in acute and chronic forms.

- **Acute FPIES:** Characterized by profuse vomiting 1 to 4 hours after ingestion of the trigger food, without typical IgE-mediated allergic skin or respiratory symptoms. It may be accompanied by extreme lethargy, pallor, diarrhea, hypotension, or hypothermia, and may warrant medical intervention.
- **Chronic FPIES:** Presentation is more variable; manifests as intermittent and often progressive vomiting and/or diarrhea, usually accompanied by poor weight gain and, in more severe instances, dehydration and metabolic acidosis.[14]

Management of both acute and chronic FPIES involves avoidance of the trigger food. Most children outgrow FPIES by school age. Resolution is assessed via oral food challenge, typically under medical supervision with intravenous access. Treatment options for an FPIES reaction include ondansetron to control vomiting, rehydration, and/or emergency care when indicated.

The most common FPIES triggers in children include cow's milk, soy, rice, and oat, although reactions to all types of foods have been reported, and FPIES reactions to egg and peanut have been increasingly reported.[15] Approximately 60% of children have a single FPIES food trigger, 33% have two to three triggers, and 10% have multiple triggers.[16]

FPIES is often diagnosed during a critical developmental window when complementary foods and textures are typically first offered. Dietary restrictions due to FPIES diagnosis, combined with caregiver hesitation to introduce new foods after a severe reaction, can put children with FPIES at risk of nutritional deficiency, poor growth, and feeding difficulties. Support from a dietitian is highly recommended for identifying safe foods, advancing food textures, and preventing nutritional deficiencies and feeding challenges. With the guidance of a dietitian, infants just starting complementary foods can be introduced first to lower risk FPIES foods such as broccoli, blueberry, cauliflower, millet parsnip, peach, plum, strawberry, and quinoa, followed then by more moderate and eventually higher risk FPIES foods (see Table 25.6).[14] While the number of tolerated foods may be low, developmentally appropriate texture

TABLE 25.6 FOOD PROTEIN-INDUCED ENTEROCOLITIS SYNDROME FOOD INTRODUCTION

FOOD GROUP	LOWER RISK	MODERATE RISK	HIGHER RISK	HIGHEST RISK
Vegetables	Broccoli, cauliflower, cucumber, kale, onions, mushrooms, parsnip, pumpkin, spinach, Swiss chard	Carrot, squash, white potato, string bean	Sweet potato, peas	
Fruits	Blueberry, cantaloupe, mango, papaya, peach, plum, prune, raspberry, strawberry, watermelon	Apple, pear, orange	Banana, avocado	
Proteins/Fats	Tree nut butters and seed butters[a] (almond butter, sunflower seed butter, tahini), canola oil, coconut oil, olive oil, lamb, beef[b]	Black beans, kidney beans, pinto beans, white beans, lentils, chickpeas[b] peanuts	Chicken,[b] turkey,[b] eggs, fish[b]	Milk, soy
Grains/Grain like foods	Millet, quinoa flakes (flakes can be made into hot cereal), amaranth	Corn, corn grits,[b] wheat, cream of wheat,[a] barley, white potato		Rice, oats

[a]Nut and seed butters should be thinned with water and added to purees for younger infants.
Adapted from the International FPIES consensus guidelines and clinical experience.
[b]Iron-rich/iron-fortified foods. Breast-fed infants should be introduced to iron-rich foods at age 6 months.

advancement is encouraged and can be facilitated by serving tolerated foods in various textures (e.g., pureed peach, fresh peach in a silicone feeder, freeze-dried peach, canned peach, ripe peach).

Atopic Dermatitis

Atopic dermatitis (AD) is a chronic, immunologic disease characterized by pruritic eczematous inflammatory skin lesions, affecting 10% to 20% of children. An estimated 20% to 30% of children with AD also have IgE-mediated food allergies.[5] While dietary elimination may slightly reduce AD symptoms, this should be weighed against the potential risks of empiric dietary elimination, including possible IgE-mediated allergic reaction upon food reintroduction,[17,18] impaired growth (lower weight, height, head circumference, mid-upper arm circumference, and body mass index),[19] and nutritional deficiencies. Patients with AD should be assessed for adequate nutrient intake, including those important for the skin, including vitamin D, vitamin A, zinc, and omega-3-fatty acids.

Food Protein-Induced Allergic Proctocolitis

Food protein-induced allergic proctocolitis (FPIAP), also commonly referred to as milk/soy protein intolerance or allergic colitis, is a non-IgE-mediated condition typically diagnosed in early infancy. Infants with FPIAP typically present with blood and/or mucus in stools, and may also have loose stools, constipation, fussiness, or reflux, but are otherwise overall well appearing. FPIAP is thought to be related to ingestion of specific food proteins; the most commonly implicated dietary trigger is cow's milk protein, followed by egg and soy protein.[20] Elimination of one or more of these foods, either by maternal dietary elimination for infants receiving human milk or by transition to an extensively hydrolyzed formula, leads to symptom resolution in the majority of infants with FPIAP. For exclusively human milk–fed infants, continued human milk use should be encouraged while the offending food is eliminated from the maternal diet. For formula-fed infants, cow's milk- or soy-based formulas should be replaced with an extensively hydrolyzed formula. Soy-based formula is not a generally recommended alternative due to risk of cross-reactivity but may be trialed if hypoallergenic formulas are inaccessible. For cow's milk elimination, all dairy products, including foods containing "casein" and "whey," and mammalian milk should be eliminated due to the high risk of cross-reactivity.[21] Given the overall benign course of FPIAP, in otherwise well-appearing infants, an alternative approach of watchful waiting without dietary restriction may be considered by some.[23] If this approach is taken, shared decision-making and close follow-up between the family and their medical team is essential.

Outside of observation for clinical improvement after elimination of presumed food trigger from the diet, there is variability in guidelines for the diagnosis of FPIAP. Although a trial of reintroduction of the suspected FPIAP trigger food shortly after symptom resolution is recommended in order to confirm FPIAP diagnosis, it is rarely done in real life practice.[22] Fecal occult blood testing (FOBT) is sensitive but nonspecific for the diagnosis of FPIAP and has a high false positive rate. For this reason, routine monitoring of FOBT in FPIAP is not recommended. For infants with FPIAP, reintroduction is typically trialed around 9 to 12 months of age, although exact protocols for reintroduction vary.[5]

EDUCATION AND PSYCHOSOCIAL BURDEN OF FOOD ALLERGIES

Ongoing education and support are critical for families managing food allergies. Dietitians should work closely with families to ensure adequate, age-appropriate, and balanced nutrition from a variety of allowed foods. Continued monitoring is recommended given the risk of micronutrient deficiencies, malnutrition, and stunted growth when an elimination diet is incomplete.

Education about food allergy management should be an ongoing process. Avoiding food allergens requires families to find alternatives to common foods, adjust recipes, and make appropriate substitutions (see Table 25.5). Safe practices in home, school, and social settings must be followed to prevent accidental exposure to food allergens (see Table 25.7). Advanced planning for food-inclusive events reduces anxiety and empowers participation in daily life.[13] Additional patient education and support information for food allergies can be found in Table 25.8.

Mental health concerns, including anxiety around having a reaction and living with food allergies, have been reported in a large proportion of children with food allergies.[24] While some degree of anxiety may be helpful in terms of taking appropriate precautions and being vigilant, conversely, hypervigilance can be associated with maladaptive behaviors (e.g., restrictive eating) affecting quality of life. Dietitians should screen for maladaptive behaviors and refer to a mental health provider when indicated.

TABLE 25.7 PRACTICAL TIPS FOR LIVING WITH FOOD ALLERGIES

At Home

- Cook the allergen-free meal first.
- Designate areas in the pantry, refrigerator, and cabinets for allergen-free foods.
- Keep an extra supply of "safe" foods frozen for quick meals.
- Be aware that cooking fumes from fish during frying and steaming can result in an allergic reaction from inhalation.
- Use squeeze top condiments rather than those requiring utensils.

At School

- Provide the food for a school celebration or snack time for the entire class.
- Keep favorite treats individually wrapped in the freezer for easy access on celebration days.
- Recommend nonedible treats for classroom parties (i.e., stickers, colorful pencils, or other child-friendly collectibles).
- Pack a lunch of "safe" foods.
- Encourage child not to trade foods at lunch or snack time.
- Encourage good handwashing practices for all students, especially after meal and snack time.
- Allergens can be removed from surfaces with commercial cleaning wipes.

Dining Out

- Speak to the manager to explain food allergies and go to restaurants at off hours and days when the restaurant is less busy.
- Order foods "naked" without sauces or gravies.
- Bring your own safe salad dressing, margarine, or condiments.
- Fried foods may contain protein from other foods cooked in the same oil (i.e., French fries cooked in oil that was previously used to fry fish).
- Provide a "chef card" to the manager and chef, personalized with the individual's allergies listed.
- Focus on what your child can have on the menu.
- Ask about food preparation techniques and remind staff about possible sources of cross-contamination.

An estimated one in two adults and children require treatment for food allergy in the emergency department at some point in their lifetime.[25] An anaphylaxis emergency action plan is essential and should be constructed with the allergist. Fatalities related to food allergies, while rare, are often associated with delayed treatment with epinephrine and are more common in adolescents and young adults with asthma and previously diagnosed food allergies. Early recognition of symptoms and treatment can be lifesaving.

Nutritional Adequacy of the Diet

Elimination of multiple foods can increase the risk of growth failure, micronutrient deficiencies, and shorter-than-average stature.[26] Inadequate intake of micronutrients, including calcium, phosphorus, magnesium, zinc, iodine, vitamin A, vitamin D, vitamin E, and riboflavin, may be seen in the setting of cow's milk allergy and/or multiple food allergies. Specific nutrients that are provided by the common food allergens are shown in Table 25.9.

TABLE 25.8 FOOD ALLERGY RESOURCES

Organizations:

The Food Allergy Research and Education

www.foodallergy.org

The Asthma and Allergy Foundation of America (AAFA)

www.aafa.org

Allergy Home

www.allergyhome.org/

Kids with Food Allergies

https://kidswithfoodallergies.org/

American Partnership for Eosinophilic Disorders (APFED)

www.apfed.org

American Academy of Allergy Asthma and Immunology (AAAAI)

www.aaaai.org

Patient and Family Education Materials

Food Allergy Management

- Food Allergy Stages Handouts
  - https://www.aaaai.org/tools-for-the-public/conditions-library/allergies/food-allergy-stages-handouts
- Living Confidently with Food Allergies
  - https://www.allergyhome.org/handbook/
- Food Allergy Travel Translation Cards
  - https://equaleats.com
  - www.selectwisely.com
- Elimination Diets
  - https://www.foodallergy.org/living-food-allergies/food-allergy-essentials/common-allergens

Food Allergy Prevention

- Food Allergy Canada
  - https://foodallergycanada.ca/wp-content/uploads/Eat-Early-Eat-Often.pdf
- FARE, Food Allergy Research & Education
  - https://foodallergyprevention.org/
- National Allergy Council (Australia)
  - https://preventallergies.org.au/

TABLE 25.9 MOST COMMON ALLERGENS AND THE NUTRIENTS THEY PROVIDE

ALLERGEN	NUTRIENTS
Milk	Protein, vitamins A and D, riboflavin, pantothenic acid, vitamin B_{12}, calcium, and phosphorus
Egg	Protein, vitamin B_{12}, riboflavin, pantothenic acid, biotin, and selenium
Soy	Protein, thiamin, riboflavin, pyridoxine, folate, calcium, phosphorus, magnesium, iron, and zinc and B_{12} if the product is fortified
Wheat	Thiamin, riboflavin, niacin, iron, and magnesium and folate if the product is fortified
Peanut/ Tree nuts	Protein, vitamin E, niacin, magnesium, manganese, and chromium and zinc
Fish	Protein, omega-3 fatty acids, vitamins A, D, and B_{12}

TABLE 25.10 NUTRIENTS IN PLANT-BASED "MILK"[a]

BEVERAGE (240 ML)	CALORIES	PROTEIN	FAT	ADDED SUGAR (TSP[b])	CALCIUM	VITAMIN D
Whole milk (cow)	150	8	8	0	275	124
Camel milk	108	5	5	0	280	–
Soy "milk"	70-150	6-9	3.5-5	0 -4	10-350	80-200
Oat "milk"	45-160	1-4	0.5-9	0-4	17-350	0-160
Coconut "milk"	45-90	0	0-7	0-2.5	40-470	0-100
Pea "milk"	80-140	4-8	4.5-8	0-4	320-455	184-240
Nut "milk"	25-130	0-5	1.5-11	0-5	0-470	0-200
Hemp "milk"	60-140	3-4	4.5-6	0-3	260-270	80
Flax "milk"	25	0	2.5	0	270	90

[a]Varies based on product and information provided on nutrition facts label.
[b]1 teaspoon sugar = 4 g.

Children eliminating cow's milk from their diet require an age-appropriate nutrient-dense calcium-fortified beverage or formula:

- Human milk (for children under 2 years, when available)
- Hypoallergenic, extensively hydrolyzed formula or amino acid-based formula
- Complete, plant-based formula (for children over 1 year, under the guidance of a dietitian)

Commercially available plant-based "milk" (e.g., almond, coconut, rice) are not nutritionally complete and should never be used as a primary source of nutrition for young children. Inappropriate use of plant-based "milk" has been associated with rickets, metabolic alkalosis, failure to thrive, anemia, and scurvy.[27] If used, plant-based "milk" should contain a micronutrient and macronutrient profile similar to that of cow's milk (Table 25.10). Plant-based "milk" can be considered in children greater than 1 year of age provided volume is limited to approximately less than 16 fl. oz. per day, with 2/3 of the child's intake coming from a variety of complementary foods rich in protein and fat, and nutritional status is monitored.[28]

For the majority of children with food allergies who are consuming human milk, the lactating parent need not restrict their diet if the child is asymptomatic.[21] The exception to this is in FPIAP, where restriction is often indicated, but rechallenging to confirm the diagnosis may be recommended. When the lactating parent does require a restricted diet, ongoing monitoring and supplementation with an allergen-free vitamin and mineral supplement may be necessary to ensure nutritional adequacy.

REFERENCES

1. Savage J, Sicherer S, Wood R. The natural history of food allergy. *J Allergy Clin Immunol Pract*. 2016; 4(2):196-203.
2. Gupta RS, Warren CM, Smith BM, et al. The public health impact of parent-reported childhood food allergies in the United States. *Pediatrics*. 2018;142(6):e20181235.

3. U.S. Food and Drug Administration. The FASTER Act: sesame is the ninth major food allergen. U.S. Food and Drug Administration. Published September 4, 2024. Accessed December 13, 2024. https://www.fda.gov/food/food-allergies/faster-act-sesame-ninth-major-food-allergen
4. Lee ECK, Trogen B, Brady K, Ford LS, Wang J. The natural history and risk factors for the development of food allergies in children and adults. *Curr Allergy Asthma Rep*. 2024;24(3):121-131.
5. Venter C, Groetch M, James JM, Sicherer SH. *Health Professional's Guide to Nutrition Management of Food Allergies*. Academy of Nutrition and Dietetics; 2022.
6. Wood RA, Sicherer SH, Vickery BP, et al. The natural history of milk allergy in an observational cohort. *J Allergy Clin Immunol*. 2013;131(3):805-812.
7. Sicherer SH, Wood RA, Vickery BP, et al. The natural history of egg allergy in an observational cohort. *J Allergy Clin Immunol*. 2014;133(2):492-499.e8.
8. Greer FR, Sicherer SH, Burks AW; American Academy of Pediatrics Committee on Nutrition; American Academy of Pediatrics Section on Allergy and Immunology. Effects of early nutritional interventions on the development of atopic disease in infants and children: the role of maternal dietary restriction, breastfeeding, timing of introduction of complementary foods, and hydrolyzed formulas. *Pediatrics*. 2008;121(1):183-191.
9. Perkin MR, Logan K, Tseng A, et al. Randomized trial of introduction of allergenic foods in breast-fed infants. *N Engl J Med*. 2016;374(18):1733-1743.
10. Toit GD, Roberts G, Sayre PH, et al. Randomized trial of peanut consumption in infants at risk for peanut allergy. *N Engl J Med*. 2015;372(9):803-813.
11. Fleischer DM, Chan ES, Venter C, et al. A consensus approach to the primary prevention of food allergy through nutrition: guidance from the American Academy of Allergy, Asthma, and Immunology; American College of Allergy, Asthma, and Immunology; and the Canadian Society for Allergy and Clinical Immunology. *J Allergy Clin Immunol Pract*. 2021;9(1):22–43.e4.
12. Schaible A, Kabourek J, Elverson W, Venter C, Cox A, Groetch M. Precautionary allergen labeling: avoidance for all? *Curr Allergy Asthma Rep*. 2024;24(3):81-94.
13. Nowak-Węgrzyn A, Chehade M, Groetch ME, et al. International consensus guidelines for the diagnosis and management of food protein–induced enterocolitis syndrome: executive summary—workgroup report of the Adverse Reactions to Foods Committee, American Academy of Allergy, Asthma & Immunology. *J Allergy Clin Immunol*. 2017;139(4):1111-1126.e4.
14. Rotella K, Lee ASE, Lopes JP, Sicherer SH, Kattan JD, Baker MG. Food protein-induced enterocolitis syndrome (FPIES) to peanut: characteristics and long-term outcomes of a large cohort. *J Allergy Clin Immunol Pract*. 2024;12(3):768770.
15. Cianferoni A. Food protein-induced enterocolitis syndrome epidemiology. *Ann Allergy Asthma Immunol*. 2021;126(5):469477.
16. LeBovidge JS, Elverson W, Timmons KG, et al. Multidisciplinary interventions in the management of atopic dermatitis. *J Allergy Clin Immunol*. 2016;138(2):325-334.
17. Oykhman P, Dookie J, Al-Rammahy H, et al. Dietary elimination for the treatment of atopic dermatitis: a systematic review and meta-analysis. *J Allergy Clin Immunol Pract*. 2022;10(10):2657-2666.e8.
18. Low DW, Jamil A, Md Nor N, Kader Ibrahim SB, Poh BK. Food restriction, nutrition status, and growth in toddlers with atopic dermatitis. *Pediatr Dermatol*. 2020;37(1):69-77.
19. Lake AM. Food-induced eosinophilic proctocolitis. *J Pediatr Gastroenterol Nutr*. 2000;30:S58-S60.
20. McWilliam V, Netting MJ, Volders E, et al. World Allergy Organization (WAO) Diagnosis and Rationale for Action against Cow's Milk Allergy (DRACMA) guidelines update – X – breastfeeding a baby with cow's milk allergy. *World Allergy Organ J*. 2023;16(11):100830.
21. Martin VM, Virkud YV, Seay H, et al. Prospective assessment of pediatrician-diagnosed food-protein induced allergic proctocolitis by gross or occult blood. *J Allergy Clin Immunol Pract*. 2020;8(5):1692-1699.e1.
22. Martin VM, Virkud YV, Phadke NA, et al. Increased IgE-mediated food allergy with food protein-induced allergic proctocolitis. *Pediatrics*. 2020;146(3):e20200202.
23. Casale TB, Warren C, Gupta S, et al. The mental health burden of food allergies: insights from patients and their caregivers from the Food Allergy Research & Education (FARE) Patient Registry. *World Allergy Organ J*. 2024;17(4):100891.
24. Warren CM, Jiang J, Gupta RS. Epidemiology and burden of food allergy. *Curr Allergy Asthma Rep*. 2020;20(2):6.
25. Meyer R. Nutritional disorders resulting from food allergy in children. *Pediatr Allergy Immunol*. 2018;29(7):689-704.
26. Merritt RJ, Fleet SE, Fifi A, et al. North American Society for Pediatric Gastroenterology, Hepatology, and Nutrition position paper: plant-based milks. *J Pediatr Gastroenterol Nutr*. 2020;71(2):276-281.
27. Groetch M, Venter C. Nutritional management of food allergies. *J Food Allergy*. 2020;2(2):131-141.

CHAPTER 26

Gastrointestinal Diseases

Kayla E. Hope, Wendy Elverson, and Denis Chang

Most pediatric gastrointestinal diseases require nutritional assessment and therapy to augment medical therapy; in some diseases, nutrition therapy is the primary treatment. In this chapter, we will review the nutritional management of common gastrointestinal diseases: gastroesophageal reflux disease, celiac disease, inflammatory bowel disease, eosinophilic esophagitis, constipation, diarrheal diseases, lactose intolerance, and disorders of the gut-brain interaction.

GASTROESOPHAGEAL REFLUX

Gastroesophageal reflux (GER) is the effortless movement of gastric contents into the esophagus and is considered a normal physiologic process. GER may occur with or without regurgitations and/or bothersome symptoms. Physiologic regurgitation occurs due to transient relaxations of the lower esophageal sphincter (LES) and is characterized as postprandial, lasting a few minutes, and not associated with other symptoms. As many as 50% of healthy infants have several physiologic regurgitations daily in early infancy. Infant regurgitations resolve over the first several months of life without treatment.[1]

GASTROESOPHAGEAL REFLUX DISEASE

A diagnosis of gastroesophageal reflux disease (GERD) is made when the presence of troublesome symptoms or complications of multiple reflux episodes occur.[1] Children at higher risk for GERD include those with neurologic disorders, hypotonia, repaired esophageal atresia, repaired achalasia, congenital diaphragmatic hernia, hiatal hernia, cystic fibrosis, lung transplantation, short bowel syndrome, obesity, and a family history of GERD.[1] Multiple physiologic factors are thought to be responsible for GERD, including a decreased LES tone, delayed esophageal peristalsis, and delayed gastric emptying, which lead to esophageal mucosal irritation from hydrochloric acid, pepsin, and possibly bile acid exposure.

Most commonly, a diagnosis of GERD is made on history and physical exam alone. Symptoms of GERD vary by age group, and regurgitation and vomiting associated with crying and food refusal may not be a specific indicator of GERD in infants and toddlers. GERD in toddlers and young children (1-6 years) tends to present with food refusal, regurgitation, vomiting, and abdominal pain. In older children (6-17 years), regurgitation or vomiting is associated with epigastric pain, heartburn, or cough. See Table 26.1 for signs and symptoms typically associated with GERD.

Diagnostic tests for evaluating for GERD and its complications include pH-metry and esophagogastroduodenoscopy (upper GI endoscopy), respectively.[1] Esophageal pH monitoring combined with multiple intraluminal impedance testing (MII) allow

TABLE 26.1 SIGNS AND SYMPTOMS ASSOCIATED WITH GASTROESOPHAGEAL REFLUX DISEASE IN CHILDREN

Symptoms	Signs
General	*General*
Irritability in infants	Anemia
Feeding refusal/poor weight gain	Dental erosion
Dystonic neck posturing (Sandifer syndrome)	
Gastrointestinal	*Gastrointestinal*
Recurrent regurgitation with/without vomiting	Esophagitis
Heartburn or chest pain	Esophageal stricture
Epigastric pain	Barrett esophagus
Hematemesis	
Dysphagia/Odynophagia (difficulty/painful swallowing)	
Extra-esophageal	*Extra-esophageal*
Wheezing	Apnea spells
Stridor	Asthma
Cough	Recurrent pneumonia (due to aspiration)
Hoarseness	Recurrent otitis media

From Rosen R, Vandenplas Y, Singendonk M, et al. Pediatric gastroesophageal reflux clinical practice guidelines: joint recommendations of the North American Society for Pediatric Gastroenterology, Hepatology, and Nutrition and the European Society for Pediatric Gastroenterology, Hepatology, and Nutrition. *J Pediatr Gastroenterol Nutr*. 2018;66(3):516-554.

for assessing symptom correlation with acid or nonacid reflux events. Endoscopy can reveal erosions (mucosal breaks) in the distal esophagus and can be used to survey for rare complications associated with chronic acid reflux, such as Barrett esophagus.[1]

Treatment for GERD may include both dietary and lifestyle modifications, in addition to pharmacologic therapies. However, evidence for efficacy of diet and lifestyle changes is limited (Table 26.2). In infancy, milk protein allergy can present with similar symptoms of GERD, including excessive crying, regurgitation, or vomiting, and a trial of an extensively hydrolyzed (or free amino acid in severe cases) infant formula or withdrawal of cow milk from the maternal diet if exclusively breastfed for 2 to 4 weeks can be considered.[1] Thickening of formula (or use of a commercial antiregurgitation formula) decreases the height of reflux in the esophagus, thus visible regurgitation, but the impact on nonregurgitation symptoms is unclear.[1] The addition of rice cereal to thicken infant formula increases the energy density of the formula and may displace calories (see Table 26.2). Additionally, rice cereal may be less efficacious in thickening hydrolyzed and amino acid–based formulas. In an infant with poor weight gain, a trial of higher calorie formula with education to caregivers on the required volume of formula needed to meet nutritional needs for growth is recommended in addition to hydrolyzed and thickened formula. Large-volume feedings can promote regurgitation, and, thus, smaller frequent feedings may reduce regurgitation. In older children, evidence to support dietary modification for GERD is lacking; however, expert opinion suggests small, frequent lower fat meals, with the avoidance of carbonation, caffeine, chocolate, and spicy foods if they provoke symptoms. In severe cases, transpyloric

TABLE 26.2 DIET/LIFESTYLE INTERVENTIONS FOR INFANTS, CHILDREN, AND ADOLESCENTS WITH GASTROESOPHAGEAL REFLUX DISEASE

Dietary interventions in infancy and children with gastroesophageal reflux disease (GERD):

Thicken feedings: 1 tsp rice cereal to 1 oz formula (25 cal/oz formula)—*not effective with amino acid–based formula, use commercial thickener with breastmilk or amino acid—based formula*
Formula change: 2-4 wk trial of an extensively hydrolyzed or free amino acid formula (to evaluate for milk or soy protein allergy)

Dietary changes to consider in infancy:

Change formulas: Trial of whey predominant (to assist gastric emptying)
Change feeding schedule: Smaller, more frequent feeding schedule, Bolus better tolerated than continuous in many cases

Dietary changes in infants/children with poor weight gain or enteral nutrition support:

Concentrate formula: Increase caloric density per ounce and decrease total volume.

Dietary interventions in children and young adults with GERD:

Limited evidence for dietary changes in GERD

- Avoidance of high-fat, acidic, spicy foods
- Avoidance of carminatives (spearmint and peppermint)
- Avoidance of caffeinated beverages or foods (tea, coffee, cola, chocolate)

Avoidance of late-night eating and large-volume meals helpful in obese adults

Weight reduction may help if obesity exists.

Lifestyle interventions in infants with GERD:

Change positioning: Supine positioning recommended birth to 1 y (due to increased SIDS risk) while sleeping. After 1-y, prone or left-sided positioning may reduce amount of esophageal exposure.
Avoidance of cigarette smoke exposure

Lifestyle interventions in children and young adults with GERD:

Elevate head of bed and sleep in left lateral decubitus position.
Avoidance of excessive alcohol and smoking (adult studies).

feeding may be trialed; however, in children with reflux, transpyloric feeding did not eliminate reflux episodes.[2] In addition, in children with gastrostomy tubes, feeding modality (continuous vs. bolus vs. no feeds) was not associated with differences in the frequency of reflux episodes as measured by pH impedance.[3]

Lifestyle interventions for GERD (Table 26.2) include positioning during sleep and avoidance of exposure to cigarette smoke.[4] While prone (on stomach) positioning after feeds may reduce esophageal acid exposure, given the higher risk of sudden infant death syndrome (SIDS), all infants from birth to 12 months of age should sleep in the supine (on back) position on a flat surface and not on an incline.[1] After 1 year of age, prone and left-sided sleeping can be considered to help reduce reflux episodes.

Pharmacologic therapy, including antacids, H_2 receptor antagonists, and proton pump inhibitors (PPI), are used if dietary and lifestyle changes do not alleviate symptoms, especially in school-aged children.[1] There is insufficient evidence to support the routine use of PPI in infancy, and it is not recommended as a diagnostic test for GERD in this population[1]; PPI use in infancy may increase the risk of allergies, anaphylactic reactions, lower respiratory tract infections, diarrhea, and necrotizing enterocolitis (NEC).[5] A 2 to 4-week trial of a PPI is recommended in adolescents with GERD symptoms with continuation to 3 months if applicable. There is insufficient evidence to support the use of prokinetic agents (metoclopramide, erythromycin, bethanechol, domperidone) with the exception of prucalopride to treat GERD in children.[6] Surgery (e.g., Nissen fundoplication) is considered if severe GERD refractory to medical management is present or if life-threatening complications of GERD exist.[1]

CELIAC DISEASE

Celiac disease (CeD) is a chronic, immune mediated enteropathy triggered by the ingestion of gluten in genetically susceptible individuals.[7] CeD affects 1% of the general population, although individuals with certain comorbid conditions are at higher risk: Type 1 diabetes mellitus (3%-12%), trisomy 21 (5%-12%), autoimmune thyroid disease (4%-7%), Turner syndrome (3%-4%), Williams syndrome (2%-4%), IgA deficiency (2%-8%), Sjogren syndrome (4%-12%), Addison disease (5%), and first-degree relatives with CeD (2%-20%).[7]

Clinical manifestations of CeD require exposure to dietary gluten, and the immunologic response to gluten causes cellular damage to the small intestinal villi, leading to the malabsorption of nutrients. Thus, children with failure to thrive, especially if they manifest symptoms of malabsorption (diarrhea, bloating, abdominal pain), should be evaluated for CeD. Symptoms, however, may be highly variable and can be gastrointestinal or extraintestinal (see Table 26.3). Examples of extraintestinal symptoms include headaches, fatigue, dermatitis herpetiformis, dental enamel defects, iron deficiency anemia, osteoporosis, delayed puberty, and short stature. Some individuals present without symptoms; screening should be considered in certain high-risk groups, even in the absence of symptoms.[8]

TABLE 26.3 CLINICAL MANIFESTATIONS OF CELIAC DISEASE

Gastrointestinal	Extraintestinal
Abdominal pain/distension	Anemia (iron deficiency)
Constipation	Delayed puberty
Diarrhea	Dental enamel defects
Growth retardation (in children)	Dermatitis herpetiformis
Nausea/vomiting	Elevated liver enzymes
Poor weight gain/weight loss	Fatigue (chronic)
	Headaches (recurrent)
	Neuropathy
	Osteoporosis
	Recurrent aphthous ulcers
	Short stature

From Husby S, Koletzko S, Korponay-Szabo I, et al. European Society Paediatric Gastroenterology, Hepatology and Nutrition guidelines for diagnosing coeliac disease 2020. *J Pediatr Gastroenterol Nutr*. 2020;70(1):141-156.

The recommended initial test for screening is a tissue transglutaminase IgA antibody (tTG IgA) given its high sensitivity and specificity.[8] A total IgA level should also be assessed as the tTG IgA may be falsely low in individuals with IgA deficiency. In IgA deficient individuals, IgG-based tests (antitissue transglutaminase IgG, anti-deamidated gliadin IgG, or anti-endomysial antibody (EMA) IgG) should be performed, although an intestinal biopsy is required to establish a diagnosis since IgG-based celiac serology tests are less specific.[8]

Current guidelines in children and adults recommend confirmation of a positive serologic screen with a small intestinal biopsy since the presence of characteristic histologic features (flattened villi, crypt hyperplasia, and intraepithelial lymphocytes) is considered the gold standard for diagnosis.[8] Individuals should be on a gluten-containing (unrestricted) diet at the time of the endoscopy as gluten elimination can result in mucosal healing, impacting diagnostic accuracy and clarity.

The European Society of Pediatric Gastroenterology, Hepatology, and Nutrition guidelines allow for the diagnosis of CeD to be made in certain children without undergoing an intestinal biopsy if specific serologic criteria are met—an initial tTG IgA is greater than 10 times the upper limit of normal, and an EMA IgA level is positive on a second, separate blood draw.[9] However, as of 2025, the North American Society of Pediatric Gastroenterology, Hepatology, and Nutrition guidelines continue to recommend histologic confirmation and have yet to endorse serologic criteria, citing the variation in interassay performance as well as the potential for missed pathology if endoscopy is foregone.[8]

Treatment

Currently, the only treatment for CeD is a lifelong, strict gluten-free diet (GFD). Gluten is the common name for the storage proteins (prolamins) in many cereal grains. The toxic prolamins that damage the small intestine in individuals with CeD are gliadin (in wheat), secalin (in rye), and hordein (in barley). While the prolamin, avenin, in oats has been found to be safe and well tolerated in most individuals with CeD, only purity protocol oats (grown, harvested, processed, stored, and manufactured under a dedicated system) or those that are labeled gluten-free are considered safe due to the risk of gluten cross-contamination of oats that occurs if harvested and milled with barley and wheat.

A GFD that involves complete elimination of wheat, barley, and rye and its derivates is the primary treatment for individuals with CeD and results in the resolution of symptoms, normalization of celiac serology, and mucosal/intestinal healing in most individuals.[8] Persistent symptoms may be due to nonadherence to the diet, ongoing (unintentional) gluten exposure in those on a GFD or another gastrointestinal condition, such as irritable bowel syndrome (IBS), secondary lactase deficiency or constipation due to lack of dietary fiber.[10] If secondary lactose intolerance exists, a 1-month trial of a lactose-free diet while initiating a GFD may allow mucosal healing before lactose is reintroduced.

A variety of foods can be included in the GFD, including all fresh fruits and vegetables, all fresh meats, poultry, fish and other animal meats, and a variety of grains that are naturally gluten free. Avoiding obvious dietary gluten is not sufficient to manage this disease. All sources of gluten must be identified to ensure that the diet is gluten free as gluten is often hidden in many food additives or preservatives such as hydrolyzed vegetable protein (HVP), modified food starch, malt flavoring, broth, seasonings, and medications. Table 26.4 highlights grains to be avoided in the GFD. Table 26.5 highlights safe grains to be included in a GFD. Table 26.6 provides a list of additives and ingredients to question in the GFD.

The Food Allergen Labeling and Consumer Protection Act of 2006 required that manufacturers identify on their food labels if the food contains any of eight common food allergens, including wheat. While this makes it easier for individuals with CeD to identify wheat in a product, the absence of wheat does not necessarily indicate the absence of gluten since barley or rye may be in the product. If there is any question about ingredients on the label, the manufacturer should be contacted to assure that the ingredients are gluten free before consuming the food. In 2014, the U.S. Food and Drug Administration (FDA) enacted a rule that foods marketed as gluten free must contain less than 20 parts per million (ppm) or 20 mg/kg of gluten, which is considered to be safe for individuals with CeD. As ingredients and food labels often change, parents and caretakers must keep abreast of changes in ingredients by food manufacturers, and all food labels need to be checked on a regular basis.

The increasing diagnosis of CeD and the subsequent awareness and use of the GFD by the general public for "gluten intolerance" has led to the increased availability of gluten-free foods sold in stores and served in restaurants. Gluten-free foods can be found in mainstream grocery stores, health food stores, ethnic markets, or can be ordered online from a variety of companies specializing in gluten-free foods.

TABLE 26.4 GRAINS AND STARCHES TO AVOID IN THE GLUTEN-FREE DIET

Atta	Malt (extract, flavoring, syrup, vinegar)
Barley	Matzoh
Brewer yeast	Modified wheat starch
Brown rice syrup (if made from malt)	Oat bran
Bulgur	**Oats**[b]
Cereal binding	Orzo
Couscous	Pasta (unless from gluten-free grains)
Dinkel	Rusks
Durum	**Rye**
Eikorn[a]	Semolina
Emmer[a]	Spelt
Farina	Triticale
Farro[a]	Udon
Gluten or gluten flour	**Wheat** (bran, flour, enriched flour, germ, starch, protein, stabilizers)
Graham flour	
Kamut[a]	
Kasha	

[a]Types of wheat.
[b]Cross-contamination of oats with wheat and or barley is a concern; therefore, oats are not recommended unless manufactured using GF practices.

TABLE 26.5 GRAINS AND STARCHES ALLOWED IN THE GLUTEN-FREE DIET

Amaranth	Potato flour, starch
Arrowroot	Quinoa seed, quinoa flour
Buckwheat	Rice (all forms brown, white, wild, basmati, jasmine, bran)
Corn (bran, flour, grits, hominy)	Rice flour (brown, sweet, white)
Flax	Sago
Legume/bean flours (garbanzo/chickpea, fava, lentil, pea)	Seed flours (sesame)
Millet	Soy flour
Mesquite flour	Sorghum
Montina flour (Indian Rice Grass)	Tapioca (manioc, cassava, yucca)
Nut flours (almond, hazelnut, pecan)	Teff (Tef) grain, flour
Oats (uncontaminated with wheat, barley, rye)	

Vitamin and Minerals in Celiac Disease

The nutritional status of the person with a new diagnosis CeD can vary depending on the length of undiagnosed CeD, the degree of villous damage, and the extent of malabsorption. Iron, folate, vitamin B_{12}, calcium, magnesium, and fat-soluble vitamin (A, D, E, and K) deficiencies may be found in patients with untreated CeD.[11] The GFD

TABLE 26.6 ADDITIVES AND INGREDIENTS TO QUESTION IN A GLUTEN-FREE DIET

Alcohol	Groats	Modified food starch
Baking powder	Hydrolyzed plant protein (HPP)	Miso
Brown rice syrup (made from barley)	Hydrolyzed vegetable protein (HVP)	Nondairy creamer
Beer (most made with barley or wheat)	Textured vegetable protein (TVP)	Nuts, dry roasted
Bran	Malt, malt extract, malt flavoring, malt syrup	Preservatives
Brewer Yeast (if by-product of beer)	Mono- and di-glycerides	Seafood analogs
Caramel color/flavoring[a]		Seasoning (powder, cubes)
Clarifying agents[a]		Stabilizers
Dextrins[a]		Starch[b]
Emulsifiers		Soy sauce
Fat replacers		Tocopherols
Flavorings (natural and artificial)		Vegetable gum
		Vegetable protein

[a]Caramel color and dextrin in North American products are almost always made from corn.
[b]Starch in food products is usually from cornstarch, but medications often contain gluten containing starch.

alone and subsequent healing of the intestine improving absorption may correct these deficiencies, but supplementation with a gluten-free multivitamin with minerals at diagnosis should be considered. Individual dosing for severe deficiencies, particularly of the fat-soluble vitamins, may be warranted. Given the high risk of bone disease in CeD and to improve bone mineral density, strict adherence to the diet coupled with adequate consumption of calcium and vitamin D is essential.[11] Bone densitometry measured by DEXA bone scan is recommended at diagnosis by some.[11]

With careful planning, the GFD can meet all of the nutrient needs of the individual. However, since gluten-based fortified grain products (cereals, breads, pasta) comprise a majority of children's intake of iron, fiber, zinc, folic acid, and B vitamins and most gluten-free alternatives are not fortified, intake of these nutrients may be low on the GFD.[11] Children on the diet may also require additional calcium and vitamin D supplementation, particularly if they have a secondary lactase deficiency, given the risk for bone disease in this population. The GFD shown here (Table 26.7) provides guidelines for the GFD recommended at Boston Children's Hospital.

INFLAMMATORY BOWEL DISEASE

Inflammatory bowel disease (IBD) is a general name for diseases that cause chronic intestinal inflammation. The two most recognized forms of IBD are Crohn disease (CD) and ulcerative colitis (UC). It is estimated that approximately 2.39 million US citizens suffer from IBD.[12] IBD manifests during childhood or adolescence in at least 25% of patients.[12] The rates of pediatric diagnosis of IBD are increasing and being seen in regions not previously noted to have a high prevalence of pediatric IBD. CD is characterized by transmural granulomatous intestinal inflammation and can involve the entire gastrointestinal tract, including the colon, small intestine, stomach, esophagus, and mouth. In contrast, UC is characterized by mucosal inflammation limited to the large intestine. Both forms of IBD are manifested by exacerbations and remissions of gastrointestinal symptoms, including abdominal pain, bloody diarrhea, rectal bleeding, fever, arthritis, and skin rashes.

The incidence of IBD has increased in the last 60 years and is attributed in part to changes in dietary habits of populations toward a more "Westernized" diet that is higher in fat, particularly in the ratio of omega-6 fatty acids to omega-3 fatty acids as well as ultra-processed foods.[13] Fruits, vegetables, fiber, and breastfeeding may be protective against the development of CD.[14]

Children and adolescents with IBD often present with malnutrition. Poor nutrient intake and malabsorption of nutrients associated with gastrointestinal exacerbations contribute to the weight loss, growth failure (decreased height velocity leading to short stature), and nutrient deficiencies seen in the IBD pediatric population. Growth failure is seen in 15% to 40% of all children and adolescents with CD and in about 3% to 10% with UC. Protein-energy malnutrition is seen in 20% to 85% of patients with CD and is the third most common symptom besides abdominal pain and diarrhea.[14] Factors contributing to the nutritional complications in pediatric IBD patients include inadequate energy and nutrient intake, increased nutrient requirements secondary to elevated resting energy expenditure, malabsorption with enteric leakage of protein, blood, vitamins, minerals, electrolytes, and trace elements from the bowel during periods of inflammation, and long-term corticosteroid use.[15] The etiology of reduced dietary intake (anorexia) is multifactorial

TABLE 26.7 GLUTEN-FREE DIET GUIDELINES

FOOD ITEM	FOODS RECOMMENDED	FOODS TO QUESTION[a]	FOODS NOT RECOMMENDED
Grains and flours	• Almond, arrowroot starch, artichoke, amaranth, buckwheat, corn starch, cornmeal, corn bran, corn flour, flax, legume flours (peas, lentils, beans), millet, Montina' flour, potato starch and flour, quinoa, rice bran, rice flours, sago, sorghum, soy flour, sesame, sunflower, tef, tapioca	• Safe flours in bulk bins in health food stores • Some buckwheat or millet flour mixes	• Low gluten flours • All flours containing wheat, rye, barley, or oats such as • Durham wheat, all-purpose flour, white enriched flour, wheat flour, wheat germ, whole wheat flour, wheat starch, wheat bran, oat bran, bulgur, graham, kasha, kamut, spelt, triticale, matzo and matzo meal, rusks, semolina, farina, einkorn, emmer, farro
Breads	• Specially prepared breads using only allowed flours (100% corn, rice, tapioca, soy, bean, nut, amaranth, buckwheat, millet, quinoa, teff and sorghum, etc.) • Commercial gluten-free baking mixes	• Buckwheat mixes (ensure they are manufactured in a dedicated facility)	• All breads, rolls, etc., made with wheat, rye, oats, barley, or unsafe flours
Cereals	• Hot and cold • Puffed amaranth, puffed corn, puffed millet, puffed rice, cornmeal, cream of buckwheat, cream of rice, hominy grits, soy grits, rice flakes, soy flakes, quinoa flakes, soy cereal.	• Hot and cold • Rice and corn cereals (may have malt flavoring)	• Hot and cold • Cereals containing wheat, wheat starch, rye, barley, oats, bran, graham, wheat germ, malt, kasha, bulgur, matzo, Durham wheat, rusks, triticale • Cereals made with malt flavoring
Noodles, pastas, potatoes, and other starches	• Macaroni, spaghetti, and noodles made from allowed flours • Rice, wild rice, and oriental rice noodles • White or sweet potatoes, yams • Corn tacos, corn tortillas	• French fries • Commercial rice or pasta mixes	• Macaroni, spaghetti, noodles, and pastas made from wheat, wheat starch, and other gluten containing grains • Scalloped potatoes (containing wheat flour) • Couscous • Tabbouleh

(continued)

TABLE 26.7 GLUTEN-FREE DIET GUIDELINES (*continued*)

FOOD ITEM	FOODS RECOMMENDED	FOODS TO QUESTION[a]	FOODS NOT RECOMMENDED
Crackers and snack foods	• Corn chips (plain) • Rice cakes (plain) • Popcorn (plain) • Crackers made with allowed flours • Potato chips (plain) • Plain nuts and soy nuts	• All containing malt • Flavored potato chips, rice cakes, and tortilla chips • Rice crackers	• All containing wheat, wheat starch, rye, barley, oats, bran, graham, wheat germ, bulgur, matzo, Durham wheat, rusks, triticale • Pretzels • Rice crackers made with brown rice syrup • Flour tortillas
Milk	• Plain milk products: • fresh, dry, evaporated, or condensed • Cream • Plain Yogurt	• Sour cream • Whip cream • Flavor/fruited yogurts • Nondairy creamers • Commercially prepared milkshakes and chocolate drinks • Frozen yogurt and ice cream • Soy and rice milks	• All milk products containing ingredients not allowed • Malted milk
Cheese	• Aged cheeses • Cottage cheese • Cream cheese	• Cheese sauces • Cheese spreads • Imitation cheese products • Low-fat or fat-free cheese • Ricotta cheese	• Cheese products containing ingredients not allowed • Blue cheese

Meat and meat alternatives	• Fresh meat, fish, poultry, and eggs • Plain nuts or soy nuts • Dried beans and peas • Fish canned in oil, water, or brine • Plain peanut butter	• Soybean and other meat substitutes • Luncheon meats, frankfurters, sausages, and bacon without fillers • Egg substitutes, dried eggs, egg whites • Dry roasted nuts • Imitation meat and fish • Canned soups, chillies, stews	• Any meat or meat product containing wheat, rye, barley, and oat fillers or stabilizers • Bread containing meat products; Swiss steak, meatballs, pot pies, croquettes, most vegetable burgers, meatloaf, etc. • Meats or fish injected with HVP (hydrolyzed vegetable protein) or HPP (hydrolyzed plant protein) • Tuna canned with HVP
Fruits and fruit juices	• Most fresh, frozen, and canned fruit	• Thickened or prepared fruits and pie fillings • Dried fruits	• Fruit products containing ingredients not allowed
Vegetables	• Most plain, fresh, frozen, or canned vegetables • Dried beans, peas, and lentils • Tomato puree and paste	• Vegetables in sauces prepared commercially • Baked beans	• Battered dipped vegetables
Fats	• Butter, margarine • Vegetable oil • Lard • Shortening	• Salad dressing • Mayonnaise	• Packaged suet
Desserts	• Special gluten-free cakes, cookies and baking mixes • Honey, coconut, chocolate (plain), gelatin, meringues, pure cocoa, hard candies, sherbet	• Ice cream, frozen yogurt • Pudding/custard mixes • Candy, jelly and jam, frozen desserts, icing, powdered sugar, marshmallows, molasses, ices	• Most commercially prepared cakes, cookies, and other baked goods • Instant and bread puddings • Ice cream cones • Licorice

(continued)

TABLE 26.7 GLUTEN-FREE DIET GUIDELINES (*continued*)

FOOD ITEM	FOODS RECOMMENDED	FOODS TO QUESTION[a]	FOODS NOT RECOMMENDED
Soups	• Homemade broth and soups made with allowed ingredients • Special gluten-free commercial soups or broth	• Canned soups, soup mixes, bouillon, bouillon cubes/ powder	• Soups or bouillon cubes containing ingredients not allowed
Beverages	• Plain tea, plain brewed coffee, hot chocolate made with pure cocoa powder, fruit juice, most carbonated drinks, cider	• Some soy and rice beverages • Instant tea, coffee and hot cocoa mixes, flavored fruit drinks, root beer • Distilled alcohol: wine, brandy, rum	• Beer, ale, and lager • Malted beverages • Ground coffee with added grains
Miscellaneous	• Vinegar (apple cider, rice, balsamic, wine) • Plain pickles, olives, relish • Ketchup, mustard, salt, black or red pepper, pure herbs, pure spices, pure flavoring extracts, soy sauce (wheat free), monosodium glutamate (MSG) • Pure baking chocolate, • Yeast, cream of tartar, baking soda • Distilled alcohol	• Curry powder, distilled white vinegar, dry seasoning mixes, gravy extracts and meat sauces, yeast flakes, extracts, imitation flavoring, mustard powder, baking powder	• Imitation pepper • Soy sauce • Worcestershire sauce • Malt vinegar • Communion wafers

[a]**Foods to Question:** Contact manufacturers to ensure the product does not contain any gluten.

and may include gastritis and esophagitis, cytokine-mediated anorexia, fear of eating secondary to diarrhea, and reduced taste sensation due to micronutrient deficiencies (e.g., zinc deficiency).[15] Treatment with antibodies to tumor necrosis factor (TNF)–α may help reduce the frequency and severity of secondary malnutrition in CD.[14]

Patients with IBD, particularly those with CD, present with deficiencies of vitamins, minerals, and trace elements as a result of inadequate intake or increased losses. Deficiency of the water-soluble vitamin folic acid can occur as a result of the interference of sulfasalazine and methotrexate with folate metabolism and is relatively common.[16] Vitamin B_{12} deficiency may occur in patients with CD or ileal resection and may be suspected in the presence of macrocytic anemia or if anemia does not respond to iron supplementation.[16] Patients with IBD are at an increased risk for developing fat-soluble vitamin deficiencies likely reflective of disease activity.[15] Vitamin D deficiency is found in about 35% of children and young adults with UC and appears to be more prevalent in those with darker skin, with CD with upper gastrointestinal involvement and in the winter months. Iron deficiency anemia is common in patients with IBD and may be caused by gastrointestinal blood loss and/or impaired utilization of iron with chronic disease. Inflammation and corticosteroids can increase urinary excretion of vitamin C, potassium, calcium, magnesium, phosphorus, zinc, and sulfur, and prolonged corticosteroid use can affect the metabolism of vitamin D. Low blood zinc levels occur in up to 50% of patients with active IBD.[15] Routine monitoring and supplementation of water- and fat-soluble vitamins and trace minerals is recommended. Table 26.8 provides guidelines on routine and therapeutic supplementation. See Chapter 20 for assessment and treatment of fat-soluble vitamin deficiencies.

Low bone mineral density is seen in approximately 25% of children with IBD and may be associated with the combined effects of chronic inflammation, corticosteroid use, excessive calcium urine loss, vitamin D malabsorption, decreased calcium intake, and cytokine-mediated bone resorption.[15] Early identification of children at risk of osteopenia through monitoring plasma 25-OH vitamin D levels, urinary calcium excretion, and bone density scans is recommended. Adequate intake of calcium and vitamin D following the recommendations by the Dietary Reference Intakes (DRI) is important for normal growth and development. CD patients who present with vitamin D deficiency may benefit from therapeutic supplementation with vitamin D_2 or D_3 (Table 26.8).

Management of children with IBD often requires a combination of nutritional therapy, pharmacologic agents, surgical consultations, and psychological intervention. The primary nutritional therapy goals are to replace nutrient losses, to correct specific nutrient deficiencies, and to provide sufficient nutrients to promote energy and nitrogen balance for the restoration of normal growth and maturation.[15,16] Nutritional therapy may also help to achieve and maintain remission by modifying the mucosal cytokine profiles and reducing inflammation in the gut.[14] While no studies have shown that nutritional intervention can induce remission in patients with UC, controlled studies have shown that the exclusive enteral nutrition (EEN) with the use of medical nutrition supplements, whether orally or via enteral feeding tube or both, is at least as effective as corticosteroids in inducing remission in CD, particularly in children. Remission rates in children with CD treated with polymeric enteral formulas is as high as 79%, and in newly diagnosed children is greater than 80%.[14] EEN, whether via elemental or polymeric formula, is also associated with better growth outcomes than corticosteroids.[17] No added benefit has been found in the use of elemental versus

TABLE 26.8 NUTRITION RECOMMENDATIONS AND SUPPLEMENTATION FOR THE PEDIATRIC INFLAMMATORY BOWEL DISEASE PATIENT

ROUTINE SUPPLEMENTATION	COMMENTS
Energy and protein	Schofield or WHO equation multiplied by activity factor and goal weight Protein needs while in remission are the same as a healthy child of the same age. Protein needs while in an active disease flare are increased by 25%-50%.
Vitamins and minerals	One serving of age-appropriate multivitamin with minerals per day
Calcium	Dietary Guidelines for age for calcium 1-3 y old: 700 mg/d 4-8 y old: 1000 mg/d 9-18 y old: 1300 mg/d Ca+ supplementation is indicated with steroid use
Vitamin D	10-25 μg/d
THERAPEUTIC SUPPLEMENTATION	
Vitamin D (Ergocalciferol [D_2])	Children with normal absorption: 25-125 μg/d × 6-16 wk Children with malabsorption: 250-625 μg/d until normal
Iron	2-6 mg elemental Fe/kg/d or every other day
Zinc	100%-200% DRI; stool losses may be high during acute exacerbations of disease
Vitamin B_{12}	1000 μg/d orally OR 100-1000 μg IM monthly if terminal ileum resected or diseased
Folate	100%-200% DRI; sulfasalazine and methotrexate may interfere with metabolism

DRI, dietary reference intakes; IM, intramuscular.

polymeric formulas in CD,[18] and the improved taste and reduced expense of the latter may make it the better choice for EEN.

The major advantages of using EEN include the avoidance of corticosteroids, increased growth velocity, nutritional repletion, and decreased disease activity in children with IBD. However, long-term compliance of EEN remains difficult for children and their families. If successful supplementation by mouth is not achieved, providing nutritional supplementation nocturnally via nasogastric or gastrostomy feedings can be done. The length of use of EEN varies between centers, but a period of 6 to 8 weeks to achieve remission and growth is often used.[18] Biologic therapy, such as anti-TNF or monoclonal antibodies, for the treatment of IBD is growing in use in an effort to achieve and maintain corticosteroid-free remission. EEN or partial EN (PEN) is used as an adjunct therapy to biologic use in CD when remission is not achieved by biologic therapy alone.[19] The nutritional effect of biologic therapy is not known at this time.

Patients with IBD often make use of supplements including glutamine, fish oil, short chain fatty acids, and pre- and probiotics, but data are currently insufficient to allow specific recommendations regarding their use. Insufficient data exist for the benefits of adding anti-inflammatory agents, such as transforming growth factor-β (TGF-β) and pre- and probiotic in enteral formulas.[14] Enteral nutrition is the preferred choice in the treatment of IBD, although parenteral nutrition may be necessary when there is stricture, feeding intolerance, or immediately postsurgery.

There is emerging evidence of success of other prescribed diets in IBD, including PEN, Crohn Disease Exclusion Diet (CDED), Anti-inflammatory diet (IBD-AID), Autoimmune protocol diet (AIP), CD-TREAT diet, and the Specific Carbohydrate Diet (SCD). While each of these vary, the primary goal is to limit dietary intake of nutrients that may contribute to dysbiosis. Patients who are interested in pursuing dietary therapy as part of their IBD management should do so under the guidance of an RD as many of these diets require elimination phases that may result in inadequate intake of certain nutrients and require careful reintroduction of many food items.

The first general approach to providing nutritional supplementation is to increase caloric intake with an unrestrictive high-calorie, high protein diet. Minor food sensitivities and intolerances may occur during a flare but generally do not persist and are not important enough to warrant elimination from the child's diet. On occasion, a low-fiber or lactose-restricted diet may be necessary when reintroducing food after active colitis if there is a stricture in the intestinal lumen or with widespread mucosal disease. However, dietary restrictions should be well justified and made on an individual basis.

Nutritional support and monitoring are essential in the pediatric patient with IBD in order to minimize malnutrition and maximize growth. The use of EEN versus pharmaceutical therapy continues to be widely debated, but EEN provides some added advantages, as discussed previously. Currently, the combination of nutritional and drug therapy remains the standard of care.

■ EOSINOPHILIC GASTROINTESTINAL DISEASES, INCLUDING EOSINOPHILIC ESOPHAGITIS

Eosinophilic gastrointestinal diseases (EGIDs) are chronic, immune-mediated disorders characterized by eosinophilic infiltration of one or more portions of the gastrointestinal tract. The most common EGID is eosinophilic esophagitis (EoE), with a global prevalence of 40 cases per 100,000 inhabitant-years.[20] Males are affected at higher rates than females, and atopic comorbidities (e.g., food allergies/anaphylaxis, asthma, eczema, chronic rhinitis, and environmental allergies) are frequent in children with EoE.[21]

Symptoms of EoE vary widely based on age; infants and young children may present with feeding difficulty, poor growth, and vomiting, while heartburn, dysphagia, and food impactions are more common in adolescents and adults. Since children may engage in behaviors to reduce symptoms, parents and clinicians should watch for compensatory behaviors such as avoidance of highly textured foods, refusal to accept previously preferred foods, need to cut food into small pieces, lubricating foods with liquid or fats before eating, extensive chewing of foods, washing food down with liquids, and prolonged mealtimes.

The diagnosis is established based on findings of eosinophilic infiltration (>15 eosinophils per high-powered field) on esophageal mucosal biopsies obtained during endoscopy and when they are accompanied by signs of esophageal dysfunction.[21] Esophageal eosinophilia can be seen in other conditions (e.g., GERD), so these must be excluded prior to establishing the diagnosis.

Treatment of Eosinophilic Esophagitis

Treatment goals in EoE include improvement of clinical symptoms, resolution of esophageal eosinophilia, adequate growth and nutrient intake, and improved quality of life. Often patients with EoE are under the care of an allergist and gastroenterologist. A referral to a registered dietitian is recommended when diet therapy is prescribed.[22]

Effective pharmacologic and diet-based treatment options are available for EoE. Current available medications include PPI, swallowed corticosteroids (budesonide, fluticasone, mometasone), and biologics, such as dupilumab, an interleukin-4 and interleukin-13 inhibitor.[21]

Dietary therapies can result in near-complete resolution of both clinical and histologic symptoms and are classified into three categories: elemental, targeted (or test directed) elimination diets and empiric elimination diets. In general, empiric diet therapy involves a stepwise approach, starting with a more restrictive (4- or 6-food elimination diet [FED]) or a less restrictive (1FED) diet and increasing or decreasing foods eliminated based on both clinical and histologic response (Table 26.9). Chang et al. summarized current data on treatment efficacy based on available dietary treatment in addition to advantages and disadvantages between starting with a more stringent (6FED) or a less restrictive (1FED) diet.[23] A multisite randomized trial found similar remission rates in 63 children randomly assigned to either a 1FED (milk) or a 4FED (milk, egg, soy, wheat).[24] Foods proven to cause EoE symptoms should be restricted indefinitely from the diet if dietary therapy continues to be the shared decision-making therapy of choice. Those foods not proven to be antigenic can be reintroduced with careful observation for symptom recurrence.

TABLE 26.9 DIETARY STRATEGIES TO TREAT EOSINOPHILIC ESOPHAGITIS

EMPIRIC DIET	FOODS ELIMINATED	POOLED RESPONSE RATE[a]
6 Food Elimination Diet (6FED)	Milk, soy, egg, wheat, peanut/tree nuts, fish/shellfish	40%-73%
4 Food Elimination Diet (4FED)	Milk, soy, egg, wheat	41%-60%
2 Food Elimination Diet (2FED)	Milk, wheat	43%
1 Food Elimination Diet (1FED)	Milk	34%-65%

[a]Adapted from Chang JW, Kliewer K, Haller E, et al. Development of a practical guide to implement and monitor diet therapy for eosinophilic esophagitis. *Clin Gastroenterol Hepatol*. 2023;21(7):1690-1698.

Considerations for Dietary Therapy

Decisions regarding whether to prescribe diet therapy should include a comprehensive nutrition assessment and shared decision-making between family, patient, and providers. Diet therapy may not be the best initial treatment in settings of malnutrition, pediatric feeding disorder, limited repertoire of accepted foods, food refusal of key nutrient dense substitutions, family lifestyle, lack of social support, and food insecurity. Although exclusive amino acid–based elemental diets have been shown to be effective, they are rarely used as a first line of dietary treatment and should be prescribed with caution due to their effects on quality of life and potential interference with the development of feeding skills in infants and young children.[21,22]

Comprehensive nutrition assessment and ongoing nutrition monitoring are necessary; children with EoE often have compromised nutrient intake and nutritional status related to feeding difficulties, maladaptive feeding behaviors, and preexisting IgE-mediated food allergies. Education on eliminating food allergens and specific foods to avoid, the proper reading of food labels and ingredient lists, and the appropriate food substitutions to avoid nutrient deficiencies must be conducted to prevent nutritional deterioration and increase adherence. Children under 2 years of age on a cow's milk–free diet should receive hypoallergenic formula or human milk. However, for children above 1 year of age, a plant-based beverage may be a consideration when the child can meet their nutrition needs from complementary foods and a fortified plant-based beverage. See Chapter 25 for more information on the appropriate use of plant-based beverages, under the guidance of a dietitian.

Regular follow-ups with a registered dietitian will offer support to both the child and the family to reduce the risk of prolonged inadequate nutrient intake.[22] In cases where adequate protein or calories are a concern, for example, in the setting of feeding difficulties and/or high energy needs for sport or rehabilitative nutrition, an amino acid–based formula can be used to supplement the diet. Hypoallergenic vitamins may be prescribed when indicated for inadequate intake or deficiencies. Further discussion of food allergen elimination, including nutritional risk in the setting of elimination diets, baking and cooking substitutions, dining out, food labeling laws, and resources, are covered in Chapter 25.

Management

EoE may significantly impact patients' health-related quality of life, resulting in impairment of an individual's social and psychological functioning. Untreated EoE over a prolonged period can result in chronic inflammation, esophageal scarring, and stricture formation.[21] As clinical symptoms do not always correlate with mucosal healing (endoscopic or histologic), a follow-up endoscopy is required to assess disease activity/response to treatment and to document remission.[21] Given the chronic nature of the disease, long-term adherence to dietary and/or medical therapy is generally required.

■ CONSTIPATION

Constipation is a common medical condition in children characterized by infrequent and painful defecation, hard or large caliber stools, fecal incontinence, and abdominal pain.[23] The clinical presentation of constipation may include abdominal distension, early satiety, vomiting, poor appetite, and irritability. Although functional constipation is a common cause of childhood constipation, the differential diagnosis varies widely and includes anatomic, neuromotor/motility, inflammatory, metabolic, and medication-associated etiologies.[25] The presence of alarm signs or symptoms, such as failure to pass meconium within the first 48 hours of life, bilious vomiting, severe abdominal distension, or abnormal physical exam findings, should prompt testing to identify possible underlying conditions.

Medical treatment options for constipation includes osmotic laxatives (PEG 3350, milk of magnesia, lactulose), stimulant laxatives (senna, bisacodyl), along with a behavioral stool sitting regimen.[5] The use of suppositories (glycerin, bisacodyl) or enemas may be necessary if the patient is not tolerating oral intake and stool burden in the rectal vault is high (i.e., fecal impaction). There is increasing evidence to support the use of secretagogues (linaclotide, lubiprostone) in children as young as 2 years of age with functional constipation.[26]

Dietary and other nonpharmacologic therapies are often utilized in conjunction with or in lieu of medications; however, more data to support its efficacy are needed.[27] While an increase in fiber and fluid intake is often recommended for treatment, there is insufficient evidence to show the advantage of supplemental fluid, the use of probiotics, or fiber supplementation in the treatment of constipation.[25] Consequently, normal fiber and fluid intake is recommended. There is emerging evidence on the use of prebiotic and fiber mixtures as well as other nonpharmacologic therapies, although additional research is required prior to revising current guidelines.[27]

■ ACUTE DIARRHEA

Acute diarrhea is defined as three or more loose or watery bowel movements during a 24-hour period that typically lasts less than 7 days and no more than 14 days.[28] Any change in stool consistency may be indicative of diarrhea over the number of stools, in the first year of life and in breastfed babies. Appropriate therapy for acute diarrhea consists of rehydration with a reduced osmolarity oral rehydration solution (ORS) (Table 26.10) and continued feeding.[29] Common household beverages, such as apple juice or carbonated drinks, may be inappropriate due to their high osmolarity and inadequate electrolyte composition. The immediate use of oral rehydration therapy (ORT, defined as ORS plus nutritional support) is effective for acute diarrhea. Table 26.11 offers guidance on the use of ORT. If oral rehydration is not feasible, then nasogastric tube feeding is as effective as if not better than intravenous fluids.[28] Substantial data support the use of early feeding during diarrheal disease, which has been shown to improve gastrointestinal function, as well as anthropometric, biochemical, and clinical outcomes.[29,30] Feeding should not be withheld longer than 4 to 6 hours after the start of rehydration.[28] Although children with acute diarrhea commonly suffer anorexia, it is crucial to maintain adequate hydration and nutrient intake (Table 26.11).

Recommendations for diet therapy in acute diarrhea may vary by age, nutritional status, and the medical history of the patient. Breastfed infants should continue nursing on demand. Formula-fed infants can remain on full-strength formula and do not usually need a lactose-free version. Soy infant formulas or hydrolyzed protein formulas do not provide an added benefit. Dilution of infant formula or a gradual introduction of feeding is not recommended. Children receiving solid foods should continue on their regular diet with the exception of foods high in simple sugars (i.e., carbonated

TABLE 26.10 AVAILABLE ORAL REHYDRATION SOLUTIONS (ORS)

NAME (MANUFACTURER)	CARBOHYDRATE (G/L)	NA (MMOL/L)	K (MMOL/L)	BASE (MEQ/L)	OSMOLALITY (MOSM/L)	COMMENTS
ORS (WHO—2005)	13.5	75	20	10	245	Solution recommended by the World Health Organization & UNICEF (WHO—2005)
Pedialyte (Abbott)	19.5	47	20	10	250 (unflavored) 270 (flavored)	Available in liters, single-servings (8 oz), and freezer pops Available unflavored and in multiple flavors 7.8 mg zinc/L
Enfalyte (Mead Johnson)	30	50	25	11	160	Rice-syrup solids is carbohydrate source.
CeraLyte 70 (Cera Products)	40	70	20	30	220	Rice-syrup solids is carbohydrate source. Available in multiple flavors.

TABLE 26.11 ORAL REHYDRATION THERAPY FOR ACUTE DIARRHEA

DEGREE OF DEHYDRATION	REHYDRATION THERAPY	REPLACEMENT OF LOSSES	NUTRITION
None	None needed	<10 kg: 60-120 mL ORS for each diarrheal stool or vomiting episode >10 kg: 120-240 mL ORS for each diarrheal stool or vomiting episode	Regular diet for age A. Breastmilk or full-strength formulas for infants, and B. Complex carbohydrates, fresh fruits, vegetables, and lean meats for older children.
Some	ORS, 50-100 mL/kg over 3-4 h	As above	As above
Severe	Lactated Ringer solution 20 mL/kg IV route until perfusion and mental status improve, then 100 mL/kg of ORS over 4 h	As above; administer via nasogastric tube if unable to drink.	As above; NB: children with a history of severe dehydration may have a higher likelihood of lactose-intolerance during recovery

Adapted from: King CK, Glass RI, Bresee JS, Duggan C. Managing acute gastroenteritis among children: oral rehydration, maintenance and nutritional therapy. *MMWR Recomm Rep.* 2003;52(rr-16):1-16.

soft drinks, juice, and gelatin desserts) since the osmotic load of these foods may exacerbate diarrhea.[28] Although some fatty foods may be poorly absorbed, a diet moderate in fat is recommended in order to maintain adequate caloric intake.[29] Undiluted cow's milk and cow's milk–based formulas can safely be given to most children with acute diarrhea. A minority of children will have clinically significant lactose intolerance and a significant increase in stool output requiring a lactose-free diet following acute diarrheal illness.[28] Highly restrictive diets, like the BRAT diet (bananas, rice, applesauce, and toast), do not offer any benefit and may worsen the child's nutritional status.

Supplemental zinc therapy is effective in treating and preventing diarrheal disease, particularly in the malnourished patient.[28] Zinc supplementation may reduce the severity and frequency of childhood diarrhea. UNICEF/WHO recommend zinc supplementation as standard treatment for all children with diarrhea, although studies supporting the role of zinc in reducing diarrheal disease have largely been performed in children at risk of inadequate dietary zinc intake, and recommended doses range from 5 to 20 mg/d for 10 to 14 days.[31] Limited data on zinc supplementation in children living in industrialized countries have been published.[28]

Probiotics may have a role in the treatment of acute diarrhea, in conjunction with ORT. The benefits include reduction in the duration of diarrhea or volume of stool. Several studies have shown a benefit from using *Lactobacillus rhamnosus* and *Saccharomyces boulardii* strains, while other strains (*Lactobacillus reuteri, Lactobacillus acidophilus* LB) may also be beneficial.[28] Safety issues with the use of probiotics may be a concern in children with chronic disease or immune disorders; due to the risk of bacterial translocation, we do not recommend their use in patients with indwelling central venous catheters. Antiemetics, such as ondansetron and metoclopramide, may reduce the need for intravenous rehydration therapy in children with vomiting and acute diarrhea, but increased diarrhea may occur.[28,32]

■ CHRONIC/PERSISTENT DIARRHEA

An episode of diarrhea that lasts for 14 days or more is termed chronic or persistent diarrhea.[33] In low-resource countries, the cycle of persistent diarrhea, malabsorption, anorexia, and malnutrition is one of the leading causes of death in children less than 5 years of age. Nutritional and medical management centers on treating infection, correcting acidosis and dehydration, gradually reintroducing enteral nutrition, and correcting micronutrient deficiencies. Culturally acceptable and cost-effective formulas have been employed with great success.

In industrialized countries, diarrhea and malnutrition should prompt an evaluation for malabsorption or systemic illness (Table 26.12). In the cases of persistent diarrhea due to extensive gastrointestinal mucosal disease (e.g., allergic disease, CeD, or other malabsorptive conditions), nutritional management may be undertaken with a wide range of enteral formulas. These are generally lactose-free (to avoid lactose malabsorption), protein hydrolysate or peptide-based (to treat possible protein sensitivities) and isotonic (to prevent osmotic loads worsening diarrhea) (see Chapter 16). Occasionally, parenteral nutrition is indicated, although the enteral route is preferred.

Chronic, nonspecific diarrhea (CNSD), often called toddlers' diarrhea, is characterized by two or more loose, odoriferous, voluminous stools per day and generally occurs between 6 and 36 months of age. The diarrhea lasts more than 4 weeks and is not associated with significant abdominal pain, fever, or growth failure. The etiology of the diarrhea is unknown, although it may be initiated by an acute infection. Nutritional management of CNSD centers on normalizing the diet as much as possible in order to avoid iatrogenic malnutrition. The prognosis of CNSD is excellent, with the majority of children improving by the age of 4 years.

Chronic diarrhea may also include congenital diarrhea and enteropathies, which are rare monogenic disorders that lead to chronic diarrhea in infancy, including: tufting enteropathy, microvillus inclusion disease, and trichohepatic enteric syndrome, among others.[33] Dietary management of these conditions often requires parenteral nutrition support during the early years of life; depending on the diagnosis, however,

TABLE 26.12 CHRONIC/PERSISTENT DIARRHEA IN INDUSTRIALIZED COUNTRIES

Weight Loss Present	Normal Nutritional Status
• Cystic fibrosis or other causes of pancreatic insufficiency • Hepatobiliary diseases • Protein-losing enteropathy • Inflammatory bowel disease (Crohn disease or ulcerative colitis) • AIDS or other immunodeficiencies • Celiac disease or allergic disorders • Congenital enteropathy	• Infection (e.g., *Giardia*) • Lactose intolerance • Chronic nonspecific diarrhea • Excessive juice intake

enteral autonomy and the ability to wean parenteral nutrition and transition to full enteral or oral diets may be achieved in the future. In each case, the dietary therapy is tailored to each individual and their underlying diagnosis.[34]

LACTOSE INTOLERANCE

Lactose intolerance refers to the inability to digest lactose, the main carbohydrate in milk. Clinical symptoms of lactose intolerance include abdominal pain, bloating, diarrhea, or flatulence. The severity of symptoms and the amount of lactose that will cause symptoms varies between individuals and depends on the degree of lactase deficiency, how much lactose is consumed, the mixture of lactose with other foods, gastric emptying rate, and colonic scavenge of malabsorbed carbohydrate.[35]

Lactose malabsorption is attributed to a relative deficiency of the disaccharidase lactase, which can be primary, secondary, congenital, or developmental. Primary lactase deficiency is a condition in which lactase activity falls after weaning and can happen at any point in childhood, adolescence, or adulthood. Onset is subtle and gradually progressive. Race, ethnic origin, and age will influence the presence of lactose intolerance. Primary lactose intolerance is prevalent in African American, Hispanic, Native American, and Asian populations (from 60% to 100% of these populations) and is less common in Northern Europeans and certain African and Indian populations.[35]

Secondary lactose intolerance is usually due to mucosal injury associated with disease (e.g., infectious diarrhea, CD, short bowel syndrome, untreated CeD). Congenital lactose deficiency is very rare. Developmental lactase deficiency is defined as lactase deficiency seen among preterm infants of less than 34 weeks' gestation.[35]

The diagnosis of lactose intolerance can be made using a good clinical history and on observing whether symptoms develop after lactose ingestion. If suspected, improvement with a trial of a lactose-free diet for 2 weeks can reveal this causal relationship. If symptoms are more subtle, a hydrogen breath test can be administered. A dose of lactose (2 g/kg to a maximum of 25 g) is ingested, and expired hydrogen is measured over 2 to 3 hours. An increase greater than 20 PPM of hydrogen expiration in 60 minutes indicates lactose malabsorption. Factors that may influence the results include consumption of a high-fiber diet before the test as well as use of antimicrobial agents and probiotics, lack of hydrogen-producing bacteria, bacterial overgrowth in the intestine, and disorders of intestinal motility.[35]

The treatment of lactose intolerance involves the removal of lactose from the diet. Lactose deficiency secondary to primary lactase deficiency is very rare before 2 to 3 years of age and any suspected lactose malabsorption before these ages should trigger an evaluation of other etiologies.[35] Lactose restriction is not usually necessary in secondary lactose intolerance since resolution of the underlying issue will reverse the lactose intolerance.[35] However, in infants less than 3 months of age or malnourished children, lactose intolerance can influence the course of their illness, and lactose restriction may be considered.[35]

Lactose is a common ingredient in many foods, including milk and milk products but also breads, crackers, soups, cereals, cookies, granola bars, chocolate, candy, salad dressings, luncheon meats, margarine, and baked goods. See Table 26.13 for common ingredient labeling terms, which indicate lactose.

Eliminating or reducing lactose-containing ingredients from the diet is usually adequate to relieve symptoms of lactose intolerance. Individuals with primary lactose intolerance may tolerate varying amounts of lactose but may require a permanent dietary

TABLE 26.13 LACTOSE-CONTAINING INGREDIENTS

Butter	Ghee
Buttermilk	Lactose
Cheese	Margarine
Cream	Milk (malted, liquid, evaporated, powder, condensed)
Curds	Sweet or sour cream
Dry milk solids	Whey

change. Individuals with secondary lactose intolerance should eliminate all lactose from their diets for a short period of time (2-6 weeks). If symptoms resolve, lactose may be reintroduced slowly, as tolerated by the individual. The amount of lactose that an individual can tolerate is highly variable. In fact, including dairy products in the diet has been shown to improve tolerance to lactose for some individuals.[36] Many children can tolerate small amounts of lactose, particularly yogurt or hard cheese, without discomfort.

For individuals who choose to restrict lactose in their diets, a variety of lactose-free and low-lactose food choices are available. Lactose-reduced products, containing 70% to 100% less lactose than standard foods, may be purchased commercially. Individuals may also choose to consume lactose-containing foods with lactase enzyme tablets or drops.

A lactose-free diet can provide adequate amounts of all essential nutrients when a varied diet is consumed. However, children maintained on a strict lactose-free diet may not meet their recommended calcium and vitamin D requirements and may require supplementation. Table 26.14 provides a list of low-lactose foods, which are high in calcium.[35] Table 26.15 provides a list of some commercially available lactose-free calcium supplements.

DISORDERS OF GUT-BRAIN INTERACTION

Disorders of gut-brain interaction (DGBI), previously known as "functional gastrointestinal disorders" encompass a wide array of GI symptoms, including IBS, functional abdominal pain, and functional dyspepsia. These disorders occur in the absence of inflammatory and mechanical complications of the GI tract but rather as a result of a combination of genetics, microbiome differences, mental health status, early childhood events, and environmental factors.[37] Symptoms often persist for months to years and treatment requires a multidisciplinary rehabilitation approach (biopsychosocial model). It is estimated that more than 40% of persons globally experience some degree of symptoms due to a DGBI that impacts their quality of life.[38]

Diagnosis of DGBIs often relies on clinical history and reported symptoms as lab results, imaging, and endoscopic findings are often normal. The criteria used for diagnosis (Rome IV criteria) include symptoms that last for a minimum of 8 weeks, impact daily activity and quality of life, and in some cases, the frequency of the symptoms.[37]

Nutritional management of DGBI primarily revolves around identifying dietary triggers that may contribute to or worsen GI symptoms. Certain elimination diets may be prescribed, such as a low FODMAP (fermentable oligosaccharides, disaccharides, monosaccharides, and polyols) diet, the most evidence-based diet for treating IBS.[39]

TABLE 26.14 HIGH-CALCIUM LOW-LACTOSE FOODS

FOOD ITEM	MILLIGRAMS OF CALCIUM/SERVING
Milk/Dairy Products	
Lactose-free Milk	300
Cheddar cheese, 1 oz.	200-260
Cottage cheese (1% milk), ½ cup	70
Sherbet, 1 cup	80
Protein	
Salmon, canned with bones, 3 oz.	210
Beans, cooked, 1 cup	90
Soybeans, cooked, 1 cup	175
Tofu, firm, 1 cup	507
Vegetables	
Broccoli, cooked, 1 cup	60
Kale, cooked, 1 cup	94
Spinach, cooked, 1 cup	245
Fruits	
Orange Juice (Calcium fortified) 8 fl. oz.	~500
Miscellaneous	
Fortified soymilk, rice milk, almond milk, hemp milk, 8 fl. oz.	250-300
Black strap molasses, 1 tbsp.	180

TABLE 26.15 LACTOSE-FREE COMMERCIAL CALCIUM SUPPLEMENTS

PRODUCT	MANUFACTURER	ELEMENTAL CALCIUM PER SERVING (MG)	VITAMIN D PER SERVING (μG)	ALSO CONTAINS
Citracal Maximum Plus	Bayer	650	25	Zinc, copper, manganese, sodium
Citracal Petites	Bayer	400	12.5	Sodium
Citracal Slow Release 1200	Bayer	1200	25	Magnesium, sodium
Citracal Calcium Gummies	Bayer	500	25	Phosphorus, sodium
Caltrate 600 + D_3	Haleon	600	20	Sodium
Caltrate 600 + D_3 Soft Chews	Haleon	600	20	Sodium
Caltrate Gummy Bites	Haleon	500	20	Phosphorus, sodium
Caltrate 600 + D_3 Minerals	Haleon	600	20	Magnesium, zinc, copper, manganese

TABLE 26.15 LACTOSE-FREE COMMERCIAL CALCIUM SUPPLEMENTS (*continued*)

PRODUCT	MANUFACTURER	ELEMENTAL CALCIUM PER SERVING (MG)	VITAMIN D PER SERVING (μG)	ALSO CONTAINS
Caltrate 600 + D_3 Plus Minerals Chewables	Haleon	600	20	Magnesium, zinc, copper, manganese
Caltrate 600 + D_3 Plus Minerals Minis	Haleon	600	40	Magnesium, zinc, copper, manganese
Kirkman's Calcium with Vitamin D_3 Capsule	Kirkman	200	2	Sodium, magnesium
Kirkman's Calcium with Vitamin D_3 Powder	Kirkman	1000	4.4	
TUMS Chewy Bites	Haleon	300	0	
TUMS Smoothies	Haleon	410	0	Magnesium, sodium
TUMS Naturals	Haleon	410	0	Magnesium, sodium
TUMS Ultra Strength	Haleon	410	0	Magnesium, sodium
TUMS Extra Strength	Haleon	300	0	sodium
TUMS Regular Strength	Haleon	200	0	sodium
Calcium with Vitamin D_3 Softgels	Nature Made	600	10	Soybean oil
Calcium with Vitamin D_3 Gummies	Nature Made	500	25	Phosphorus, sodium, sugar water (8 g CHO)
L'il Critters Calcium + D_3 Gummy Bear	Church & Dwight Co., Inc.	110	4	Phosphorus, glucose syrup (2 g CHO)
L'il Critters Bone Support Gummy Supplement	Church & Dwight Co., Inc.	110	4	Phosphorus, glucose Syrup (2 g CHO)

Given the restrictive nature of the diet, a low-FODMAP diet should be initiated with the guidance of a registered dietitian knowledgeable of the diet. Once initiated, patients are monitored for improvement in symptoms, with the goal of reintroducing foods that are not associated with symptoms.[39] Since patients with DGBI may develop restrictive eating practices due to fear of GI symptoms, providers should monitor for signs/symptoms of disordered eating, such as Avoidant restrictive food intake disorder (ARFID).

TABLE 26.16 DIETARY REFERENCE INTAKES FOR FIBER

Children	
1-3 y old	14 g/d
4-8 y old	28 g/d
Boys	
9-13 y old	14 g/d
14-18 y old	28 g/d
Girls	
9-13 y old	28 g/d
14-18 y old	28 gm/d

In patients for whom an elimination diet may not be feasible, other dietary guidelines include small frequent meals at regular intervals; emphasis on adequate hydration; avoidance of caffeine, carbonated beverages, insoluble fiber, resistant starches, and sugar alcohol; and limiting fresh fruit intake. Soluble fiber may be effective in treating global symptoms of IBS.[39] The current Dietary Reference Intakes (DRI) set forth by the Food and Nutrition Board of the Institute of Medicine can be much higher than a child's usual intake[40] (Table 26.16); thus, if fiber is increased in the diet, it is important to increase slowly based on symptoms and to provide adequate fluids in order to ensure the effectiveness of the fiber. Table 26.17 provides a guide on the fiber content of common foods. If it is difficult to increase fiber from food sources in the diet, commercially available fiber supplements may be used. Table 26.18 provides a list of such supplements.

In cases where symptoms become severe and impede an oral intake, temporary enteral access (e.g., nasogastric tube) is recommended in order to receive enteral nutrition while continuing to work on functional rehabilitation. Standard, polymeric formulas are appropriate for use, although an individual's current diet should be considered—if following a dairy-free diet for symptom management, this should be continued when selecting an appropriate formula. Parenteral nutrition is rarely indicated or appropriate. Micronutrients of concern for patients with DGBI include vitamin D and calcium (due to the frequency of dairy avoidance), in addition to thiamine and B_{12} (due to the common elimination of grains). Individuals with DGBIs should have their dietary intake evaluated by a registered dietitian to assess the need for micronutrient supplementation.

TABLE 26.17 DIETARY FIBER CONTENTS OF FOODS

	LITTLE (<0.5 G)	LOW (1 G)	MODERATE (2 G)	HIGH (3 G)	HIGHEST (≥4 G)
Dairy	Cheese				
	Ice cream				
	Milk				
	Pudding				
	Yogurt				
Protein	Beef		2 tbsp. peanut butter		½ cup
	Chicken				Chickpeas (6)
	Eggs				Kidney beans (6)
	Fish				Lentils (8 g)
	Pork				Lima beans (5)
	Turkey				Navy beans(5)
					Northern beans(4)
					Pork and beans (6)

(*continued*)

TABLE 26.17 DIETARY FIBER CONTENTS OF FOODS (*continued*)

	LITTLE (<0.5 G)	LOW (1 G)	MODERATE (2 G)	HIGH (3 G)	HIGHEST (≥4 G)
Fruit	Fruit juice	½ cup canned	Fresh	Fresh	Fresh
	Watermelon	Fruit cocktail	3 apricots	1 apple	½ avocado (4)
		Peaches	½ grapefruit	1 banana (6-7")	1 pear (5)
		Pears	1 peach	3 dates	½ cup
		Pineapple	½ cup	1 orange	Raspberries (4)
		½ cup	blueberries	3 plums	
		Applesauce	strawberries	¼ cup dried apricots, apples, prunes, raisins,	
		Cherries			
		Grapes (fresh)			
		Mango			
Vegetables		½ cup	½ cup cooked green beans	Broccoli	1 baked potato with skin (4)
		Cabbage	Peas	Carrots	½ cup cooked
		Cauliflower	Spinach	Corn	Sweet potato
		Celery		Potato salad	
		Cucumber			
		Lettuce			
		Spinach			
		Tomato			
		Tomato juice			

Breads and cereals	**Bread** 1 slice French bread Italian bread Raisin bread White bread 1 each Pancake Doughnut ½ plain bagel **Cereals** ½ cup Cheerios Corn flakes Frosted flakes Lucky charms	**Bread** 1 slice Cracked wheat Pumpernickel Rye 1 whole wheat Pancake 1 corn tortilla **Cereals** ½ cup Oatmeal Life cereal Nutrigrain Wheaties Total Honey nut shredded wheat	**Bread** 1 slice 100% whole wheat 3 oz bran muffin 2 Eggo multigrain waffles 1 (42 g) whole wheat flour tortilla **Cereals** ½ cup Shredded wheat Granola Crispy wheat-n raisins Wheat Chex	**Cereals** ½ cup Bran flakes Kashi Heart to Heart Raisin bran 2 tbsp. Wheat germ **Crackers** 1 rye crisp	**Bread** 1 slice Sprouted wheat breads (4) **Cereals** ½ cup 100% bran (14) All Bran (13) Fiber One (14) Grape nuts (7) Kashi (5) Steel-cut oats ¼ cup Unprocessed wheat bran (7)

(*continued*)

TABLE 26.17 DIETARY FIBER CONTENTS OF FOODS (*continued*)

	LITTLE (<0.5 G)	LOW (1 G)	MODERATE (2 G)	HIGH (3 G)	HIGHEST (≥4 G)
	Pasta	**Pasta**	**Pasta**		**Pasta**
	½ cup	½ cup	½ cup		½ cup
	Macaroni	Egg Noodles	Brown rice		Whole wheat
	Crackers	White rice	**Crackers**		Spelt
	Goldfish	**Crackers**	3 Harvest Wheat		Quinoa
	Saltines	2 graham	3 Triscuit		**Crackers**
	Ritz	16 Wheat Thins	2 TLC Kashi		2 Metamucil Wafers
		1 granola bar			
Desserts	Chocolate chip	Oatmeal cookies	Fig Newtons	Fresh fruit salad	
	Cookies				
Misc.	Beverages	1 cup	¼ cup	¼ cup	¼ cup
	Fats	Popcorn	Cashews	Almonds	Coconut
	Sweets		Pecans	Peanuts	
				Walnuts	

TABLE 26.18 COMMERCIAL FIBER SUPPLEMENTS

PRODUCT	FIBER/SERVING	CONSIDERATIONS
Benefiber Novartis Consumer Health, Inc www.benefiber.com	4 g/2 tsp powder 3 g/3 chewable tablets or caplets 3 g/1 stick pack packet	• Wheat dextrin (meets FDA criteria for gluten-free food) • Sugar-free, gluten-free • Available in powder, chewable tablets, stick packs, caplets • Available flavored and unflavored • Not recommended for carbonated beverages
Citrucel with SmartFiber GSK Corp. www.citrucel.com	2g per dose 1 g per caplet	• Methylcellulose • Sugar-free, clear mix, caplets available
FiberCon Wyeth www.fibercon.com	0.5 mg insoluble fiber per caplet	• Calcium polycarbophil • Caplets only • 224 mg calcium per 2 caplets
Metamucil Proctor & Gamble www.metamucil.com	3 g/1 tbsp. or packet 2 g/5 capsules 5 g/3 gummies	• Psyllium fiber • Clear and Natural—inulin fiber • Available in capsules, powder, or wafers • Available flavored and unflavored
Vitafusion Fiber Gummies www.vitafusion.com	5 g/2 gummies	• Polydextrose (soluble fiber) • Gluten free, peanut free, dairy free, soy free • Natural food colors

REFERENCES

1. Rosen R, Vandenplas Y, Singendonk M, et al. Pediatric gastroesophageal reflux clinical practice guidelines: joint recommendations of the North American Society for Pediatric Gastroenterology, Hepatology, and Nutrition and the European Society for Pediatric Gastroenterology, Hepatology, and Nutrition. *J Pediatr Gastroenterol Nutr*. 2018;66(3):516-554.
2. Rosen R, Hart K, Warlaumont M. Incidence of gastroesophageal reflux during transpyloric feeds. *J Pediatr Gastroenterol Nutr*. 2011;52(5):532-535.
3. Mahoney LB, Liu E, Rosen R. Continuous feedings are not associated with lower rates of gastroesophageal reflux when compared with bolus feedings. *J Pediatr Gastroenterol Nutr*. 2019;69(6):678-681.
4. van der Pol R, Smite M, Benninga MA, van Wijk MP. Non-pharmacological therapies for GERD in infants and children. *J Pediatr Gastroenterol Nutr*. 2011;53(suppl 2):S6-S8.
5. Tan J, Jeffries S, Carr R. A review of histamine-2 receptor antagonist and proton pump inhibitor therapy for gastroesophageal reflux disease in neonates and infants. *Pediatr Drugs*. 2023;25(5):557-576.
6. Rosen R. Gastroesophageal reflux treatment in infancy through young adulthood. *Am J Gastroenterol*. 2023;118(3):452-458.
7. Lindfors K, Ciacci C, Kurppa K, et al. Coeliac disease. *Nat Rev Dis Primers*. 2019;5(1):3.
8. Hill ID, Fasano A, Guandalini S, et al. NASPGHAN clinical report on the diagnosis and treatment of gluten-related disorders. *J Pediatr Gastroenterol Nutr*. 2016;63(1):156-165.
9. Husby S, Koletzko S, Korponay-Szabo I, et al. European Society Paediatric Gastroenterology, Hepatology and Nutrition guidelines for diagnosing coeliac disease 2020. *J Pediatr Gastroenterol Nutr*. 2020; 70(1):141-156.
10. Veeraraghavan G, Therrien A, Degroote M, et al. Non-responsive celiac disease in children on a gluten free diet. *World J Gastroenterol*. 2021;27(13):1311-1320.
11. Pinto-Sanchez MI, Blom JJ, Gibson PR, Armstrong D. Nutrition assessment and management in celiac disease. *Gastroenterology*. 2024;167(1):116-131.e1.

12. Lewis JD, Parlett LE, Jonsson Funk ML, et al. Incidence, prevalence, and racial and ethnic distribution of inflammatory bowel disease in the United States. *Gastroenterology*. 2023;165(5):1197-1205.e2.
13. Lo CH, Khandpur N, Rossato SL, et al. Ultra-processed foods and risk of Crohn's disease and ulcerative colitis: a prospective cohort study. *Clin Gastroenterol Hepatol*. 2022;20(6):e1323-e1337.
14. Alastair F, Emma G, Emma P. Nutrition in inflammatory bowel disease. *JPEN J Parenter Enteral Nutr*. 2011;35(5):571-580.
15. Kleinman RE, Baldassano RN, Caplan A, et al. Nutrition support for pediatric patients with inflammatory bowel disease: a clinical report of the North American Society for Pediatric Gastroenterology, Hepatology and Nutrition. *J Pediatr Gastroenterol Nutr*. 2004;39(1):15-27.
16. Mallon DP, Suskind DL. Nutrition in pediatric inflammatory bowel disease. *Nutr Clin Pract*. 2010;25(4):335-339.
17. Heuschkel R, Salvestrini C, Beattie RM, Hildebrand H, Walters T, Griffiths A. Guidelines for the management of growth failure in childhood inflammatory bowel disease. *Inflamm Bowel Dis*. 2008;14(6):839-849.
18. Whitten KE, Rogers P, Ooi CY, Day AS. International survey of enteral nutrition protocols used in children with Crohn's disease. *J Dig Dis*. 2012;13(2):107-112.
19. Wang J, Tang Z, Li J, et al. Treatment of Vedolizumab with exclusive enteral nutrition in adult patients with moderate to severe Crohn's disease (Crohn Exclusive Enteral Nutrition study). *Clin Transl Gastroenterol*. 2024;15(11):e00759.
20. Hahn JW, Lee K, Shin JI, et al. Global incidence and prevalence of eosinophilic esophagitis, 1976-2022: a systematic review and meta-analysis. *Clin Gastroenterol Hepatol*. 2023;21(13):3270-3284.e77.
21. Amil-Dias J, Oliva S, Papadopoulou A, et al. Diagnosis and management of eosinophilic esophagitis in children: an update from the European Society for Paediatric Gastroenterology, Hepatology and Nutrition (ESPGHAN). *J Pediatr Gastroenterol Nutr*. 2024;79(2):394-437.
22. Groetch M, Venter C, Skypala I, et al. Dietary therapy and nutrition management of eosinophilic esophagitis: a work group report of the American Academy of Allergy, Asthma, and Immunology. *J Allergy Clin Immunol Pract*. 2017;5(2):312-324.e29.
23. Chang JW, Kliewer K, Haller E, et al. Development of a practical guide to implement and monitor diet therapy for eosinophilic esophagitis. *Clin Gastroenterol Hepatol*. 2023;21(7):1690-1698.
24. Kliewer KL, Abonia JP, Aceves SS, et al. One-food versus 4-food elimination diet for pediatric eosinophilic esophagitis: a multisite randomized trial. *J Allergy Clin Immunol*. 2025;155(2):520-532.
25. Tabbers MM, DiLorenzo C, Berger MY, et al. Evaluation and treatment of functional constipation in infants and children: evidence-based recommendations from ESPGHAN and NASPGHAN. *J Pediatr Gastroenterol Nutr*. 2014;58(2):258-274.
26. Di Lorenzo C, Robert J, Rodriguez-Araujo G, et al. Safety and efficacy of linaclotide in children aged 2-5 years with functional constipation: Phase 2, randomized study. *J Pediatr Gastroenterol Nutr*. 2024;79(3):510-518.
27. Wegh CAM, Baaleman DF, Tabbers MM, Smidt H, Benninga MA. Nonpharmacologic treatment for children with functional constipation: a systematic review and meta-analysis. *J Pediatr*. 2022;240:136-149.e5.
28. Guarino A, Ashkenazi S, Gendrel D, et al. European Society for Pediatric Gastroenterology, Hepatology, and Nutrition/European Society for Pediatric Infectious Diseases evidence-based guidelines for the management of acute gastroenteritis in children in Europe: update 2014. *J Pediatr Gastroenterol Nutr*. 2014;59(1):132-152.
29. King CK, Glass R, Bresee JS, Duggan C. Managing acute gastroenteritis among children: oral rehydration, maintenance, and nutritional therapy. *MMWR Recomm Rep*. 2003;52(rr-16):1-16.
30. Gregorio GV, Dans LF, Silvestre MA. Early versus delayed refeeding for children with acute diarrhoea. *Cochrane Database Syst Rev*. 2011;2011(7):Cd007296.
31. Dhingra U, Kisenge R, Sudfeld CR, et al. Lower-dose zinc for childhood diarrhea—a randomized, multicenter trial. *N Engl J Med*. 2020;383(13):1231-1241.
32. Fedorowicz Z, Jagannath VA, Carter B. Antiemetics for reducing vomiting related to acute gastroenteritis in children and adolescents. *Cochrane Database Syst Rev*. 2011;2011(9):CD005506.
33. Thiagarajah JR, Kamin DS, Acra S, et al. Advances in evaluation of chronic diarrhea in infants. *Gastroenterology*. 2018;154(8):2045-2059.e6.
34. Avitzur Y, Jimenez L, Martincevic I, et al. Diet management in congenital diarrheas and enteropathies—general concepts and disease-specific approach, a narrative review. *Am J Clin Nutr*. 2024;120(1):17-33.
35. Heyman MB. Lactose intolerance in infants, children, and adolescents. *Pediatrics*. 2006;118(3):1279-1286.
36. Pribila BA, Hertzler SR, Martin BR, Weaver CM, Savaiano DA. Improved lactose digestion and intolerance among African-American adolescent girls fed a dairy-rich diet. *J Am Diet Assoc*. 2000;100(5):524-528; quiz 529-530.

37. Drossman DA. Functional gastrointestinal disorders: history, pathophysiology, clinical features, and Rome IV. *Gastroenterology*. 2016;150(6):1262-1279.e2.
38. Sperber AD, Bangdiwala SI, Drossman DA, et al. Worldwide prevalence and burden of functional gastrointestinal disorders, results of Rome Foundation Global Study. *Gastroenterology*. 2021;160(1):99-114.e3.
39. Chey WD, Hashash JG, Manning L, Chang L. AGA clinical practice update on the role of diet in irritable bowel syndrome: expert review. *Gastroenterology*. 2022;162(6):1737-1745.e5.
40. Institute of Medicine. *Dietary Reference Intakes for Energy, Carbohydrate, Fiber, Fat, Fatty Acids, Cholesterol, Protein, and Amino Acids*. The National Academies Press; 2005.

SUGGESTED RESOURCES

GENERAL RESOURCES ON GASTROINTESTINAL CONDITIONS

1. Academy of Nutrition and Dietetics
   120 South Riverside Plaza, Suite 2000
   Chicago, Illinois 60606-6995
   Website: www.eatright.org
2. American Society for Pediatric Parenteral and Enteral Nutrition
   8630 Fenton Street, Suite 412
   Silver Spring, MD 20910
   Website: http://www.nutritioncare.org/
3. North American Society Pediatric Gastroenterology, Hepatology and Nutrition
   Resources available on Celiac disease, Eosinophilic Esophagitis, Inflammatory Bowel Disease, GERD
   NASPGHAN
   PO Box 6
   Flourtown, PA 19031
   Website: http://www.naspghan.org/

NATIONAL SUPPORT GROUPS

1. Celiac Disease/Gluten Related Disorders:
   Beyond Celiac
   PO Box 544
   Ambler, PA 19002
   Website: https://www.beyondceliac.org/
2. Celiac Disease Foundation
   13251 Ventura Blvd., #1
   Studio City, CA 91604
   Website: www.celiac.org/
3. National Celiac Association
   1329 Highland Ave., Ste 2
   Needham, MA 02492
   Website: https://nationalceliac.org/
4. Inflammatory Bowel Disease:
   Crohn's and Colitis Foundation
   733 Third Avenue, Suite 510
   New York, NY 10017
   Website: https://www.crohnscolitisfoundation.org/
5. Eosinophilic Esophagitis/EGID:
   American Partnership for Eosinophilic Disorders
   PO Box 29545
   Atlanta, GA 30359
   Website: https://apfed.org/

CHAPTER 27

Malnutrition and Growth Failure

Mollie Studley and Sarah Fleet

"Malnutrition," for the purposes of this chapter, refers to undernutrition and describes children whose weight or length/height is not increasing at a rate consistent with a growth reference or growth standard.[1,2] The terms "weight faltering" or "growth faltering" can also be used to emphasize concerns around weight gain and are perceived to be less critical of parents or caregivers.[3,4] "Failure to thrive" was previously used to describe these growth changes, but is now considered an archaic term that lacks a precise definition.[2]

Commonly used definitions of malnutrition are reviewed in Chapter 2. See Chapter 2 for definitions of underweight, stunting, and wasting, as well as criteria for assessing these subtypes of malnutrition as moderate or severe. Other terms in the literature of severe malnutrition include marasmus (which occurs after severe deprivation primarily of energy and is characterized by growth retardation and wasting of muscle and subcutaneous fat[5]) and kwashiorkor (which is marked by edema accompanying muscle wasting resulting from acute protein deprivation and/or infectious or inflammatory stress).[6] Symptoms of these include indifference, lethargy, fatigue, and psychological alterations. Severe anorexia, apathy, and irritability make children with these conditions difficult to feed and manage. Many of the clinical signs (changes in hair and skin) lack specificity and are identical to symptoms of other nutrient deficiencies listed in Table 3.1.

The morbidity and mortality associated with malnutrition are more closely correlated with the degree of malnutrition than with sex, age, or specific clinical factors, although some studies show a higher mortality rate in infancy than in older age groups. A higher mortality rate is seen with kwashiorkor than with marasmus; electrolyte and fluid imbalances, increased risk of infections, and underlying disease increase the death rate significantly.

ASSESSMENT OF GROWTH PATTERN

The growth pattern of a child is best assessed with serial measurements plotted on a growth chart, as a single point on the growth chart will not reflect growth fluctuations or a child's growth pattern. For most children, the two growth charts used in the United States are the Centers for Disease Control and Prevention (CDC) growth reference and the World Health Organization (WHO) growth standards (see Chapter 2 for more information on growth charts). The CDC and the American Academy of Pediatrics (AAP) recommend that the WHO growth charts be used for all children from birth to 2 years of age, with 2000 CDC growth charts used for children older than

TABLE 27.1 PATHOGENESIS OF MALNUTRITION

INADEQUATE INTAKE	INADEQUATE ABSORPTION	INCREASED METABOLISM
Mechanical feeding problems • Oromotor or swallowing dysfunction • Congenital anomalies • Chronic vomiting or gastroesophageal reflux	Gastrointestinal disease • Pancreatic insufficiency • Celiac disease • Inflammatory bowel disease • Cystic fibrosis • Biliary atresia or liver disease • Short bowel syndrome • Allergic enterocolitis	Acute and chronic disease • Congenital or acquired heart disease • Chronic pulmonary disease • Hyperthyroidism • Renal failure • Cancer
Reduced appetite (anorexia)		Hypertonia
Dietary factors • Breastfeeding difficulties • Improper formula mixing • High intake of low-calorie foods • Excessive fruit juice consumption		Acute and chronic infection • Sepsis or other disseminated infection • GI infection • Pneumonia • Human immunodeficiency virus infection • Tuberculosis
Behavioral factors • Disordered feeding techniques • Altered mental status • Sensory-based food aversions, ARFID		Critical illness
Inadequate access to food		
Neglect or abuse		

ARFID, avoidant restrictive food intake disorder; GI, gastrointestinal.
Source: Adapted from Woo Baidal JA, Huh SY. Failure-to-thrive: growth failure in the outpatient setting. In: Duggan C, Watkins JB, Koletzko B, Walker WA, eds. *Nutrition in Pediatrics: Basic Science, Clinical Applications*. 5th ed. People's Medical Publishing House; 2016; and Homan G. Failure to thirve: a practical guide. *Am Fam Physician*. 2016;94(4):295-299.

2 years.[3,7] For children younger than 2 years, the WHO growth charts were developed using longitudinal data from infants who were all breastfed for the first year of life, contrasting with the cross-sectional data from predominantly formula-fed infants used for the 2000 CDC growth charts. Breastfed infants show a greater growth velocity than formula-fed infants during the first few months of life but subsequently have lower rates of weight gain in infancy.[7] Data on U.S. children suggest that use of WHO charts is likely to reduce the prevalence of growth failure diagnoses in early childhood,[7,8] but may increase the prevalence of growth failure diagnoses in the first 6 months of life.[6] For children with certain medical conditions or genetic syndromes (e.g., trisomy 21), syndrome-specific growth charts may be available. However, these should be used with caution when assessing growth, as they are often more descriptive in nature, compiled from small sample sizes, and may not represent optimal growth patterns.

In the first 2 years of life, it is common for healthy children to exhibit shifting of growth percentiles. A U.S. study estimated that 39% of healthy children between birth and 6 months of age, 6% to 15% of children between 6 and 24 months of age, and 1% to 5% of children between 24 and 60 months of age crossed two major weight-for-age percentiles in either direction.[5] For weight-for-length/height, 62% of children between birth and 6 months of age, 20% to 27% of children between 6 and 24 months of age, and 6% to 15% of children between 24 and 60 months of age crossed two major percentiles in either direction.[5] The authors speculated that the shifts in growth percentile could be due to genetic predisposition and regression to the mean (e.g., a large infant born to slim parents, who crosses weight percentiles downward), to measurement error, or to random variation.

Malnutrition should be differentiated from normal variations in growth pattern, including genetic short stature and constitutional growth delay. The classic pattern for malnutrition is a decline in weight percentile, followed in sequence by a decline in linear and head circumference growth percentiles. Children who cross percentiles downward due to genetic predisposition will maintain normal linear growth velocity once they reach their genetically appropriate height percentile, and bone age will generally match chronologic age. See Chapter 2 for calculating genetic height potential. Children with constitutional growth delay are generally born with a normal birth size but begin crossing height and sometimes weight percentiles downward in the first 2 to 3 years, followed by a normal linear growth velocity. In children with constitutional growth delay, bone age will be delayed compared to the chronologic age, and they will tend to have later puberty than their peers, resulting in a normal adult height.[9,10] The difference between constitutional growth delay and malnutrition is often not clear until a child's growth has been monitored for a number of years.

ETIOLOGY

Malnutrition results from condition(s) that cause inadequate energy intake, malabsorption, excessive caloric expenditure, or defective utilization of nutrients (see Table 27.1). Most children with malnutrition are not consuming or not retaining sufficient calories to meet their energy needs.[2] The *Diagnostic and Statistical Manual of Mental Health Disorders* (DSM) released their fifth edition in 2013 (updated to *DSM 5-TR* in 2022) and proposed changes to expand the diagnostic criteria for disordered eating. "Feeding disorder of infancy and childhood" was replaced with avoidant/restrictive food intake disorder (ARFID) to better capture an eating or feeding disturbance associated with weight loss, nutritional deficiency, dependency on enteral feeding or oral formula supplements, and/or marked interference with psychosocial functioning[11,12] (see Chapter 23). Frequently, physiologic, psychological, and social factors contribute to a child's malnutrition and thus a comprehensive biopsychosocial approach is useful in planning evaluation and treatment.

MANAGEMENT OF MALNUTRITION

Effective management of malnutrition in a young child often benefits from a multidisciplinary team approach. The team can include a physician, registered dietitian, feeding specialist (speech and language pathologist), behavioral psychologist, nurse, and social worker. Each team member has specific roles to play.

The Role of the Physician

The physician collects a detailed past and present medical history. Collected information should include prenatal, birth, developmental, and family history, including parental heights and onset of puberty. A comprehensive physical examination should be conducted to identify physical features consistent with a genetic syndrome or underlying medical condition contributing to growth failure; to identify signs of child abuse or neglect; and to determine the severity and complications associated with undernutrition.[2,3]

If the history and physical examination findings suggest specific underlying etiologies or complications related to malnutrition, targeted laboratory testing can be considered. Screening tests may include a complete blood count, albumin, erythrocyte sedimentation rate, lead concentration, urinalysis, and thyroid studies. Screening for celiac disease (tissue transglutaminase immunoglobulin A [IgA] along with total serum IgA) should be considered. If malabsorption is suspected, stool studies can help to determine the etiology, and a sweat test for cystic fibrosis may also be indicated. For toddlers consuming excessive cow's milk, breast milk, or juice, iron studies are also indicated.[3] If indicated, the physician may prescribe medical therapies for appetite stimulation, or control of reported gastrointestinal (GI) symptoms that may be contributing to the malnutrition.

The Role of the Dietitian

The dietitian completes a detailed nutrition assessment, including relevant feeding history, as well as capturing intake on a typical day or 24-hour dietary recall. Once the pattern of eating, estimated volumes, and variety have been captured, the dietitian can make recommendations around micronutrient testing that can complement the physician's laboratory testing. The next section provides more detail regarding nutrition management.

The Role of the Speech and Language Pathologist

Observation of an oral feeding at the clinic, home, or by video recording by a feeding specialist is helpful in identifying any oral-motor problems affecting chewing or swallowing. The clinician can also complete an exam of the oral cavity. A modified barium swallow is helpful if aspiration or mechanical feeding problems are suspected.

The Role of the Behavioral Psychologist

A feeding observation at the clinic, home, or by video recording is also helpful for the psychologist to understand the family dynamics and environmental interactions affecting child feeding. Key details of the feeding observation can include the following:[11,12]

- Parental behaviors: anxious, inattentive to child, force feeding, bothered by food messes, does not allow child to participate in feeding, props bottle, ignores child's feeding signals
- Child's behaviors: cries, spits up, gags, vomits or ruminates, holds food in mouth, arches, plays with food or toys at mealtime, takes more than 30 minutes to eat, refuses to stay seated

The Role of the Social Worker

The social worker collects psychosocial information, including the parents' education, financial status, household living conditions, and psychological and mental health status of the caregivers. Screening for food insecurity should be completed at each visit, based on the understanding of the social and cultural context, in order to help identify families at risk for nutritional deficits.[4] A social worker can use the collected information to identify supports for the family, as well as clinical counseling to address parental mental health.

NUTRITIONAL MANAGEMENT

Nutritional Assessment

In addition to evaluating the child's growth pattern (see section Assessment of Growth Pattern), the anthropometric data need evaluation and, when appropriate, should be used to diagnose varying degrees and acuity of malnutrition. See Chapter 2 for details.

Feeding History

A detailed feeding history from birth will help determine whether feeding has progressed along a normal developmental spectrum. Key features of the feeding history include:

- Breastfeeding/chestfeeding: initiation and duration, latch, frequency, nighttime feedings
- Formula feeding: formula type(s), tolerance, recipe mixing accuracy
- Mixed feedings: preference for bottle versus breast/chest, if any
- Food intake: age at which solids or table foods were introduced, types and texture of preferred or rejected foods
- Use of bottle or cup for beverages and other utensils for food
- Feeding schedule: daytime and nighttime feeding schedule, meal duration
- Feeding atmosphere: where meals or snacks are eaten and with whom, presence of distractions (TV, toys, phone)
- Feeding-related behaviors: child's expression of hunger and satiety, feeding control (self vs. force feeding), positive (bribing or rewards) or negative (withholding toys, punishment) strategies.

The small quantities of food consumed by young children and the common presence of multiple caregivers render accurate assessment of energy and nutrient intake a challenging task. For breastfed/chestfed infants, estimation of the volume of human milk intake requires the use of a scale sufficiently sensitive to detect a difference in an infant's pre- and postfeeding weights, and is typically completed in the clinical setting rather than at home. Assessment of food intake can use the following methods:

- Food record: Caregivers record the type and amount of food and beverages consumed by the child for 3 to 7 days. Parents should be instructed to note both the amount served and the amount eaten.
- 24-hour recall: Dietitian asks caregiver to recall types and amounts of food and beverages consumed by the child over a 24-hour period. Because caregivers are relying on their memory, they may under- or overestimate intake.

A computerized nutrient analysis program such as Cronometer (Revelstoke, British Columbia, Canada) can be used to estimate energy as well as macro- and micronutrient intake from a food record or 24-hour recall.

Estimation of Energy Needs for Catch-Up Growth

Daily energy needs can be calculated using prediction equations, coupled with an estimated stress and activity factor (see Chapter 5). In a study that compared predictive equations against resting energy expenditure (REE), the weight- and height-based Schofield equation was least likely to underestimate REE in children with growth failure under age 3.[13,14]

To promote weight gain, additional calories to allow for catch-up growth can be calculated by using the following formula:[15]

1. Determine the child's dietary reference intakes (DRIs) for age, calculating the estimated energy required (EER): REE × activity/stress factor (using standards for estimated degree of activity and/or known conditions that impact the metabolic rate).
2. Determine the child's ideal weight-for-height or ideal weight-for-age (50th percentile on the sex- and age-specific growth chart).
3. Multiply DRI for age by ideal weight.
4. Divide by the child's actual weight.

Equation: EER for age × Ideal weight-for-height (kg)/Actual weight (kg)

Alternatively, calculating REE and then adding stress factors of ×1.5 to 2.0 is also appropriate for assessing the higher energy needs required for catch-up growth.

Nutrition and Feeding Interventions

For mild-to-moderate malnutrition, ad libitum oral feedings using energy-dense foods are appropriate (see Table 27.2). For severe malnutrition, a dietitian should be consulted early, and energy intake should be advanced slowly to prevent complications associated with refeeding syndrome (see Chapter 14). Treatable etiologies of malnutrition should be addressed, and treatment should be tailored to the type of feeding disorder, if present. Consultation with a physician regarding the potential use of cyproheptadine, an antihistamine appetite stimulant, can be considered. If access to food is a concern, a social worker can help identify food resources such as the Special Supplemental Nutrition Program for Women, Infants, and Children (WIC), the Supplemental Nutrition Assistance Program (SNAP), and food pantries, as well as local support systems to minimize parental stress (see Chapter 12). If oral feedings are unsuccessful in increasing the rate of weight gain, then enteral feedings may be necessary (see Chapter 16).

■ INFANTS

Breastfeeding/chestfeeding should be supported as it provides many other health benefits beyond nutrients to the infant. Inadequate intake of human milk may be due to insufficient milk production, which can result from improper latching to the breast or a weak suck. Increasing the frequency of breastfeeding/chestfeeding or pumping can increase a lactating parent's milk supply. If necessary, formula powder can be added to expressed human milk to increase the energy density of the human milk. Prior to supplementing human milk with formula, the infant's growth failure should be verified using the WHO growth charts, and consultation with a lactation consultant

TABLE 27.2 CALORIE-DENSE FOODS

Powdered whole milk: 40 calories/tbsp Stir into mashed potatoes, soups, eggs, ground meats, cooked cereals, puddings, yogurt, shakes, smoothies, creamy sauces, canned soups, and other foods with milk.	***Cooked meats/poultry/fish: 50-75 calories/oz*** Add cooked or diced meats, poultry, shrimp, or fish to salads, soups, casseroles, cooked noodles, and sauces.
Granola: 30 calories/tbsp Add to cereals, yogurt, and ice cream. Combine with mixed nuts.	***Canned coconut milk/cream: 55-90 calories/oz*** Add to soups, curries, sauces, and cooked cereals. Blend into shakes and smoothies. Blend with fruit and pour into popsicle molds for a frozen treat.
Hummus: 30 calories/tbsp Spread on crackers, wraps, or sandwiches, or use as a dip with chips, pretzels, and vegetables.	***Nuts/seeds: 50-100 calories/tbsp*** Add to hot or cold cereals, stir-fried meats and vegetables, stuffing, baked goods, salads, granola, ice cream, or just eat plain as a snack. ***Note:*** *Not recommended for children under age 3.*
Shredded coconut: 30 calories/tbsp Top hot or cold cereals and granola. Add to trail mix. Bake into granola bars, quick breads, and muffins.	***Avocado: 80 calories for ¼ avocado*** Add sliced to sandwiches, quesadillas, tacos, and wraps. Mash and spread on toast, crackers, or sandwiches.
Sour cream: 30 calories/tbsp Add to potatoes, beans, squash, and carrots. Use to make a dip or dressing. Add to sauces/gravies and casseroles.	***Tahini: 90 calories/tbsp*** Add to salad dressings, marinades, and dips. Blend into shakes and smoothies. Bake into quick breads and muffins.
Butter, margarine, oil, ghee: 45 calories/tsp Add to soups, gravies/sauces, mashed potatoes, cooked cereals, vegetables, rice, and pasta. Spread on crackers, breads, muffins, and sandwiches.	***Cheese: 100 calories/oz*** Melt cheese on vegetables, casseroles, fish, meats, eggs, pasta, and rice. Add slices of cheese to crackers, breads, and sandwiches. Mix into mashed potatoes and add extra when making macaroni and cheese.
Cream cheese: 50 calories/tbsp Spread on toast, crackers, bagels, breads, muffins, and fruits. Try it on a sandwich with jelly or peanut butter. Add to mashed potatoes and macaroni and cheese.	***Nut and seed butters: 100 calories/tbsp*** Spread on toast, bread, crackers, cookies, vegetables like carrots or celery, or fruits such as apples or bananas. Add to yogurt, ice cream, cooked cereals, shakes, and smoothies. Try sunflower seed butter or soy nut butter as a peanut and tree nut alternative.
Heavy cream: 50 calories/tbsp Add to hot chocolate, cooked cereals, mashed potatoes, desserts, eggs, cream soups, milk (in a cup to drink or in a bowl of cereal), shakes, and smoothies.	***Mayonnaise: 100 calories/tbsp*** Mix into salad dressings and dips. Use on sandwiches, wraps, hamburgers, and chicken sandwiches.

should be considered to assess problems with breastfeeding/chestfeeding technique or human milk supply. The diet of older infants should be supplemented with nutrient-dense age-appropriate foods, with a particular emphasis on iron-rich choices (meats, beans, iron-fortified infant cereal)[14] (see Chapter 7).

Irritability associated with feedings, with or without reflux or vomiting, may be indicative of a food protein–induced allergic enteritis or proctocolitis (cow's milk protein allergic colitis), gastroesophageal reflux, or dysphagia. Such symptoms may warrant an empiric trial of a parental and infant milk elimination diet or a trial of thickened liquids. Medications to treat gastroesophageal reflux should be considered with caution. Acid suppressant medications have mixed evidence of efficacy in infants and known long-term risks to bone health and other morbidities.[16]

For formula-fed infants who require additional calories, powdered formula offers a convenient way to increase energy density without increasing the feeding volume. Most infant formulas are mixed to provide 20 kcal/oz or 0.67 kcal/mL. The energy density can be advanced up to 28 kcal/oz by adjusting the mixing ratio by adding a smaller amount of water than typically recommended for a standard preparation without exceeding the recommended renal solute load for infants. Commercially available modulars such as Duocal and household ingredients such as canola oil can be used to further increase the energy density of the formula, up to a typical maximum of 30 kcal/oz. Care must be taken to ensure that an infant's hydration status is monitored and fluid requirements are met.

■ TODDLERS AND PRESCHOOL-AGED CHILDREN

Meals and snacks should be spaced 2 to 3 hours apart to foster the child's recognition of hunger and satiety cues.[17] Parents should be encouraged to offer foods that are both energy as well as nutrient dense. Paring a grain, fruit, or vegetable with a protein at snack time is recommended to boost the energy density of a snack. Fruit juice or sugar-sweetened beverages should be limited to less than 4 oz per day and replaced with milk and/or plain water.[18] Calorie enhancers can be added to foods (see Table 27.3). Commercially available oral nutrition supplements should be considered to supplement both macro- and micronutrient intake if needed. However, parents should be counseled to hold these supplements until after solid foods, without sipping or grazing in between meals and snacks.

A meal pattern consisting of three meals and two to three snacks between meals is recommended. Offering food before breastfeeding/chestfeeding is recommended, and the frequency of feeding at the breast/chest may need to be reduced if it resembles "grazing" throughout the day and night. Frequent overnight feeding can impact appetite not only in the morning, but throughout the day.

When addressing concerns about poor oral intake, care should be taken to avoid exacerbating behavior problems around mealtimes (see Table 27.3). As toddlers strive to become independent, mealtimes can be quite stressful for parents, especially if the child has growth concerns. The concept of division of feeding responsibilities proposed by Satter is helpful in explaining to parents how to avoid battles at mealtime.[17] The parent chooses food that is safe and appropriate for the child and offers it in a safe and supportive manner. The child is responsible for deciding how much and whether

TABLE 27.3 STRATEGIES TO PROMOTE HEALTHY EATING BEHAVIORS IN PRESCHOOL-AGED CHILDREN

TIPS FOR GOOD EATING BEHAVIOR: PREPARING FOR MEALTIME

- **Sit down at a table to eat meals and snacks.** Have meals and snacks 2-3 h apart, with only water in between eating times. This way, your toddler will come to the table ready to eat. They will feel hungry, but not too hungry, tired or cranky.
- **Arrange for a quiet time before meals** to help your child pay attention to eating.
- **Seat your child** in a highchair with a foot rest that reaches their feet, booster seat, or children's table.

During Meals and Snacks: Feeding Environment

- **Eat at a table as a family** as often as possible.
- **Avoid distractions** like TV, video games, or radio so your child can pay attention to eating.
- **Give your child their own small fork and spoon.** Cut food into bite-size pieces or serve soft finger foods. Children often enjoy feeding themselves.
- **Give your child enough time to enjoy the meal (20-30 min).** If your child is finished earlier or starts acting up, excuse them from the table.
- **Take your child's food away when they lose interest in eating.** If they stop eating, push the food away or remove the food from the table.

During Meals and Snacks: Your Child's Plate

- **Offer 2-3 foods** at each meal.
- **Give your child small servings.** A serving is about a tablespoon for every year of age for each food. For example, a 3-y-old might eat 3 tablespoons of brown rice, 3 tablespoons of broccoli, and 3 tablespoons of chicken.
- **Give your child some kinds of food they have had before and some new ones.** It is normal for your child not to want new foods. Just give them this new food again another time. It can take many tries before a child accepts a new kind of food.
- **Wait for your child to ask for seconds before giving them more.** Children know when they are finished! Allow them to practice this at an early age.
- **Never force or pressure your toddler to eat or finish** a certain amount of food.
- **Do not give your child something else to eat if they are not eating what you serve.** Good nutrition can add up over several days. Remember: As a parent or caregiver, you decide what your child eats, and your child decides whether to eat it. It gets better over time!
- **Choose whole fruit over juice.** Your child does not need juice to be healthy. If you do give juice, limit it to 4 oz a day. You can try mixing it with water.

Setting Limits and Giving Praise

- **Your child will learn how to behave by eating with you** and your family at the table.
- **Praise your child for good eating behavior,** but do not make them the center of attention.
- **Do not punish your child if they refuse to eat.** Instead, take your child away from the table and do not offer other food until the next meal/snack time, except for water. Remember, they will get enough nutrition over the next few days.
- **Do not reward or bribe your child with food.** For example, do not say, "If you eat your broccoli, you can have ice cream." This teaches them that some foods are better than others.

they eat. Parents should not force a child to drink or eat predetermined amounts of liquids or foods prescribed by the child's clinicians. Force feeding can worsen feeding disorders or cause posttraumatic stress disorder. Parents should be encouraged to notify the child's clinician if they find that their child is not able to drink or eat the recommended goal amount.

PROGNOSIS

The majority of children with malnutrition will show improved intake and weight gain with appropriate intervention. Some children with "picky eating" or food refusal may continue to have feeding problems into childhood, especially if untreated,[17] and some may be diagnosed with anxiety or other psychiatric disorders.[1,19] A small percentage of children, particularly those with underlying medical conditions and neurologic disorders, may require ongoing supplemental nutrition by enteral tube feeding. The first 2 years of life are considered the most essential time period for optimizing long-term cognition and linear growth, as well as minimizing nutrition-related mortality risk.[2] A multidisciplinary approach that addresses the biologic, psychological, and social factors underlying a child's malnutrition is important to ensure optimal long-term health outcomes.

REFERENCES

1. Woo Baidal JA, Huh SY. Failure-to-thrive: growth failure in the outpatient setting. In: Duggan C, Watkins JB, Koletzko B, Walker WA, eds. *Nutrition in Pediatrics: Basic Science, Clinical Applications*. 5th ed. People's Medical Publishing House; 2016.
2. Tang MN, Adolphe S, Rogers SR, Frank DA. Failure to thrive or growth faltering: medical, developmental/behavioral, nutrition, and social dimensions. *Pediatr Rev*. 2021;42(11):590-603.
3. Homan G. Failure to thirve: a practical guide. *Am Fam Physician*. 2016;94(4):295-299.
4. Lezo A, Baldini L, Asteggiano M. Failure to thrive in the outpatient clinic: a new insight. *Nutrients*. 2020;12:2202.
5. Mei Z, Grummer-Strawn LM, Thompson D, Dietz WH. Shifts in percentiles of growth during early childhood: analysis of longitudinal data from the California Child Health and Development Study. *Pediatrics*. 2004;113(6):e617-e627.
6. Mei Z, Grummer-Strawn LM. Comparison of changes in growth percentiles of US children on CDC 2000 growth charts with corresponding changes on WHO 2006 growth charts. *Clin Pediatr.* 2011;50(5):402-407.
7. Grummer-Strawn LM, Reinold C, Krebs NF. Use of World Health Organization and CDC growth charts for children aged 0-59 months in the United States. *MMWR Recomm Rep*. 2010;59(RR-9):1-15.
8. Mei Z, Ogden CL, Flegal KM, Grummer-Strawn LM. Comparison of the prevalence of shortness, underweight, and overweight among US children aged 0 to 59 months by using the CDC 2000 and the WHO 2006 growth charts. *J Pediatr.* 2008;153(5):622-628.
9. Halac I, Zimmerman D. Evaluating short stature in children. *Pediatr Ann*. 2004;33(3):170-176.
10. Rogol AD, Hayden GF. Etiologies and early diagnosis of short stature and growth failure in children and adolescents. *J Pediatr*. 2014;164(5 suppl):S1-S14.e6.
11. Ornstein R, Katzman D. Child and adolescent feeding and eating disorders and the DSM-5: a brave New World. *Adolesc Med*. 2014;25(2):360-376.
12. Brown K. Evolution of pediatric feeding disorders. *Mathews J Pediatr*. 2024;9(1):36.
13. Sentongo TA, Tershakovec AM, Mascarenhas MR, Watson MH, Stallings VA. Resting energy expenditure and prediction equations in young children with failure to thrive. *J Pediatr.* 2000;136(3):345-350.
14. Cooke R, Goulet O, Huysentruyt K, et al. Catch-up growth in infants and young children with faltering growth: expert opinion to guide general clinicians. *J Pediatr Gastroenterol Nutr*. 2023;77(1):7-15.
15. Becker P, Carney LN, Corkins MR, et al. Consensus statement of the Academy of Nutrition and Dietetics/American Society for Parenteral and Enteral Nutrition: indicators recommended for the identification and documentation of pediatric malnutrition (undernutrition). *Nutr Clin Pract*. 2015;30(1):147-161.

16. Rosen R, Vandenplas Y, Singendonk M, et al. Pediatric gastroesophageal reflux clinical practice guidelines: Joint Recommendations of the North American Society for Pediatric Gastroenterology, Hepatology, and Nutrition and the European Society for Pediatric Gastroenterology, Hepatology, and Nutrition. *J Pediatr Gastroenterol Nutr*. 2018;66(3):516-554.
17. Satter E. *Child of Mine: Feeding With Love and Good Sense*. Bull Publishing Company; 2000.
18. Lott M, Callahan E, Welker Duffy E, Story M, Daniels S. Healthy beverage consumption in early childhood: recommendations from key National Health and Nutrition Organizations. Consensus statement. Healthy Eating Research. 2019. http://healthyeatingresearch.org
19. Chatoor I. *Diagnosis and Treatment of Feeding Disorders in Infants, Toddlers, and Young Children*. Zero to Three; 2009.

CHAPTER 28

Hepatobiliary Diseases

Leanna Shea and Andrew Wehrman

Nutritional complications are common in pediatric liver disease. In acute liver failure, most patients present with adequate nutritional status and may require only short-term, uncomplicated strategies to meet nutritional goals. In contrast, children with chronic liver disease often develop some degree of malnutrition, with reported prevalence ranging from 33% to 64% depending on the severity of disease and extent of liver dysfunction.[1] Early nutrition intervention to address malnutrition is paramount, especially in chronic liver disease, as poor nutritional status prior to liver transplantation can negatively impact outcomes following transplant and may contribute to delayed neurocognitive development and faltering long-term growth.[2,3] The pathophysiology of malnutrition in liver disease is multifactorial, including inadequate energy intake, malabsorption, and altered nutrient metabolism.[1] Depending on disease severity, infants and children with chronic liver disease may have increased energy needs due to infections, abnormal macronutrient metabolism, circulating proinflammatory cytokines, and increased respiratory effort from abdominal competition.[3,4] For example, infants and children with chronic liver disease can have increased energy requirements of up to 130% to 150% compared to those without liver disease.[1,2,5] Indirect calorimetry, if available, can be used to measure the resting energy expenditure (REE) to more accurately guide nutrition goals. Table 28.1 highlights clinical manifestations and etiologies of nutritional deficiencies seen in pediatric liver disease.

The underlying etiology of liver dysfunction largely determines the potential nutritional complications. The majority of hepatobiliary disease in infants and children is cholestatic in nature, such as biliary atresia, Alagille syndrome, alpha-1-antitrypsin deficiency, and progressive familial intrahepatic cholestasis (PFIC). In these conditions, obstruction of biliary flow or impaired bile formation and transport, results in decreased luminal bile concentration, causing impaired digestion and absorption of long chain fats and fat-soluble vitamins.[6] This can lead to energy losses from malabsorption, essential fatty acid deficiency, and fat-soluble vitamin deficiencies. Intestinal congestion from portal hypertensions or medications used to bind bile salts may worsen these effects. Irreversible impairment in liver function resulting in cirrhosis presents additional nutritional issues as the liver disease progresses. Early satiety, nausea/vomiting, and increased energy requirements may occur from ascites and organomegaly. Hypoglycemia risk is present, particularly in infants, due to reduced glycogen stores and impaired gluconeogenesis.

Tables 28.2 and 28.3 highlight nutritional monitoring and assessment techniques specific to pediatric liver disease. In addition to standard nutrition assessment (see Chapters 1-4), physical exam and review of growth trends should be carefully considered, as weight gain from ascites and organomegaly can be misleading. In these circumstances,

TABLE 28.1 CLINICAL MANIFESTATIONS AND ETIOLOGIES OF COMMON NUTRITIONAL PROBLEMS IN PEDIATRIC LIVER DISEASE

NUTRIENT AFFECTED	MANIFESTATION	ETIOLOGY
Protein	Stunting, muscle wasting, motor developmental delay	Protein energy malnutrition, negative nitrogen balance, decreased IGF-1 synthesis resulting in growth hormone resistance
	Ascites or peripheral edema	Impaired plasma protein synthesis
	Coagulopathy	Alteration of synthesis in clotting factors
	Hepatic encephalopathy	Impaired aromatic amino acid metabolism resulting in abnormal BCAA/AAA ratio
Fat	Steatorrhea, essential fatty acid deficiency, fat-soluble vitamin deficiencies (see below)	Impaired intestinal digestion of long-chain triglycerides, reduced dietary intake of essential fatty acids, bile salt binding medications (cholestyramine), inefficient elongation of essential fatty acid precursors by dysfunctional hepatocytes, and enhanced peroxidation of lipids
	Hypercholesterolemia, hypertriglyceridemia, xanthomas	Impaired hepatic clearance
Carbohydrate	Hyperglycemia	Impaired carbohydrate use and insulin resistance
	Fasting hypoglycemia	Decreased glycogen stores and capacity for gluconeogenesis due to hepatocellular dysfunction. Infants more vulnerable
Vitamin A	Night blindness, xerophthalmia, degeneration of retina, Bitot spots, poor growth	Impaired intestinal absorption due to decreased bile salt delivery to intestine, reduced dietary intake, reduced transport due to impaired synthesis of retinol-binding protein
Vitamin D	Osteopenia, rickets, hepatic osteodystrophy	Impaired intestinal absorption due to decreased bile salt delivery to intestine, inactivity, and decreased hydroxylation of vitamin D
Vitamin E	Peripheral neuropathy, myopathy, ataxia, hemolytic anemia, vision impairment	Impaired intestinal absorption due to decreased bile salt delivery to intestine, reduced dietary intake
Vitamin K	Coagulopathy	Impaired intestinal absorption due to decreased bile salt delivery to intestine and may be exacerbated by lactulose use
Trace elements and minerals	Low serum iron, zinc, magnesium, calcium	Impaired intestinal absorption due to binding with unabsorbed fatty acids and low vitamin D status (calcium and magnesium), gastrointestinal bleeding and frequent blood draws (iron), low circulating albumin levels (zinc)

BCAA/AAA, branched-chain amino acid/aromatic amino acid; IGF-1, insulin-like growth factor-1.

TABLE 28.2 SPECIFIC NUTRITIONAL MONITORING IN LIVER DISEASE

NUTRIENT	MONITORING
Energy	Diet recall, energy expenditure (indirect calorimetry if available), changes in growth parameters over time (weight, length/height, weight-for-length, BMI, head circumference, soft tissue anthropometrics
Protein	Mid-upper arm circumference (MUAC), albumin, prealbumin, clotting factor levels, ammonia, muscle wasting on physical exam
Fat	Triceps skin fold, fat wasting on physical exam, essential fatty acid panel, including triene-tetraene ratio and mead acid, triglycerides, total cholesterol
Carbohydrate	Serum glucose
Vitamin A	Vitamin A to retinol-binding protein ratio; deficiency defined as <0.07-0.08, ophthalmology exam, retinol dose response
Vitamin D	25-OH vitamin D level, calcium, phosphorus, parathyroid hormone, alkaline phosphatase, bone density scan (DEXA)
Vitamin E	Vitamin E level, α-tocopherol to total lipid (triglycerides, phospholipids, and total cholesterol) ratio if available
Vitamin K	PT/INR, PIVKA-II
Iron	Iron, total iron-binding capacity, ferritin, transferrin saturation, MCV, hemoglobin, hematocrit
Zinc	Serum zinc, alkaline phosphatase
Copper	Serum copper, ceruloplasmin, 24-h urine copper excretion

BMI, body mass index; DEXA, dual-energy x-ray absorptiometry; MCV, mean corpuscular volume; PIVKA-II, proteins induced by vitamin K absence or antagonist-II; PT/INR, prothrombin time/international normalized ratio.

TABLE 28.3 SPECIAL CONSIDERATIONS OF NUTRITIONAL ASSESSMENT

Diet history

- Total energy intake
- Total macronutrient intake and source (example LCT vs. MCT)
- Total fluid intake and fluid status
- Sodium intake
- Medications with potential effects on nutritional status
- Stool consistency, pallor, steatorrhea
- Functional capacity and physical activity

Physical examination and assessment

- Evidence of edema or ascites
- Jaundice
- Hepatomegaly or splenomegaly
- Fat and muscle stores
- Height, weight, BMI, head circumference (if <2 y old)
- Arm anthropometrics (MUAC and TSF)

BMI, body mass index; LCT, long-chain triglyceride; MCT, medium-chain triglyceride; MUAC, mid-upper arm circumference; TSF, triceps skinfold thickness.

anthropometric techniques such as mid-upper arm circumference (MUAC) and triceps skinfold thickness (TSF) are useful and more sensitive to malnutrition than weight-for-length z-scores.[1,4] Serial anthropometric measurements are recommended at a frequency of every 2 weeks to 3 months depending on the severity of malnutrition and frequency of nutrition intervention changes. In addition to typical diet history, symptoms of liver disease should also be assessed as a potential impact to adequacy of oral intake or may help inform degree of malabsorption, such as steatorrhea and stool color/consistency. In reviewing laboratory data, it is important to note that all fat-soluble vitamin levels are sensitive to inflammation and adequacy of carrier proteins and may appear falsely depleted. Serum retinol levels alone may not accurately represent vitamin A status. Retinol-binding protein and C-reactive protein should also be assessed to assist in interpretation of fat-soluble vitamins levels.[7]

Table 28.4 addresses special aspects of nutritional management in hepatobiliary diseases. To compensate for the increased metabolic demand in both infants and children with liver disease, high-calorie diets or supplemental enteral nutrition may be necessary to ensure adequate energy delivery to prevent or treat malnutrition. Infants often require caloric fortification by medium-chain triglycerides (MCTs)–rich formula or modulars and may benefit from feeding smaller volumes more frequently, including

TABLE 28.4 SPECIAL ASPECTS OF NUTRITIONAL MANAGEMENT IN CHRONIC HEPATOBILIARY DISEASES

Overview:

- Daily energy and protein requirements:
  - Energy needs: 130%-150% of requirement for age. Use indirect calorimetry if available.
  - Protein needs: 130%-150% of requirement for age
- Use gut if possible; initiate enteral nutrition (EN) if inadequate energy intake by mouth
- Parenteral nutrition (PN) may be necessary if unable to tolerate enteral nutrition or growth failure despite optimizing enteral nutrition.

Enteral product selection:

Infant formulas for fat malabsorption:

Alfamino Infant (Nestle)—43% fat calories as MCT
Alimentum (Abbott)—33% fat calories as MCT
Extensive HA (Nestle)—49% fat calories as MCT
Pregestimil (Mead Johnson)—53% fat calories as MCT

Pediatric formulas for fat malabsorption:

Peptamen Junior 1.0 or 1.5 (Nestle)—60% fat calories as MCT
Pediasure Peptide 1.0 or 1.5 (Abbott)—60% fat calories as MCT
Kate Farms Pediatric Peptide 1.5 or 1.5 (Kate Farms)—50% fat calories as MCT

Modulars:

MCT oil (Nestle)—7.7kcal/mL
Liquigen (Nutricia)—emulsified MCT oil, 4.5kcal/mL

Postliver transplantation:

- Age-appropriate diet with food safety considerations in setting of immunosuppression
- Tube feeding may be necessary to ensure optimal calories and protein
- Short-term PN may be necessary if oral or EN is contraindicated

MCT, medium-chain triglyceride.

overnight. Diets in older children may be similar in composition to healthy children; however, these will likely depend on type of liver disease and disease severity. When necessary, higher energy provision can be achieved with increased portion sizes, calorically dense snacks, high-calorie additives, and oral nutrition supplements. MCT oil can be used as supplementation directly to solid foods. Ascites or hepatosplenomegaly can lead to anorexia and nausea, and older children may therefore also benefit from smaller, frequent meals. Restrictive diets are not typically necessary and may pose additional challenges for adequate intake. Low-sodium or no-added salt diet may be necessary for those with refractory ascites despite diuretic management.[8] Protein restriction below the Recommended Dietary Allowance (RDA) should not be implemented for infants and children, even in cases of hepatic encephalopathy, since inadequate protein provision will lead to consumption of endogenous muscle protein.[3-5]

If oral nutrition is not feasible or adequate, enteral nutrition via nasogastric or nasojejunal tube should be considered. Hepatosplenomegaly, ascites, and portal hypertension may limit the feasibility of placing a permanent feeding tube. Table 28.4 highlights enteral formulas and modulars rich in MCT to support absorption in the absence of bile for those with cholestatic liver diseases. Presence of long chain fats remains an important component of enteral formulas in order to avoid essential fatty acid deficiency with long-term use.

Parenteral nutrition (PN) may be required if patients are unable to achieve adequate nutrition and growth with enteral nutrition due to intolerance, gastrointestinal bleeding, or fluid limitations. Despite known risk of hepatotoxicity with long-term PN use, it is safe to use in children with hepatobiliary diseases under these circumstances, and sometimes the only option to provide sufficient nutrition. PN prior to liver transplant has been shown to improve soft tissue anthropometrics in malnourished patients with biliary atresia, which, in turn, was associated with improved post-transplant outcomes.[9] Standard parenteral amino acid solutions are appropriate to use. The utility of branched-chain amino acids is not well supported by the literature, particularly in children, and are therefore not routinely used as a method to prevent hepatic encephalopathy.[2,4,5] Special attention should be paid to fluid balance, electrolyte provision (particularly sodium, potassium, and phosphorus), glucose infusion rate, choice of lipid emulsion, and micronutrient supplementation (especially with long-term use).

Fat-soluble vitamin deficiencies are common in hepatobiliary diseases, particularly cholestatic liver disease, due to the dependence on adequate bile salts for digestion and absorption of these micronutrients. The degree of malabsorption typically correlates with the severity of cholestasis and may be prevalent in 20% to 35% of patients, developing as soon as in the first 6 to 12 weeks of life.[2,5] Clinical manifestations of fat-soluble vitamin deficiencies are described in Table 28.1 and laboratory monitoring in Table 28.2. Frequency of monitoring depends on severity and persistence of cholestasis, from every 3 to 4 weeks if the child is receiving repletion for a deficiency, or every 3 to 6 months once deficiency has been corrected. Table 28.5 provides recommendations for management of fat-soluble vitamin deficiencies.[1]

Successful liver transplantation is usually associated with improved nutrition outcomes, including linear growth, weight gain, soft tissue anthropometrics, and developmental outcomes; however, outcomes are impacted by preoperative nutritional status.[2] Following liver transplantation, oral or enteral feeds should be started as soon as possible to optimize energy provision in the postoperative catabolic state, but

TABLE 28.5 TREATMENT OF FAT-SOLUBLE VITAMIN DEFICIENCIES IN CHRONIC LIVER DISEASE

DEFICIENCY	RECOMMENDATION	ADDITIONAL CONSIDERATIONS
Vitamin A	Water-miscible vitamin A *<10 kg: 5000 IU* *>10 kg: 10,000 IU*	Intramuscular (IM) supplementation may be necessary with severe, refractory deficiency
Vitamin E	Water-miscible vitamin E (TPGS) *15-25 IU/kg/d*	Doses ≥50 IU/kg/d may be necessary
Vitamin D	Cholecalciferol or ergocalciferol *30-100 μg/d*	Increase to 100-200 μg/d if deficiency persists after 1 mo Consider need for 1,25-OH_2 vitamin D (Calcitriol) starting at 0.05-0.2 μg/kg/d in cases of rickets or osteoporosis
Vitamin K	Vitamin K_1 *2-10 mg (IM/IV) as needed* *and/or 2-5 mg (oral) daily*	IM or IV repletion as needed based on INR. Anaphylactoid reactions have been reported with IV vitamin K. Oral vitamin K may not be well absorbed.

INR, international normalized ratio; IV, intravenous; TPGS, D-α-tocopheryl polyethylene glycol 1000 succinate

short-term PN may be safely used while awaiting return of bowel function. Children with oral aversion due to symptoms of liver disease prior to transplant may require tube feeds until oral intake is sufficient. Nutritional requirements change after liver transplantation, including an eventual reduction in energy needs closer to age-appropriate guidelines. MCT-rich formulas are no longer indicated once bile production/flow has been reestablished, and children can transition to standard formulas or diets. Bone disease is a common comorbidity both before and after transplantation due to reduced physical activity, fat-soluble vitamin malabsorption, steroid use, and other factors. With high prevalence of vitamin D deficiency in transplant recipients, serum levels should be closely monitored and treated accordingly.[1] Table 28.6 lists other common medications prescribed for patients with chronic liver disease and their many nutritional implications.

In summary, children with liver disease have many risk factors and a high prevalence for malnutrition. The etiology of malnutrition can be complex and multifactorial; therefore, specialized nutrition approaches are necessary and should be tailored to type of liver disease, age, and barriers to sufficient growth and nutrition. Treatment is aimed at minimizing the impact of disease-related symptoms, increasing energy provision to meet the high metabolic demand in this population, and maximizing intestinal absorption of fat and micronutrients.

TABLE 28.6 MEDICATIONS COMMONLY USED IN CHRONIC LIVER DISEASE

MEDICATION	SELECTED SIDE EFFECTS RELEVANT TO NUTRITION
Medications commonly used in cholestasis	
Cholestyramine	Fat-soluble vitamin deficiency, hyperchloremic metabolic acidosis, constipation
Ursodiol	Nausea, vomiting
Rifampin	Red discoloration of body fluids
IBAT inhibitors	Diarrhea, fat-soluble vitamin deficiency
Naltrexone	Diarrhea, nausea, abdominal pain
Medications commonly used for hepatic encephalopathy	
Lactulose	Diarrhea, cramping, electrolyte abnormalities
Neomycin	Diarrhea, nausea, vomiting, kidney injury
Medications commonly used following liver transplantation	
Corticosteroids	Edema, hypertriglyceridemia, hyperglycemia, decreased bone mineral density, Cushing syndrome
Tacrolimus	Hypomagnesemia, hypophosphatemia, hypertriglyceridemia, hyperglycemia
Mycophenolate	Diarrhea, electrolyte abnormalities

IBAT, ileal bile acid transporter.

REFERENCES

1. Mouzaki M, Bronsky J, Gupte G, et al. Nutrition support of children with chronic liver diseases: a joint position paper of the North American Society for Pediatric Gastroenterology, Hepatology, and Nutrition and the European Society for Pediatric Gastroenterology, Hepatology, and Nutrition. *J Pediatr Gastroenterol Nutr.* 2019;69(4):498-511.
2. Yang CH, Perumpail BJ, Yoo ER, et al. Nutritional needs and support for children with chronic liver disease. *Nutrients*. 2017;9(10):1127.
3. Menon J, Shanmugam NP. Nutrition in pediatric liver disease. *Indian J Pediatr*. 2024;91(4):366-373.
4. Nightingale S, Ng, V. Optimizing nutritional management in children with chronic liver disease. *Pediatr Clin North Am*. 2009;56:1161-1183.
5. Young S, Kwarta E, Azzam R, et al. Nutrition assessment and support in children with end-stage liver disease. *Nutr Clin Pract*. 2013;28:317-329.
6. Feldman A, Sokol J. Neonatal cholestasis: updates on diagnostics, therapeutics, and prevention. *Neoreviews*. 2021;22(12):e819-e836.
7. Berger M, Shenkin A, Schweinlin A, et al. ESPEN micronutrient guideline. *Clin Nutr*. 2022;41:1357-1424.
8. Lane E, Hsu E, Murray K. Management of ascites in children. *Expert Rev Gastroenterol Hepatol*. 2015;9(10): 1281-1292.
9. Sullivan J, Sundaram S, Pan Z, et al. Parenteral nutrition supplementation in biliary atresia patients listed for liver transplantation. *Liver Transpl*. 2012;18(1):120-128.

CHAPTER 29

Inborn Errors of Metabolism

Suzanne Hollander and Daniel Pomerantz

Inborn errors of metabolism are inherited disorders caused by a defect in the enzymes required to metabolize protein, carbohydrate, or fat. The inheritance of most metabolic disorders is autosomal recessive. Many of the disorders result in severe clinical manifestations that appear soon after birth. Rapid diagnosis and treatment are essential to prevent neurologic damage, intellectual disability, and possible death. Newborn screening using tandem mass spectrometry allows for early detection of over 20 metabolic disorders, often before clinical symptoms occur.

Nutrition therapy is central to the management of metabolic disorders. The overall goal of nutrition therapy is to correct the metabolic imbalance while providing adequate nutrients for normal growth and development. Frequent monitoring of growth, nutrient intake, and laboratory values is necessary to evaluate the adequacy of the diet. Dietary management often involves small, frequent adjustments to ensure metabolic stability. Treatment is based on the specific metabolic defect and includes reducing substrate availability through dietary restriction, supplementing the product of the blocked pathway, supplementing enzymatic cofactors in vitamin-responsive enzyme defects, and/or using medications that facilitate excretion or utilization of toxic metabolites.

Selected metabolic disorders are discussed briefly in what follows, with guidelines for these and additional disorders presented in Table 29.1. Detailed protocols on the nutritional management of specific metabolic disorders are available.[1,2] Resources for nutritional products used to treat these disorders are listed at the end of the chapter.

■ DISORDERS OF AMINO ACID METABOLISM

Disorders of amino acid metabolism and the affected amino acids associated with each include phenylketonuria (phenylalanine), tyrosinemia (tyrosine, phenylalanine), homocystinuria (methionine), and maple syrup urine disease (leucine, isoleucine, valine). Nutritional management of amino acid disorders involves restricting one or more essential amino acids to the minimum requirement through a low-protein diet and supplementing all other essential nutrients through the use of medical foods (formulas), which are age and diagnosis specific. A medical food is administered orally or enterally under the supervision of a physician and registered dietitian. These formulas provide a major portion of the daily intake of protein, calories, vitamins, and minerals. Formulas are often composed of L-amino acids. Since these amino acids are absorbed and oxidized more rapidly than amino acids derived from digestion of whole protein, recommended protein and calorie intakes for children with metabolic disorders are often higher than the Dietary Reference Intakes (DRI).[1,2]

Intact protein intake must be limited to supply only the minimum amount of amino acids required for growth. For infants, intact protein is supplied by human milk

TABLE 29.1 INHERITED METABOLIC DISORDERS

DISORDER	ENZYME AFFECTED	BIOCHEMICAL FINDINGS	CLINICAL FEATURES	NUTRITIONAL MODIFICATION	VITAMIN THERAPY
Amino Acid Disorders					
Phenylketonuria: Severe (classical), Moderate (atypical), Mild (hyperphenylalaninemia)	Phenylalanine hydroxylase	Increased blood phenylalanine Severe: >1200 μmol/L Moderate: 360-1200 μmol/L Mild: 120-360 μmol/L	If untreated, intellectual disability, seizures, hyperactivity and eczema; normal development with proper treatment Untreated PKU in a pregnant woman can cause intellectual disability, congenital heart disease, low birth weight, and microcephaly in offspring.	Phenylalanine restriction, ±tyrosine supplementation	None
Hyperphenylalaninemia (pterin defect)	Dihydropteridine Reductase; GTP cyclohydrolase	Mild to moderate Hyperphenylalanin-emia (see above)	Psychomotor retardation, tonicity disorders, hyperthermia, hypersalivation, difficulty swallowing	±Phenylalanine restriction ±Tyrosine supplementation	Tetrahydropterin 2 mg/kg/d orally ± Neurotransmitter supplements
Tyrosinemia type I	Fumarylacetoacetate hydrolase	Increased blood phenylalanine and tyrosine; increased α-fetoprotein; urinary succinylacetone	Liver failure; renal tubular acidosis, failure to thrive, vomiting, diarrhea, rickets, porphyria-like crises, hepatic carcinoma	Phenylalanine and tyrosine restriction (diet used in conjunction with NTBC or until liver transplantation is possible)	None
Tyrosinemia type II	Tyrosine aminotransferase	Increased blood phenylalanine and tyrosine	Intellectual disability, photophobia, palmar keratosis	Phenylalanine and tyrosine restriction	None

(continued)

TABLE 29.1 INHERITED METABOLIC DISORDERS (*continued*)

DISORDER	ENZYME AFFECTED	BIOCHEMICAL FINDINGS	CLINICAL FEATURES	NUTRITIONAL MODIFICATION	VITAMIN THERAPY
Homocystinuria (pyridoxine nonresponsive)	Cystathionine ß-synthase	Homocystine in blood and urine, increased methionine, and decreased cystine in blood	Dislocated lenses, Marfanoid-like skeletal changes, intravascular thromboses, intellectual disability, osteopenia	Methionine restriction; cystine, betaine, B_{12}, and folate supplementation	Betaine 100 mg/kg/d orally, B_{12} and folate supplementation to achieve DRI
Homocystinuria (pyridoxine responsive)	Cystathionine ß-synthase	Same as above	Same as above	Methionine restriction only if tHcy >50 µmol/L after pyridoxine response	Pyridoxine 25-500 mg/d orally
Maple syrup urine disease	Branched-chain keto-acid dehydrogenase complex	Elevated blood, urine, and CSF leucine, isoleucine, valine, alloisoleucine	Neonatal form: poor feeding, fluctuating tone, apnea, seizures, death, developmental delay Variant forms: milder ketoacidosis triggered by protein load or illness	Valine, isoleucine, and leucine restriction	Only in variant forms where 100-300 mg/d oral thiamin may enhance residual enzyme activity
Organic Acidemias					
Glutaric acidemia type I	Glutaryl-CoA dehydrogenase	Elevated blood, urine and CSF glutaric acid and 3-OH-glutaric acid, metabolic acidosis	Acute metabolic crisis (vomiting, acidosis) and neurologic deterioration triggered by illness; macrocephaly, ataxia, choreoathetosis, developmental delay	Lysine and tryptophan restriction; carnitine supplementation	May have partial response to riboflavin 100-300 mg/d orally.

Glutaric acidemia type II	Multiple acyl-CoA dehydrogenase	Elevated blood, urine and CSF glutaric acid and 2-OH glutaric acid, metabolic acidosis, hyperammonemia, hypoglycemia (± ketones) Impaired fatty acid oxidation	Malformations in most severe form, hypotonia, hepatomegaly, developmental delay	Mild protein and fat restriction; fasting avoidance, ± carnitine supplementation	±Riboflavin 100-300 mg/d orally
Isovaleric acidemia	Isovaleryl-CoA dehydrogenase	Elevated blood, urine and CSF isovaleric acid; metabolic acidosis Hyperammonemia, hypoglycemia	Poor feeding, vomiting, sweaty-feet body odor Seizures, coma, death if untreated	Leucine restriction; glycine and carnitine supplementation	None
Methylmalonic academia	Methylmalonyl-CoA mutase	Metabolic acidosis, ketonuria, hypoglycemia Hyperammonemia, hyperglycinemia	Lethargy, failure to thrive, vomiting, hepatomegaly, hypotonia, coma, death if untreated	Isoleucine, methionine, valine, threonine restriction; carnitine supplementation	None
Methylmalonic academia	Cobalamin processing defect (hydroxycobalamin or adenosyl-cobalamin)	Metabolic acidosis Ketonuria, ± homocystine in urine and blood, ± folate deficiency	Lethargy, failure to thrive, vomiting, hepatomegaly, hypotonia, coma, death if untreated	Carnitine supplementation	Hydroxocobalamin 1-2 mg daily to weekly intramuscularly
Propionic acidemia	Propionyl-CoA carboxylase	Metabolic acidosis, ketonuria, hyperglycinemia, hypoglycemia, hyperammonemia	Poor feeding, vomiting, lethargy, hypotonia, seizures, coma, death if untreated Developmental delay	Isoleucine, methionine, valine, threonine restriction; carnitine supplementation	None
Urea Cycle Disorders					
Carbamyl phosphate synthetase deficiency	Carbamyl phosphate synthetase	Hyperammonemia Respiratory alkalosis	Lethargy, vomiting, apnea, coma, and death if untreated	Protein restriction; essential amino acid and arginine supplementation; sodium phenylbutyrate	None

(*continued*)

TABLE 29.1 INHERITED METABOLIC DISORDERS (*continued*)

DISORDER	ENZYME AFFECTED	BIOCHEMICAL FINDINGS	CLINICAL FEATURES	NUTRITIONAL MODIFICATION	VITAMIN THERAPY
Ornithine transcarbamylase deficiency	Ornithine transcarbamylase	Hyperammonemia, respiratory alkalosis	Lethargy, vomiting, apnea, coma and death if untreated Developmental delay	Protein restriction; essential amino acid and arginine supplementation; sodium phenylbutyrate	None
Citrullinemia	Argininosuccinic synthetase	Hyperammonemia, respiratory alkalosis	Lethargy, vomiting, apnea, coma, and death if untreated; developmental delay	Protein restriction; essential amino acid and arginine supplementation; sodium phenylbutyrate	None
Argininosuccinic aciduria	Argininosuccinic lyase	Hyperammonemia, respiratory alkalosis	Lethargy, vomiting, apnea, coma, and death if untreated; cirrhosis, developmental delay	Protein restriction; essential amino acid and arginine supplementation; sodium phenylbutyrate	None
Arginemia	Arginase	±Hyperammonemia	Spastic diplegia, intellectual disability	Restrict protein; essential amino acid supplementation; sodium phenylbutyrate	None
Hyperornithinemia-Hyperammonemia-Homocitrullinuria	Defect in mitochondrial transport of ornithine	Hyperornithinemia, hyperammonemia, homocitrullinuria, hyperglutaminemia, hyperalaninemia	Ataxia, lethargy, vomiting, choreoathetosis, seizures, coma, developmental delay	Protein restriction; arginine supplementation	None
Ornithine transcarbamylase deficiency	Ornithine transcarbamylase	Hyperammonemia, respiratory alkalosis	Lethargy, vomiting, apnea, coma and death if untreated; developmental delay	Protein restriction; essential amino acid and arginine supplementation; sodium phenylbutyrate	None

Citrullinemia	Argininosuccinic synthetase	Hyperammonemia, respiratory alkalosis	Lethargy, vomiting, apnea, coma and death if untreated; developmental delay	Protein restriction; essential amino acid and arginine supplementation; sodium phenylbutyrate	None
Argininosuccinic aciduria	Argininosuccinic lyase	Hyperammonemia, respiratory alkalosis	Lethargy, vomiting, apnea, coma and death if untreated; cirrhosis, developmental delay	Protein restriction; essential amino acid and arginine supplementation; sodium phenylbutyrate	None
Arginemia	Arginase	±Hyperammonemia	Spastic diplegia, intellectual disability	Restrict protein; essential amino acid supplementation; sodium phenylbutyrate	None
Hyperornithinemia-Hyperammonemia-Homocitrullinuria	Defect in mitochondrial transport of ornithine	Hyperornithinemia, hyperammonemia, homocitrullinuria, hyperglutaminemia, hyperalaninemia	Ataxia, lethargy, vomiting, choreoathetosis, seizures, coma, developmental delay	Protein restriction; arginine supplementation	None
Disorders of Carbohydrate Metabolism					
Galactosemia	Hepatic and erythrocyte Epimerase	Galactose in blood and urine	Hepatomegaly, jaundice, vomiting	Restrict galactose; calcium and vitamin D supplementation	None
Galactosemia	Galactokinase	Galactose in blood and urine	Cataracts	Restrict galactose; calcium and vitamin D supplementation	None
Galactosemia	Galactose-1-phosphate uridyl transferase	Galactose in blood and urine; renal Fanconi syndrome	Cataracts, diarrhea, failure to thrive, hepatomegaly, jaundice, vomiting, *E. coli* sepsis	Restrict galactose; calcium and vitamin D supplementation	None

(continued)

TABLE 29.1 INHERITED METABOLIC DISORDERS (*continued*)

DISORDER	ENZYME AFFECTED	BIOCHEMICAL FINDINGS	CLINICAL FEATURES	NUTRITIONAL MODIFICATION	VITAMIN THERAPY
Pyruvate dehydrogenase complex deficiency	Pyruvate dehydrogenase	Elevated blood pyruvate and lactate, elevated blood alanine	Hypotonia, failure to thrive, seizures, ±dysmorphism, developmental delay	Restrict carbohydrate, provide high-fat diet (50% of energy) or ketogenic diet	Thiamin 50-100 mg/d orally
Disorders of Fatty Acid Oxidation					
Medium Chain acyl-CoA dehydrogenase deficiency	Medium-chain acyl-CoA dehydrogenase	Hypoketotic hypoglycemia, mild hyperammonemia and metabolic acidosis	Metabolic decompensation with fasting (lethargy, vomiting, coma), hepatomegaly	Fasting and MCT avoidance; ± fat restriction (30% of energy); ±carnitine	None
Carnitine uptake deficiency	Short-chain acyl-CoA dehydrogenase; short-chain hydroxyacyl-CoA dehydrogenase	Hypoketotic hypoglycemia, ±hyperammonemia,	Poor feeding, vomiting, failure to thrive; cardiac arrhythmia	Fasting avoidance; ±Carnitine	None
Very long-chain acyl-CoA dehydrogenase deficiency, carnitine palmitoyltransferase II deficiency, carnitine-acylcarnitine translocase deficiency	Very long-chain acyl-CoA dehydrogenase	Hypoketotic hypoglycemia, rhabdomyolysis ±Hyperammonemia	Cardiomyopathy, failure to thrive, rhabdomyolysis, hypotonia, hepatomegaly, lethargy, coma (brain malformations in CPTII)	Fasting avoidance; ± long-chain fat restriction (10%-25% of energy); MCT oil or triheptanoin, ±carnitine, and ± essential fatty acid supplementation	None
Long-chain 3-hydroxyacyl-CoA dehydrogenase deficiency, Mitochondrial trifunctional protein deficiency	Long-chain hydroxyacyl-CoA dehydrogenase/mitochondrial trifunctional protein	Hypoketotic hypoglycemia, rhabdomyolysis ±Hyperammonemia	Cardiomyopathy, retinopathy, failure to thrive, hypotonia, hepatomegaly, lethargy, coma	Fasting avoidance; ± long-chain fat restriction (10%-25% of energy); MCT oil or triheptanoin, ±carnitine, and ± essential fatty acid supplementation	None

GLYCOGEN STORAGE DISORDERS					
Type 0 (hepatic glycogen synthase deficiency)	Glycogen synthase	Fasting hypoglycemia and ketosis, postprandial hyperglycemia and glucosuria	Failure to thrive, no hepatomegaly	High-protein diet (2-4 g/kg or 25% calories); reduced simple sugars in favor of complex carbohydrates; frequent feeding every 3 h during day; use of uncooked cornstarch (UCCS) to achieve up to 6 h of overnight fasting, daytime UCCS supplementation if euglycemia not achieved with high-protein diet alone	None
Type Ia (Von Gierke Disease, Hepatorenal Glycogenosis)	Glucose-6-phosphatase	Severe hypoglycemia, elevated production of lactic acid, triglycerides, and uric acid	Hepatomegaly, failure to thrive, distended abdomen, delayed motor development	Infants: lactose-free formula every 2 h during day and every 3 h overnight, continuous overnight enteral feeds or more frequent daytime feeds as needed to achieve euglycemia; 6 mo and older: UCCS (1.6 g/kg ideal body weight) every 3 h during the day and every 3-4 h at night, 60%-70% CHO, 15%-20% protein, 20% fat, fructose and galactose restricted	Multivitamin with minerals; calcium and vitamin D if not consuming fortified milk alternative

(continued)

TABLE 29.1 INHERITED METABOLIC DISORDERS (*continued*)

DISORDER	ENZYME AFFECTED	BIOCHEMICAL FINDINGS	CLINICAL FEATURES	NUTRITIONAL MODIFICATION	VITAMIN THERAPY
Type Ib (Von Gierke Disease, Hepatorenal Glycogenosis)	Glucose-6-phosphate transporter	Severe hypoglycemia, elevated production of lactic acid, triglycerides and uric acid, constant or cyclic neutropenia, IBD	Hepatomegaly, failure to thrive, distended abdomen, delayed motor development	As in type 1a	As in type 1a
Type III (Cori disease, Forbes disease, debrancher deficiency)	Amylo-1, 6-glucosidase (AGD)	Fasting hypoglycemia with ketosis, hyperlipidemia, profound elevation of serum transaminases, elevated creatine kinase	Hepatomegaly in childhood, myopathy (usually more prominent in adulthood)	Small, frequent feedings and avoidance of fasting; CS 1.0-1.6 g/kg q4h during the day and overnight; high-protein diet (2-4 g/kg), limited simple sugars	Based on individual need
Type IV (Andersen disease, amylopectinosis, brancher deficiency)	Glycogen-branching enzyme	Hepatic presentation: elevated serum transaminase levels, hypoglycemia with advanced cirrhosis Neuromuscular presentation: increased CK	Hepatic presentation: failure to thrive, hepatosplenomegaly, cirrhosis, portal hypertension, esophageal varices and ascites; neuromuscular presentation: myopathy	Frequent meals, snacks, and CS as needed to maintain normal blood glucose levels and provide sufficient nutritional intake in order to improve liver function and muscular strength	None
Type V (McArdle disease, muscle phosphorylase deficiency)	Muscle phosphorylase	Elevated serum creatine kinase; uric acid may be elevated	Muscle weakness and cramping with exercise, myoglobinuria	Provide a high-protein diet; moderate exercise; glucose or fructose ingestion during early stage exercise to achieve second wind; studies of ketogenic or modified ketogenic diets are ongoing	Vitamins B_6 and creatine supplement

Type VI (Hers disease, liver phosphorylase deficiency)	Liver phosphorylase	Mild fasting ketotic hypoglycemia, mild hypertriglyceridemia, and elevated serum transaminase levels	Hepatomegaly, distended abdomen, growth retardation, delayed motor development; muscle involvement may occur	Small, frequent feedings with avoidance of fasting; high-protein diet 2-3 g/kg; UCCS as needed, starting with low dose and up to 1g/kg every 4-8 h during overnight fast; reduced simple sugars in favor of complex carbohydrates totaling 40%-50% calories	None
Type VII (Tarui disease, muscle phosphofructokinase deficiency)	Muscle phosphofructokinase	Elevated serum creatine kinase, hemolytic anemia, myoglobinuria, and hyperuricemia (postexercise)	Muscle weakness and cramping with exercise, myoglobinuria	Diet should be high in protein (45% CHO, 25% protein, 30%, fat), moderate exercise	None
Type IX (phosphorylase kinase deficiency)	Phosphorylase kinase	Symptomatic hypoglycemia and ketosis with prolonged fasting or strenuous exercise; mild hypertriglyceridemia, hypercholesterolemia, and elevated serum transaminases	Hepatomegaly, growth retardation, mild delayed motor development	As in type VI	None
Type XI (Fanconi-Bickel syndrome)	Lactate dehydrogenase	Elevated serum creatine kinase, elevated pyruvate	Myoglobinuria, myalgia, excessive fatigue	Avoid intense exercise; case reports of success with galactose- and glucose-restricted diet	None

CHO, carbohydrate; CK, creatine kinase; CSF, cerebrospinal fluid; DRI, dietary reference intake; GTP, guanosine triphosphate; IBD, inflammatory bowel disease; MCT, medium-chain triglyceride; PKU, phenylketonuria; UCCS, uncooked cornstarch.

or standard infant formula. In older children, table foods with low to moderate protein content provide intact protein. Overrestriction of protein or specific amino acids is harmful and can impair growth. Personalized protein prescriptions must consider the specific disorder as well as an individual's age, growth rate, and degree of enzyme activity. Close monitoring of plasma amino acids is key to assessing individual protein and amino acid needs. Adequate energy intake from nonprotein sources is essential for growth and to limit tissue catabolism leading to metabolic instability.

Recommended vitamin and mineral intakes follow the DRI guidelines. In low-protein diets where special metabolic formulas provide the majority of protein intake, medical food is the primary source of vitamins and minerals. Intake of vitamins and minerals should be monitored, especially when formula intake is suboptimal. Recommendations for clinical, nutritional, and laboratory monitoring of children on amino acid and protein-restricted diets are found in Table 29.2.

Phenylketonuria

Phenylketonuria (PKU) is the most common amino acid disorder, caused by a defect in the enzyme phenylalanine hydroxylase, which converts phenylalanine to tyrosine. The recommended diet is restricted in phenylalanine and supplemented with tyrosine. Early treatment of PKU prevents severe intellectual disability. Treatment should be continued throughout life to prevent learning difficulties and behavioral problems that appear in childhood as well as emotional and executive functioning difficulties that present in later adolescence and adulthood.[3]

PKU severity ranges from benign hyperphenylalaninemia, which requires no treatment, to mild, moderate, and classical/severe forms of PKU, which require progressively more treatment to lower blood phenylalanine levels into the target treatment range. For children with moderate or classical PKU, formula provides the primary source of protein, calories, vitamins, and minerals. Formula options are selected based on age, protein/calorie content, and palatability. Glycomacropeptide (GMP)-based formulas can be a more palatable option for some patients.

A prescribed amount of phenylalanine is allowed from food. High-protein foods, such as meat, poultry, fish, milk, cheese, dairy products, nuts, soy, and legumes, must be avoided. Bread and cereal products, pasta, rice, and starchy vegetables are allowed in limited amounts. Adequate energy intake from nonprotein sources is essential for growth and to minimize tissue catabolism that can lead to metabolic instability. Inadequate energy intake may result from diet restrictions that severely limit food choices, unpleasant taste of medical foods, and poor appetite. Fruits, vegetables, and special low-protein foods (e.g., pastas, breads, baked items) may be eaten in larger quantities, supplemented with concentrated sweets and fats. Detailed food lists and online tools are available to assist in estimating phenylalanine intake from foods.[4,5]

Phenylalanine intake is counted in milligrams of phenylalanine or grams of protein. For many children with classical PKU, daily intake of phenylalanine is limited to approximately 300 mg (5-6 g of intact protein).

Adherence to diet is monitored by following blood phenylalanine concentrations:

- Infants/children: less than or equal to 360 μmol/L (United States[3] and Europe[6])
- Adults: less than or equal to 360 μmol/L (United States[3]) and 120 to 600 μmol/L (Europe[6])

TABLE 29.2 MONITORING OF NUTRITIONAL THERAPY

	AMINO ACID DISORDERS	ORGANIC ACIDEMIAS	UREA CYCLE DISORDERS	GALACTOSEMIA	FATTY ACID OXIDATION DISORDERS
Anthropometrics:					
Length/height	X	x	x	x	x
Weight					
Head circumference					
BMI					
Nutritional intake:					
Energy	X	x	x	x	x
Protein					
Fat					
Vitamins/minerals					
Laboratory indices:					
Plasma amino acids	X	x	x		
Hemoglobin	X	x	x	x	x
Hematocrit					
Serum ferritin	X	x	x		
Transferrin saturation					
Total iron-binding capacity					
Vitamin B_{12}[a]	X	x	x		
RBC folate[a]	X	x	x		

(continued)

TABLE 29.2 MONITORING OF NUTRITIONAL THERAPY (*continued*)

	AMINO ACID DISORDERS	ORGANIC ACIDEMIAS	UREA CYCLE DISORDERS	GALACTOSEMIA	FATTY ACID OXIDATION DISORDERS
Serum zinc[a]	X	x	x		
25-Hydroxy vitamin D	X	x	x	x	x
Essential fatty acid profile[b]	X	x	x		x
Organic acids (urine/plasma)		x			
Acylcarnitines		x			x
Carnitine		x			x
Ammonia		x	x		
Galactose-1-phosphate				x	
Urine galactitol					
DXA	X	x	x	x	
Urine ketones	x[c]	x			

BMI, body mass index; DXA, dual-energy x-ray absorptiometry.
[a]If metabolic formula intake is suboptimal.
[b]If dietary fat intake is low and/or metabolic formula contains no fat.
[c]Monitor urine ketones only in MSUD.

The PKU diet is very restrictive, and maintaining the recommended plasma phenylalanine concentrations with diet alone is difficult. Children must develop the knowledge and skills necessary to manage their diet successfully as they develop increasing independence.

In older adolescents and adults unable to sustain standard dietary treatment, large neutral amino acid (LNAA) therapy may be used, which may reduce uptake of phenylalanine across the blood-brain barrier but does not lower blood phenylalanine concentrations.[7]

Three blood phenylalanine lowering medications are currently available—tetrahydrobiopterin (sapropterin or BH_4)[3], sepiapterin which is a precursor to BH_4, and phenylalanine ammonia lyase (PAL or palynziq).[8] Individuals must have some functioning PAH enzyme activity to respond to sepiapterin or sapropterin, both of which are approved for all ages. Individuals with any type of PKU may respond to PAL after an initial dose escalation phase; however, this medication is approved only for adolescents and adults. PAL blood phenylalanine reduction is typically significant enough that individuals are able to consume an unrestricted protein diet without formula. Guidelines for nutritional management of BH_4 and PAL therapy are available.[2,9]

Infants born to pregnant women with PKU who had pregnancy blood phenylalanine levels greater than 360 μmol/L are at an increased risk for low birth weight, microcephaly, cardiac anomalies, and intellectual disability. Strict dietary control alongside pharmacotherapy before conception and during pregnancy can prevent these complications.[3]

Maple Syrup Urine Disease

Maple syrup urine disease (MSUD) is caused by a deficiency of branched-chain α-ketoacid dehydrogenase, an enzyme in the metabolic pathway of branched-chain amino acids (BCAA). Leucine is the primary toxic metabolite, and the recommended diet is restricted in leucine, isoleucine, and valine. In classic MSUD, infants present within the first 2 weeks of life with poor feeding, lethargy, dystonia, ketoacidosis, encephalopathy, and life-threatening brain edema. Immediate treatment is necessary to correct metabolic imbalances in these infants.

During acute metabolic decompensation, the treatment goal is rapid removal of toxic metabolites, reduction of catabolism, and promotion of anabolism. Nutrition therapy includes aggressive enteral nutrition via BCAA-free formula (up to 150% of maintenance calorie needs), adequate BCAA-free protein, as well as replenishment of fluids and electrolytes. Levels of BCAAs and electrolytes are closely monitored to assess for possible cerebral edema. Isoleucine and valine often drop faster than leucine and must be supplemented to restore balance and support protein synthesis. Parenteral nutrition using BCAA-free amino acids, glucose, and lipids may be used for acutely ill patients who are unable to tolerate adequate enteral feedings.[10]

The goal of long-term nutritional management in MSUD is to maintain plasma concentrations of leucine, isoleucine, and valine as close to the normal range as possible while providing adequate nutrients for growth and development. A BCAA-free metabolic formula containing all other essential nutrients and amino acids is supplemented with small amounts of intact protein, with the prescribed intact protein based on leucine tolerance. Supplemental isoleucine and valine are prescribed to maintain plasma concentrations slightly above the normal range.[10] Growth, nutrient intake, and plasma amino acids are monitored. At times of illness, urine may be checked for ketoacids.

Guidelines are available for the nutritional management of MSUD in pregnancy.[10] Nutritional needs are similar to those of pregnant women without MSUD, but with protein intake maintained through use of a BCAA-free formula with intact protein providing an amount of leucine to maintain plasma leucine concentrations at 100 to 300 μmol/L and supplemental isoleucine and valine to maintain blood concentrations of these amino acids in the upper range of normal (200-400 μmol/L).[10] Metabolic decompensation of the pregnant individual requires aggressive treatment, with special attention needed during labor and delivery and for at least 6 weeks postpartum as these are periods of significant catabolism.

Liver transplantation is a treatment alternative to the traditional BCAA-restricted diet for MSUD. Liver transplantation eliminates the risk of metabolic decompensation and decreases plasma BCAA concentrations, so dietary restriction is no longer needed.

ORGANIC ACIDEMIAS

Organic acidemias are inherited enzyme deficiencies that affect the catabolic pathways of amino acids, resulting in accumulation of intermediary metabolites (organic acids). The organic acidemias and the affected amino acids associated with each include glutaric acidemia (lysine, tryptophan), isovaleric acidemia (leucine), and propionic acidemia and methylmalonic acidemia (isoleucine, methionine, threonine, valine). In these disorders, excessive protein intake or catabolic stress, such as infection or prolonged fasting, produces an accumulation of organic acids, resulting in ketoacidosis, hypoglycemia, and hyperammonemia.

Propionic Acidemia and Methylmalonic Acidemia

The disorders propionic acidemia (PROP) and methylmalonic acidemia (MMA) are caused by defects in the enzymes propionyl-CoA carboxylase and methylmalonyl-CoA mutase, respectively. Clinical symptoms of organic acidemias include vomiting and dehydration, poor feeding, growth failure, hypotonia, metabolic ketoacidosis, and hyperammonemia; severe brain damage or coma leading to death may occur without immediate treatment to correct metabolic imbalances. During illnesses contracted throughout childhood, acute metabolic decompensation can occur due to catabolism, causing metabolic acidosis, hyperammonemia, and ketonuria.[11]

The treatment goal during both illness and well states is to reduce toxic concentrations of organic compounds and promote anabolism. The recommended diet is moderate in protein and focused on adequate caloric intake to prevent catabolism.

During illness with risk of metabolic decompensation, nutritional therapy consists of short-term, 24- to 48-hour protein reduction/elimination while providing adequate glucose and fluids to suppress catabolism and assist in urinary removal of abnormal metabolites. Energy intake goals are 120% of usual maintenance needs and may be achieved with a combination of intravenous dextrose, intravenous lipids, and/or a high-calorie, protein-restricted enteral formula. Protein is restricted for no more than 24 to 48 hours before it is gradually reintroduced. Inadequate energy intake or use of a protein-free diet for more than 2 days can lead to protein catabolism and rebound ketoacidosis and hyperammonemia. Parenteral nutrition may be used when enteral feedings are not tolerated, with protein supplied through specially formulated amino acid mixtures or with a standard solution providing 0.5 g of protein per kg/d and increasing in increments of 0.25 g/kg/d as tolerated.[12]

Ongoing nutritional management of PROP and MMA in the well state involves a moderate protein restriction. Individuals may metabolically tolerate adequate protein through an intact source to achieve the recommended dietary allowance (RDA) or more; however, if adequate protein is not well tolerated, then MMA/PROP specific medical food may be used.[12] This medical food is restricted in valine, methionine, isoleucine, and threonine. Overuse of medical food may result in amino acid imbalance, with an excessive ratio of leucine to valine and/or isoleucine, that can cause decreased plasma levels of valine and isoleucine and predicts impaired brain uptake of multiple essential amino acids.[13] Adequate nonprotein energy is essential to prevent tissue catabolism and optimize growth, and extended periods of fasting should be avoided. Constipation presents commonly in children with MMA and PROP, leading to poor nutritional intake and tolerance that compromises metabolic stability.[12]

Information on long-term outcomes is limited. Medical complications may include growth retardation, neurologic impairment, chronic renal failure in MMA, as well as pancreatitis, diabetes, and cardiomyopathy in PROP. Liver transplantation may reduce the risk of severe metabolic decompensation and improve quality of life, but it does not eliminate the need for a modified diet.[11]

Glutaric Acidemia Type 1

Glutaric acidemia type 1 (GA1) is an organic acid disorder caused by the deficiency of glutaryl Co-A dehydrogenase, the enzyme involved in metabolizing the essential amino acids lysine and tryptophan. Infants with GA1 are usually healthy at birth and may be macrocephalic. Other symptoms usually occur between 2 months and 4 years of age and are triggered by an acute infection, prolonged fasting or other stress. If untreated, metabolic acidosis ensues, and severe and permanent neurologic problems may result, including dystonia, choreoathetosis, and seizure disorders. During acute crises, metabolic acidosis may lead to brain edema, coma, and death. The most critical component of care is the early and aggressive treatment of illnesses to prevent a metabolic crisis. Intravenous glucose, insulin, and L-carnitine are often recommended in the setting of illness, vomiting, and/or decreased appetite.[14]

Individuals are typically diagnosed and treated with diet presymptomatically after identification through newborn screening. These individuals are treated with diet to help prevent the onset of symptoms. Chronic treatment includes the restriction of protein and use of medical foods that are low in lysine and tryptophan and supplemented with arginine. Carnitine is supplemented to aid in removing the toxic accumulation of compounds. Arginine supplementation in formula serves to competitively reduce blood-brain barrier transport of lysine. Prolonged fasting must be avoided to prevent catabolism. Dietary strategies have been shown to dramatically reduce the risk of striatal injury and neurodevelopmental issues. Efficacy of treatment beyond age 6 is uncertain, so dietary protein intake is often liberalized, and medical food intake is reduced in later childhood.[15]

UREA CYCLE DISORDERS

Urea cycle disorders result from a defect in one of the enzymes involved in the conversion of ammonia to urea in the liver. Hyperammonemia is common to all the disorders to varying degrees and most prominent in disorders of the proximal urea cycle. The enzyme defects include carbamyl phosphate synthetase (CPS) deficiency, ornithine transcarbamylase (OTC) deficiency, argininosuccinic acid synthetase deficiency (citrullinemia), argininosuccinic acid lyase deficiency (argininosuccinic aciduria), and arginase deficiency. Infants with neonatal onset present with hyperammonemia, poor feeding, vomiting, and hypotonia, which may progress rapidly to seizures, coma, and death. Plasma ammonia concentrations at presentation are often greater than 1000 μmol/L. Rapid diagnosis and treatment are essential as neurologic outcome is related to the duration of severe hyperammonemia and coma. Older infants and children may present with later onset and potentially less severe hyperammonemia, often induced by illness-related catabolism.

Catabolism during diagnosis and illness can lead to life-threatening hyperammonemia. Nutritional therapy during acute metabolic crisis consists of reducing protein and providing intravenous fluids and glucose to correct dehydration, provide energy, and suppress catabolism. Intravenous dextrose in combination with lipid or protein-free formula is used for 24 to 48 hours to maximize energy intake and decrease ammonia concentrations; protein is then gradually reintroduced. Inadequate energy intake or use of a protein-free diet for more than 1 to 2 days can lead to protein catabolism and rebound hyperammonemia. Parenteral nutrition can be used when enteral feedings are not tolerated, with protein supplied through a standard solution providing 0.5 g of protein/kg/day and progressing in small g/kg increments as tolerated.[16]

The long-term goals of nutritional therapy are to reduce ammonia levels to normal, to provide sufficient nitrogen for optimal growth, and to provide adequate calories to prevent catabolism. Protein intake goals depend on disorder severity as well as age and growth. The goal for dietary protein intake is to achieve as close to the RDA as possible, without causing hyperammonemia or other toxic abnormalities. Essential amino acids are less ureagenic than nonessential amino acids; therefore, essential amino acid medical foods may constitute 25% to 50% of the dietary protein intake in order to provide sufficient amino acid intake without increasing ammonia levels.[16]

Supplementation of L-arginine is required in all of the urea cycle defects except arginase deficiency; in CPS and OTC deficiency, L-citrulline may be substituted for arginine. Sodium phenylbutyrate or sodium benzoate and sodium phenylacetate are used to provide alternate pathways for waste nitrogen excretion. These drugs should optimally be taken 4 times each day, with dosing linked to meals. Vitamin and mineral supplementation is required either separately or within medical foods; the protein restriction leads to a diet limited in many nutrients, including iron, vitamin B_{12}, and zinc. Special low-protein foods help provide additional calories and variety in the diet. Growth, nutrient intake, plasma amino acids, and ammonia should be monitored routinely; plasma glutamine is generally considered a better marker for chronic management than ammonia. Dietary management may be complicated by poor appetite and feeding difficulties. Long-term outcomes and intellectual development in urea cycle disorders are variable depending on the severity of the disorder and the number of acute metabolic episodes.

Liver transplantation is a treatment option that can improve outcomes for some patients, especially those with severe phenotypes who are prone to frequent episodes of hyperammonemia. Liver transplantation corrects the metabolic defect, and thus no further protein restriction is needed after transplantation.

Women with urea cycle disorders require monitoring during pregnancy and in the postpartum period, when catabolic stress increases decompensation risk. Dietary modifications, as well as ammonia scavenging medications, may be necessary during pregnancy. The postpartum period is an especially vulnerable time due to the high rate of catabolism, so additional caloric support and protein restriction are necessary for at least 6 weeks postpartum.[17]

DISORDERS OF CARBOHYDRATE METABOLISM

Galactosemia

Classical galactosemia is an inherited disorder of galactose metabolism. The most common defect is in the galactose-1-phosphate uridyltransferase (GALT) enzyme. If untreated, symptoms of vomiting, diarrhea, failure to thrive, jaundice, hepatomegaly, cataracts, and *Escherichia coli* sepsis are seen within the first 2 weeks of life. Galactosemia is treated by restricting dietary galactose. Because lactose is hydrolyzed into galactose and glucose, the primary emphasis of diet modification is lactose elimination. Therefore, breastfeeding is completely contraindicated. Dietary lactose restriction should be followed for life.[18]

Infants with classical galactosemia are fed lactose-free formulas, which are often soy-based. Older children must avoid milk products as well as incidental sources of lactose found in prepared foods and medications. Individuals must avoid ingredients such as whey, casein, nonfat dry milk, milk solids, lactose, lactoglobulin, lactalbumin, caseinate, and hydrolyzed protein. Food ingredients that are unacceptable on this diet are listed in Table 29.3. Certain fruits, vegetables, and legumes may also contain

TABLE 29.3 INGREDIENTS TO AVOID ON A GALACTOSE-RESTRICTED DIET

Butter	Lactoglobulin
Buttermilk	Lactose
Buttermilk solids	[a]Margarine
Casein	Milk
Cheese	Milk chocolate
Cream	Milk solids
Curds	Nonfat dry milk
Dry milk	Nonfat dry milk solids
Dry milk protein	Nonfat milk
Garbanzo beans	[b]Organ meats (liver, heart, kidney, brain)
Ghee	[c]Sherbet
[d]Hydrolyzed protein	Sour cream
Ice cream	Whey and whey solids
Lactalbumin	Yogurt

[a]margarines do not contain any milk products and are acceptable. Check labels before using any brand.
[b]Organ meats are often listed on labels as meat by-products.
[c]Sherbet contains nonfat dry milk. However, many brands of sorbet do not and are acceptable.
[d]Hydrolyzed protein is unacceptable if it is made from casein or whey.
Reproduced with permission from: Gleason L, Raspberry M, van Calcar S. *Understanding Galactosemia: A Diet Guide*. Abbott Nutrition; 2010.

substantial amounts of galactose; however, the contribution of galactose from these foods is considered minimal compared to endogenous galactose production and other dietary sources. While these foods were historically restricted in galactosemia, they are now considered safe. Most cheeses are not considered safe; however, certain aged cheeses are low enough in lactose to be considered safe and must be selected with caution.[18]

Early treatment with a galactose-restricted diet prevents neonatal sepsis, corrects liver disease, and causes regression of cataracts. Even with optimal dietary treatment, many have speech and visual-perception problems. Growth may be stunted, and primary ovarian failure is seen in most females. Endogenous galactose production may account for these difficulties, but the etiology remains unknown. Growth, nutrient intake, bone density, plasma galactose-1-phosphate, and urine galactitol are monitored. Calcium and vitamin D supplements are usually required.[18]

Hereditary Fructose Intolerance

Hereditary fructose intolerance (HFI) is an autosomal recessive disorder secondary to deficient enzymatic activity of aldolase B. If untreated, HFI causes hypoglycemia, liver dysfunction, renal tubular acidosis, gastrointestinal distress, disseminated intravascular coagulation (DIC) and can progress to potentially fatal seizures and coma. Dietary management involves avoidance of fructose, which is found in fruit, sucrose (table sugar), sorbitol, and high fructose corn syrup. Breastmilk contains no fructose. Some infant formulas do contain fructose in the form of sucrose and must be avoided. As many fructose-containing foods are key sources of vitamin C, supplementation may be required in older children.[19]

FATTY ACID OXIDATION DISORDERS

Fatty acid oxidation disorders (FAODs) are inborn errors in β-oxidation of fatty acids. Defects in the breakdown of fatty acids of specific carbon chain lengths lead to impaired production of ketones as an energy source for the brain and other organs. FAODs are identified by elevated fatty acid acylcarnitine profiles by newborn screening. More severe forms may present clinically in the neonatal period or following a period of fasting, febrile illness, or increased muscle activity. Features include hypoketotic hypoglycemia, liver dysfunction, episodic vomiting, rhabdomyolysis, muscle weakness, cardiomyopathy, and risk of sudden death. Age of presentation varies, but severe forms of the disorders often present during early infancy.[20]

Defects in fatty acid oxidation and their specific treatment strategies are included in Table 29.1. The treatment goal for all FAODs is to avoid dependence on long-chain fat as an energy source. Metabolic decompensation can be triggered by illness and/or prolonged fasting because of the inability to properly metabolize lipid stores. During acute illness, treatment with intravenous dextrose is often necessary to correct hypoglycemia and rhabdomyolysis.[20]

Medium-chain acyl-CoA dehydrogenase deficiency (MCADD) is the most common FAOD and has been identified as the leading known cause of sudden infant death syndrome (SIDS) due to catastrophic hypoketotic hypoglycemia. Long-term management involves avoiding extended periods of fasting and providing increased intake of carbohydrate calories during periods of increased energy demand (illness or exercise).

Meals and snacks that include carbohydrates should be included in regular intervals during the day, and a mixed nutrient snack may be required prior to the longer fasting interval before bedtime.[20] Dietary fat intake should be based on standard-for-age recommendations. Dietary fat restriction is not required; however, very high-fat diets and extended periods of fasting must both be avoided as the body cannot adequately produce ketones.

Long-chain FAODs (LC-FAODs) are disorders of the metabolism of long-chain fatty acids. They include very long-chain acyl-CoA dehydrogenase deficiency (VLCADD), long-chain 3-hydroxyl CoA dehydrogenase deficiency (LCHADD), trifunctional protein deficiency (TFPD), carnitine acyl-CoA translocase (CACT), carnitine palmitoyltransferase type Ia and type II (CPT-Ia and CPT II). Hypoketotic hypoglycemia, rhabdomyolysis, and cardiomyopathy are key concerns of management in LC-FAODs.[20,21]

Dietary management typically requires restriction of long-chain fatty acids with the addition of medium-chain triglyceride (MCT) supplementation to make up remaining total fat requirements since MCT is able to be utilized despite the metabolic defect. MCT requirement is calculated on the basis of percentage of calories from fat needed with the goal of total long-chain fat tolerance + MCT supplement providing 100% of estimated dietary fat needs. Overrestriction of long-chain fat is detrimental and can lead to poor growth and essential fatty acid deficiency. To prevent essential fatty acid deficiency, linoleic acid and α-linolenic acid should provide 3% and 1% of total energy, respectively.[21] Oils available to supplement essential fatty acid intake are listed in Table 29.4.

Most MCT supplementation is provided as C8 or C10. Triheptanoin (C7) is an alternative MCT. Because of its odd number of fatty acids, C7 metabolism promotes anaplerosis, unlike traditional MCT oil. Further study is required to determine what degree of clinical outcome improvements exist with the use of C7 in LC-FAODs.[22]

GMDI/SERN Nutrition Management Guidelines have been developed for the dietary management of VLCADD.[21] Broadly, these guidelines focus on the length of fasting intervals, calorie and protein goals, restriction of long-chain fatty acids, as well as composition of MCT and essential fatty acid supplementation. These guidelines

TABLE 29.4 ESSENTIAL FATTY ACID CONTENT OF SELECTED OILS

OIL[a]	LINOLEIC ACID G/100G[b]	LINOLENIC ACID G/100G[c]
Canola	20.3	9.3
Cod liver	0.9	0.9
Corn	58.0	0.7
Flaxseed	14.0	35.1
Safflower	14.4	0
Soybean	40.2	5.1
Sunflower	3.6	0.2
Walnut	52.9	10.4

[a]One teaspoonful of oil contains 4.5 g fat, 0 g carbohydrate, 0 g protein, and 40 kcal.
[b]Linoleic acid = C18:2; (*n*–6) Recommended intake for infants >3% of energy.
[c]Linolenic acid= C18:3; (*n*–3) Recommended intake for infants 0.3% to 1% of energy.

are further stratified based on disease severity phenotype (mild, moderate, severe), history of symptomatology, age, gender, acute illness and pregnancy/lactation status.

GLYCOGEN STORAGE DISEASES

Glycogen storage diseases (GSDs) are a group of inherited disorders caused by enzyme deficiencies of glycogen metabolism, leading to abnormal accumulation or structure of glycogen in tissues. Depending on the enzyme defect, GSDs may predominantly present in the liver, in the muscles, or both. In hepatic GSDs, hypoglycemia is the primary symptom. In muscle GSDs, weakness, muscle cramps, and reduced exercise tolerance are present. Other systems that can be affected include heart, kidney, and blood cells.

The most common GSD is type I, which is subdivided into types Ia and Ib. GSD type Ia (80% of GSD I) occurs due to a glucose-6-phosphatase enzyme deficiency, whereas GSD type Ib occurs due to a defect of the glucose-6 phosphate transporter. Both enzyme defects lead to an inability to release glucose from glycogen stores and result in hypoglycemia and an inability to utilize fructose and galactose. Symptoms of GSD I include hepatomegaly, hypoglycemia, growth retardation, and an abnormal biochemical profile, including elevated blood lipids, lactate, and uric acid.[23] GSD type Ib may additionally present with neutropenia and inflammatory bowel disease characteristics. More recently, medical management for GSD Ib sometimes includes SGLT-2 inhibitors, such as empagliflozin, which may have an impact on dietary therapy and nutritional outcomes.[24]

Because the body cannot utilize carbohydrates from glycogen, the main component of nutritional management for GSD I includes limiting fasting intervals in order to provide consistently available dietary carbohydrates with the goal of achieving euglycemia. Symptomatic diagnosis can occur in infancy or early toddlerhood, and symptoms commonly present initially when the infant begins to extend their sleeping interval through the night, undergoing longer intervals between feeds.

Infants diagnosed with GSD I are treated with a lactose- and fructose-free infant formula, with feeds every 2 to 3 hours. During overnight periods when fasting intervals tend to be longer, continuous nocturnal feeds via gastrostomy tube are used at least until individuals develop the enzymes necessary to digest uncooked cornstarch (UCCS). To allow longer periods of fasting as the child grows older, UCCS therapy may be used because it is slowly digested and absorbed into the circulation, allowing euglycemia. The UCCS should be initiated only after 6 months of age, at the earliest, and titrated up slowly in older infants and toddlers; amylase concentrations mature over this time period and allow for UCCS digestion.[23]

Recommendations for using UCCS are as follows:

- Mixed with formula or water in a 1:2 starch/liquid ratio (sugar-free juice can be used for older children and adults).
- Measure UCCS on a gram scale to ensure proper amounts. Excess UCCS contributes to excess weight gain and insulin response.
- Use starting UCCS dose of 0.25 g/kg body weight; then slowly increase to ensure euglycemia. Initially, low dosing and slow progression of UCCS allows for monitoring of side-effects such as bowel distension, flatulence, and loose stools.

In addition to standard UCCS, there is a modified extended-release cornstarch product available (Glycosade, Vitaflo NA, Nestle) approved for use for ages 5 years and older in the United States and from 2 years of age in Canada. This extended-release cornstarch product extends fasting tolerance and may allow some individuals to sleep through the night without waking for cornstarch therapy and without continuous enteral feeds. Extended-release cornstarch must be dosed using the same method as UCCS; however, the total dose per administration will be larger given the increase in total number of hours the extended-release cornstarch is intended to release glucose into the bloodstream.

The formula to calculate the basal glucose production rate can be used as an estimate for minimum glucose needs for UCCS or extended-release cornstarch therapy:

$$Y = 0.0014\,(wt^3) - 0.214\,(wt^2) + 10.411\,(wt) - 9.084$$

(Y = mg Glucose per minute, wt = Body weight in kilograms)[53]

Adjustments to cornstarch dosing must take into account individual response to current therapy and should be titrated slowly. Both overtreatment and undertreatment can be harmful. Dosing adjustments must be made in response to regular blood glucose monitoring, which can be achieved through fingerstick blood glucose meters with levels prior to every cornstarch dose and through continuous glucose monitoring (CGM) systems. CGM offers a way for individuals with GSD and clinicians to monitor trends but has limited accuracy within the tight and often lower end blood glucose range that is experienced in GSDs. Therefore, CGM systems should be used alongside traditional meters.

Diet therapy for GSD type I involves following a low fructose and galactose diet as the enzyme defect prevents the body from converting these sugars to glucose and results in unusable glycogen stores and lactic acid. Calcium fortified milk alternatives can be used in place of dairy milk, and fruit intake is limited to approximately 1/2 a serving per day. Carbohydrates should comprise approximately 60% to 70% of the daily calories, with at least 50% of those from cornstarch. Protein, essential fatty acids, and micronutrients should be monitored. Sugar-free multivitamin with mineral supplements and/or essential fatty acid supplementation may be warranted. Overweight and obesity are common due to the high reliance on frequent feeding intervals and intolerance to fasting.

In GSD types 0, III, VI, and IX, a higher protein diet typically alongside UCCS therapy is recommended. Approximately 45% carbohydrate, 25% protein (~2-4 g/kg), and 30% fat is often recommended in the clinical setting. The extra protein provides a substrate for gluconeogenesis and muscle repair.[25,26] For patients with difficulty consuming high quantities of protein through food, protein powders or supplements should be used. There is typically decreased reliance on UCCS to maintain euglycemia compared to GSD type I; however, hypoglycemia is still often present with standard fasting intervals in individuals with these GSD types, and UCCS is often needed before an overnight fasting interval. UCCS dosing and adjustment guidelines, along with blood glucose testing recommendations, are similar to GSD I.

Additional treatment guidelines are available for types III, VI, and IX.[25,26] Various types of GSDs with guidelines are presented in Table 29.1.

REFERENCES

1. Acosta PB, Yannicelli S. *The Ross Metabolic Formula System Nutrition Support Protocols*. 4th ed. Ross Products Division, Abbott Laboratories; 2001.
2. Singh R, Rohr F, Frazier D, et al. Management guidelines portal. GMDI/SERN Nutrition Management Guidelines. Accessed December 11, 2024. https://managementguidelines.net/
3. Smith WE, Berry SA, Bloom K, et al. Phenylalanine hydroxylase deficiency diagnosis and management: a 2023 evidence-based clinical guideline of the American College of Medical Genetics and Genomics (ACMG). *Genet Med*. 2025;27(1):101289.
4. Schuett VE. *Low Protein Food List for PKU*. 3rd ed. Hemlock Printers; 2010.
5. How Much PHE. Accessed December 11, 2024. howmuchphe.org
6. van Spronsen FJ, van Wegberg AM, Ahring K, et al. Key European guidelines for the diagnosis and management of patients with phenylketonuria. *Lancet Diabetes Endocrinol*. 2017;5(9):743-756.
7. Van Spronsen FJ, de Groot MJ, Hoeksma M, Reijngoud DJ, van Rijn M. Large neutral amino acids in the treatment of PKU: from theory to practice. *J Inherit Metab Dis*. 2010;33:671-676.
8. Thomas J, Levy H, Amato S, et al. Pegvaliase for the treatment of phenylketonuria: results of a long-term phase 3 clinical trial program (PRISM). *Mol Genet Metab*. 2018;124(1):27-38.
9. Cunningham A, Rohr F, Splett P, et al. Nutrition management of PKU with pegvaliase therapy: update of the web-based PKU nutrition management guideline recommendations. *Orphanet J Rare Dis*. 2023;18(1):155.
10. Frazier DM, Allgeier C, Homer C, et al. Nutrition management guideline for maple syrup urine disease: an evidence- and consensus-based approach. *Mol Genet Metab*. 2014;112(3):210-217.
11. Forny P, Hörster F, Ballhausen D, et al. Guidelines for the diagnosis and management of methylmalonic acidaemia and propionic acidaemia: first revision [published correction appears in *J Inherit Metab Dis*. 2022;45(4):862]. *J Inherit Metab Dis*. 2021;44(3):566-592.
12. Jurecki E, Ueda K, Frazier D, et al. Nutrition management guideline for propionic acidemia: an evidence- and consensus-based approach. *Mol Genet Metab*. 2019;126(4):341-354.
13. Myles JG, Manoli I, Venditti CP. Effects of medical food leucine content in the management of methylmalonic and propionic acidemias. *Curr Opin Clin Nutr Metab Care*. 2018;21(1):42-48.
14. Boy N, Mühlhausen C, Maier EM, et al. Recommendations for diagnosing and managing individuals with glutaric aciduria type 1: third revision. *J Inherit Metab Dis*. 2023;46(3):482-519.
15. Strauss KA, Williams KB, Carson VJ, et al. Glutaric acidemia type 1: treatment and outcome of 168 patients over three decades. *Mol Genet Metab*. 2020;131(3):325-340.
16. Singh RH. Nutritional management of patients with urea cycle disorders. *J Inherit Metab Dis*. 2007;30(6):880-887.
17. Stepien KM, Langendonk JG, Dao M, et al. The management and clinical outcomes of pregnancies in women with urea cycle disorders: a review of the literature and results of an international survey. *J Inherit Metab Dis*. 2024;47(6):1239-1259.
18. Bernstein LE, van Calcar S. Nutrition management of galactosemia. In: Bernstein LE, Rohr F, van Calcar S, eds. *Nutrition Management of Inherited Metabolic Diseases: Lessons from Metabolic University*. 2nd ed. Springer International Publishing; 2022:339-347.
19. Úbeda F, Santander S, Luesma MJ. Clinical practice guidelines for the diagnosis and management of hereditary fructose intolerance. *Diseases*. 2024;12(3):44.
20. Rohr F. Nutrition management of fatty acid oxidation disorders. In: Bernstein LE, Rohr F, van Calcar S, eds. *Nutrition Management of Inherited Metabolic Diseases: Lessons from Metabolic University*. 2nd ed. Springer International Publishing; 2022:325-335.
21. Van Calcar SC, Sowa M, Rohr F, et al. Nutrition management guideline for very-long chain acyl-CoA dehydrogenase deficiency (VLCAD): an evidence- and consensus-based approach. *Mol Genet Metab*. 2020;131(1-2):23-37.
22. Vockley J, Burton B, Berry G, et al. Effects of triheptanoin (UX007) in patients with long-chain fatty acid oxidation disorders: results from an open-label, long-term extension study. *J Inherit Metab Dis*. 2021;44(1):253-263.
23. Kishnani PS, Austin SL, Abdenur JE, et al. Diagnosis and management of glycogen storage disease type I: a practice guideline of the American College of Medical Genetics and Genomics. *Genet Med*. 2014;16(11):e1.
24. Veiga-da-Cunha M, Wortmann SB, Grünert SC, Van Schaftingen E. Treatment of the neutropenia associated with GSD1b and G6PC3 deficiency with SGLT2 inhibitors. *Diagnostics (Basel)*. 2023;13(10):1803.

25. Kishnani PS, Austin SL, Arn P, et al. Glycogen storage disease type III diagnosis and management guidelines [published correction appears in *Genet Med.* 2010;12(9):566]. *Genet Med.* 2010;12(7):446-463.
26. Kishnani PS, Goldstein J, Austin SL, et al. Diagnosis and management of glycogen storage diseases type VI and IX: a clinical practice resource of the American College of Medical Genetics and Genomics (ACMG). *Genet Med.* 2019;21(4):772-789.

SELECTED RESOURCES

■ PRODUCTS FOR NUTRITIONAL THERAPY

- Abbott Nutrition (abbottnutrition.com)
- BioMarin Pharmaceutical Inc. (hcp.biomarin.com/en-us/palynziq/; kuvan.com/hcp/)
- Cambrooke Foods (cambrookefoods.com)
- Lil's Dietary Shop (lilsdietary.com)
- Mead Johnson Nutrition (meadjohnson.com)
- Nutricia North America (nutricia-na.com)
- PKU Perspectives (pkuperspectives.com)
- PKU GoLike (https://www.pkugolike.com/)
- Solace Nutrition (solacenutrition.com)
- Ultragenyx (dojolvi.com/)
- Vitaflo North America (vitaflousa.com)

■ OTHER RESOURCES

- Fatty Oxidation Disorders Family Support Group (fodsupport.org)
- Flok (flok.org)
- Genetic Metabolic Dietitians International (gmdi.org)
- MSUD Family Support Group (msud-support.org)
- National PKU Alliance (npkua.org)
- National Organization for Rare Diseases (rarediseases.org)
- National Urea Cycle Disorders Foundation (nucdf.org)
- New England Consortium of Metabolic Programs (newenglandconsortium.org)
- Organic Acidemia Association (oaanews.org)
- Parents of Galactosemia Children (galactosemia.org)
- United Mitochondrial Disease Foundation (umdf.org)

CHAPTER 30

Intestinal Failure

Kathleen M. Gura, E. Reese, Brittany Depaula, Margaret Murphy, and Christopher P. Duggan

Intestinal failure (IF) in children has been defined as a condition characterized by the "reduction of functional intestinal mass below [that] which can sustain life, resulting in dependence on supplemental parenteral support for a minimum of 60 days within an interval of 74 consecutive days."[1] Three main types of IF include short bowel syndrome (due to acquired or congenital disorders of the gastrointestinal tract), intestinal motility disorders (where intestinal length is preserved but function is limited), and intestinal epithelial defects (such as microvillus inclusion disorder, tufting enteropathy, and others). These latter two classes of IF are substantially less common than IF due to surgical treatment of congenital or acquired anomalies, and much of the literature is based on clinical experience with so-called surgical short bowel syndrome (SBS). This chapter will therefore generally refer to care of patients with this type of IF.

IF can lead to malabsorption of macronutrients and micronutrients, electrolyte abnormalities, dehydration, and, ultimately, malnutrition. Table 30.1 lists common etiologies of SBS in children. The frequency of SBS increases in an inverse relationship with birth weight; the incidence of SBS in infants weighing 401 to 1000 g was 1.1% (61/5657), nearly twice that in infants with a birth weight of 1001 to 1500 g (28/6659; 0.4%).[2] The prognosis of IF depends on several factors, including (1) the length and portion of small and/or large bowel affected by a disease process and/or surgically resected, (2) the presence or absence of the ileocecal valve (ICV), (3) the adaptive and functional capacity of the remaining bowel, and (4) the health of other organs that assist with digestion and absorption. Enteral autonomy is considered the maintenance

TABLE 30.1 COMMON CAUSES OF SHORT BOWEL SYNDROME IN INFANTS AND CHILDREN

- Necrotizing enterocolitis (NEC)
- Intestinal atresia
- Gastroschisis
- Midgut volvulus
- Crohn disease
- Tumors
- Radiation enteritis
- Ischemic injury
- Total intestinal aganglionosis

of normal growth, nutrition and hydration status by means of enteral support without the use of parenteral support for a period of greater than 3 consecutive months.[1]

LENGTH AND PORTION OF SMALL BOWEL RESECTED

Normal small intestine length has been estimated at 70 cm in infants at 24 to 26 weeks' gestational age and ~143 cm in infants at 36 to 38 weeks with broad ranges around these estimates. At term, mean length is reported to be 157 to 240 cm and continues to increase with age, weight, and linear growth. The large intestine is ~33 cm at full-term birth, growing to 122 cm by 5 years of age (Figure 30.1).[3]

Loss of intestinal length can limit digestion by reducing exposure of nutrients to brush border hydrolytic enzymes, as well as pancreatic and biliary secretions. Many studies have examined the relationship between length of residual small intestine and successful weaning from parenteral nutrition (PN). It appears that infants require approximately 10 to 30 cm of small intestine, with intact ICV, to avoid lifelong dependence on PN. If the ICV is not present, 30 to 50 cm of small intestine is generally needed for successful weaning of PN.[4] These anatomic estimates, however, are mere "rules of thumb" and individual results can and do vary substantially. Because of new management strategies combined with a multidisciplinary team approach, the majority of patients will wean from PN despite short intestinal length.[5]

In one retrospective from a single-center academic institution, the cumulative probability of weaning from PN with at least 50 cm of small intestine was 96% after 24 months and for those with less than 50 cm, 71% after 57 months.[5] Residual small intestinal length was found to be the primary predictor of the ability to achieve enteral autonomy.

PORTION OF SMALL BOWEL RESECTED

The location of resected bowel has an impact on nutrient loss in IF. Duodenal resection may result in iron or folate malabsorption. Calcium absorption may be impaired with proximal small bowel resection. The jejunum has long, large villi, extensive absorptive surface area, highly concentrated digestive enzymes, and many transport carrier proteins and is the primary digestive and absorptive site for most nutrients. Loss of jejunum is also associated with reduction of cholecystokinin and secretin levels, which secondarily impairs pancreatic and biliary secretion, causing subsequent malabsorption of fat- and fat-soluble vitamins. Loss of the terminal ileum results in malabsorption of bile acids. Steatorrhea, fat-soluble vitamin malabsorption, and the formation of lithogenic bile may ensue. The terminal ileum is also the primary site for vitamin B_{12} absorption, so resection there can lead to B_{12} deficiency. The ileum secretes hormonal substances that slow gastrointestinal motility in response to fat malabsorption. The antimotility effect of fat in the ileum is known as the ileal brake and is important in ensuring adequate fat absorption from the small intestine.[6] The ileum and proximal colon also secrete glucagon-like peptide-2, a hormone that helps maintain and augment intestinal villus and crypt structure.

Intestinal transit time is faster following small bowel resection. Changes in transit time will vary depending on the area of intestine removed. Normally, motility in the distal ileum is considerably slower than in the jejunum. Consequently, ileal resection reduces intestinal transit time more than proximal bowel resection. Gastric emptying

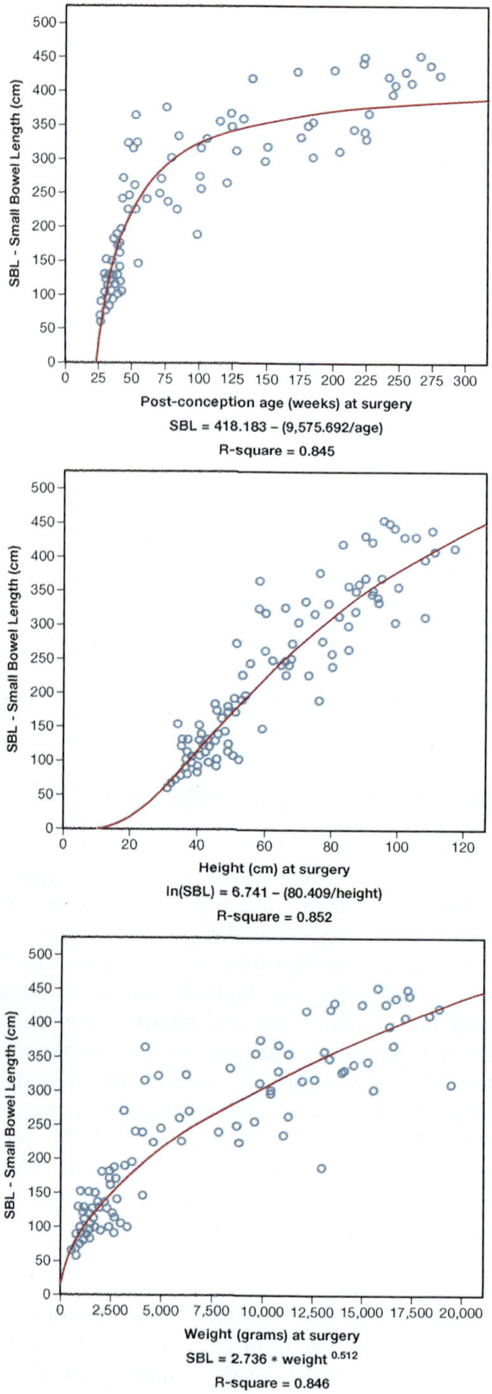

Figure 30.1 Small bowel length varies with age, weight, and height in children. (From Struijs MC, Diamond I, de Silva N, Wales P. Establishing norms for intestinal length in children. *J Ped Surg*. 2009; 44:933-938.)

tends to be more rapid following ileal resection but can be normalized if the colon is retained. In patients with ileal or colonic resection, cells that release peptide YY are missing, resulting in a loss of inhibition on gastric emptying and faster intestinal transit time. Following jejunal resection, gastric emptying is more rapid; however, intestinal transit time may remain normal due to the ileal brake.[6] In patients with residual bowel in continuity, gastric emptying is slower and similar to normal controls. Colon resection is associated with delays in bowel adaptation and loss of energy from malabsorption of short-chain fatty acids.[4] The colon has an important role in the control of fluids and electrolyte losses, and thus resection of the colon will speed transit time further.

■ PRESENCE OR ABSENCE OF THE ILEOCECAL VALVE

The ileocecal valve (ICV) serves to regulate the flow of enteric contents from the small bowel into the colon. The absence of an ICV reduces gastrointestinal transit time and increases fluid and nutrient losses. In a cohort of children with IF followed during their wean from PN, resection of the ICV was a significant risk factor for having at least one vitamin deficiency.[7] In the absence of the ICV, colonic bacteria may "overgrow" into the small intestine (termed "small intestine bacterial overgrowth [SIBO]"). SIBO may cause deconjugation of bile acids and an inflammatory response that damages small bowel mucosa. This leads to exacerbation of the malabsorptive state,[6] particularly dietary fat, fat-soluble vitamins, and B_{12}. A rotating schedule of oral antibiotics is commonly used to treat SIBO (Table 30.2). Due to product design limitations, oral administration of injectable products may be necessary.

One important, but relatively rare, consequence of SIBO is D-lactic acidosis. The inability of humans to metabolize the D- (as opposed to the L-) dimer of lactic acid synthesized by intestinal bacteria leads to a variety of associated symptoms, including headache, drowsiness, stupor, confusion, behavioral disturbance, ataxia, blurred vision, ophthalmoplegia, or nystagmus.[8] D-Lactic acidosis should be suspected when there is an acidosis with an unexplained anion gap accompanied with by behavioral changes in the child.

■ ADAPTIVE AND FUNCTIONAL CAPACITY OF THE REMAINING SMALL INTESTINE

Following extensive resection, the remaining intestine has an ability to compensate, but this depends on the area of resection and other trophic stimuli. The ileum appears to be more able to adapt and compensate for loss of proximal small intestine. Intestinal adaptation refers to the gross anatomic and histologic changes that occur after significant intestinal resection. These adaptive changes begin 12 to 24 hours after massive intestinal resection and likely continue for years after resection.[6] These changes include lengthening of the villi, an increase in intestinal absorptive surface area, and gradual improvements in absorptive function.

Enteral nutrition is an important stimulant of mucosal adaptation. This is thought to be a result of direct contact of nutrients with epithelial cells; stimulation of gastric, pancreatic, and biliary secretions; as well as stimulation of trophic hormone production. Much research has been directed at examining whether specific nutrients promote adaptation more than others, but to date no rigorously designed study has defined these for children.

TABLE 30.2 COMPARISON OF AGENTS USED FOR TREATMENT OF BACTERIAL OVERGROWTH (TYPICAL COURSE 7-10 DAYS)

MEDICATION	PEDIATRIC DOSE	ADULT DOSE	COMMENTS	% ORALLY ABSORBED	% RENALLY EXCRETED
Amphotericin	<5 y: 100 mg bid 5-12 y: 250 mg bid	500 mg bid	Injection given orally	9	40% (2%-5% active)
Augmentin	10 mg/kg/dose bid	500 mg bid		Complete (amoxicillin)	30%-40%
Bactrim (TMP/SMX)	2 mg TMP/kg/dose d	1 Single Strength (SS) tablet daily Each tablet: Sulfamethoxazole 400 mg/trimethoprim 80 mg		Almost completely, 90%-100%	Sulfamethoxazole, 10%-30%; Trimethoprim, 50%-75%
Ciprofloxacin	20-40 mg/kg/d bid	500 mg bid		50%-80%	30%-50%
Clindamycin	10-30 mg/kg/d Divided tid/qid	300 mg tid		90%	10%
Colistin	<5 y: 25 mg 2-4 times per day 5-12 y: 50 mg 2-4 times per day	100 mg 2-4 times per day	Injection given orally	insignificant	75% in 24 h
Doxycycline	Children >8 y 100 mg bid	100 mg bid		100%	23%
Gentamicin	2 mg/kg/dose bid Others: 2.5 mg/kg/dose tid not to exceed 300 mg/d	2-2.5 mg/kg/dose tid Not to exceed 300 mg	Injection given orally	None	100%

Metronidazole	10 mg/kg/dose bid Others: 5 mg-10 mg/kg/dose bid-tid	250 mg-500 mg tid-qid		90%	10%
Neomycin	50 mg/kg/d divided every 6 h	500 mg bid 500 mg-2 g every 6-8 h	Available as tablets only	3%	0.9%-1.5%
Tetracycline	Children >8 y: 25-50 mg/kg/d in divided doses every 6 h	500 mg tid		75%	60%
Tobramycin	<5 y: 10 mg 2-4 times per day 5-12 years: 40 mg 2-4 times per day	80 mg 2-4 times per day	Injection given orally	Poor	90%-95%
Rifaximin	Not established, 20-30 mg/kg/d has been used	400 mg tid		<0.4%	<1%
Vancomycin	125 mg every 6 h (10 mg/kg/dose qid) Max total daily dose 2 g/d	125 mg-500 mg every 6 h Max total daily dose 2 g/d		Poor	Oral doses primarily via feces

TMP-SMX, Trimethoprim-Sulfamethoxazole.
All meds given enterally.
Online Formulary, Boston Children's Hospital, 2025.

HEALTH OF OTHER ORGANS THAT ASSIST WITH ABSORPTION AND DIGESTION

Hepatic complications can occur in patients with IF. Intestinal failure–associated liver disease (IFALD) is a clinical spectrum ranging from mild steatosis, cholestasis, and fibrosis progressing to liver failure and cirrhosis, portal hypertension, and coagulopathies. The relationship between PN use and cholestasis is likely multifactorial and includes the risk factors of sepsis, prematurity, mucosal atrophy, and bacterial overgrowth.[9] It can be stabilized or reversed with appropriate early modification of management strategies and promotion of intestinal adaptation; otherwise, it may progress to hepatic dysfunction and end-stage liver disease. Strategies used to prevent or reverse IFALD include prevention of sepsis, cycling the PN infusion, and the use of alternative lipid injectable emulsions (ILE). Data suggest the provision of soy-based intravenous fat emulsions is associated with the development of IFALD due to the presence of hepatoxic phytosterols and high omega-6 content. Decreasing the dose of pure soybean oil or using ILE products rich in omega-3 fatty acids in the form of fish oil may reduce cholestasis.[9] Furthermore, the establishment of interdisciplinary intestinal rehabilitation programs (IRP) has improved the care of IF patients considerably through the use of nutritional, pharmacologic, and surgical modalities.[10] Every effort should therefore be made to reduce the risk of IF–associated liver disease (Table 30.3).

SPECIAL ASPECTS OF NUTRITIONAL THERAPY IN INTESTINAL FAILURE

The goals of nutrition therapy in IF are to maintain normal growth, promote intestinal adaptation, and avoid complications associated with intestinal resection and PN.

TABLE 30.3 STEPS TO REDUCE THE RISK OF INTESTINAL FAILURE–ASSOCIATED LIVER DISEASE

METHOD	COMMENTS
Avoid overfeeding	Provide adequate kcals for desired growth • Infants: 90-100 kcal/kg from PN • Children: Consider measuring resting energy expenditure and titrating energy intake to achieve normal growth
Limit exposure to soy-based fat emulsions	Reduce risk of hepatocellular damage induced by exposure to phytosterols and inflammatory mediators
Cycle PN off at least 2-6 h/d	Promotes cyclic release of GI hormones Mimic age-appropriate feeding patterns when considering time free from PN
Aggressively treat and prevent infections	Meticulous Central Venous Line (CVC) care Treat bacterial overgrowth
Push enteral nutrition	The ultimate goal of therapy

GI, gastrointestinal; PN, parenteral nutrition.

What to Feed

Fluid, Electrolytes, and Parenteral Nutrition

During the early postoperative phase, fluid and electrolyte balance is the goal of therapy. Large fluid losses are common and tend to be high in sodium content. Parenteral solutions with at least 80 to 100 mEq/L of sodium are often required to maintain sodium balance. Meticulous attention needs to be paid to the fluid and electrolyte status of IF patients. This includes daily weights; careful measurement of urine, stool, and ostomy losses; and frequent laboratory monitoring of electrolytes. PN is indicated in the management of IF until small bowel growth and adaptation permit growth on enteral nutrition alone.

Because day-to-day variations in fluid loss are common, it is often advantageous to place the patient on a stable PN solution with fluid and electrolytes appropriate for age, growth requirements, and metabolic considerations while subsequently replacing abnormal losses with a separate solution comparable in fluid and electrolyte content. Ostomy sodium concentration can be quantified and replacement fluids prescribed based on the assessment of the output. When losses have stabilized and/or use of additional hydration becomes habitual in nature, the fluid and electrolyte content of the patient's PN should be altered to compensate for chronically elevated gastrointestinal losses.

Enteral Nutrition

Once the patient's fluid and electrolyte status has stabilized and postoperative ileus has resolved, a slow introduction of enteral feedings should be started. Mothers of newborns with IF should be referred to a lactation consultant to encourage continued human milk (HM) production. Human milk has special immunologic and anti-infective properties that are especially advantageous to the infant having undergone intestinal resection, although the transition from parenteral to full enteral feedings may take weeks to months to years. Human milk from mothers of premature infants with IF may require fortification to meet the child's unique nutritional needs (see Chapter 35). Human milk also contains growth factors, nucleotides, glutamine, and other amino acids that may play an important role in assisting intestinal adaptation. If parental HM is unavailable, consider use of pasteurized donor milk.[11]

If neither parental nor donor HM is available, the selection of enteral formula remains somewhat controversial. The choice of formula should consider age, functional anatomy of the remaining small bowel, and the capacity for digestion and absorption. Premature infants have special needs that must also be considered (see Chapter 35). Studies suggest that complex nutrients that require more work for digestion and absorption tend to stimulate intestinal adaptation more effectively.[12] However, limited mucosal surface area can lead to lactose, protein, and long-chain fatty acid malabsorption with the use of intact formulas. If this malabsorption is severe, fluid, electrolyte, and energy balance can be difficult to achieve. At the initial stage of feeding, it is customary to use an amino acid-based formula that is lactose free, and this may include medium-chain triglycerides (MCTs) to facilitate nutrient absorption.

Protein is generally tolerated well and is least affected by decreased intestinal absorptive surface area. Intact protein contributes little to osmotic load. It appears that there may not be a significant absorptive advantage from the use of hydrolysate or amino acid-based formulas, particularly with older children.[13] However, infants and young children with bowel inflammation may be at risk for secondary intestinal allergic disease and may therefore benefit from the use of protein hydrolysate or amino acid-based formulas.[11]

MCTs are more water soluble than long-chain triglycerides (LCTs) and are better absorbed in the presence of bile acid loss or pancreatic insufficiency. However, MCT fats have a slightly lower caloric density and exert a greater osmotic load in the small intestine. Animal studies suggest that LCTs have a trophic effect by stimulating gut adaptation after intestinal resection. Although fat tends to be poorly absorbed in IF, it is a dense calorie source relative to carbohydrate or protein. Considering the relative adverse effect of carbohydrate on osmotic diarrhea, it is usually advantageous for patients with IF to include at least moderate amounts of fat in their diets. A mixture of both LCT and MCT may be beneficial, especially as MCT is void of essential fatty acids. Although pancreatic insufficiency is seldom present in patients with IF, use of pancreatic enzyme replacement therapy or immobilized lipase cartridges may improve fat absorption in some patients through ex-vivo hydrolysis of fats in formula or food.[14]

Carbohydrates may be poorly tolerated as they are broken down by gastrointestinal bacteria into small, osmotically active organic acids that can exert a significant osmotic load in the distal small intestine and colon. Glucose may be absorbed without hydrolysis, but its small molecular weight increases solution osmolality. Carbohydrate may be given in the form of glucose polymers to reduce the osmotic load. Lactose may be restricted initially after intestinal resection. In general, lactose-containing foods should be restricted only when intolerance is demonstrated or when there is significant resection of proximal small intestine. Fiber supplementation via modulars, food-based or other fiber-containing formulas may be helpful in older children with IF who have an intact colon. Some fermentation of the fiber will occur, producing trophic short-chain fatty acids (SCFAs), which are an important fuel for the colonocyte. Because SCFAs stimulate sodium and water absorption, a decrease in stool output and sodium losses may be expected as well. See Table 30.4 for a comparison of commonly used enteral formulas in the pediatric IF patient. Fiber can also add bulk to stool, and soluble fiber may slow intestinal transit time, resulting in improved stool consistency.[12]

How to Feed

Enteral Considerations

Continuous enteral feedings via a nasogastric or gastrostomy tube is advantageous in the child with IF since they permit constant saturation of carrier transport proteins, thus taking full advantage of the absorptive surface area available. Postpyloric feeding via nasojejunal or gastrojejunostomy tube can be used when indicated. However, these devices bypass some length of the already foreshortened bowel, require more significant intervention to replace, and pose a higher risk of complications than their gastric-terminating equivalents. Routinely reassess for ongoing indication of use throughout the patient's clinical course.

Enteral feedings are slowly advanced by volume while PN calories, volume, and hours are adjusted to maintain nutritional status, control fluid losses, and ensure intestinal adaptation. If a patient demonstrates sensitivity to enteral volume advancement, consider increasing energy density of the formula. However, higher concentration formula presents a higher osmotic load. Therefore, it is recommended to do so in smaller,

TABLE 30.4 COMMON ENTERAL FORMULAS USED IN PEDIATRIC SHORT BOWEL SYNDROME MANAGEMENT

	INFANT			CHILD		
Formula Type	Product	Calories per Ounce[a] (Osmolality mOsm/kg H_2O)	Notable Characteristics	Product	Calories per Ounce[a] (Osmolality mOsm/kg H_2O)	Notable Characteristics
Isomeric	Human milk	20 (300)	First choice for all infants with IF	Pediasure[b]	30 (335)	Also available with fiber
				Boost Kid Essentials[b]	30 (475)	
Protein Hydrolysate	Pregestimil[b]	20 (290-320)	55% of fat as MCT	Compleat Pediatric Peptide 1.0 and 1.5	30-45 (480-720)	40%-50% of fat as MCT
	Alimentum[b]	20 (370)	Ready to feed is corn-free	Kate Farms Pediatric Peptide 1.0 and 1.5	30-45 (280-326)	Plant-based (pea protein hydrolysate) Free of the top 9 allergens
	Pepticate[b]	20 (300)	15% of fat as MCT Contains prebiotic fiber	Pediasure Peptide 1.0 and 1.5[b]	30-45 (390-450)	60% of fat as MCT
				Peptamen Jr 1.0 and 1.5[b]	30-45 (260-450)	1.0 is available with or without fiber
Amino Acid Based	EleCare	20 (330-350)	33% of fat as MCT	EleCare Jr	30 (487)	33% of fat as MCT
				Neocate Junior	30 (600)	
				Alfamino Junior	30 (627)	65% of fat as MCT
	Neocate Infant			Essential Care Jr	30 (750)	Does not contain corn or corn syrup solids High protein (40 g/L)
	PurAmino			Neocate Splash	30 (670-790)	Ready to feed
	Alfamino Infant		43% of fat as MCT	Vivonex Pediatric	24 (413)	25% of kcals from fat, 70% of fat as MCT

(continued)

TABLE 30.4 COMMON ENTERAL FORMULAS USED IN PEDIATRIC SHORT BOWEL SYNDROME MANAGEMENT (*continued*)

	INFANT			CHILD		
Calorically Dense Useful for patients with fluid restriction or high energy demand				Pediasure 1.5[b]	45 (390)	Also available with fiber
				Boost Kid Essentials 1.5[b]	45 (620)	
Probiotic-containing Contraindicated in children with central venous access	Neocate Syneo Infant	20 (360)	33% of fat as MCT Also contains prebiotic fiber	Neocate Syneo Junior	30 (600)	34% of fat as MCT Also contains prebiotic fiber
	Nutramigen with Probiotic LGG[b]	20 (300)				
	Extensive HA[b]	20 (220)	49% of fat as MCT Does not contain corn syrup solids			
Plant-based				Kate Farms Pediatric Standard 1.2	36 (270-320)	40% of fat as MCT Pea protein Free of the top 9 allergens
				Compleat Pediatric Standard 1.0 and 1.4	30-42 (410-650)	Pea protein Free of the top 9 allergens and corn

Food-based	Compleat Pediatric Original 1.0, 1.5 and Reduced Calorie	18-45 (310-840)	
	Compleat Pediatric Organic Blends	36 (710-720)	
	Kate Farms Pediatric Blended Meals	30 (440-560)	Pouches can connect directly to some feeding tube adapters
	Nourish and Nourish Peptides	34-44 (460-553)	

MCT, medium-chain triglyceride.
[a] Based on standard preparation/dilution.
[b] These products should be used only in the patient with known mucosal adaptation and tolerance to milk protein.

incremental steps toward the goal concentration, closely monitoring stool output, symptoms, and biochemical data with each change.

The rate of advancement of enteral feeds should be determined by multiple factors, including stool or ostomy output, perianal skin breakdown, hydration and electrolyte status, and weight gain. We have generally employed the scheme in Table 30.5. In general, it is acceptable for infants to have up to 10 watery stools per day as long as urine output, labs, skin integrity, and growth remain stable. If intolerance occurs soon after an increase in rate or concentration of the formula, a return should be made to the previously tolerated regimen. Once tolerance is established, advancement can be attempted again. Frequent setbacks are not unusual. Enteral feedings may eventually be transitioned to oral/bolus feedings or combination oral/bolus and nocturnal feedings to allow more freedom from the feeding pump.

Excessive fluid and electrolyte losses may continue to complicate advancement of enteral feedings, particularly in patients with high output jejunostomies. Oral rehydration solutions with a sodium concentration of 75 to 90 mEq/L should be used to

TABLE 30.5 SUGGESTED GUIDELINES FOR ENTERAL FEEDING ADVANCEMENT IN THE INFANT WITH INTESTINAL FAILURE

A. **Feeding Initiation:**

1. *Assess bowel function*
   - Audible bowel sounds?
   - Functioning ostomy (if applicable)?
   - NG/GT clamped?

   No → Continue IVF/PN/NPO
   Yes → Evaluate for contraindications to feeding.

2. *Contraindications*
   - Paralytic or drug-induced ileus
   - Grossly bloody stools or ostomy output and/or radiologic changes of intestinal ischemia
   - Shock/poor perfusion due to cardiac or respiratory insufficiency
   - Bilious and/or persistent vomiting (defined as more than three episodes of emesis in 12 h)
   - Clinical suspicion of obstruction or ileus (severe abdominal distension, decreased ostomy or stool output, and/or radiologic changes of obstruction or ileus)

   Yes → Continue IVF/PN/NPO
   No → Start feeds (NG/NJ/G-tube/J-tube)

   - Day 1: Human milk (full strength) or amino acid-based formula (20 kcal/oz) at 10-20 mL/kg/d continuously* × 24 h

B. **In-Patient Feeding Advancement:**

Principle 1: Quantify feeding intolerance primarily by stool or ostomy output and secondarily by hydration, electrolyte status, and perianal skin integrity
Principle 2: Tolerance assessed ≤2× per 24 h; no more than one advancement per 24 h period
Principle 3: Ultimate goals: 150-200 mL/kg/d, 100-140 kcal/kg/d
Principle 4: If ostomy/stool output precludes advancement at 20 kcal/oz for 7 d, then increasing caloric density of the formula can be performed.
Principle 5: Isocaloric reductions in PN support should be undertaken simultaneously with feeding advancement

TABLE 30.5 SUGGESTED GUIDELINES FOR ENTERAL FEEDING ADVANCEMENT IN THE INFANT WITH INTESTINAL FAILURE (*continued*)

1. **Stool output**
   If <10 g/kg/d or <10 stools/d → Advance rate by 10-20 mL/kg/d.
   If 10-20 g/kg/d or 10-12 stools/d → No change
   If >20 g/kg/d or >12 stools/d → Reduce rate or hold feeds.[a]
2. **or Ileostomy output**
   If <2 g/kg/h → Advance rate by 10-20 mL/kg/d.
   If 2-3 g/kg/h → No change
   If >3 g/kg/h → Reduce rate or hold feeds.[a]
3. **Signs of dehydration or electrolyte abnormalities:**
   If absent → Advance feeds per stool or ostomy output.
   If present → Reduce rate or hold feeds.[a]
4. **Perianal skin integrity**
   If absent → Advance feeds per stool or ostomy output.
   If mild/moderate → No change
   If severe → reduce rate or hold feeds.[a]

C. **In-patient transition to oral bolus feeds:**
- Begin when infant is developmentally ready to feed by mouth.
- Offer 1 hour's worth of continuous feed volume 1-3 times per day, pausing the continuous feeds.
- More than 1 hour's worth of continuous feed volume can be offered once the infant has reached full volume continuous feeds *OR* at least 7 d have passed on the feeding advancement protocol.

D. **Outpatient Feeding Advancement:**
Principle 1: Feeding advancement should be paused leading up to discharge.
Principle 2: Feeding advancement can resume at a lower frequency of 1-2× per week if clinically stable at the first outpatient visit.

GT, gastrostomy tube; IVF, intravenous fluid; J-tube, jejunostomy tube; NG, nasogastric tube; NJ, nasojejunal; PN, parenteral nutrition.
[a]Feeds should generally be held for 8 h, then restarted at 3/4 the previous rate.

replace losses (see Chapter 26 for a list of commercially available oral rehydration solutions). Children who have persistently high fluid and electrolyte losses may benefit from a rice-based oral rehydration solution.

Oral Feeding

It is important to initiate oral feedings early in the infant's course to stimulate sucking and swallowing and to minimize the risk of oral aversion, a common morbidity among infants with a history of critical illness in the neonatal period. We commonly employ a regimen of both continuous and oral bolus feeding by pausing the continuous enteral infusion for 1 hour, during which the volume equivalent is offered via bottle.[12] Oral bolus volumes can be gradually advanced as tolerated. If the patient is fed via postpyloric enteral tube or cannot be fed for other anatomic reasons, consider "sham" feedings: nonnutritive oral feedings with the gastrostomy tube to drainage. Older children and adults have a better capacity to regulate gastric emptying and therefore tolerate gastric bolus or oral bolus feedings better than infants.

Solid foods should be introduced at developmentally appropriate stages unless medically contraindicated. Evaluation of readiness for solids should be considered on a regular basis by the dietitian, speech language pathologist (SLP) and medical team. Solids are typically initiated as pureed vegetables, proteins, or grains. New foods should be introduced one at a time to allow for identification of poor tolerance. Volume of solids and frequency of feedings should be incrementally advanced as tolerated. Delayed introduction of allergens is generally not indicated, although cow's milk is often poorly tolerated and introduced later.

Tolerance of more complex textures is an important step in oral feeding development, so infants with IF should progress to lumpy purees, dissolvable solids, and soft table foods when appropriate. The SLP plays an important role in assessing patients for early signs of feeding difficulties and can help provide appropriate intervention to prevent long-term development of pediatric feeding disorder.[15]

Mineral Supplementation in Intestinal Failure

Mineral supplementation requires an individualized plan for each patient. For those with cholestasis who are dependent on PN, the provision of manganese and copper should be carefully considered given their dependence on enterohepatic circulation for excretion and risk of toxicity with cholestasis. Cholestatic patients are at risk of manganese accumulation and potentially damaging effects to the developing basal ganglia. Copper toxicity may also be seen in cholestasis, although copper requirements can increase in the setting of increased gastrointestinal losses. Copper deficiency manifests as a microcytic anemia unresponsive to iron supplementation and may also negatively impact proper bone development. Similarly to copper, zinc deficiency is common in the patient with high-volume gastrointestinal (GI) losses. The need for additional supplementation is common, and serum values should be assessed periodically given the risk of growth failure with zinc deficiency. Selenium status should be carefully assessed in the PN patient given the risk of cardiomyopathies associated with deficiency.[16] Abnormal values should be carefully assessed and applied to the current clinical picture to assess if supplementation or treatment of toxicity is required. If parenteral selenium is not available, enteral supplementation should be considered, when possible.

For IF patients receiving both parenteral and enteral nutrition, close monitoring of electrolyte status is crucial due to the high concentration of electrolytes in gastrointestinal secretions. Many IF patients may require supplementation of sodium, potassium, and magnesium based on routine laboratory assessment and/or clinical findings. Magnesium deficiency frequently occurs in patients with jejunocolic anastomosis or those with jejunostomies due to hyperaldosteronism secondary to sodium depletion and dehydration.[7] Once sodium and fluid status are corrected, ongoing magnesium supplementation is often necessary. Adequate intake of calcium, phosphorus, and magnesium should also be encouraged for adequate bone mineralization. The IF patient remains at risk of decreased bone mineral density and delayed linear growth secondary to metabolic bone disease associated with long-term PN exposure as well as malabsorption of calcium and vitamin D that accompanies fat maldigestion. Bone mineral density should be routinely monitored. Iron deficiency can result from loss of duodenal-jejunal absorptive area and has been shown to impact upward of 50% of PN dependent IF patients and 30% enterally autonomous IF patients.[17]

Vitamin Deficiencies

Children with IF, especially those with hepatic disease, are at risk for developing a variety of fat-soluble vitamin deficiencies related to fat malabsorption and/or inadequate dietary intake. The frequency of vitamin deficiencies in the IF population is rather marked as reflected by studies identifying ≥88% of children on PN and >70% children off PN as having at least one vitamin deficiency.[17] The risk for vitamin deficiencies increased with discontinuation of PN support, loss of the ICV or the absence of multivitamin supplementation.[17] Even patients receiving glucagon-like peptide 2 (GLP-2) analogs that increase villus height and crypt depth in the small intestine, despite improving fluid and nutrient absorption and enteral autonomy from PN, experience significant micronutrient deficiencies unless carefully monitored and supplemented.[18]

Table 30.6 contains dosing recommendations of fat-soluble vitamins in children with malabsorption and/or cholestasis. Low serum vitamin A concentrations are present in children with cholestatic liver disease receiving routine vitamin supplementation.[17] Altered hepatic synthetic function may also decrease retinol binding protein synthesis, suggesting that unbound vitamin A concentrations could be elevated in liver failure. Remarkably, vitamin E levels generally remain normal in this population, although unsupplemented infants and children continue to demonstrate deficiencies.[7,17] Even with supplementation, children with mild to moderate cholestatic liver disease are at risk for developing vitamin K deficiency. Traditional supplemental doses of oral vitamin K may be inadequate for more than half of children with IF.[19] Patients with ileal resection should be monitored carefully for vitamin B_{12} deficiency. Deficiencies should be corrected by either the nasal, sublingual, or intramuscular route.

The method of micronutrient supplementation in IF patients will vary based on the patient's anatomy, degree of malabsorption, and routes of nutrition. Vitamin and mineral preparations are available for patients dependent on PN (see Chapter 17), allowing provision of multiple micronutrients in a single product. The provider should be aware of the concentrations of vitamins and minerals in these products and dose appropriately to meet the patient's needs. While the provision of intravenous micronutrients is a valuable tool for the patient unable to fully absorb vitamins and minerals enterally, recent findings have demonstrated micronutrient deficiencies in patients receiving PN fortified with these preparations, pointing toward the need for routine monitoring of micronutrients, even when provided parenterally.[17]

For the patient who continues to experience maldigestion following PN weaning and/or has a history of ileal resection, the use of a complete water-miscible multivitamin with mineral supplement (e.g., DEKAs Plus) is warranted. Providing fat-soluble vitamins in a water-soluble form, enhances absorption of these key nutrients. These products should be reserved for patients with known risk factors for micronutrient deficiencies and/or malabsorption since they are costly and may not be covered by private insurance. For the patient with minimal malabsorption and an intact terminal ileum, use of an over-the-counter complete pediatric multivitamin with minerals supplement may be sufficient (see Chapter 11). In either case, routine monitoring of micronutrient blood concentrations is indicated, and doses of vitamin and mineral products should be modified based on these laboratory findings and clinical presentation.

TABLE 30.6 SUGGESTED DOSING OF FAT-SOLUBLE VITAMINS FOR INTESTINAL FAILURE PATIENTS

VITAMIN	DEFICIENCY	RECOMMENDED FORMULATIONS	RECOMMENDED DOSE IN IF	COMMENTS
Vitamin A	Night blindness, xerophthalmia, keratomalacia, Bitot spots	Retinol (water soluble) palmitate injection, 50,000 units/mL (15 mg retinol/mL)	Prophylaxis: children ≥8 y and adults, 10,000-15,000 units/d water-miscible product orally Suggested dose for infants with cholestasis receiving enteral feedings is 3,000 units/d (provided in 2 mL of infant multivitamin drops)	Adjust dose according to levels, check levels regularly in prolonged therapy Patients receiving doses >25,000 units/kg should be closely monitored for toxicity Injectable form may be given orally 1 USP vitamin A unit = 0.3 μg of all-trans isomer of retinol, 1 RE (retinol equivalent) = 1 μg of all-trans retinol
Vitamin D	Rickets, osteomalacia, dental caries, hypocalcemia, hypophosphatemia, phosphaturia, aminoaciduria	Ergocalciferol (vitamin D_2, calciferol, Drisdol)	Suggested dose for infants with cholestasis receiving enteral feedings is 1200 units per day (provided by 2 mL of infant multivitamin drops plus 400 units additional)	1.25 mg ergocalciferol provides 50,000 units of vitamin D activity.
Vitamin E	Anemia, hemolysis, neurologic deficits (wide-based gait, decreased deep tendon reflexes (DTRs))	α-Tocopherol polyethylene glycol succinate (water soluble)	Full-term neonates: 5 units/L of formula PO; chronic cholestasis (oral): 50 units/kg/d, and increase in 50 unit/kg/d increments to 150-300 units/d Alternative dosage for infants with cholestasis receiving enteral feedings is 50 units PO daily	1 unit vitamin E = 1 mg DL-tocopherol acetate Necrotizing enterocolitis is reported with oral administration of large dosages (>200 units/d) of hyperosmolar vitamin E preparations in low-birthweight infants. Adjust dose according to blood levels.
Vitamin K	Coagulopathy, prolonged PT, abnormal bone matrix synthesis	**Phytonadione, vitamin K1**	Suggested dose for infants with cholestasis receiving enteral feedings is 2.5 mg PO QOD or 1 mg SQ q/wk.	Severe reactions resembling anaphylaxis/hypersensitivity were reported during or immediately after IV administration. Chronically ill children receiving long-term antibiotics may require larger doses.

PT, prothrombin time.
Online Formulary, Boston Children's Hospital, 2025.

COMPLICATIONS OF INTESTINAL FAILURE

In patients with steatorrhea, long-chain fatty acids (LCFAs) combine with magnesium and calcium, leaving calcium unavailable for the formation of calcium oxalate. Unabsorbed bile salts in the colon are thought to increase mucosal permeability to oxalate. These two factors combine to increase enteric oxalate absorption, which, in turn, increases the risk of oxalate renal stones.[8] Hyperhydration, dietary oxalate restriction, and oral calcium supplementation may help in the prevention of calcium oxalate renal stones.[20]

An increased presence of gallstones, both among patients with ileal resection and among those without an ICV, has been noted.[8] It is assumed that precipitation of cholesterol occurs due to the low concentration of bile salts following ileal resection, causing an interruption of the enterohepatic circulation.[6]

As long-term patient outcomes continue to improve, IF can now be considered a chronic illness. Although enteral autonomy is the goal outcome in intestinal rehabilitation, reliance on the gastrointestinal tract for absorption of all nutrients and fluids often requires extensive and complicated regimens of enteral nutrition and micronutrient supplements on top of a robust oral diet. The efforts required to maintain such regimens can have negative impacts on patient quality of life beyond those reported by patients who remain dependent on PN support.[21] Furthermore, enteral autonomy in one stage of life does not guarantee against the indication for resuming PN support in another stage. Patients able to wean from PN in their childhood years may again require intravenous nutrition support throughout their pubertal growth period to achieve optimal development and linear growth.

PHARMACOLOGIC MANAGEMENT OF INTESTINAL FAILURE

Patients with IF often require unique therapies to assist in bowel adaptation. Depending on the patient, they may require prokinetic, antimotility, and or antisecretory agents. Due to the complexities of IF, dosage recommendations are often quite different from established norms. Table 30.7 summarizes medications often used in IF management.

Intolerance to enteral nutrition is a hallmark of IF with nausea, vomiting, and abdominal distention presenting as common signs and symptoms. Prokinetic agents such as metoclopramide, erythromycin, and cisapride have been shown to promote gastrointestinal motility in these patients.[22] Side effects, however, have limited their usefulness. Prucalopride may be helpful.

Loperamide is often used in IF patients to reduce transit rate and enhance fluid and nutrient absorption. By slowing intestinal motility, water and sodium loss can be reduced by approximately 20% to 30% from an ileostomy.[22] Loperamide is an opioid-receptor agonist that inhibits peristalsis by acting directly on the musculature of both the small and large intestine. At extremely excessive doses (i.e., more than 100-200 mg/d), loperamide can cross the blood-brain barrier and produce effects like those associated with centrally acting opioids like heroin, hydrocodone, or morphine. Loperamide overdoses have been associated with serious cardiac complications, including arrhythmias, loss of consciousness or fainting, and myocardial infarction. Moreover, even standard doses of loperamide may interact with medications that can cause QT prolongation such as azole antifungal drugs and macrolide antibiotics.[23] Loperamide should generally not

TABLE 30.7 EXAMPLES OF MEDICATIONS USED IN PEDIATRIC INTESTINAL FAILURE PATIENTS

INDICATION	MEDICATION	TYPICAL DOSE	COMMENTS
Antimotility agents	**Loperamide**	Usual doses: Infants ≥2 mo and Children: Oral: 0.08-0.24 mg/kg/d in divided doses every 8-12 h; maximum dose: 2 mg/dose Typical max doses used in IF: 0.8 mg/kg/d or 24 mg/d	Cases of torsades de pointes, cardiac arrest, and death have been reported with the use of a higher than recommended dosage of loperamide. Use tablets, avoid liquid formulations. Propylene glycol content may increase output.
Prokinetics	**Erythromycin**	Note: Most commonly reported salt form in studies was erythromycin ethylsuccinate (when reported). Preterm neonates: Postnatal age (PNA) ≥14 d: Note: Treatment duration is typically 7-14 d. *Low-dose regimen*: Oral: 1.5-2.5 mg/kg/dose every 6 h or 1 mg/kg/dose every 8 h *Intermediate-dose regimen*: Oral: 5 mg/kg/dose every 6 to 8 h. *High-dose regimen*: Oral: 10-12.5 mg/kg/dose every 6-8 h.; after 2 d, may decrease dose to 4 mg/kg/dose every 6 h for 5 additional days. *Note: High-dose regimens not recommended due to risk of adverse effects and the possibility that therapeutic effects may be reduced.* **Infants, Children, and Adolescents:** Response determination during gastric emptying study: IV: 2.8 mg/kg infused over 20 min; maximum dose: 250 mg/dose Treatment: Oral: 3 mg/kg/dose 4 times daily; may increase as needed to effect up to 10 mg/kg/dose; maximum dose: 250 mg/dose	Involved in many drug interactions; prokinetic at low dose but causes gastric antral spasm and delayed gastric emptying at high doses; oral route preferred; serious cardiac complications, including arrest, have occurred with IV administration

	Azithromycin	Azithromycin use as a prokinetic agent has not been widely researched. Median dose of azithromycin was 3.97 mg/kg has been used.	Risk of antimicrobial resistance Risk of tachyphylaxis, cardiac arrhythmia Azithromycin may be an equal alternative to erythromycin. Unlike erythromycin, azithromycin is not extensively metabolized by CYP3A4, may decrease cardiac risk associated with increased blood levels secondary to enzyme inhibition
Miscellaneous	**Octreotide**	Wide dosing variation exists IV, subcutaneous: begin with 1-10 g/kg every 12 h and increase by 0.3 g/kg/dose at 3-d intervals	• Dose titrated to stool output • May cause hyper- or hypoglycemia • Based on animal data, suppression of growth hormone may be of concern when used as long-term therapy in children
	Ursodeoxycholic acid (urso, ursodiol)	Infants and children: 30 mg/kg/d in 3 divided doses **Parenteral nutrition–induced cholestasis:** Treatment: Preterm and term neonates: Oral: 10-30 mg/kg/d in 3 divided doses Prevention: Preterm neonates: Oral: 20-25 mg/kg/d in 2-4 divided doses Infants and Children: Oral: 30 mg/kg/d in 3 divided doses **Pruritus secondary to cholestasis** Infants, Children, and Adolescents: Oral: 15-20 mg/kg/d once daily or in divided doses twice daily; doses up to 30 mg/kg/d may be necessary in some patients	May cause diarrhea; liquid formulation must be specially compounded.

(continued)

TABLE 30.7 EXAMPLES OF MEDICATIONS USED IN PEDIATRIC INTESTINAL FAILURE PATIENTS (*continued*)

INDICATION	MEDICATION	TYPICAL DOSE	COMMENTS
	Cholestyramine	**Diarrhea secondary to intestinal failure, short bowel syndrome:** Children and Adolescents: Oral: 240 mg/kg/d in 2-3 divided doses; maximum daily dose: 8 g/d has been suggested **Pruritus secondary to cholestasis**: Dosages are expressed in terms of anhydrous resin: Children ≤10 y: Oral: 240 mg/kg/d in 2 or 3 divided doses administered in the morning around breakfast and, if necessary, the third dose at lunch; may titrate dose to effect. Typical maximum daily dose of 4 g/d; however, higher doses have been reported to treat pruritus patients, higher doses were associated with increased steatorrhea and required dosage reduction. Children > 10 y and Adolescents: Oral: 240 mg/kg/d administered in the morning before breakfast; may titrate dose to effect. Some experts have suggested a maximum daily dose of 8 g/d; in adult patients, the AASLD guidelines recommend an initial dose of 4 g/d; may titrate up to 16 g/d	Interacts with ursodeoxycholic acid. Administer 1 h after ursodiol doses. Therapeutic effect may differ among products due to excipients (e.g., sorbitol, sucrose), which could potentially worsen diarrhea. Significant drug interactions exist.
	Teduglutide	Children and Adolescents weighing ≥10 kg: Subcutaneous: 0.05 mg/kg/dose once daily	Reduce dose in renal dysfunction (<60 mL/min/1.73 m^2). Rotate injection site between thighs, abdomen, upper arm. Development of colorectal polyps reported. Monitor fluid and electrolyte status. REMS drug http://www.gattexrems.com/

AASLD, American Association for the Study of Liver Diseases; IV, intravenous.
Online Formulary, Boston Children's Hospital, 2025.

be used in patients with slow transit times, those with refractory small bowel bacterial overgrowth, or patients with acute GI infections, including *Clostridium difficile*. The liquid formulation should not be used unless confirmed to be both a sugar-free and alcohol-free formulation to avoid the side effect of osmotic diarrhea. Other opioid derivatives, such as codeine and tincture of opium, should be avoided in children with IF–associated diarrhea. Severe side effects have been observed in children receiving codeine, especially if they are "ultra-rapid metabolizers." Because atropine can cross the blood-brain barrier, diphenoxylate/atropine is not recommended as the high doses needed to manage diarrhea have been associated with systemic effects.

Immediately after extensive gastrointestinal resection, gastrin secretion is increased, resulting in excess gastric acid secretion.[6] Hyperacidic secretions impair carbohydrate and protein digestion, micelle formation, and lipolysis, resulting in malabsorption and diarrhea. Acid blockers can be used to decrease gastric acid and improve absorption. H_2 antagonists and proton-pump inhibitors have both been used for this purpose as acid blockade can reduce jejunostomy output. Parenteral administration may be preferred, especially in those patients with extremely short bowel as the patient's capacity for enteral absorption may be insufficient to achieve a therapeutic effect. Since there is a potential link between acid blockade and an increased risk in infections, including SIBO, weaning the patients from this class of medications as soon as possible is preferred. Hypomagnesemia can also occur with the use of PPIs.

In 2019, the U.S. FDA-approved teduglutide, an analog of glucagon-like peptide 2, an endogenous protein associated with intestinal epithelial cell proliferation, for use in children with IF dependent on parenteral support. Experience with this medication has shown promising results in terms of weaning children from parenteral support and increasing dietary energy absorption.[24]

Dosage Form Considerations

Managing drug therapy using orally administered medication in patients in whom significant amounts of small bowel are resected or nonfunctional is a critical but often overlooked component of patient care. Even in a healthy individual without IF, the exact location within the intestinal tract where a medication is absorbed is not known, nor are the specific factors that can impact it, thus making it particularly challenging to determine drug response in a patient with dysmotility or an intestinal resection. The function of the remaining bowel, the presence (or absence) of terminal ileum, and the pH within the intestine can all be altered, each factor further influencing the extent of medication absorption. Moreover, the type of an orally administered dosage form can also impact drug response in an IF patient. For example, if an IF patient is prescribed a sustained release dosage form, drug response tends to be unreliable due to the variability in drug absorption, which is both unpredictable and erratic. To avoid this, the medication should be converted into the equivalent immediate-release dosage form.

Most medications contain excipients, inactive substances that are combined with the active ingredient. Excipients are used to enhance the drug's therapeutic properties such as improving drug absorption, enhancing solubility, increasing stability, or altering the smell or taste of an otherwise unpalatable medication. These additives are used in products designed for oral administration; they are not designed for administration via a feeding tube. There are significant differences between oral administration and delivery of a medication through a feeding tube. Solid dosage forms such as tablets and capsules have coatings to reduce shelf degradation from moisture and to improve the passage of the medication through the alimentary tract. These coatings reduce surface tension to allow the drug to slide down the throat when administered with water. This type of coating, however, also acts as an adhesive with other tablets when mixed with an insufficient volume of water, causing the tablets to clump.[25] Moreover, when the crushed tablets are administered down an enteral feeding tube, clogging can result.

In addition to obstructing the device, patients using enteral feeding tubes are distinctively sensitive to concentrated medications possessing high osmolarity. Most liquid medications have an osmolarity of more than 1000 mOsm/L. Unfortunately, the tolerable osmolarity of the GI tract is about 285 mOsm/L, and, thus, hypertonic medications require dilution to improve tolerance. This may result in large volumes of water to dilute the dose to a tolerable concentration.[25] Furthermore, the location exit site of the enteral feeding tube within the GI tract must also be considered. Administration of a liquid medication into the stomach allows its residual fluid volume to help dilute the high osmolarity of the medication, thus improving tolerance.

CENTRAL LINE–ASSOCIATED BLOODSTREAM INFECTIONS (CLABSI) PREVENTION AND TREATMENT

Due to their reliance on PN and the need for a central venous catheter (CVC), patients with IF are at risk of CLABSIs and life-threatening infections. CLABSIs occur when bacteria or fungi enter the bloodstream through the CVC or during periods of bacteremia due to bacterial translocation, osteomyelitis, urinary tract infections, or others. SIBO, leading to intestinal translocation and skin contamination, can result in different organisms causing CLABSIs in the IF patient. In addition to good hand hygiene and strict aseptic technique when managing the CVC, locking solutions are often used. Concentrated antibiotic solutions are instilled into the CVC lumen and allowed to dwell for a defined period (at minimum 2 hours) with the goal of maintaining drug concentrations within the CVC that are high enough to penetrate the biofilm and kill the bacteria within the device.[26] When treating a CLABSI, systemic antibiotics are used along with the antibiotic lock. Ethanol has been used as an alternative agent as it possesses both bactericidal and fungicidal properties. Unfortunately, ethanol is not compatible with all types of CVC materials and may increase the risk for catheter occlusion and breakage.[27] Ethanol is also not compatible with heparin and, if injected through the CVC rather than aspirated, may cause a disulfiram-like reaction in patients receiving metronidazole. Table 30.8 summarizes commonly used locking solutions.[28]

SUMMARY

The nutritional management of IF is a multistage process that may take years. Aggressive use of enteral nutrition to stimulate intestinal adaptation, as well as recognition and treatment of possible complications, can significantly improve prognosis. Multidisciplinary care has been associated with better outcomes.[10]

TABLE 30.8 CATHETER LOCK SOLUTIONS

AGENT	MOA	COMMENTS
Heparin	Binds to antithrombin and inactivates thrombin and other coagulation factors This prevents the formation of clots and prolongs blood clotting time. Does not have fibrinolytic activity; it will not lyse existing clots	Considered the gold standard. May not be any better than Normal Saline (NS) lock (Cochrane Collaboration, Lopez-Briz, 2014) Only product with an FDA-labeled indication for VAD locking As much as 20% may leak into system circulation due to parabolic flow within the catheter Can predispose patient to HIT (heparin-induced thrombocytopenia) If dosed too low, increase risk of thrombosis. May induce biofilm formation in the presence of *Staphylococcus aureus* Higher heparin concentrations also increase rate of biofilm formation.
Ethanol Lock	*No anticoagulant activity.* Nonspecific protein denaturation Can penetrate and sterilize biofilms	No FDA-approved indication (off-label use of an FDA-approved product) Demonstrated efficacy for preventing/treating CLABSI Typically, 70% concentration used—requires compounding Frequency and dwell times vary (daily, weekly; 15 min-24 h) ***Not compatible with all CVC materials*** Polyurethane changes when exposed to ethanol Increased wall thickness Reduced elasticity Elution of catheter materials Increases risk of catheter rupture/splitting **Compatible with silicone**

(continued)

TABLE 30.8 CATHETER LOCK SOLUTIONS *(continued)*

AGENT	MOA	COMMENTS
Citrate Locks	Prevents activation of calcium-dependent coagulation pathways (chelates calcium)	4% citrate at least as effective as heparin Antimicrobial properties at high concentrations Adverse effects Metallic taste, perioral or peripheral paresthesia, one case of fatal cardiac arrhythmia High concentrations can lead to protein precipitation in hemodialysis (HD) catheters leading to PE Problem in U.S. market: available only in 250 mL or 500 mL bags (used in plasmapheresis)
Sodium Bicarbonate Locks	Has both anti-infective and anticoagulation properties	Fairly safe Alternative to citrate containing triCitrasol or heparin locks Inexpensive *Initially used in hemodialysis catheters, used at U.S. sites without access to ethanol* 7.5%-8.4% $NaHCO_3$ used = pH 7-8.5
4% Tetrasodium Ethylenediamine-tetraacetic Acid (T-EDTA)	Improves catheter patency by working as an in vitro anticoagulant with in vitro antimicrobial activity Active against biofilm-forming Gram positive and negative bacteria, fungi, and yeast EDTA—anticoagulant	Dilution of EDTA in sterile water for injection Approved by Health Canada in 2016 as a Class II Medical Device Also approved for use in Europe and Australia Not approved in the United States Available through compassionate use protocols

Taurolidine and Heparin	Heparin binds to antithrombin and inactivates thrombin and other coagulation factors; does not have fibrinolytic activity; will not lyse existing clots. Taurolidine is an antimicrobial; its methylol groups bind irreversibly to the cell walls of bacteria, fungi, and some viruses, causing cell death; also has anti-inflammatory properties	Currently approved only for patients with kidney failure receiving chronic HD through a central venous catheter Taurolidine 13.5 mg/mL and heparin 1000 USP Units/mL Taurolidine/heparin is **not** intended for systemic administration.May cause HIT

CLABSI, Central Line–Associated Bloodstream Infections; CVC, central venous catheter; PE, pulmonary embolism; VAC, Vascular Access Device.
From Coyne S, Gura KM. Pharmacologic challenges in pediatric intestinal failure: a review. *Intest Fail*. 2024;4:100039.

REFERENCES

1. Modi BP, Galloway DP, Gura K, et al. ASPEN definitions in pediatric intestinal failure. *JPEN J Parenter Enteral Nutr*. 2022;46(1):42-59.
2. Cole CR, Hansen NI, Higgins RD, et al. Very low birth weight preterm infants with surgical short bowel syndrome: incidence, morbidity and mortality, and growth outcomes at 18 to 22 months. *Pediatrics*. 2008;122:e573-e582.
3. Struijs MC, Diamond I, de Silva N, Wales P. Establishing norms for intestinal length in children. *J Ped Surg*. 2009;44:933-938.
4. Quiros-Tejeira RE, Ament ME, Reyen L, et al. Long-term parenteral nutrition support and intestinal adaptation in children with short bowel syndrome: a 25-year experience. *J Pediatr*. 2004;145:157-163.
5. Fallon EM, Mitchell PD, Nehra D, et al. Neonates with short bowel syndrome: an optimistic future for parenteral nutrition independence. *JAMA Surg*. 2014;149(7):663-670.
6. Carlson SJ, Chang MI, Nandivada P, Cowan E, Puder M. Neonatal intestinal physiology and failure. *Seminars in Ped Surg*. 2013;22:190-194.
7. Ching YA, Gura K, Modi B, Jaksic T. Pediatric intestinal failure: nutrition, pharmacologic, and surgical approaches. *Nutr Clin Pract*. 2007;22:653-663.
8. Nightingale JM. The medical management of intestinal failure: methods to reduce the severity. *Proc Nutr Soc*. 2003;62:703-710.
9. Tabone T, Mooney P, Donnellan C. Intestinal failure-associated liver disease: current challenges in screening, diagnosis, and parenteral nutrition considerations. *Nutr Clin Pract*. 2024;39(5):1003-1025.
10. Belza C, Wales PW. Impact of multidisciplinary teams for management of intestinal failure in children. *Curr Opin Pediatr*. 2017;29(3):334-339.
11. Puoti MG, Köglmeier J. Nutritional management of intestinal failure due to short bowel syndrome in children. *Nutrients*. 2022;15(1):62.
12. Olieman J, Kastelijn W. Nutritional feeding strategies in pediatric intestinal failure. *Nutrients*. 2020;12(1):177.
13. Ksiazyk J, Piena M, Kierkus J, et al. Hydrolyzed versus nonhydrolyzed protein diet in short bowel syndrome in children. *J Pediatr Gastroenterol Nutr*. 2002;35:615-618.
14. Sainath NN, Bales C, Brownell JN, et al. Impact of pancreatic enzymes on enteral fat and nitrogen absorption in short bowel syndrome. *J Pediatr Gastroenterol Nutr*. 2022;75(1):36-41.
15. Hopkins J, Merritt R. Strategies to promote success in oral feedings in infants and children with intestinal failure due to short bowel syndrome. *Gastroenterol Clin N Am*. 2024;53:330-341.
16. Berger MM, Shenkin A, Schweinlin A, et al. ESPEN micronutrient guideline. *Clin Nutr*. 2022;41(6):1357-1424.
17. Yang CF, Duro D, Zurakowski D, Lee M, Jaksic T, Duggan C. High prevalence of multiple micronutrient deficiencies in children with intestinal failure: a longitudinal study. *J Pediatrics*. 2011;159(1):39-44.
18. Lam K, Schwartz L, Batisti J, Iyer KR. Single-enter experience with the use of teduglutide in adult patients with short bowel syndrome. *JPEN J Parenter Enteral Nutr*. 2018;42(1):225-230.
19. Dao DT, Anez-Bustillos L, Finkelstein AM, et al. Trends of INR and fecal excretion of Vitamin K during cholestasis reversal: implications in the treatment of neonates with intestinal failure-associated liver disease. *JPEN J Parenter Enteral Nutr*. 2020;44(5):951-958.
20. Bao Y, Tu X, Wei Q. Water for preventing urinary stones. *Cochrane Database Syst Rev*. 2020;2020(2):CD004302.
21. McCaig JK, Henry OS, Stamm DA, et al. Generic and disease-specific health-related quality of life in pediatric intestinal failure. *J Pediatr Gastroenterol Nutr*. 2021;73(3):338-344.
22. Karamanolis G, Tack J. Promotility medications: now and in the future. *Dig Dis*. 2006;24:297-307.
23. Wu PE, Juurlink DN. Clinical review: loperamide toxicity. *Ann Emerg Med*. 2017;70(2):245-252.
24. Lambe C, Talbotec C, Kapel N, et al. Long-term treatment with teduglutide: a 48-week open-label single-center clinical trial in children with short bowel syndrome. *Am J Clin Nutr*. 2023;117(6):1152-1163.
25. Klang MG. Developing guidance for feeding tube administration of oral medications. *JPEN J Parenter Enteral Nutr*. 2023;47(4):519-540.
26. Daoud DC, Wanten G, Joly F. Antimicrobial locks in patients receiving home parenteral nutrition. *Nutrients*. 2020;12(2):439.
27. Fligor SC, Hirsch TI, Tsikis ST, et al. Ethanol lock therapy increases mechanical catheter complications in a pediatric intestinal failure population: a retrospective cohort study. *JPEN J Parenter Enteral Nutr*. 2023;47(5):662-669.
28. Coyne S, Gura KM. Pharmacologic challenges in pediatric intestinal failure: a review. *Intest Fail*. 2024;4:100039.

CHAPTER 31

Ketogenic Therapies

Heidi Pfeifer and Stacey Tarrant

Over a century ago, researchers observed that fasting reduced seizure frequency in individuals with epilepsy. This led to the development of the ketogenic diet (KGD) in the 1920s, designed to mimic those biochemical changes associated with starvation to provide seizure control. Nutritional ketosis occurs when carbohydrate intake is significantly restricted and fat intake increased, while protein remains adequate to support growth and development. In this metabolic state, the ketone bodies β-hydroxybutyrate, acetoacetate, and acetone replace glucose as the primary energy source.[1]

Initially regarded as a treatment of last resort, ketogenic therapy is now recognized as an effective, broad-spectrum treatment for epilepsy. It is typically recommended after the failure of two antiseizure medications (ASMs), and earlier initiation should be considered for certain epilepsy syndromes or when surgery is not an option. The diet is particularly effective for Doose syndrome, West syndrome, Dravet syndrome, infantile spasms, Rett syndrome, and tuberous sclerosis.[2-6] Ketogenic therapies are also the primary treatments for some disorders of carbohydrate metabolism, specifically, glucose transporter type 1 deficiency syndrome (Glut1DS) and pyruvate dehydrogenase deficiency (PDHD). Ketogenic treatments are contraindicated in disorders of fat metabolism (Table 31.1).[7]

Systematic reviews and meta-analyses provide consistent evidence supporting the effectiveness of ketogenic therapies for infants, children, and adolescents with epilepsy

TABLE 31.1 INDICATIONS AND CONTRAINDICATIONS OF KETOGENIC TREATMENTS

INDICATIONS	ABSOLUTE CONTRAINDICATIONS
• Failed 2 or more appropriate antiseizure medications • FIRES[a]/NORSE[b] • Glucose transporter-1 deficiency (Glut-1) • Pyruvate dehydrogenase deficiency (PDHD) • Infantile spasms • Dravet syndrome • Enterally fed via gastrostomy tubes • Angelman syndrome • Tuberous sclerosis	• Primary carnitine deficiency • Carnitine palmitoyl transferase (CPT) I or II deficiency • Carnitine translocase deficiency β-oxidation defects • Short-chain acyl dehydrogenase deficiency (SCAD) • Medium-chain acyl dehydrogenase deficiency (MCAD) • Long-chain acyl dehydrogenase deficiency (LCAD) • Medium-chain 3-hydroxyacyl-CoA deficiency • Long-chain 3-hydroxyacyl-CoA deficiency • Pyruvate carboxylase deficiency

[a]Febrile Infection-Related Epilepsy Syndrome.
[b]New-Onset Refractory Status Epilepticus.
From Kossoff EH, Zupec-Kania BA, Auvin S, et al. Optimal clinical management of children receiving dietary therapies for epilepsy: updated recommendations of the International Ketogenic Diet Study Group. *Epilepsia Open*. 2018;3(2):175-192.

in terms of reduced seizure activity.[8] For some patients with epilepsy, additional benefits include improvement in cognitive development and behavioral disorders.[8] Despite the availability of newer ASMs, about 30% of patients remain drug resistant.[8]

In an effort to continue to liberalize the restrictiveness of the KGD, the low–glycemic index treatment (LGIT) and modified Atkins diet (MAD) were developed in the early 2000s. Randomized controlled trials show these alternatives can have comparable efficacy to the classic KGD, with LGIT showing greater tolerability and increased compliance.[9,10]

Although the precise mechanisms of action of the KGD remain unknown, the diet's therapeutic effects are thought to be multifactorial. Proposed mechanisms include direct antiseizure effects of ketone bodies, neurotransmitter modulation, improved bioenergetics and mitochondrial changes, the anti-inflammatory effect of β-hydroxybutyrate, glucose restriction, and increases in polyunsaturated fatty acids. Some patients maintain seizure control after the diet is withdrawn, suggesting neuroprotective and/or antiepileptogenic properties.[11]

PATIENT EVALUATION

Before initiating ketogenic therapy, a multidisciplinary team should evaluate the patient's medical, nutritional, and psychosocial suitability. The evaluation should include a comprehensive diet history, with special attention to any history of food allergies, feeding or swallowing difficulties, gastrointestinal problems, and assessment of anthropometric measurements and nutritional status. A detailed food record can be useful for estimation of baseline daily energy intake. In addition, standard energy estimation equations such as Schofield, WHO, or estimated energy requirements (EER) may be used. Minimum protein requirement is based on the recommended dietary allowance (RDA) for protein (see Chapter 5). The full assessment guides the selection of the appropriate ketogenic therapy.

MEDICATION AND PRODUCT REVIEW

The carbohydrate content of all medications must be considered and calculated as part of the total daily carbohydrate allotment.[12] All medications must be reviewed for their carbohydrate content, especially children's liquid medications, which may contain sugars or sugar alcohols. Whenever possible, liquid medications should be changed to nonchewable tablets or capsules, which are the lowest carbohydrate forms. Alternatively, some medications may be compounded in carbohydrate-free solutions by specialty compounding pharmacies. Products that may be ingested by mouth, such as toothpastes and lip balms, should contain zero or minimal carbohydrate. The extent to which carbohydrates from topical products such as lotions and sunscreens absorb into the skin and might affect ketosis is not known. However, low-carbohydrate versions of these products may be recommended as a precaution.

CLASSIC AND MODIFIED KETOGENIC DIETS

Classic (CKD) and modified ketogenic diets (MKD) are expressed in terms of a ketogenic ratio, which is defined as grams of fat to grams of protein plus carbohydrate combined. CKDs generally refer to diets with 3:1 or higher ratios, while MKDs refer to those with ratios starting at 1:1 but less than 3:1. Food intake is usually divided into three meals per day and up to three snacks per day, with all meals and snacks calculated in the prescribed ketogenic ratio to minimize variation in the level of ketosis throughout the day. Intake other than the calculated meals and snacks is restricted to foods and liquids providing little or no carbohydrates, such as carbohydrate-free and calorie-free beverages, water, and limited amounts of nuts, avocado, iceberg lettuce, and olives. All foods and formula components are measured on a digital gram scale. Strict adherence to the diet is essential since a small variation in dietary intake can affect the maintenance of ketosis and thus seizure control.

Individualized meal plans are calculated by a registered dietitian to provide the determined amounts of carbohydrate, protein, and fat per meal according to the diet prescription (see Table 31.2), taking into account food allergies and/or intolerances. The KGD prescription consists of the ketogenic ratio, total daily calories and protein requirements, goal fluid intake (typically one times maintenance fluids), and vitamin and mineral supplements needed to meet 100% of the Dietary Reference Intake (DRI) for age. Table 31.3 illustrates a sample one-day meal plan for an individual on CKD. Specialty ketogenic formulas, including milk-, soy-, plant-, peptide-, and whole-food–based formula, may be used for patients requiring tube feeding or a liquid diet. Keto Diet Calculator, supported by the Charlie Foundation (ketodietcalculator.org), is a web-based program that can be used for accurate and efficient calculation of meal plans and formula recipes.

Whether a CKD or MKD is initiated in an inpatient or outpatient setting varies among different ketogenic programs. Either option may be considered based on the circumstances of the individual patient and family preference. Considerations for inpatient or outpatient diet initiation may include the patient's age, medical complexity, nutritional status, those who may benefit from rapid induction of ketosis, and access to emergency medical care. Initiation in the inpatient setting allows for close monitoring of acute diet-related side effects such as hypoglycemia, dehydration, and/or acidosis

TABLE 31.2 SAMPLE KETOGENIC DIET CALCULATION

1. Calculate daily calories needed.
[Example: 11-kg toddler × 82 kcal/kg/d = 900 kcal/d]

2. Calculate the daily number of dietary units needed.[a]
[Example: (900 kcal/d)/(31 kcal/unit) = 29 units/d]

3. Calculate the number of grams of fat needed per day.

4. The remainder of the calories will be provided by protein and carbohydrate.
[Example: 900 kcal/d–783kcal/d from fat = 117 kcal/d (29.25 g)]

5. Provide at least the 2005 RDA for protein.
[Example: 1.05 g/kg/d × 11 kg = 11.55 g/d protein]

6. The remaining grams are allotted to daily carbohydrate intake.
[Example: 29.25–11.55 = 17.7]

7. Divide the allotments over the number of meals desired each day.

RDA, recommended dietary allowance.

[a] A dietary unit represents the caloric value of one unit of the ketogenic ratio. For example, a 3:1 ratio means that there are 3 g of fat for every 1 g protein and carbohydrate combined. Since fat provides 9 kcal/g and protein and carbohydrate both provide 4 kcal/g, one dietary unit for a 3:1 ratio has 31 kcal [(9 kcal/g of fat × 3 g fat = 27) + (4 kcal/g of protein + carbohydrate × 1 g = 4)] = 31 kcal/dietary unit.

TABLE 31.3 SAMPLE MENU FOR AN 8-YEAR-OLD GIRL

Diet: 1500 kcal, 4:1 ratio, 3 meals per day, 0 snacks per day

Per meal: 50.0 g fat, 7.4 g protein, 5.1 g carbohydrate

BREAKFAST	LUNCH	DINNER
50 g egg	29 g tuna fish	48 g hot dog
32 g orange	18 g celery	36 g broccoli
23 g butter	23 g apple	5 g no-sugar ketchup
9 g oil	37 g mayonnaise	26 g mayonnaise
45 g heavy cream	49 g heavy cream	47 g heavy cream

that may occur with an abrupt metabolic shift into ketosis. Full calories are provided throughout the admission, and the ratio is advanced based on diet tolerance and response. In-depth diet education is provided to parents and caretakers during the hospitalization. Alternatively, initiation of CKD and MKD has been shown to be both safe and effective in the outpatient setting when started at a low ratio, and diet is advanced no more frequently than weekly.[13] Prior to initiation, the ketogenic dietitian may provide in-depth education to the family during an in-person visit (in the outpatient setting) or via telehealth. The diet is initiated at a low ketogenic ratio (e.g., 1:1 or 1.5:1), with frequent follow-up and lab monitoring as the diet ratio is slowly advanced. An advantage of this method is the opportunity to assess diet efficacy at lower ketogenic ratios. If seizure control can be achieved at a lower ratio, the diet will be more palatable and better tolerated. Patients may also experience fewer acute side effects.

■ MODIFIED ATKINS DIET

Developed in 2003 at John's Hopkins by Dr. Eric Kossoff and his team to provide a more palatable and flexible alternative to the CKD and MKD, MAD involves carbohydrate restriction of 10 to 20 g/d net carbohydrate (total carbohydrate minus fiber), encourages liberal amounts of fat eaten with each meal, and allows unrestricted protein, although it should not replace fat. Sugar alcohols are used sparingly or avoided altogether.[14] Portions of carbohydrate-containing foods are estimated using standard household measurements to maintain carbohydrate restriction. MAD provides approximately 70% of calories from fat (a 1:1 ratio), although this may be higher or lower depending on the amount of fat versus protein consumed. As with the other ketogenic therapies, a complete multivitamin and calcium supplement must be taken to avoid deficiencies, and plenty of carbohydrate-free fluid should be consumed.

■ LOW–GLYCEMIC INDEX TREATMENT

Developed in 2002 by Heidi Pfeifer, RD, LDN, and Dr Elizabeth Thiele at Massachusetts General Hospital,[15] the LGIT restricts total carbohydrate intake to 40 to 60 g/d (~10% of calories) spread evenly throughout the day. LGIT emphasizes low–glycemic index foods (GI less than 50) to promote more stable blood sugar levels and prevent blood sugar spikes. Foods are measured using household units, not by weight. The LGIT provides approximately 60% to 70% of calories from fat and approximately 20% to 30% of calories from protein. The increased amounts of carbohydrate included in the treatment allow for a higher micronutrient intake, but the need for micronutrient supplementation remains.

Neither MAD nor LGIT is intended for exclusively tube-fed patients or infants, as ketogenic formula is easy to use, and infants require especially close nutrition supervision. Both are initiated outpatient and require an increased amount of caregiver independence for meal planning. Regardless of the diet treatment selected, all ketogenic therapies for epilepsy require medical supervision by a neurologist and dietary counseling by a dietitian with expertise in this area.

■ MEDIUM-CHAIN TRIGLYCERIDE OIL

Medium-chain triglycerides (MCTs) are fats with 6- to 12-carbon chain lengths. Caprylic (C8) and Capric (C10) are more readily used during ketogenic treatment due to their ability to produce higher ketones and provide increased antiseizure benefits relative to other sources of fat. MCT can be added to any ketogenic treatment to increase the level of ketosis. It is also used as an additional treatment for constipation, which is one of the most common side effects occurring during treatment. Care should be taken to increase doses slowly as it can lead to diarrhea and abdominal pain.

■ VITAMIN AND MINERAL SUPPLEMENTATION

Due to the extreme carbohydrate limitation of ketogenic treatments, vitamin and mineral intake is also limited, highlighting the need for consistent supplement use as directed by the dietitian. Risk of deficiencies of calcium, ferritin, folate, iron, magnesium, pantothenic acid, phosphorus, selenium, thiamine, and vitamins C and D are higher when higher therapeutic ketogenic ratios are utilized.[16,17] Carnitine deficiency is also possible due to increased utilization.[18] Certain seizure medications (e.g., barbiturates, valproic acid, carbamazepine, phenytoin, levetiracetam) can exacerbate risk of deficiencies.[19]

■ MONITORING AND FOLLOW-UP

Ketogenic therapy requires regular outpatient follow-up by a multidisciplinary team including registered dietitian, nurse, neurologist, and social worker. Ongoing family commitment, is essential for success of ketogenic therapy. Typical visit intervals include 2 weeks and 6 weeks after the initial hospitalization and then every 3 months thereafter. At each outpatient visit, biochemical monitoring, anthropometrics, and appropriateness of the current calorie level, ratio, and supplementation is assessed. The diet may need to be adjusted following initiation. If seizures persist, possible adjustments include decreasing energy intake in cases of excess weight gain, adding a bedtime snack to support overnight ketone production, or optimizing the ketogenic ratio.

One of the benefits of the KGD is that its use may allow the reduction or discontinuation of antiepileptic medications, which often have adverse side effects. Still the diet itself may result in a number of short-term and long-term complications, for which all patients should be carefully monitored.[20-24] Table 31.4 reviews possible side effects

TABLE 31.4 POSSIBLE ACUTE AND CHRONIC COMPLICATIONS OF KETOGENIC DIET THERAPY

COMPLICATION	PREVENTION OR THERAPY
Dehydration	Encourage fluids Dextrose-free IV fluids may be necessary during inpatient initiation of CKD or during an acute illness
Hypoglycemia	Metabolic screen prior to diet initiation During inpatient CKD initiation, check dextrose sticks every 6 h and consider giving 10-15 mL juice if blood glucose is less than 40 mg/dL and child is symptomatic, and recheck glucose level May need to decrease diet ratio
Acidosis	Encourage adequate fluids Monitor serum bicarbonate levels Consider oral citrate supplementation Avoid or reduce zonisamide and topiramate if possible
Vomiting	Encourage carb-free beverages, diluted bouillon, and diluted formula, or ketogenic liquid meal as tolerated Monitor closely for dehydration Dextrose-free IV fluids may be indicated
Medication toxicity	Monitor antiepileptic medication levels as some can change with initiation of ketogenic therapy
Diarrhea	Encourage carb-free electrolyte replacement fluids and diluted bouillon Increase soluble fiber intake Monitor hydration status May need dextrose-free IV fluids If using MCT oil, decrease amount
Food refusal	Adjust meals to increase variety Limit mealtime to 20 min, avoid negative reinforcement, and encourage setting of limits at mealtimes and a positive feeding relationship Encourage mixing together components of a meal so that if the meal is not finished, at least the food is consumed in the proper ratio Try to make family meals similar to ketogenic meals Include child in meal planning and preparation
Nephrolithiasis	Encourage allowed fluids Monitor spot urine calcium-to-creatinine ratio (<0.3 is normal) Consider oral citrate Renal ultrasound, decrease in diet ratio, and referral to a nephrologist may be indicated

TABLE 31.4 POSSIBLE ACUTE AND CHRONIC COMPLICATIONS OF KETOGENIC DIET THERAPY (*continued*)

COMPLICATION	PREVENTION OR THERAPY
Decreased growth velocity	Ensure adequate calorie, protein, vitamin, and mineral provision
Hypoproteinemia	Monitor serum albumin and prealbumin levels Assess for protein loss in the urine or stool Increase dietary protein if needed Assess for protein allergy Ensure vitamin/mineral supplements provide 100% of DRI
Carnitine deficiency	Monitor blood carnitine levels and supplement as needed
Constipation	Encourage adequate fluid intake Increase use of high-fiber vegetables, avocado, and ground flaxseed Incorporate MCT oil Medication may be necessary (Miralax, senna tabs, and Phillips brand Milk of Magnesia are carbohydrate free)
Hyperlipidemia	Monitor fasting lipid profiles Decrease saturated fat in the diet and increase unsaturated fats by using more oils, avocados, seeds, and nuts Incorporate MCT oil
Vitamin and mineral deficiencies	Ensure intake of 100% of the DRI of vitamins and minerals Check vitamin and mineral levels as indicated
Osteopenia	Ensure adequate calcium, vitamin D, phosphorus, and magnesium provision Encourage weight-bearing activity
Exacerbation of gastroesophageal reflux disease	Decrease size and increase frequency of meals and snacks Provide fluid separate from food Gastroenterology evaluation may be indicated
Lethargy or irritability	Ensure adequate calorie provision Evaluate serum and urine ketone levels Assess for acidosis A decrease in ratio may be indicated
Pancreatitis	Check serum triglyceride levels Monitor serum amylase and lipase levels Change some long-chain fat to MCT oil Decrease diet ratio or change to MAD or LGIT Discontinuation of diet may be indicated

CKD, classic ketogenic diet; DRI, dietary reference intake; IV, intravenous; MCT, medium-chain triglyceride, MAD, modified Atkins diet; LGIT, low glycemic index treatment.

of ketogenic therapy and suggests steps for their prevention and treatment. Most side effects can be treated without the need for diet discontinuation.

During acute illness, children on ketogenic therapy are at risk for dehydration, acidosis, excessive ketosis, and hypoglycemia. At home, caregivers should offer carbohydrate-free fluids and diluted formula, along with carbohydrate-free pain relievers as needed. Diluted bouillon can be offered to provide electrolytes in the setting of diarrhea. Caregivers should be educated to recognize warning signs of dehydration, excess ketosis, and hypoglycemia and know when to seek medical attention. If a child is hospitalized for an acute illness or planned surgery, intravenous fluid with added electrolytes should be provided without dextrose. Close monitoring for acidosis and hypoglycemia is essential if the child is not eating.

Children typically remain on the diet as long as it provides seizure control without adverse effects. For glucose transporter type 1 deficiency and PDHD, lifelong therapy is indicated. Reasons for weaning include seizure freedom, unacceptable seizure control, medical complications, or behavioral complications. No standardized weaning protocols exist; however, children who have been on the diet for a short period of time (less than 2-3 months) without apparent decrease in seizure frequency or intensity may be weaned off the diet relatively quickly. Children who have been responsive to the diet should be weaned off the diet more slowly, with monitoring of seizure control at each step.

REFERENCES

1. Wheless JW. History of the ketogenic diet. *Epilepsia*. 2008;49(s8):3-5.
2. Caraballo RH, Cersosimo RO, Sakr D, Cresta A, Escobal N, Fejerman N. Ketogenic diet in patients with myoclonic-astatic epilepsy. *Epileptic Disord*. 2006;8(2):151-155.
3. Caraballo RH, Fejerman N. Dravet syndrome: a study of 53 patients. *Epilepsy Res*. 2006;70(Suppl 1): S231-S238.
4. Liebhaber GM, Riemann E, Baumeister FA. Ketogenic diet in Rett syndrome. *J Child Neurol*. 2003;18(1):74-75.
5. Prezioso G, Carlone G, Zaccara G, Verrotti A. Efficacy of ketogenic diet for infantile spasms: a systematic review. *Acta Neurol Scand*. 2018;137(1):4-11.
6. Kossoff EH, Thiele EA, Pfeifer HH, McGrogan JR, Freeman JM. Tuberous sclerosis complex and the ketogenic diet. *Epilepsia*. 2005;46(10):1684-1686.
7. Kossoff EH, Zupec-Kania BA, Auvin S, et al. Optimal clinical management of children receiving dietary therapies for epilepsy: updated recommendations of the International Ketogenic Diet Study Group. *Epilepsia Open*. 2018;3(2):175-192.
8. Ruan Y, Chen L, She D, Chung Y, Ge L, Han L. Ketogenic diet for epilepsy: an overview of systematic review and meta-analysis. *Eur J Clin Nutr*. 2022;76(9):1234-1244.
9. Sharawat IK, Panda P, Dawman L, Gupta D, Panda PK. Modified Atkins Diet versus low glycemic index treatment in children with drug-resistant epilepsy: a systematic review and meta-analysis. *Seizure*. 2024;131(4).
10. Sondhi V, Agarwala A, Pandey RM, et al. Efficacy of ketogenic diet, modified atkins diet, and low glycemic index therapy diet among children with drug-resistant epilepsy: a randomized clinical trial. *JAMA Pediatr*. 2020;174(10):944-951.
11. Rho JM. How does the ketogenic diet induce anti-seizure effects? *Neurosci Lett*. 2017;637:4-10.
12. McGhee B, Katyal N. Avoid unnecessary drug-related carbohydrates for patients consuming the ketogenic diet. *J Am Diet Assoc*. 2001;101(1):87-101.
13. van der Louw E, Olieman J, Poley MJ, et al. Outpatient initiation of the ketogenic diet in children with pharmacoresistant epilepsy: an effectiveness, safety and economic perspective. *Eur J Paediatr Neurol*. 2019; 23(5):740-748.
14. Kossoff EH. The modified atkins diet for epilepsy: two decades of an "alternative" ketogenic diet therapy. *Pediatr Neurol*. 2023;147:82-87.

15. Pfeifer HH, Thiele EA. Low-glycemic-index treatment: a liberalized ketogenic diet for treatment of intractable epilepsy. *Neurology*. 2005;65(11):1810-1812.
16. Joshi C, Stillman C, Criteser S, et al. Yield of laboratory testing in pediatric ketogenic diet patients: critical assessment of abnormal results and impact on clinical care. *Epilepsy Res*. 2019;149:70-75.
17. Kang HC, Chung DE, Kim DW, Kim HD. Early- and late-onset complications of the ketogenic diet for intractable epilepsy. *Epilepsia*. 2004;45(9):1116-1123.
18. Neal EG, Zupec-Kania B, Pfeifer HH. Carnitine, nutritional supplementation and discontinuation of ketogenic diet therapies. *Epilepsy Res*. 2012;100(3):267-271.
19. Gupta S, Sahu JK. Vitamin D deficiency in children on long-term antiseizure medications: where do we stand? *Indian J Pediatr*. 2022;89(6):533.
20. Couch SC, Schwarzman F, Carroll J, et al. Growth and nutritional outcomes of children treated with the ketogenic diet. *J Am Diet Assoc*. 1999;99(12):1573-1575.
21. Acharya P, Acharya C, Thongprayoon C, et al. Incidence and characteristics of kidney stones in patients on ketogenic diet: a systematic review and meta-analysis. *Diseases*. 2021;9(2):39.
22. Kwiterovich PO Jr, Vining EP, Pyzik P, Skolasky R Jr, Freeman JM. Effect of a high-fat ketogenic diet on plasma levels of lipids, lipoproteins, and apolipoproteins in children. *JAMA*. 2003;290(7):912-920.
23. Sankar R, Sotero de Menezes M. Metabolic and endocrine aspects of the ketogenic diet. *Epilepsy Res*. 1999;37(3):191-201.
24. Vining EP, Pyzik P, McGrogan J, et al. Growth of children on the ketogenic diet. *Dev Med Child Neurol*. 2002;44(12):796-802.

SUGGESTED RESOURCES

COMPUTER PROGRAM

- KetoDietCalculator. Supported by The Charlie Foundation and available at ketodietcalculator.org

FOR PARENTS AND PRACTITIONERS

- Martenz DM, Cramp, L. *The Keto Cookbook; Innovative Delicious Meals for Staying on the Ketogenic Diet*. Demos Health Publishing; 2012.
- *Martenz DM, Zupec-Kania B. The Modified Keto Cookbook; Quick, Convenient, Great-Tasting Recipes for Following a Low Ratio Ketogenic Diet. Demos Health Publishing; 2015.*
- *Kossoff E, Turner Z, Cervenka MC, Barron BJ. Ketogenic Diet Therapies for Epilepsy and Other Conditions. 7th ed. Demos Health Publishing; 2020.*
- *Zupec-Kania B, Vanatta L, Johnson M. Ketogenic Diet Therapies for Neurological Disorders Pocket Guide. 5th ed. The Charlie Foundation for Ketogenic Therapies; 2024.*

INTERNET RESOURCES

- Charlie Foundation for Ketogenic Therapies
  https://www.charliefoundation.org/
- *Matthew's Friends*
  http://www.matthewsfriends.org
- *USDA Food Data Central*
  https://fdc.nal.usda.gov/

CHAPTER 32

Lipid Disorders

S. Skylar Griggs and Anna Maynes

Extensive research has established that serum cholesterol is a key contributor to cardiovascular disease (CVD), the leading cause of death and morbidity in the United States.[1] Research also indicates that cholesterol levels during childhood contribute to early vascular abnormalities.[2] The National Heart Lung and Blood Institute recommended that lipid disorders be identified during childhood to enable early nutritional and pharmacologic intervention.[3] This chapter will cover lipids and lipoproteins, lipoprotein disorders of lipid metabolism in childhood, screening in childhood, normal pediatric ranges, nutrition assessment, nutrition treatment, and indications for pharmacotherapy for lipid disorders in pediatrics.

PHYSIOLOGY OF LIPIDS AND LIPOPROTEINS

There are two major forms of lipids circulating in the body: triglycerides (TG) and cholesterol. Cholesterol and TG are insoluble in the plasma and require lipoproteins, phospholipids, and apolipoproteins (apoproteins) for transport.[4] Physiologically, lipoproteins have an outer core of cholesterol, phospholipids, and apoproteins, and their inner core is composed of TG and cholesterol ester (CE). The five major lipoproteins[4,5] are:

- *Chylomicrons:* Large particles that carry dietary lipids, mostly TG; chylomicrons contain multiple apolipoproteins, including A-I, A-II, A-IV, B-48 (essential for the assembly, secretion, and metabolism of chylomicrons), C-I, C-II, C-III, and E.
- *Very low-density lipoproteins (VLDL):* Transports endogenous TG and some cholesterol from the liver; apolipoproteins associated with VLDL are B-100 (LDL-C receptor ligand), C-I, C-II, C-III, and E.
- *Intermediate-density lipoproteins (IDL-C):* Carries CE and TG; transitional particle between VLDL and LDL-C. IDL-C is associated with apolipoproteins B-100, C-III, and E.
- *Low-density lipoproteins (LDL-C):* The major cholesterol carrier; associated with apolipoprotein B-100. Its value on a fasting lipid panel must be calculated using the Friedewald equation: LDL-C = Total cholesterol (TC) − HDL-C − TG/5.[4,5] This equation fails if TG >400 mg/dL. LDL-C can also be measured directly in the nonfasting state; however, treatment decisions are generally based on the fasting calculation if possible because the direct measurement assays give results that differ from the calculated number.
- *High-density lipoproteins (HDL-C):* Carries cholesterol; its role is antiatherogenic; HDL-C is associated with apolipoproteins A-I, A-II, C-I, C-II, C-III, D, and E. Apolipoprotein A-I (ApoA-I) is the primary protein component of HDL-C, produced in the liver and intestines.[4,5]

TABLE 32.1 ACCEPTABLE, BORDERLINE-HIGH, AND HIGH/LOW PLASMA LIPID, LIPOPROTEIN, AND APOLIPOPROTEIN CONCENTRATIONS (MG/DL) FOR CHILDREN AND ADOLESCENTS

CATEGORY	ACCEPTABLE	BORDERLINE	HIGH+
TC	<170	170-199	>200
LDL-C	<110	110-129	>130
Non-HDL-C	<120	120-144	>145
ApoB	<90	90-109	>110
TG			
0-9 y	<75	75-99	>100
10-19 y	<90	90-129	>130
CATEGORY	**ACCEPTABLE**	**BORDERLINE**	**LOW+**
HDL-C	>45	40-45	<40
ApoA-I	>120	115-120	<115
ApoB	>30	30-50	>50
Lp(a)	14-30 mg/dL 75-125 nmol/L	75-125	<75

ApoB, Apoliprotein B, ApoA-I, Apoliprotein A-I HDL, high-density lipoprotein; LDL, low-density lipoprotein; TC, total cholesterol; TG, triglyceride.
From Daniels SR, et al. Integrated guidelines for cardiovascular health and risk reduction in children and adolescents. *Pediatrics*. 2011.

TGs are the major form of fat in the body. TGs are produced by the body and are influenced greatly by recent dietary and alcohol intake. TG levels should be obtained in the fasting state for 8 to 12 hours prior to measurement. Lipoprotein (a) [Lp(a)] is considered an independent risk factor for heart disease. Normal values are below 30 mg/dL (milligrams per deciliter) or 75 mmol/L.[6] Acceptable, borderline-high, and high plasma concentrations for children and adolescents of other lipids, lipoproteins, and apolipoproteins are shown in Table 32.1.

■ DISORDERS OF LIPID METABOLISM IN PEDIATRICS

Abnormal levels of circulating lipids can lead to cholesterol accumulation in arterial walls, which contributes to plaque formation and increases CVD risk. Elevated TG levels, particularly in the form of chylomicrons, also increase the risk for pancreatitis.

Lipid disorders can be primary (genetic) or secondary (related to lifestyle, medications, or medical conditions). Primary, or familial, lipid disorders are typically more severe, present earlier in life, and often require more aggressive interventions and lifelong management.[3] A summary of major primary lipid disorders in children and adolescents is shown in Table 32.2.[3,7,8-11] Additional information about more common familiar lipid disorders is included in what follows.

TABLE 32.2 SUMMARY OF MAJOR PRIMARY LIPID DISORDERS IN CHILDREN AND ADOLESCENTS

PRIMARY LIPID DISORDERS	INHERITANCE	LIPID/LIPOPROTEIN ABNORMALITY	CLINICAL FINDINGS	TREATMENT	DIETARY RECOMMENDATIONS
Familial hypercholesterolemia (homozygous)	Autosomal dominant; LDL receptor mutation	↑↑ LDL-C (400-1000 mg/dL)	Xanthomas, arcus cornea, xanthelasmas, early CAD	Lipid-lowering medications; apheresis or liver transplant in homozygous FH	Heart-healthy, low-saturated fat, low-cholesterol diet
Familial hypercholesterolemia (heterozygous)	Autosomal dominant; LDL receptor mutation	↑ LDL-C (160-400 mg/dL)	Xanthomas, arcus cornea, xanthelasmas, early CAD	Lipid-lowering medications; soluble fiber or plant sterol supplements may be beneficial	Heart-healthy, low-saturated fat, low-cholesterol diet
Familial defective apolipoprotein B	Autosomal dominant	↑ LDL-C	Similar to heterozygous FH but milder	Lipid-lowering medications	Heart-healthy, low-saturated fat, low-cholesterol diet
Familial combined hyperlipidemia	Polygenic or autosomal dominant	Type IIa: ↑ LDL-C Type IV: ↑ VLDL-C, ↑ TG Type IIb: ↑ LDL-C, ↑ VLDL-C, ↑ TG Types IIb and IV often with ↓ HDL-C	Increased risk of premature CHD	Lipid-lowering medications or omega-3s	Heart-healthy, low-saturated fat, low-cholesterol diet, reduced simple carbohydrate intake
Polygenic hypercholesterolemia	Polygenic	↑ LDL-C	Usually asymptomatic	Lipid-lowering medication, if needed	Heart-healthy, low-saturated fat, low-cholesterol diet

Familial hypertriglyceridemia	Autosomal dominant	↑ VLDL-C ↑ TG (200-1000 mg/dL)	Usually asymptomatic	Medications or high-dose omega-3 supplements may be used, as clinically indicated	Limit added sugars and simple carbohydrates, increase complex carbohydrates, dietary sources of omega-3, and fiber, pair carbohydrate with protein or fat.
Severe hypertriglyceridemia	Multifactorial	↑ Chylomicrons ↑ VLDL-C ↑↑ TG (≥ 1000 mg/dL)	Complications may include pancreatitis, liver damage, and neuropathy.	Medications or high- dose omega-3 supplements may be used, as clinically indicated.	Low-fat diet may be needed, limit added sugars and simple carbohydrates, increase complex carbohydrates.
Familial hypoalphalipo-proteinemia	Autosomal dominant or recessive	↓ HDL-C	Increased risk of premature CAD	Manage risk factors	General heart diet, increased unsaturated fats
Dysbetalipoproteinemia	Autosomal recessive; ApoE2/E2 genotype	↑ IDL-C ↑ chylomicron remnants ↑ TC (250-500 mg/dL ↑ TG: 250-600 mg/dL)	Xanthomas	Lipid-lowering mediation, fibrates or bile acid resins may be needed	General heart-healthy diet, low fat may be considered
Elevated lipoprotein(a) [Lp(a)]	Autosomal dominant; LPA gene	↑ Lp(a)	Stable high Lp(a) levels from early childhood; family history of early CVD or stroke; may coexist with FH	No specific Lp(a)-lowering drugs currently; under development	General CVD risk reduction: heart-healthy diet and lifestyle
Sitosterolemia	Autosomal recessive; ABCG5/8 mutation	↑ TC	Elevated plant sterols, xanthomas, premature atherosclerosis	Diet plus possible pharmacologic therapy	Avoid plant sterols (e.g., shellfish, nuts, seeds, plant oils, avocados, chocolate); monitor nutrient deficiencies

(continued)

TABLE 32.2 SUMMARY OF MAJOR PRIMARY LIPID DISORDERS IN CHILDREN AND ADOLESCENTS (*continued*)

PRIMARY LIPID DISORDERS	INHERITANCE	LIPID/LIPOPROTEIN ABNORMALITY	CLINICAL FINDINGS	TREATMENT	DIETARY RECOMMENDATIONS
Familial chylomicronemia syndrome (FCS)	Autosomal recessive; LPL or related gene deficiency	↑↑ TG (≥ 1000 mg/dL)	Pancreatitis, abdominal pain, failure to thrive, eruptive xanthomas	Nutritional therapy is primary; MCT oil as needed	Very–low-fat diet (<10%-15% of calories); fat-restricted infant formula
Lysosomal acid lipase deficiency (LAL-D)	Autosomal recessive; LIPA gene mutation	↑ LDL-C, ↑ TG, ↓ HDL-C	Cholesterol ester and TG accumulation in tissues, hepatomegaly, dyslipidemia, failure to thrive (infantile form), liver dysfunction	Enzyme replacement therapy	Fat restriction (<25% of calories), cholesterol <200 mg/d; monitor fat-soluble vitamins

CAD, coronary artery disease; CHD, coronary heart disease; CVD, cardiovascular disease; FH, familial hypercholesterolaemia; HDL, high-density lipoprotein; LDL, low-density lipoprotein, TG, triglyceride; VDLD, very low-density lipoprotein.

From Daniels SR, et al. Integrated guidelines for cardiovascular health and risk reduction in children and adolescents. Pediatrics. 2011; Williams L, Baker-Smith CM, Bolick J, et al. Nutrition interventions for youth with dyslipidemia: a National Lipid Association clinical perspective. *J Clin Lipidol*. 2022; Koschinsky ML, Bajaj A, Boffa MB, et al. A focused update to the 2019 NLA scientific statement on use of lipoprotein(a) in clinical practice. *J Clin Lipidol*. 2024;18(3):e308-e319; Korbelius M, Kuentzel KB, Bradić I, Vujić N, Kratky D. Recent insights into lysosomal acid lipase deficiency. *Trends Mol Med*. 2023;29(6):425-438; Rocha VZ, Tada MT, Paula A, Chacra APM, Miname MH, Mizuta MH. Update on sitosterolemia and atherosclerosis. *Curr Atheroscler Rep*. 2023;25(5):181-187; Balasubramanian S, Aggarwal P, Sharma S. Lipoprotein Lipase Deficiency. In: StatPearls [Internet]. StatPearls Publishing; 2024. https://www.ncbi.nlm.nih.gov/books/NBK560795/.

TABLE 32.3 CAUSES OF SECONDARY DYSLIPIDEMIA

EXOGENOUS	**HEPATIC**
Alcohol	Obstructive liver disease/cholestatic conditions
Drug therapy: • Corticosteroids • Isoretinoin • Beta-blockers • Some oral contraceptives • Select chemotherapeutic agents • Select antiretroviral agents	Biliary cirrhosis Alagille syndrome
	INFLAMMATORY DISEASE
	Systemic lupus erythematosus Juvenile rheumatoid arthritis
ENDOCRINE/METABOLIC	**STORAGE DISEASE**
Hypothyroidism/hypopituitarism	Glycogen storage disease
Diabetes mellitus types 1 and 2	Gaucher disease
Pregnancy	Cystine storage disease
Polycystic ovary syndrome	Juvenile Tay-Sachs disease
Lipodystrophy	Niemann-Pick disease
Acute intermittent porphyria	**OTHER**
RENAL	Kawasaki disease
Chronic renal disease	Anorexia nervosa
Hemolytic uremic syndrome	Post solid organ transplantation
Nephrotic syndrome	Childhood cancer survivor
INFECTIOUS	Progeria
Acute viral/bacterial infection	Idiopathic hypercalcemia
Human immunodeficiency virus infection (HIV)	Klinefelter syndrome
Hepatitis	Werner syndrome

From Daniels SR, et al. Integrated guidelines for cardiovascular health and risk reduction in children and adolescents. *Pediatrics.* 2011.

Secondary lipid disorders may arise from dietary and activity habits, conditions (e.g., diabetes, thyroid abnormalities, obesity, polycystic ovary syndrome, renal disease, and eating disorders), or certain medications (e.g., retinoids, oral contraceptive pills, diuretics, β-blockers, some antidepressants). Exposure to cigarette smoke can lower HDL-C levels in children. A list of common causes of secondary lipid disorders is included in Table 32.3.

NUTRITION ASSESSMENT

The nutrition assessment begins with a detailed patient history, focusing on dietary patterns, typical intake, diet recall, and snacking habits.[12] Evaluating the family and home environment helps identify both support systems and potential barriers to success. See Table 32.4 for key components of the assessment and Table 32.5 for frequently used nutrition diagnoses in pediatric lipid disorders.[13]

TABLE 32.4 NUTRITION ASSESSMENT IN LIPID DISORDERS

PATIENT HISTORY

- Age, Sex, Race/Ethnicity
- Diagnosis (e.g., type of lipid disorder)
- Past Medical History
- History of Failure to Thrive, Small for Gestational Age, or Premature Birth
- Food Allergies
- Family History
- Medications
- Laboratory Assessments: Total cholesterol, LDL-C, HDL-C, TG, less often ApoB, ApoA-I
- Alcohol/Smoking (adolescents), Smoke Exposure
- Support System (e.g., Who does child live with? Who prepares meals? What resources are available to purchase food [supplemental nutrition programs]? What is the access to physical activity?)

FOOD- AND NUTRITION-RELATED HISTORY

- Energy intake
- Sources of carbs, proteins, and fats (e.g., whole grains versus refined grain sources)
- Sugar consumption (e.g., beverages, sweets)
- Sodium consumption
- Fiber intake (e.g., fruits, veggies, whole grains)
- Location of meals eaten (e.g., in front of the television versus at the dining room table)
- Meals outside of the home (e.g., dining out, fast food)
- Herbs, vitamins, minerals (e.g., MVI, omega-3)
- School meals
- Cultural food preferences
- Cultural response to weight
- Physical activity

PHYSICAL OBSERVATIONS

- Anthropometric data
- Overweight/obesity (waist circumference)
- Xanthomas (deposits of lipids in the skin)
- Acanthosis nigricans
- Biochemical data (e.g., lipid profile, lipoprotein(a) (Lp[a]), hemoglobin A1c (HbA1c), 25-OH vitamin D, thyroid function tests, C-reactive protein [CRP], etc.)

From American Dietetic Association. Disorders of lipid metabolism. Evidence-based nutrition practice guideline. Published 2011. Accessed October 15, 2025. https://www.andeal.org/vault/pq97.pdf.

TABLE 32.5 NUTRITION DIAGNOSIS IN LIPID DISORDERS

Problems:

Food- and nutrition-related knowledge deficit NB-1.1
Excessive carbohydrate intake NI-5.8.2
Inappropriate intake of refined carbohydrate NI-5.8.3
Excessive energy intake NI-1.5
Inadequate fiber intake NI-5.8.5
Excessive oral intake NI-2.2
Not ready for diet/lifestyle change NB-1.3
Self-monitoring deficit NB-1.4
Undesirable food choices NB-1.7
Physical inactivity NB-2.1
Limited adherence to nutrition-related recommendations NB-1.6
Undesirable food choices NB-1.7
Excessive fat intake NI-5.6.2
Inappropriate intake of saturated and/or transfats NI-5.6.3

TABLE 32.5 NUTRITION DIAGNOSIS IN LIPID DISORDERS (*continued*)

Etiology:

Hyperlipidemia (and need for heart-healthy diet)
Minimal fruit and vegetable intake
Undesirable food choices
Inability to limit or refuse offered foods
Food and nutrition compliance limitations
Denial of need to change
Lack of social support for implementing changes
Exposure to unhealthful foods
Need for continued adherence to nutrition and physical activity–related recommendations

Signs and Symptoms:

Most recent lipid panel
24-h recall and self-report
Infrequent and limited duration of physical activity
Excessive amount of sedentary activity (TV, computer, video game, tablet, smartphone)
Disinterest in selecting foods consistent with the nutrition guidelines
Verbalized disinterest in learning information
Increased body adiposity (weight gain of × kg × wk/mo/y)

American Dietetic Association. *International Dietetics and Nutrition Terminology Reference Guide*. American Dietetic Association; 2009.

NUTRITION INTERVENTION IN DYSLIPIDEMIA

Excess energy intake and poor dietary patterns are major contributors to pediatric dyslipidemia.[3] Diets rich in fruits, vegetables, and whole foods, and low in saturated fat are effective in improving serum lipids and reducing cardiovascular risk. Children and adolescents need fat in their diets for calories and adequate growth, but the quality and quantity of fat intake matter. Rather than restricting total fat, current recommendations emphasize replacing saturated fats with heart-healthy alternatives.[14] Detailed recommendations for dietary fat are included in Table 32.6. Other nutrition and lifestyle recommendations are summarized below.

Lean Proteins

Replacing high-saturated-fat foods with lean proteins can help lower the saturated fat content of the diet. Examples of lean protein sources include white meat poultry (e.g., turkey breasts, skinless chicken), fish, pork tenderloin, tofu, beans, and legumes. If red meat is consumed, choose lean cuts (e.g., round, sirloin), trim visible fat, and select ground beef that is at least 90% lean.

Low-fat Dairy

For children 12 to 24 months, reduced fat milk (2% or lower) can be used. After age 2, fat-free milk is recommended, as it optimizes the nutrient benefit without adding saturated fat. Low-fat dairy products should be encouraged to reduce overall saturated fat intake.[3]

TABLE 32.6 DIETARY FATS IN PEDIATRIC DYSLIPIDEMIA MANAGEMENT

TYPE OF FAT	RECOMMENDED INTAKE	COMMON FOOD SOURCES	CLINICAL EFFECTS	NUTRITION GUIDANCE
Total Fat	• Ages 1-3: 30%-40% of total calories • Ages 4-18: 25%-35% of total calories • **Do not restrict fat** in infants <12 mo	All food groups containing fat: oils, dairy, meats, nuts, seeds, etc.	Essential for growth, brain development, and energy	Emphasize healthy fat sources; avoid very-low-fat diets in young children.
Saturated Fat	• <10% of total calories (general) - <7% if elevated LDL-C	Red meat, full-fat dairy, butter, fried foods, baked goods	Raises LDL-C; promotes atherosclerosis	Limit; replace with mono/polyunsaturated fats
Trans Fat	Avoid entirely	Previously in margarine, shortening, processed/fried foods	Raises LDL-C, lowers HDL-C; highly atherogenic	Avoid completely; largely removed from U.S. food supply
Monounsaturated Fat	~10% of total calories	Olive oil, avocado, nuts, nut butters, canola oil	Improves lipid profile; raises HDL-C, lowers LDL-C	Encourage as a preferred fat source.
Polyunsaturated Fat	~10% of total calories	Vegetable oils (soybean, corn, safflower), seeds, walnuts, fatty fish	*Lowers LDL-C; provides* essential fatty acids	*Include as part of balanced* fat intake
Omega-3 Fatty Acids (EPA/DHA)	• Fish: 2-3 servings/wk • Supplements: 2000-4000 mg EPA/DHA if TG >200 mg/dL[a]	Salmon, sardines, mackerel, trout, herring, light tuna	Lowers triglycerides, may improve LDL particle size, anti-inflammatory; fish oil supplements used effectively in children with end-stage renal insufficiency	Include in diet; limit albacore tuna (<6 oz/wk); supplement only if needed
Dietary Cholesterol	• <300 mg/d (general) - <200 mg/d if elevated LDL-C	Egg yolks, organ meats, shellfish, full-fat dairy	Modest effect on LDL-C in some; impact less than saturated fat	Limit if hypercholesterolemia present; prioritize fat quality.

DHA, docosahexaenoic acid; EPA, eicosapentaenoic acid; LDL-C, low-density lipoprotein cholesterol.

[a] Omega-3 supplements should be used under clinical supervision in children, particularly those with hypertriglyceridemia.

Cooking Methods

Encourage heart-healthy cooking techniques, such as baking, braising, broiling, grilling, sautéing, poaching, roasting, steaming, and stir-frying. Discourage deep or pan frying and the use of heavy sauces, as they are often higher in saturated fats.

Carbohydrates and Sugar-Sweetened Beverages

High carbohydrate intake, especially from added sugars, can increase plasma TG concentrations in children, particularly in children with hypertriglyceridemia. Reducing consumption of SSBs can lower TG levels and, thereby, decrease risk of T2DM and CVD.[15,16] Ideally, the primary beverage should be water or fat-free unflavored milk.[3]

Fiber

Fiber intake supports lipid management and overall health.[17] For children under 11 years old, the recommended total dietary fiber intake from food sources is the child's age in years plus 5 g. For older children and adolescents, up to 14 g/1000 kcal is recommended. Fiber intake from fiber-rich fruits, veggies, beans, lentils, and whole grains is preferred. Fiber supplements are not generally advised for the purpose of lowering lipids.[3] Water-soluble fiber, in particular, can improve serum cholesterol levels as it helps bind cholesterol for excretion.[3] Children ages 2 to 12 with dyslipidemia are encouraged to consume at least 6 g of soluble fiber daily; 12 g/d is recommended for older children and adolescents.[7] Foods high in soluble fiber include flaxseed, beans, avocado, and broccoli.

Breastfeeding

Breastfeeding is recommended exclusively for the first 6 months of life and continued through at least 12 months of age with the introduction of complementary foods. Breastfeeding may reduce the risk of atherosclerosis later in life.[18]

Plant Sterols/Stanols

Diets supplemented with plant stanols and sterol-enriched foods (e.g., fortified spreads/margarine, orange juice, yogurt drinks) can reduce LDL-C in children by 5% to 10%. Plant sterols or stanol esters (up to 2 g/d) have been studied as replacements for usual fat sources to safely enhance LDL-C in short-term studies in children with familial hypercholesterolemia (FH). However, long-term studies on the safety and efficacy of sterols and stanols have not been performed in adults or children, and, thus, these supplements should be reserved for children who do not achieve LDL-C cholesterol goals with conventional dietary treatment alone. The largest safety concern with increased consumption of plant stanols and sterols is that fat-soluble vitamins and β-carotene absorption may be reduced. Therefore, fat-soluble vitamin status should be monitored in children receiving supplementation.

Physical Activity

Promoting physical activity in childhood supports lifelong habits and lowers coronary heart disease (CHD) risk. Children aged 3 to 5 years should be physically active throughout the day to enhance growth and development. For children aged 6 to 17 years, 60 minutes or more of moderate to vigorous physical activity per day is recommended.[4]

MONITORING AND EVALUATION

Registered dietitians (RDs) play a key role in guiding children and their families toward dietary patterns that support health, specifically, diets low in saturated fat and high in fruits, vegetables, and fiber. RDs should evaluate the patient's ability to recall nutrition goals covered in the previous session(s) and track the patient's stage of change, as understanding a patient's readiness to adopt lifestyle change allows for more tailored and effective counseling. Fasting lipid panels should be monitored every 3 months to help track progress, and regular tracking of weight, height, and body mass index can help assess growth trends and the impact of dietary changes. While weight loss is not the primary goal in nutrition counseling for lipid disorders, weight loss may accompany improvements in lipid values secondary to lifestyle medications. A moderate weight reduction has been shown to decrease insulin resistance and dyslipidemia in children and adolescents with severe obesity.[19]

REFERENCES

1. Martin SS, Aday AW, Allen NB, et al. 2025 Heart disease and stroke statistics: a report of US and Global Data from the American Heart Association. *Circulation*. 2025;151(8):e41-e660.
2. Berenson GS. Childhood risk factors predict adult risk associated with subclinical cardiovascular disease: the Bogalusa Heart Study. *Am J Cardiol*. 2002;90(10C):3L-7L.
3. Daniels SR, et al. *Expert Panel on Integrated Guidelines for Cardiovascular Health and Risk Reduction in Children and Adolescents: Full Report*. NIH Publication No. 12-7486, October 2012. https://www.nhlbi.nih.gov/files/docs/guidelines/peds_guidelines_full.pdf
4. Rohrs H. Pediatric lipid disorders in clinical practice. Published 2024. Accessed August 13, 2025. http://emedicine.medscape.com/article/1825087-overview#a0104
5. Rosenson RS. Lipoprotein classification; metabolism; and role in atherosclerosis. Published 2025. Accessed August 13, 2025. http://www.uptodate.com/contents/lipoprotein-classification-metabolism-and-role-in-atherosclerosis
6. David Zieve MM. Lipoprotein (a). MedLine Plus, US National Library of Medicine and NIH. Published 2024. Accessed August 20, 2025. http://www.nlm.nih.gov/medlineplus/ency/article/007262.htm
7. Williams, L., Baker-Smith, C. M., Bolick, J., Carter, J., Kirkpatrick, C., Ley, S. L., Peterson, A. L., Shah, A. S., Sikand, G., Ware, A. L., & Wilson, D. P. (2022). Nutrition interventions for youth with dyslipidemia: a National Lipid Association clinical perspective. *Journal of clinical lipidology, 16*(6), 776–796.
8. Koschinsky ML, Bajaj A, Boffa MB, et al. A focused update to the 2019 NLA scientific statement on use of lipoprotein(a) in clinical practice. *J Clin Lipidol*. 2024;18(3):e308-e319.
9. Korbelius M, Kuentzel KB, Bradić I, Vujić N, Kratky D. Recent insights into lysosomal acid lipase deficiency. *Trends Mol Med*. 2023;29(6):425-438.
10. Rocha VZ, Tada MT, Paula A, Chacra APM, Miname MH, Mizuta MH. Update on sitosterolemia and atherosclerosis. *Curr Atheroscler Rep*. 2023;25(5):181-187.
11. Balasubramanian S, Aggarwal P, Sharma S. Lipoprotein lipase deficiency. In: *StatPearls* [Internet]. StatPearls Publishing; 2024. https://www.ncbi.nlm.nih.gov/books/NBK560795/
12. Van Horn L, Obarzanek E, Friedman LA, Gernhofer N, Barton B. Children's adaptations to a fat-reduced diet: the Dietary Intervention Study in Children (DISC). *Pediatrics*. 2005;115(6):1723-1733.
13. American Dietetic Association. *International Dietetics and Nutrition Terminology Reference Guide*. American Dietetic Association; 2009.
14. Mietus-Snyder M, Baker AL, Neufeld EJ, et al. Effects of nutritional counseling on lipoprotein levels in a pediatric lipid clinic. *Am J Dis Child*. 1993;147(4):378-381.
15. Stanhope KL, Havel PJ. Endocrine and metabolic effects of consuming beverages sweetened with fructose, glucose, sucrose, or high-fructose corn syrup. *Am J Clin Nutr*. 2008;88(6):1733S-1737S.
16. Hu FB, Malik VS. Sugar-sweetened beverages and risk of obesity and type 2 diabetes: epidemiologic evidence. *Physiol Behav*. 2010;100(1):47-54.

17. Ruottinen, S., Lagström, H. K., Niinikoski, H., Rönnemaa, T., Saarinen, M., Pahkala, K. A., Hakanen, M., Viikari, J. S., & Simell, O. (2010). Dietary fiber does not displace energy but is associated with decreased serum cholesterol concentrations in healthy children. *The American journal of clinical nutrition, 91*(3), 651–661.
18. Martin, R. M., Ebrahim, S., Griffin, M., Davey Smith, G., Nicolaides, A. N., Georgiou, N., Watson, S., Frankel, S., Holly, J. M., & Gunnell, D. (2005). Breastfeeding and atherosclerosis: intima-media thickness and plaques at 65-year follow-up of the Boyd Orr cohort. *Arteriosclerosis, thrombosis, and vascular biology, 25*(7), 1482–1488.
19. American Dietetic Association. Disorders of lipid metabolism. Evidence-based nutrition practice guideline. Published 2011. Accessed October 15, 2025. https://www.andeal.org/vault/pq97.pdf

CHAPTER 33

Obesity

Katrina A.S. Smith and Desiree Sierra-Velez

Obesity is defined as excess accumulation of adipose tissue that can pose a risk to an individual's health. Obesity is recognized as a chronic disease by numerous professional organizations and is classified based on body mass index (BMI), or weight in kilograms divided by height in meters squared (kg/m^2). In children aged 2 to 19, this classification is dependent on BMI percentiles for age and sex (z-scores are not currently standardized for use defining overweight or obesity status). Extended BMI growth charts were published by the Centers for Disease Control and Prevention (CDC) in 2022 as previous growth charts were unable to capture significantly elevated BMI. In some circumstances (e.g., to determine eligibility for bariatric surgery), the obesity class expressed in kg/m^2 typically used for adults may also be used in adolescents. Definitions of overweight and obesity are shown in Table 33.1.

The prevalence of overweight and obesity in children has risen steadily over the last several decades, with an accelerated increase during the COVID-19 pandemic. In the United States, approximately 20% of children and adolescents have obesity, compared to 8% globally, with prevalence increasing with age. Certain populations are disproportionately affected, including Hispanic children (26.2%) and non-Hispanic Black children (24.8%). Those with lower household incomes, lower parental education, and higher incidence of adverse childhood experiences (ACEs) are also at higher risk.[1,2]

■ ETIOLOGY

Obesity is a complex, multifactorial condition resulting from the interaction of multiple genetic, epigenetic, and environmental factors.[5] In most individuals, genetic susceptibility is polygenic, meaning it arises from the combined influence of multiple risk

TABLE 33.1 DEFINITIONS OF OVERWEIGHT AND OBESITY FOR CHILDREN AGED 2 TO 19 YEARS

CATEGORY	DEFINITION
Overweight	BMI ≥85th to 95th percentile for age and sex
Obesity	BMI ≥95th percentile for age and sex
Severe obesity (Class 2)	BMI ≥120%-140% of the 95th percentile for age and sex or BMI ≥35-40 kg/m^2, whichever is lower
Severe obesity (Class 3)	BMI ≥140% of the 95th percentile for age and sex or BMI ≥40 kg/m^2, whichever is lower

BMI, body mass index.

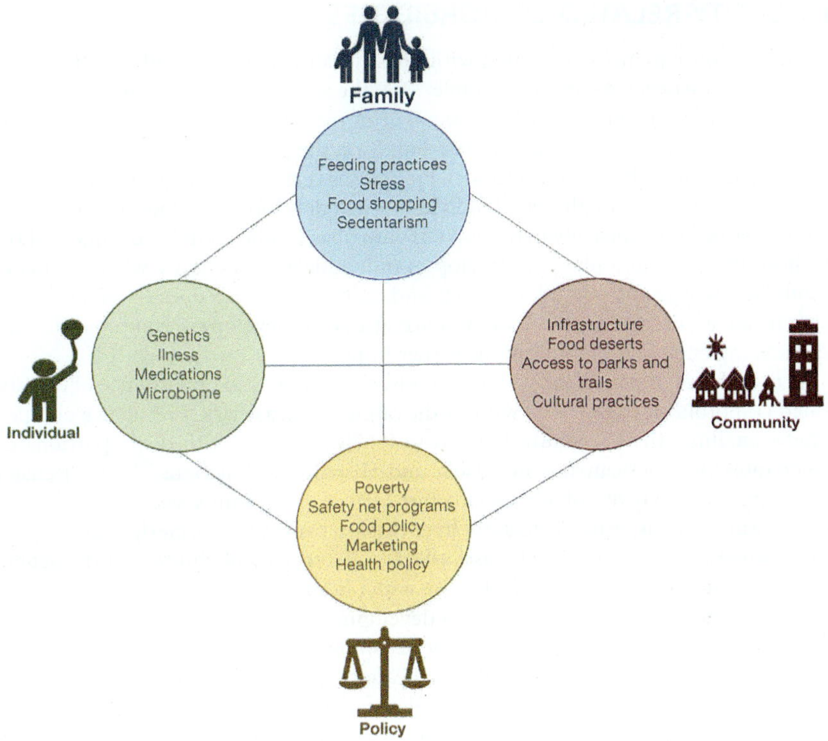

Figure 33.1 Multilevel contributors to obesity.

genes. Monogenic forms of obesity caused by mutations in a single gene (e.g., melanocortin 4 receptor deficiency, leptin receptor deficiency) are rare. Syndromic forms of obesity, which occur as part of genetic syndromes (e.g., Bardet-Biedl syndrome, Prader Willi syndrome), are also uncommon.

Epigenetic changes triggered by external influence are especially influential during the first 1000 days from conception, a critical development period. For example, maternal smoking during pregnancy has been linked to increased risk of obesity in offspring.[4] Across the lifespan, multilevel factors interact in complex and dynamic ways to increase obesity risk. The majority of these influences lie beyond an individual's control, and their effects accumulate over time (Figure 33.1).

PATHOPHYSIOLOGY OF OBESITY

The central nervous system regulates appetite by integrating signals related to hunger and satiety from the body (e.g., gut hormones) and the environment (e.g., food availability). In obesity, dysfunction in these regulatory processes result in a state of sufficient energy intake to sustain excess adiposity. When individuals with obesity lose weight, the body typically responds with compensatory mechanisms (e.g., increased energy intake, decreased energy expenditure) that favor weight regain. These physiologic responses help explain the difficulty many individuals face in sustaining weight loss.[5]

OBESITY-RELATED COMORBIDITIES

The health consequences associated with obesity can result from both metabolic and nonmetabolic aspects. As shown in Table 33.2, the state of adipose tissue dysfunction in obesity can contribute to the development of metabolic complications of obesity. Nonmetabolic complications of obesity result from the presence of excess adipose tissue mass, as well as those related to social processes (e.g., psychological consequences of weight stigma). Although not all individuals will develop comorbidities, and no comorbidities occur exclusively in individuals with obesity, obesity-related comorbidities are those that are more likely to develop in individuals with obesity when compared to individuals without obesity. Children and adolescents with obesity are also more likely to have obesity in adulthood and are at risk of developing comorbidities and experiencing end-stage complications earlier in life.[6]

As prevalence of childhood obesity has risen, so too has the prevalence of obesity-related comorbidities associated with cardiovascular disease risk. Prevalence of type 2 diabetes mellitus in U.S. youth doubled to 0.67% in 2017, with disproportionately higher rates in American Indian, Black, and Hispanic populations.[3,7] Hypertension affects approximately 4% of adolescents but 14% of those with severe obesity.[8] Metabolic dysfunction–associated steatotic liver disease (MASLD), formerly known as pediatric nonalcoholic fatty liver disease, affects 4.5% to 13% of children in the general population and an estimated 40% of those with obesity.[9]

While obesity can increase the risk of developing certain medical conditions, some medical conditions (e.g., hypothyroidism, Cushing syndrome) can contribute to the development of obesity. Use of certain medications (e.g., β-blockers, atypical antipsychotics, insulin, corticosteroids, anticonvulsants, and some selective serotonin reuptake inhibitors) are also known to contribute to weight gain. The relationship between obesity and eating disorders is bi-directional, with symptoms of disordered eating (e.g., emotional eating, loss of control eating) associated with the onset of obesity and individuals with obesity at increased risk of developing eating disorders.

TABLE 33.2 OBESITY-RELATED COMORBIDITIES

SYSTEM	COMPLICATION
Cardiovascular	Hypertension, dyslipidemia
Pulmonary	Obstructive sleep apnea, obesity hypoventilation syndrome, asthma, exercise intolerance
Gastrointestinal/hepatic	Metabolic dysfunction–associated steatotic liver disease (MASLD), gastroesophageal reflux, constipation, gallstones
Endocrine	Type 2 diabetes mellitus, polycystic ovarian syndrome, precocious puberty
Musculoskeletal	Slipped capital femoral epiphysis, Blount disease, osteoarthritis, joint pains
Neurologic	Idiopathic intracranial hypertension
Psychological	Depression, anxiety, eating disorders, low self-esteem

NUTRITIONAL ASSESSMENT

Assessing a child's nutritional status involves evaluating growth patterns and dietary intake and typically includes anthropometric measurements, evaluation of energy needs, and a thorough dietary assessment.

Anthropometric Measurements

BMI percentiles are used to classify overweight or degree of obesity in children. The z-scores in this patient population are not as helpful as large differences in BMI can correlate with only small changes in z-score. While BMI has limitations (e.g., it may not reflect true body composition), it remains useful clinically when plotted on the CDC growth charts (including extended charts) to determine a child or adolescent's growth trajectory. More precise measures of body composition, such as dual-energy x-ray absorptiometry (DEXA), are available but less commonly used in clinical settings due to cost and limited access. Older methods such as skinfold thickness and waist circumference are not widely used in clinical practice due to a lack of standardized interpretation.

Energy Requirements

Energy requirements can be estimated using equations such as Harris Benedict, estimated energy requirements (EER), and Schofield (see Chapter 5). The majority of children with obesity have basal metabolic rates equal to or greater than those without obesity, likely due to increased lean body mass.[10] However, the proportion of lean body mass associated with excess body weight is highly variable.

In hospitalized patients with obesity, resting energy expenditure (REE) should be measured by indirect calorimetry, which provides a more accurate estimate than predictive equations, which do not take into account body composition or clinical status.[11] In outpatient settings, a detailed dietary history often provides more practical insight into a child's intake, although underreporting of energy intake is common. In this setting, estimating the energy requirement may not be as necessary since focusing on dietary quality (addressed later in this chapter) and the type of counseling received may be more effective in eliciting lifestyle change compared with prescribing a specific energy intake target.

Dietary Evaluation

Assessment of a child with overweight or obesity should include a detailed nutrition and activity history to assess environmental and behavioral contributors to weight. A detailed 24-hour food recall or Food Frequency Questionnaire can be administered to help assess typical intake patterns, with a goal of understanding what, where, and how they eat on a typical day or in a typical week or month. A focused assessment of specific eating habits, physical activity, and sedentary behaviors is recommended. Additional assessment questions can reveal important context related to the food and eating environment, such as:

- Who does most of the food shopping and preparation?
- Where do you eat meals? Who is with you? Is there a screen on while you are eating?

- Do you ever worry about having enough money to afford healthy food?
- Do you ever eat in the absence of physical hunger such as when bored, stressed, or upset?
- How does your body tell you when it is hungry and full?

PREVENTION AND MANAGEMENT

Overview of Prevention

Given the rising prevalence of obesity and its associated comorbidities, effective strategies for primary prevention must target the multilevel contributors to obesity, starting as early as the first 1000 days of life (from conception through the child's second birthday). Key preventive measures include[4]:

- Maternal smoking cessation before and during pregnancy
- Preventing excessive maternal weight gain and gestational diabetes
- Exclusive breastfeeding for at least 6 months
- Promoting adequate sleep for infants

Clinically, health care providers should screen for conditions that can predispose to obesity and, when possible, select weight-neutral medications. At the family level, prevention includes fostering responsive feeding practices, which involve recognizing and heeding hunger and satiety cues and avoiding restrictive or coercive feeding practices.[12,13] Families should also receive education about the negative influence of poor sleep, excessive screen time, stress, and intake of processed foods and sugary drinks. Families should be encouraged to access necessary resources within their communities to support healthy behaviors.

Goals of Management

The primary goal of pediatric obesity management is to prevent and control obesity-related comorbidities. Weight loss is typically not appropriate for growing children. Instead, management often focuses on BMI stabilization, or slowing the rate of weight gain, to allow for normal linear growth. Comprehensive treatment requires collaboration with the child and their family to set realistic and individualized goals. These goals should not be limited to BMI stabilization or reduction and may be focused on improving or resolving comorbidities, poor quality of life, and low self-image.[6] In adolescents that are approaching or that have reached adult height, weight loss of approximately 1 kg (or 2 pounds per week) can be appropriate if done safely and with proper support, as described next.

Approach to Management

The gold standard for treatment of child and adolescent obesity is intensive health behavior and lifestyle treatment (IHBLT), which emphasizes health education, behavior modification, and counseling. Ideally, IHBLT is multidisciplinary and family-centered, with at least 26 hours of face-to-face treatment over 3 to 12 months. Topics included in IHBLTs are nutrition education, physical activity, and sleep, among others; content can be delivered to individual families, in group settings, or a combination. There is some evidence that virtual delivery can be effective, which may be an option for children that do not have access to these programs in their own community.

Motivational interviewing (MI) is recommended to support behavior change by guiding patients and their families in setting their own goals. Unlike directive approaches where the provider sets the goals and teaches the patient how to reach those goals, MI involves the provider acting as a partner and collaborator, helping to evoke the patient's own motivation for change. Information is shared only with the patient's permission, fostering autonomy and engagement.[14]

Lifestyle Change

The American Academy of Pediatrics (AAP) recommends the following behavior changes to support healthy weight management in children and adolescents:

- Reduce sugar-sweetened beverages (SSBs) such as soda and energy drinks.
- Follow a MyPlate-style eating pattern that include nutrient-dense foods and that is low in added sugar and balanced in carbohydrates and protein, without calorie restriction.
- Engage in at least 60 minutes of moderate to vigorous physical activity daily.
- Decrease sedentary behavior, including screen time.
- Avoid skipping breakfast.
- Ensure age-appropriate, adequate sleep.

Family feeding practices also strongly influence a child's relationship with food. Clinicians should counsel parents to avoid labeling foods as "good" or "bad," refrain from restricting access to foods by locking them up, and adopt an "all foods fit" approach, with a focus on nourishment and enjoyment without guilt. Similarly, parents should also avoid offering different foods to different children based on body size (e.g., giving one child fat-free yogurt and another child ice cream), as this can foster an unhealthy relationship with food and can lead to secretive eating or feelings of shame and guilt.

Families should be encouraged to prioritize foods that are nutrient-dense and higher in fiber (e.g., fruit, vegetables, beans, nuts, and whole grains) over low-nutrient options (e.g., SSBs, refined carbohydrates). To help support sustained satiety, a useful strategy is to pair a high-fiber food (fruit, vegetable, whole grain) with a protein source (dairy, egg, meat, nut, legume), such as snacking on apple with peanut butter, celery with hummus, or whole grain crackers with cheese. The low–glycemic index approach to eating is another popular method that can help families focus on foods and meals that are higher in fiber and lower in refined carbohydrates.

While popular diets such as intermittent fasting, ketogenic, paleo, or low-carbohydrate diets are often promoted in the media, these are not recommended in pediatrics. Their restrictive nature can foster an unhealthy relationship with food and promote disordered eating behaviors. Instead, the focus should be on sustainable, flexible eating patterns, guided by IHBLT and MI.

Mindful eating strategies can help children and adolescents recognize hunger and fullness cues, reduce emotional or mindless eating (especially in those who eat in response to boredom, anxiety, or stress), promote awareness during meals, and reinforce a more intuitive, less reactive approach to eating. These include:

- Avoiding eating meals or snacks in front of a screen (phone, tablet, TV, computer)
- Using a plate or bowl rather than eating directly out of a package

- Paying attention to the senses when eating (taste, feel, texture) in an effort to slow down and savor the food
- Tuning in to hunger and fullness cues by using a Hunger and Fullness scale or thermometer (widely available online)

WEIGHT STIGMA AND DISORDERED EATING

Weight stigma is highly prevalent, with children and adolescents with overweight and obesity frequently experiencing weight-based teasing, victimization, and bullying. These experiences are associated with reduced social engagement, decreased physical activity, greater risk for unhealthy weight control behaviors and binge eating, reduced quality of life, psychosocial impairment, and health care avoidance.[15]

Historically, pediatric obesity care followed a "weight centric" model, which assumed that weight was entirely within the individual's control and emphasized restrictive dieting and increasing physical activity.[16] This model has contributed to pervasive societal weight stigma, which is now recognized as a social determinant of health.

In contrast, a "weight inclusive" model shifts the focus to health and well-being, regardless of weight, and removes weight as a marker of health.[16] This approach emphasizes:

- Creating a welcoming clinical environment for children in larger bodies by providing appropriately sized gowns and chairs and displaying inclusive imagery
- Asking permission to talk about weight
- Using the patient's preferred terminology
- Avoiding moral language around food and bodies ("good" vs. "bad")
- Focusing on non-weight-based outcomes to measure progress (e.g., improvements in blood pressure, lipids, or glucose, increased energy or stamina, better quality of sleep, or improved strength)

Children may receive praise from their family and health care providers for losing weight, regardless of method, which can reinforce unhealthy or disordered behaviors. Clinicians should avoid assuming that disordered eating occurs only among children at lower weights. Eating disorders can occur across the weight spectrum. Given the high rates of disordered eating among youth with obesity, especially those who have experienced weight-based bullying, routine screening for disordered eating throughout treatment of obesity is recommended (see Chapter 23).[17] Warning signs include meal skipping or elimination of certain foods or food groups, excessive focus on weight or food tracking, exercising in a way that feels excessive, and eating in response to emotions like stress or boredom. If any disordered eating behaviors are identified, referral to an interdisciplinary team, including medical and mental health providers, is recommended.

PHARMACOTHERAPY

Until recently, treatment options for pediatric obesity management were limited to IHBLT or bariatric surgery in those with severe obesity. More recently, antiobesity medications (AOMs) have emerged as a treatment option.[18,19] In general, there are fewer U.S. Food and Drug Administration (FDA)-approved options for pediatric patients compared to adults, but the AAP supports the use of some medications in children with obesity that meet age thresholds (see Table 33.3). Importantly, these medications

TABLE 33.3 ANTIOBESITY MEDICATIONS WITH FDA APPROVAL FOR PEDIATRIC PATIENTS

MEDICATION	MECHANISM	FDA-APPROVED INDICATION FOR OBESITY	BMI REDUCTION (kg/m^2)[a]	ADVERSE EFFECTS	CONTRAINDICATIONS
Liraglutide Semaglutide	GLP-1 receptor agonist, delayed gastric emptying, increased satiety, incretin effect	12 y and older	−1.58 −5.88	Nausea, vomiting, abdominal pain, constipation	Personal or Family history of medullary thyroid cancer, multiple endocrine neoplasia (MEN) 2, pregnancy
Orlistat	Intestinal lipase inhibitor	12 y and older	−0.79	Steatorrhea, flatulence, urgency	Pregnancy, malabsorptive disease, cholestasis
Phentermine/ topiramate	NE reuptake inhibitor/ enhanced GABA activity lead to lower appetite	12 y and older	−4.57	Dry mouth, constipation, increased heart rate, insomnia, dysgeusia	MAOI use, pregnancy, glaucoma[a]; avoid if nephrolithiasis, severe anxiety
Setmelanotide	MC4R agonists—regulate hunger, satiety, and energy expenditure	6 y and older with proopiomelanocortin (POMC), proprotein convertasesubtilisin/kexin type 1 (PCSK1), Leptin receptor deficiency, Bardet-Biedl syndrome	−3.4	Nausea, injection site reaction	

GABA, gamma-aminobutyric acid; GLP-1, glucagon-like peptide-1; MAOI, monoamine oxidase inhibitors.
[a]BMI reduction time to follow up varied between 6 and 24 months.

should be used as an adjunct to IHBLT to obtain maximum benefit from these therapies. Current knowledge suggests that discontinuation of these medications will often result in weight regain, especially if lifestyle changes are not established appropriately. Long-term safety and efficacy in pediatric populations remain under investigation.

BARIATRIC SURGERY

For those with greater severity of obesity, with or without comorbidities, IHBLT often only results in modest success. In these cases, timely referral to adolescent bariatric surgery programs is warranted and supported by current guidelines from the AAP.[6] Criteria for referral to an adolescent bariatric surgery program are based on BMI thresholds and presence of obesity-related comorbidities:

- Adolescents 13 years or older with Class 2 obesity (BMI ≥120%-140% of the 95th percentile for age and sex, or 35 kg/m^2 or greater, whichever is lower) AND obesity-related comorbidities such as type 2 diabetes, obstructive sleep apnea, gastroesophageal reflux disease, idiopathic intracranial hypertension, MASLD, cardiovascular disease risks (such as hypertension and dyslipidemia), among others.
- Adolescents 13 years or older with Class 3 obesity (BMI ≥ 140% of the 95th percentile for age and sex, or 40 kg/m^2 or greater, whichever is lower) regardless of the presence of obesity-related comorbidities.

Patient readiness is an important consideration for bariatric surgery. Surgical candidates should be motivated and have a clear understanding of what surgery entails. A supportive family environment is also necessary, especially for patients with syndromic obesity or developmental delays, as these are not considered contraindications to surgery. Other considerations include psychological stability and active treatment for any mental health conditions, absence of active substance use or binge eating behaviors, adherence to all preoperative evaluations and protocols, no current or planned pregnancy, and exclusion of medically correctable causes of obesity.[20] Completion of linear growth is no longer required, as current evidence does not support a negative impact on puberty or linear growth following surgery.

The two main surgical procedures currently performed in adolescents in the United States are the Roux en Y gastric bypass (RYGB) and sleeve gastrectomy (SG). These are performed in a minimally invasive manner through laparoscopy. BMI reduction for the two procedures is comparable at 20.6% for RYGB and 19.2% for SG. Data from the Teen Longitudinal Assessment of Bariatric Surgery (Teen-LABS) show that at 10 years, rates of resolution of type 2 diabetes, hypertension, and dyslipidemia average around 55%, 57%, and 54% of individuals, respectively.[21] Although weight regain can occur, outcomes of BMI reduction, in general, match those in adults, but adolescents tend to have better and more durable rates of resolution of obesity-related comorbidities.[22] The best outcomes exist for those who continue with ongoing IHBLT postoperatively.

Presurgical preparation aligns with principles of IHBLT, including nutritional modifications and increase in physical activity. In addition, patients are educated on perioperative and postoperative diets, as well as postoperative nutritional risks, including protein and micronutrient deficiencies and risk of dehydration. A hypocaloric diet, often in the form of liquid meal replacements, is usually prescribed 2 weeks prior to surgery to promote weight loss, which can reduce hepatic fat content. This results in easier hiatal visualization during surgery due to easier mobilization of the left hepatic lobe.

Following the surgery, advancement of diet toward regular textures occurs in a stepwise fashion as surgical sites heal.

Micronutrient monitoring should occur preoperatively and, at least annually, postoperatively. Preoperatively, vitamin D and iron deficiencies are common. Micronutrient deficiencies after surgery occur due to a combination of decreased absorption due to new anatomy and inadequate intake due to lower volumes of food consumed. RYGB carries a higher risk of deficiencies than SG. The most common nutritional deficiencies that occur postoperatively include thiamine, iron, vitamin B_{12}, vitamin A, vitamin D, and zinc. Lifelong multivitamin supplementation is typically required, with some deficiencies requiring higher treatment doses than used in patients that have not had surgery. Iron and vitamin B_{12} deficiencies can require parenteral treatment; for vitamin B_{12} deficiency, supplementation via the sublingual route is also possible.[20,23,24]

ENDOBARIATRICS

Endobariatrics is an emerging field offering less invasive alternatives to pharmacotherapy or bariatric surgery in adults. These endoscopic procedures aim to reduce BMI through mechanisms including restriction (such as intragastric balloon placement or endoscopic sleeve gastroplasty), aspiration (using a gastrostomy with aspirator), and malabsorption (e.g., by placement of a duodenal-jejunal bypass liner). Total body weight loss with these procedures typically ranges from 10% to 20%.[25] Similar outcomes are reported in limited pediatric studies, although these procedures are currently not FDA approved for use in pediatric patients in the United States.

REFERENCES

1. Stierman B, Afful J, Carroll MD, et al. National Health and Nutrition Examination survey 2017-March 2020 prepandemic data files-development of files and prevalence estimates for selected health outcomes. *Natl Health Stat Report*. 2021;(158).
2. World Health Organization. Obesity and overweight. 2024. Accessed December 10, 2024. https://www.who.int/news-room/fact-sheets/detail/obesity-and-overweight
3. Perng W, Conway R, Mayer-Davis E, Dabelea D. Youth-onset type 2 diabetes: the epidemiology of an awakening epidemic. *Diabetes Care*. 2023;46(3):490-499.
4. Taveras EM, Perkins M, Woo Baidal JA, et al. The impact of the first 1,000 days on childhood obesity. Healthy Eating Research. 2016. https://healthyeatingresearch.org/wp-content/uploads/2016/03/her_1000_days_final-1.pdf
5. Garvey WT. Is obesity or adiposity-based chronic disease curable: the set point theory, the environment, and second-generation medications. *Endocr Pract*. 2022;28(2):214-222.
6. Hampl SE, Hassink SG, Skinner AC, et al. Clinical practice guideline for the evaluation and treatment of children and adolescents with obesity. *Pediatrics*. 2023;151(2):e2022060640.
7. Lawrence JM, Divers J, Isom S, et al. Trends in prevalence of type 1 and type 2 diabetes in children and adolescents in the US, 2001-2017. *JAMA*. 2021;326(8):717-727.
8. Jackson SL, Zhang Z, Wiltz JL, et al. Hypertension among youths—United States, 2001-2016. *MMWR Morb Mortal Wkly Rep*. 2018;67(27):758-762.
9. Rupasinghe K, Hind J, Hegarty R. Updates in metabolic dysfunction-associated fatty liver disease (MAFLD) in children. *J Pediatr Gastroenterol Nutr*. 2023;77(5):583-591.
10. Tamini S, Caroli D, Bondesan A, Abbruzzese L, Sartorio A. Measured vs estimated resting energy expenditure in children and adolescents with obesity. *Sci Rep*. 2023;13(1):13178.
11. Mehta NM, Skillman HE, Irving SY, et al. Guidelines for the provision and assessment of nutrition support therapy in the pediatric critically ill patient: Society of Critical Care Medicine and American Society for Parenteral and Enteral Nutrition. *JPEN J Parenter Enteral Nutr*. 2017;41(5):706-742.
12. Kittisakmontri K, Fewtrell M. Impact of complementary feeding on obesity risk. *Curr Opin Clin Nutr Metab Care*. 2023;26(3):266-272.

13. Bergamini M, Simeone G, Verga MC, et al. Complementary feeding caregivers' practices and growth, risk of overweight/obesity, and other non-communicable diseases: a systematic review and meta-analysis. *Nutrients*. 2022;14(13):2646.
14. Miller WR, Rollnick S. *Motivational Interviewing: Helping People Change*. Guilford Publications; 2012.
15. Haqq AM, Kebbe M, Tan Q, Manco M, Salas XR. Complexity and stigma of pediatric obesity. *Child Obes*. 2021;17(4):229-240.
16. Mauldin K, May M, Clifford D. The consequences of a weight-centric approach to healthcare: a case for a paradigm shift in how clinicians address body weight. *Nutr Clin Pract*. 2022;37(6):1291-1306.
17. Sonneville KR, Thurston IB, Milliren CE, Gooding HC, Richmond TK. Weight misperception among young adults with overweight/obesity associated with disordered eating behaviors. *Int J Eat Disord*. 2016;49(10):937-946.
18. Torbahn G, Jones A, Griffiths A, et al. Pharmacological interventions for the management of children and adolescents living with obesity—an update of a Cochrane systematic review with meta-analyses. *Pediatr Obes*. 2024;19(5):e13113.
19. Haqq AM, Chung WK, Dollfus H, et al. Efficacy and safety of setmelanotide, a melanocortin-4 receptor agonist, in patients with Bardet-Biedl syndrome and Alström syndrome: a multicentre, randomised, double-blind, placebo-controlled, phase 3 trial with an open-label period. *Lancet Diabetes Endocrinol*. 2022;10(12):859-868.
20. Pratt JSA, Browne A, Browne NT, et al. ASMBS pediatric metabolic and bariatric surgery guidelines, 2018. *Surg Obes Relat Dis*. 2018;14(7):882-901.
21. Ryder JR, Jenkins TM, Xie C, et al. Ten-year outcomes after bariatric surgery in adolescents. *N Engl J Med*. 2024;391(17):1656-1658.
22. Beamish AJ, Ryan Harper E, Järvholm K, Janson A, Olbers T. Long-term outcomes following adolescent metabolic and bariatric surgery. *J Clin Endocrinol Metab*. 2023;108(9):2184-2192.
23. Mechanick JI, Apovian C, Brethauer S, et al. Clinical practice guidelines for the perioperative nutrition, metabolic, and nonsurgical support of patients undergoing bariatric procedures—2019 update: cosponsored by American Association of Clinical Endocrinologists/American College of Endocrinology, The Obesity Society, American Society for Metabolic and Bariatric Surgery, Obesity Medicine Association, and American Society of Anesthesiologists. *Obesity (Silver Spring)*. 2020;28(4):O1-O58.
24. Xanthakos SA, Khoury JC, Inge TH, et al. Nutritional risks in adolescents after bariatric surgery. *Clin Gastroenterol Hepatol*. 2020;18(5):1070-1081.e5.
25. Lahooti A, Johnson KE, Sharaiha RZ. The future of endobariatrics: bridging the gap. *Gastrointest Endosc Clin N Am*. 2024;34(4):805-818.

CHAPTER 34

Oncology and Stem Cell Transplant

Lauren Oliveira, Sarah Goldman, and Erin Gordon

INTRODUCTION

It is estimated that more than 400,000 children and adolescents under the age of 20 develop cancer annually worldwide. Approximately 10% of children with cancer have a genetic predisposition; however, most childhood cancers do not have a known cause. Cancer is a leading cause of death for children and adolescents, and survival rates vary greatly depending on access to treatment. In high-income countries, survival rates are more than 80%. In low- and middle-income countries, survival rates can be less than 30%.[1] In the United States, leukemias, brain and other central nervous system malignant tumors, and lymphomas are the most common types of cancer. However, both the type and frequency of diagnosis vary by age as well as race and ethnicity.[2]

Nutritional status, including both under- and overnutrition, impacts clinical outcomes. Changes in nutritional status can occur prior to and/or during diagnosis, throughout treatment, and after treatment has concluded. Poor nutritional status can lead to increased risk of infection, altered pharmacokinetics, poor quality of life, greater risk of relapse, increased risk of comorbidities, and increased mortality.[3-5] Nutrition goals during cancer treatment and cancer survivorship should focus on the unique growth and development goals of childhood and adolescence, optimize quality of life, and prioritize patient and family-centered care while balancing the physical and emotional impacts of cancer treatment on the child.

NUTRITION RISK FACTORS OF CANCER TREATMENT

The most common types of treatments* include chemotherapy, surgery, and/or radiotherapy. Treatment for refractory or high-risk cancer may include hematopoietic stem cell transplantation (HSCT). Pending the cancer type and stage, many patients require a combination of treatment agents and approaches. Side effects of cancer treatment as well as the manifestations of the disease itself can cause nutritional complications. Disruptions in dietary intake, physical activity, and altered growth (either unintentional weight loss or weight gain) are significant risk factors that can occur.

Treatment-related side effects such as gastrointestinal (GI) toxicity resulting in mucositis, nausea, and emesis, may lead to reduced dietary intake and subsequent weight loss and/or nutrient deficiencies. Medications such as corticosteroids may result in fluid retention, changes to emotional regulation, and changes to hunger/satiety cues, resulting in unintentional weight gain. Prolonged hospitalizations and treatment/disease-related fatigue may impact a young person's ability to be physically active and engage in healthy lifestyle habits, resulting in disruptions to both physical and mental

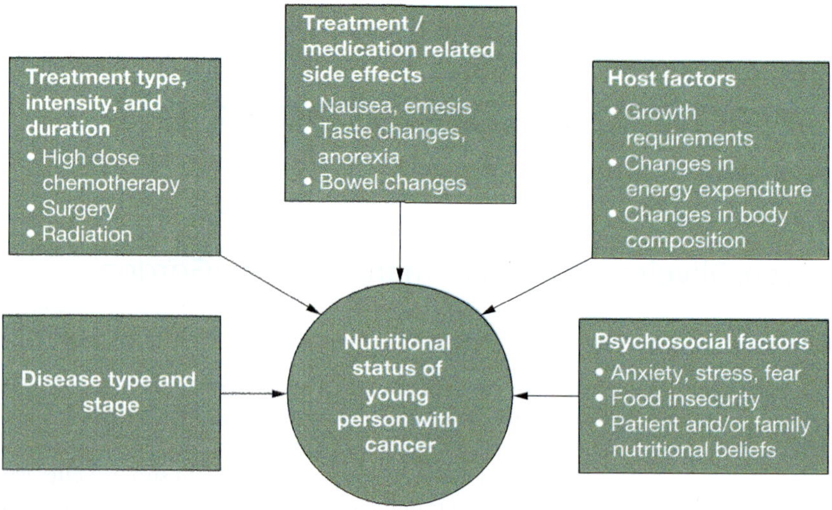

Figure 34.1 Factors impacting nutrition status in pediatric cancer.

developmental milestones. Often, these disruptions nutritional in intake and growth precipitate the need for some degree of nutrition intervention—including oral, enteral, and parenteral nutrition support, in addition to consistent nutritional education and counseling by a registered dietitian (Figure 34.1).

SPECIAL ASPECTS OF NUTRITIONAL ASSESSMENT

Conducting a Nutritional assessment (see Chapters 1-4) is a multifaceted process essential for identifying and addressing the unique dietary and metabolic needs of children and adolescents undergoing cancer treatment and/or HSCT. A comprehensive nutritional assessment should be conducted by a trained nutrition clinician and should include at minimum the following: a thorough anthropometric history, a detailed diet history including vitamin/mineral supplementation as well as use of any traditional and complementary medicine(s) (T&CM), symptom history, as well as current diagnosis and treatment status.

Biochemical assessment and nutrition-related lab work may be necessary pending the results of a detailed diet history to assess for electrolyte disorders, altered visceral protein markers, micronutrient deficiencies or inflammatory markers. A nutrition-focused physical exam (NFPE) should be performed to assess baseline muscle and fat stores, edema, and signs of micronutrient deficiencies. Fluid retention, hyperhydration, tumor mass burden, amputations, and changes in body composition due to medications can all influence weight status during treatment. As a result, monitoring mid-upper arm circumference (MUAC) provides a reliable method for assessing nutritional status. If available, assessment of body composition using tools such as bioelectrical impedance analysis (BIA), computed tomography (CT), or dual-energy X-ray absorptiometry (DEXA) may be beneficial to better assess changes.

Indirect calorimetry remains the gold standard for estimating energy needs. In the absence of indirect calorimetry, resting energy expenditure (REE) and estimated energy requirements (EER) should be calculated using pediatric comparative standard equations outlined in Chapter 5. Some children and adolescents undergoing cancer treatment may experience periods where they are hypermetabolic while some may experience hypometabolism—commonly seen, for example, in young people undergoing HSCT. Consistent evaluation of growth patterns and dietary intake in addition to frequent adjustment of EER is essential.

Patients with a new cancer diagnosis may be at risk for experiencing tumor lysis syndrome, the rapid breakdown of large numbers of cancer cells that often occurs after the initiation of cancer treatment. With tumor cell breakdown, hyperkalemia, hyperphosphatemia, hypocalcemia, and hyperuricemia can ensue, causing metabolic disturbances that can be life-threatening. Special attention is needed in the evaluation of biochemical markers to elicit what values may be nutrition related versus treatment or disease related.

SPECIAL ASPECTS OF NUTRITIONAL MANAGEMENT

Oral Nutrition

Ensuring an adequate oral diet that aligns with The Dietary Guidelines for Americans is essential for pediatric oncology patients to support age-appropriate growth and development.[6] However, the common side effects of cancer treatment often impact the ability to do so. Oral nutrition supplements can be an effective option for those who struggle to meet their nutritional needs from food alone. These supplements are specially formulated to deliver concentrated amounts of energy, protein, vitamins, and minerals, making them a valuable tool for addressing malnutrition and enhancing recovery during treatment. There are many additional strategies for improving oral intake during cancer treatment (Table 34.1).

Enteral Nutrition

If a child is unable to maintain their nutritional status through oral intake alone, enteral nutrition (EN) is the preferred method for supplementation prior to the consideration of parenteral nutrition (PN).[7] Education regarding the use of EN during cancer treatment should be discussed with the child and caregiver(s) proactively to increase acceptance of this intervention.[7]

Children with cancer may have difficulty tolerating standard/intact protein or calorically dense formulas due to GI symptoms commonly associated with treatment and may therefore benefit from extensively hydrolyzed or elemental formulas.[8] Determining feeding volume and schedule should be individualized; however, a continuous feeding regimen may be better tolerated than bolus feeds in children with GI symptoms.[8,9] Nocturnal continuous feeds in combination with daytime oral or bolus feeds may work well to meet nutrition needs while still promoting oral-motor development skills and providing a more common lifestyle pattern. If GI symptoms such as intractable nausea and/or vomiting persist, postpyloric feeds may help improve EN tolerance.[8,9] Refer to Chapter 16, for EN indications and contraindications.

TABLE 34.1 STRATEGIES FOR IMPROVING ORAL INTAKE DURING CANCER TREATMENT

Loss of Appetite and Early Satiety	• Small, frequent meals and snacks • High-calorie foods and additives incorporated into snacks, meals, and beverages
Nausea and Vomiting	• Small, frequent meals • Slow-paced eating • Dry, salty, bland foods • Cool liquids between meals • Ginger and/or lemon • Avoid strong odors
Diarrhea	• Bland (non-spicy or greasy) foods • Increase fluid intake • Cold or room temperature foods and beverages • Limit lactose and/or gas forming foods
Constipation	• Increase fluid intake • Consume fiber-rich foods • Encourage ambulation • Pharmacotherapy such as laxatives
Mucositis	• Soft, bland foods • Foods/drinks that are cool or room temperature • Moisten foods with liquids or sauces • Avoid hard, rough, salty, sour/acidic, and spicy foods
Altered Taste and Smell	• Use stronger seasonings and add sauces to foods • Use plastic utensils to eliminate potential metallic taste of metal utensils • Offer cold foods/dishes to reduce odor • Cook with exhaust fans or open windows in your home • Remove hot plate covers outside of the room
Malnutrition (Unintentional Weight Loss)	• Small, frequent meals and snacks • High-calorie and protein-rich drinks, shakes, oral nutrition supplements • Keep foods readily available • Language usage, treat food as medicine

Parenteral Nutrition

The use of PN in pediatric oncology and HSCT patients is well accepted. Common indications for PN in the oncology/HSCT population include typhlitis (neutropenic colitis), severe mucositis with associated enteral intolerance (large volume stool output and abdominal pain), and veno-occlusive disease (VOD) with associated abdominal competition and bowel obstruction. Special consideration for PN in oncology/HSCT patients include fluid status and electrolye derrangements associated with end-organ dysfunction, medication side effects, among other causes. Measures of REE in the weeks after allogeneic HSCT suggest a degree of hypometabolism, so overfeeding should be avoided. More details of PN management are outlined in Chapter 17.

TRADITIONAL AND COMPLEMENTARY MEDICINE

Many patients, families, and caregivers inquire about and/or use nutritional T&CM during their cancer journey. These may include the use of bioactive compounds, supplements, herbs, as well as dietary approaches. Commonly requested products include, but are not limited to, pre- and probiotics, antioxidants, and use of specific vitamins and/or foods such as papaya, beets, or honey. Commonly requested diets include, but are not limited to, the ketogenic or "low-sugar" diets, plant-based diets, or "whole-foods" diets. There is a lack of evidence supporting the effectiveness of these approaches in treating the side effects of the disease and/or treatment.[10] Despite the lack of evidence, many patients and families are at least interested in learning more about T&CM approaches. Unfortunately, fewer than half of families using T&CM disclose what they are using to the child's medical team.[10]

In the United States, dietary T&CM products are classified as dietary supplements and therefore have less stringent regulations, leading to increased variability in the availability, quality, and labeling of such products. Additionally, there is limited research on the use of such products and any potential interactions with chemotherapy that may result in unknown side effects, increased treatment toxicity, or reduced treatment efficacy.[10] It is important to establish rapport and trust with the patient and caregiver(s) to understand their goals, especially as it pertains to T&CM. The use of T&CM should be interdisciplinary and involve the oncologist, an oncology pharmacist, and the registered dietitian. It may be beneficial to have a member of the psychosocial team as part of these discussions as well.

HEMATOPOIETIC STEM CELL TRANSPLANT

Hematopoietic stem cell transplantation (HSCT) can be used to treat certain types of cancer, immune dysregulation, and nonmalignant hematologic disorders. Most commonly, patients will undergo either an allogeneic HSCT (donation from an individual) or an autologous HSCT (donation from self). Most HSCT patients start the "HSCT diet" on day 0 (day of transplant) or if their absolute neutrophil count (ANC) is less than 500 prior to day 0 as this is when the ANC is expected to decline and patients are at the highest risk for infection. See Table 34.2 for details. Patients undergoing an autologous transplant remain on the HSCT diet for approximately 60 days. Patients undergoing an allogenic transplant will remain on this diet for approximately 6 months. It is recommended that HSCT patients follow food safety guidelines as outlined by the Centers for Disease Control and Prevention (CDC) (Table 34.3).[11]

Human milk-fed patients who are admitted for an allogeneic transplant cannot receive unprocessed human milk beginning day –5 of conditioning. Lymphocytes in human milk could potentially cross and disrupt the GI barrier, increasing the risk of developing graft versus host disease (GVHD) in immune-compromised patients. After day –5, patients may receive irradiated human milk orally or enterally through day + 42 or discharge, whichever is first. Infants undergoing an autologous stem cell transplant are excluded from this and are able to remain on untreated human milk throughout their transplant course.

During the initial days of HSCT, while patients are awaiting engraftment, patients are often unable to meet their nutrition needs orally due to treatment-related

TABLE 34.2 FOOD PLAN AFTER HEMATOPOIETIC STEM CELL TRANSPLANT

FOOD GROUP	FOODS ALLOWED	FOODS NOT ALLOWED
Meat, Poultry, Eggs, and Seafood	• Meats, poultry, and seafood cooked to safe internal temperatures • Hot dogs, lunch, and deli meats heated until steaming hot before eating (temperature should be 165 °F/73.8 °C) • Pasteurized eggs and egg products	• Raw or undercooked meat, poultry, or seafood • Smoked meats (like salmon/lox) • Unpasteurized meat spreads or pates • Foods with raw eggs (including homemade Caesar dressing, homemade mayonnaise, homemade eggnog, and cookie dough)
Milk and Milk Products	• Pasteurized milk and milk products • Hard cheeses • Processed/pasteurized cheeses (like cheddar, mozzarella, cream cheese)	• Unpasteurized milk and milk products • Unpasteurized or soft cheeses made from (raw) milk such as queso fresco, blue-veined, feta, brie, and camembert
Fruits and Vegetables	• Washed fresh vegetables, including lettuce/salads • Cooked sprouts • Washed fruits with thin skins • Thick-skinned fruits (like oranges, melon, kiwi)	• Unwashed fresh vegetables, including lettuce/salads • Raw alfalfa and bean sprouts • Unwashed fresh fruits
Juices, Drinks, and Water	• Bottled water (recommended while in hospital) • City water, including tap water (on discharge) • Well water boiled for at least 2 min	• Unpasteurized cider or juices • Ice from communal ice machines
Other	• Restaurant food (including fast food and food from takeout, drive-through, and delivery) • Commercially packaged honey	• Prepared salads • Unpasteurized honey

TABLE 34.3 FOOD SAFETY GUIDELINES AS PER CDC RECOMMENDATIONS

- Clean: Wash hands and surfaces often.
- Separate: Separate raw meat from other foods.
- Cook: Cook to the right temperature.
- Chill: Refrigerate foods right away.
- Never buy food displayed in unclean conditions.
- Avoid buffet-style foods, including salad bars.
- Do not buy produce that is bruised or damaged.
- Do not consume canned food from cans with dents, cracks, or bulging lids (clean lids once home).
- Do not leave cooked food out of the refrigerator or oven for more than 60 min.
- Throw away leftover cooked foods after 2 days. When ordering restaurant food, do not hesitate to ask questions about how the food is prepared.

toxicities such as mucositis, nausea, and emesis. Enteral access is ideally obtained prior to the development of mucositis to support nutritional needs during this acute phase of transplant. If patients are unable to tolerate enteral feeds or have GI toxicity where EN is contraindicated, HSCT patients may require PN support. Once patients are engrafted, defined as an ANC greater than 500 for 3 consecutive days, treatment-induced mucositis and GI toxicity often improve, leading to better tolerance of oral and enteral feedings.

LATE EFFECTS AND SURVIVORSHIP

As advances continue both in treatment and supportive care options, the numbers of childhood cancer survivors (CCS) are increasing. However, the late effects of cancer treatment have led to a higher burden of chronic health conditions among CCS. The most common treatment-related late effects are endocrinopathies, including diabetes mellitus and metabolic syndrome, which, in turn, are risk factors for cardiovascular disease—one of the leading causes of late mortality in CCS.[12,13]

Diet and physical activity are major contributors to metabolic disease, type 2 diabetes mellitus, and cardiovascular disease. They are also modifiable and therefore have the potential to prevent or delay onset of these chronic diseases in CCS. All CCS should undergo regular nutritional screening as part of their survivorship care and should have access to a registered dietitian for ongoing education and counseling as needed.

CONCLUSION

The importance of nutrition during and after cancer treatment has become increasingly known. Effective and timely nutritional screening followed by comprehensive nutritional assessments and reassessments at regular intervals throughout treatment and into survivorship can help assure appropriate growth and development while optimizing quality of life. While preventing nutritional concerns before they emerge continues to be the foundation of pediatric nutrition oncology, providers must work collaboratively with the patient, family/caregiver, and interdisciplinary care team to adapt to the dynamic challenges that can occur throughout cancer treatment and into survivorship.

REFERENCES

1. World Health Organization. Childhood cancer [Fact sheet]. https://www.who.int/news-room/fact-sheets/detail/cancer-in-children
2. National Cancer Institute. Cancer in Children and Adolescents [Fact sheet]. https://www.cancer.gov/types/childhood-cancers/child-adolescent-cancers-fact-sheet
3. Rogers PC, Barr RD. The relevance of nutrition to pediatric oncology: a cancer control perspective. *Pediatr Blood Cancer*. 2020;67(suppl 3):e28213.
4. Barr RD, Stevens MCG. The influence of nutrition on clinical outcomes in children with cancer. *Pediatr Blood Cancer*. 2020;67(suppl 3):e28117.
5. Loeffen EA, Brinksma A, Miedema KG, de Bock GH, Tissing WJ. Clinical implications of malnutrition in childhood cancer patients—infections and mortality. *Support Care Cancer*. 2015;23(1):143-150.
6. U.S. Department of Agriculture and U.S. Department of Health and Human Services. *Dietary Guidelines for Americans, 2020-2025*. 9th ed. DietaryGuidelines.gov; 2020.

7. Mu Muscaritoli M, Arends J, Bachmann P, et al. ESPEN practical guideline: clinical nutrition in cancer. *Clin Nutr.* 2021;40(5):2898-2913.
8. Ladas EJ, Sacks N, Meacham L, et al. A multidisciplinary review of nutrition considerations in the pediatric oncology population: a perspective from children's oncology group. *Nutr Clin Pract.* 2005;20(4):377-393.
9. Trehan A, Viani K, da Cruz LB, Sagastizado SZ, Ladas EJ. The importance of enteral nutrition to prevent or treat undernutrition in children undergoing treatment for cancer. *Pediatr Blood Cancer.* 2020;67(suppl 3):e28378.
10. Diorio C, Kelly KM, Afungchwi GM, Ladas EJ, Marjerrison S. Nutritional traditional and complementary medicine strategies in pediatric cancer: a narrative review. *Pediatr Blood Cancer.* 2020;67(suppl 3):e28324.
11. Center for Disease Control and Prevention. Food safety: about four steps to food safety. 2024. www.cdc.gov/food-safety/
12. Cohen J, Collins L, Gregerson L, Chandra J, Cohn RJ. Nutritional concerns of survivors of childhood cancer: a "First World" perspective. *Pediatr Blood Cancer.* 2020;67(suppl 3):e28193.
13. Esbenshade AJ, Lu L, Friedman DL, et al. Accumulation of chronic disease among survivors of childhood cancer predicts early mortality. *J Clin Oncol.* 2023;41(20):3629-3641.

CHAPTER 35

Prematurity

Yvette Penner, Lindsay Boland, and Madeline Keyes

Globally, more than one in four of all live births are newborns small for gestational age, of low birthweight, or preterm, and these "small vulnerable newborns" account for more than 1 million deaths yearly. The preterm infant (<37 weeks gestation) is born with limited nutrient stores, the highest nutrient demands (per kg) in the lifecycle, and organ system immaturity that present substantial challenges for replicating in utero growth and development (Table 35.1). Complications of prematurity such as osteopenia, anemia, and respiratory distress add to metabolic demand and some, like necrotizing enterocolitis (NEC), disrupt nutrient delivery (Table 35.2). Multidisciplinary teams in neonatal intensive care units (NICU) strive to optimize growth and nutrient delivery despite these challenges to ensure optimal developmental, cardiometabolic, body composition, and overall health outcomes.[1]

NUTRITIONAL ASSESSMENT

The nutritional assessment of preterm infants begins immediately after birth with the measurements of birth weight, length, and head circumference. These anthropometrics provide the basis for nutrient needs and growth expectations (Table 35.3).

TABLE 35.1 NUTRITIONAL RISK FACTORS IN PREMATURITY

Increased nutritional demands

- Rapid growth phase
- Metabolic stresses of medical/surgical course
- Cold stress/energy demand of thermoregulation
- Lower bioavailability of enteral nutrients compared to direct placental transport

Immature organ function

- GI immaturity—intestinal hypomotility and reduced digestive enzyme activity impairs feeding tolerance and nutrient absorption
- Liver immaturity—risk for hypoglycemia and cholestasis
- Renal immaturity—urinary loss of electrolytes and bicarbonate
- Bone marrow immaturity—lower erythropoietic responsiveness to hypoxia
- Integumentary immaturity—thin skin may result in higher insensible fluid losses

Inadequate nutrient stores

- Cessation of placental nourishment interrupts fetal accretion
- Lower fat, muscle, and glycogen stores
- Iatrogenic nutrient deficits
  - Feeds held for procedures, NEC, clinical instability, blood transfusions
  - Incomplete nutrient delivery during PN/enteral feeding advancement
  - Medication-related nutrient losses

GI, gastrointestinal; NEC, necrotizing enterocolitis; PN, parenteral nutrition.

TABLE 35.2 MEDICAL RISK FACTORS OF PREMATURITY AND THEIR NUTRITIONAL IMPLICATIONS

Necrotizing enterocolitis (NEC)

- Acquired infectious/ischemic GI disease of undetermined etiology, most common in preterm infants
- Ranges from mild feeding intolerance to pneumatosis intestinalis to necrotic bowel with perforation
- Treatment includes NPO, IV antibiotics, PN, gradual re-introduction of feeds

Respiratory Distrdistress syndrome (RDS)/bronchopulmonary dysplasia (BPD)

- Chronic lung disease secondary to reduced surfactant, extended mechanical ventilation and/or O_2 support
- Can increase energy demands (especially in acute phase)
- May require fluid restriction and subsequent increase in energy density of feedings
- Steroids used in treatment may impede growth
- Increased risk of osteopenia (mineral wasting from steroids and diuretics)
- Severe/chronic disease may result in altered body composition (poor linear growth, excess adipose tissue)
- May require long-term enteral access (poor oral feeding with increased work of breathing, oral aversion with prolonged intubation)

Patent ductus arteriosus (PDA)

- Connection between pulmonary artery and aorta fails to close within 72 h of birth.
- May lead to reversed flow of oxygenated blood resulting in inadequate intestinal perfusion and pulmonary edema
- Treatment ranges from monitoring to medications to transcatheter/surgical closure.
- May require fluid restriction and subsequent increase in energy density of feedings or even NPO and PN if hemodynamically unstable

Osteopenia of prematurity

- Ranges from mild bone demineralization to nontraumatic fractures
- Due to interrupted transplacental mineral transport, inadequate provision of mineral substrate, reduced mechanical bone stimulation in the extrauterine environment
- May impair linear growth.
- Increased risk with immobility, medications that cause mineral excretion (diuretics, steroids), long-term PN (due to limited calcium/phosphorus solubility of solution and inherent aluminum content)
- May require vitamin D, calcium, and/or phosphorus supplementation

Anemia of prematurity

- Low number of red blood cells that can result in inadequate tissue oxygenation
- Due to interrupted transplacental iron transport, inadequate iron stores, iatrogenic phlebotomy, shorter lifespan of fetal hemoglobin, reduced EPO responsiveness
- Treatment involves PRBCs, iron supplementation, minimizing phlebotomy as able

Developmental delay

- Multifactorial etiology: genetic, intraventricular hemorrhage, medications, long-term hospitalization, inadequate nutrition provision/growth faltering
- Can impair oral intake; long-term enteral access may be needed

EPO, erythropoietin; GI, gastrointestinal; IV, intravenous; NPO, nil per os; O_2, oxygen; PN, parenteral nutrition; PRBC, packed red blood cell.

TABLE 35.3 PREMATURITY AND BIRTH WEIGHT CLASSIFICATIONS

Maturity by gestational age (GA)

- Preterm: <37 wk
  - Extremely—moderately preterm: <34 0/7 wk
  - Late preterm: 34 0/7-36 6/7 wk
- Term: 37 0/7-41 6/7 wk
- Postterm: >42 0/7 wk

Birth weight

- Low birth weight (LBW): <2500 g
- Very low birth weight (VLBW): <1500 g
- Extremely low birth weight (ELBW): <1000 g

Birth weight for gestational age

- Small for gestational age (SGA): <10th percentile
- Appropriate for gestational age (AGA): 10th-90th percentile
- Large for gestational age (LGA): >90th percentile

Intrauterine growth charts (Fenton or Olsen) should be used to assess whether the infant is small for gestational age (SGA), appropriate for gestational age (AGA), or large for gestational age (LGA) and can be used until at least 42 weeks postmenstrual age (PMA).[2-4] The most recent intrauterine chart was published in 2025[4]—an update to the Fenton 2013 charts.[3] The "gold standard" for postnatal growth of preterm infants remains the expected rate of weight gain seen in utero (Table 35.4).[2] However, this model does not account for physiologic auto-diuresis (the expected fluid loss and extra- to intracellular fluid shift that occurs in the first 1 to 2 weeks of postnatal life) (Table 35.5). Disregarding this expected loss of fluid weight may promote nutritional strategies that result in rapid weight gain (primarily as adipose tissue). Determining the change in weight-for-age z-score since birth augments the growth assessment by distinguishing between a "healthful" decline in z-score and growth faltering.[2] The INTERGROWTH-21st charts do take this phenomenon into account, but they are limited by a small sample size at the lowest gestational ages.[2] Weight- and length-for-age z-score changes are included as part of the neonatal malnutrition assessment;[5] however, these criteria have not yet been consistently validated to predict neurodevelopmental or neurodisability outcomes at all levels of malnutrition. Weight-for-length z-scores are not available for preterm infants. Body mass index (BMI) z-scores are

TABLE 35.4 GROWTH VELOCITY TARGETS (AFTER INITIAL DIURESIS)

WEIGHT	TARGET WEIGHT GAIN	TARGET LENGTH GAIN	TARGET HC GAIN
<2000 g	18-22 g/kg/d	1.2-1.4 cm/wk	0.9-1 cm/wk
2000-2500 g	30-35 g/d	1.2-1.4 cm/wk	0.7-0.9 cm/wk
>2500 g	30-35 g/d	1.0-1.3 cm/wk	0.5-0.8 cm/wk

After PMA of 40 weeks—weight gain may be similar to that of FT infant.
FT, full term; HC, head circumference; PMA, postmenstrual age.

TABLE 35.5 FLUID AND PARENTERAL NUTRITION IN PRETERM INFANTS

Fluid

- Preterm infants have greater ECF volumes, and body weight is a greater percentage of fluid compared with term infants.
- Initial physiologic diuresis occurs within the first week of life with 10%-15% loss of body weight for preterm infants, can be up to 20% for ELBW.
- Fluids are initiated and gradually advanced over the first 72 h of life with increasing urine output.

INITIATION AND ADVANCEMENT OF FLUIDS

BIRTH WEIGHT (G)	AGE (HOURS OF LIFE)		
	<24 h	*24-48 h*	*>72 h*
<1000 g	100-150 mL/kg/d	120-160 mL/kg/d	140-190 mL/kg/d
1000-1500 g	80-100 mL/kg/d	100-120 mL/kg/d	120-160 mL/kg/d
>1500 g	60-80 mL/kg/d	80-120 mL/kg/d	100-150 mL/kg/d

- Fluid restrictions may be required in cardiac or lung disease, PDA, neuromuscular blockade.
- Increased insensible and sensible losses may increase fluid requirements.
  - Insensible losses higher with increased skin permeability at low gestational ages, increased BSA to weight ratio, phototherapy, radiant warmer beds, respiratory distress syndrome, cold stress, and increased activity
  - Sensible fluid losses higher with vomiting, diarrhea, and ostomy, or drain output

Carbohydrate

- Initial GIR minimum to ensure adequate glucose supply is 4-6 mg/kg/min.
  - In infants <1000 g advance GIR by 1-1.5 mg/kg/min as tolerated
  - In infants >1000 g advance GIR by 1-2 mg/kg/min as tolerated
- Limit to GIR to <14 mg/kg/min to prevent overfeeding, fatty liver, CO_2 production.
- May require >14 mg/kg/min if on 1 g/kg/d IV lipid restriction to meet energy needs.

Protein

- In infants <1500 g BW: begin at 2-3 g/kg/d, advance to goal of 3.5-4 g/kg/d
- In infants >1500 g BW: begin at 2 g/kg/d, advance to goal of 3-3.5 g/kg/d

Fat

- Begin at 1 g/kg/d and advance by 1 g/kg/d to goal of 3 g/kg/d (soy and mixed oil emulsions)
- Soybean oil lipid or mixed oil emulsion if anticipated PN duration or limited EN exposure for <2-3 wk
- If anticipated PN duration or limited EN exposure is >2-3 wk, consider maintaining 1-2 g/kg/d soybean oil or a mixed lipid emulsion at 3 g/kg/d.
- For infants with established IFALD, consider switching to a fish oil lipid emulsion at 1 g/kg/d. Higher doses are under investigation.
- May run lipid via central or peripheral access, over 12-24 h.
- Monitor tolerance with serum triglycerides; serum levels <250 mg/dL are acceptable.
- EFAD may occur in <1 wk without lipid source; provide minimum 0.5 g/kg/d soy oil emulsion to prevent deficiency.

Energy

- <1000 g: 100-115 kcal/kg/d
- 1000-1500 g: 90-110 kcal/kg/d
- 1500-2000 g: 90-100 kcal/kg/d
- 2000-2500 g: 90-105 kcal/kg/d

TABLE 35.5 FLUID AND PARENTERAL NUTRITION IN PRETERM INFANTS (*continued*)

Electrolytes

	INITIAL DOSE (DAY 0)	TRANSITION DOSE	GROWING PRETERM
Sodium (mEq/kg/d)	0-1	2-5	3-5
Potassium (mEq/kg/d)	0	1-2	2-4
Calcium (mEq/kg/d)	1-2	2-3	3
Phosphorus (mmol/kg/d)	0.7-1.3	1.3-2	1.3-2
Magnesium (mEq/kg/d)	0-0.4	0.2-0.3	0.2-0.3
Chloride (mEq/kg/d)	0-1	2-7	2-7
Acetate (mEq/kg/d)		As needed	

Additional dosing considerations:

- Sodium: Infants with renal immaturity or high GI losses may need closer to 5-8 mEq/kg.
- Magnesium: If mother received antenatal magnesium sulfate, infant may have elevated levels for 5+ days of life.
- Calcium: Ca/Phos ratio of 2.2-2.6 mEq Ca: 1 mmol phos (minimum 1.6 mEq calcium: 1 mMol phos) is ideal to promote bone mineralization.
- Acetate: Preterm infants require more acetate (especially in the first week of life) due to renal or GI losses of bicarbonate.

Micronutrients[6]

Pediatric MVI:

- Nutrition Advisory Group-AMA: <2.5 kg: 2 mL/kg/d
- Manufacturer: <1 kg: 1.5 mL/d, 1-3 kg: 3.25 mL/d, > 3 kg: 5 mL/d

Trace Minerals:

- Zinc: 400 μg/kg/d—Higher dosing may be considered for infants with increased losses (e.g., high stool output, diuretics) or for wound healing.
- Copper: 20 μg/kg/d—may require increased dosing for cholestasis, high stool output
- Selenium: 2 μg/kg/d
- Manganese: 1 μg/kg/d—may be inherent "contaminant," so some facilities omit
- Chromium: 0.05-0.3 μg/kg/d—may be inherent "contaminant," so some facilities omit

Other additives:

- L- Cysteine: The addition of cysteine is recommended for infants <1000 g. It can also be utilized for patients >1000 g to optimize calcium and phosphorus provision, although solubility varies with the type of amino acid solution being utilized. Recommended dosing is 40 mg/g amino acid/d.
- Carnitine: ASPEN recommends the routine parenteral supplementation of carnitine at 2-5 mg/kg/d for preterm neonates if no enteral source is provided.

AMA, American Medical Association; ASPEN, American Society for Parenteral and Enteral Nutrition; BSA, body surface area; BW, birth weight; Ca, calcium; CO_2, carbon dioxide; ECF, extracellular fluid; EFAD, essential fatty acid deficiency; ELBW, extremely low birth weight; EN, enteral nutrition; GI, gastrointestinal; GIR, glucose infusion rate; IV, intravenous; IFLAD, intestinal failure–associated liver disease; PDA, patent ductus arteriosus; Phos, phosphorus; PN, parenteral nutrition.

available, but as with older children, BMI measures do not distinguish between fat and lean mass and the outcome significance for preterm infants is unknown.[2]

Fenton growth curves are merged with the World Health Organization (WHO) curves for term infants, which combines intrauterine growth with postnatal growth and results in a "fetal-infant" growth curve that can be used to plot the growth of preterm infants on the same chart until 50 weeks PMA.[2-4] However, transitioning to the WHO chart earlier (approximately 42-44 weeks PMA) has the added capability of assessing weight-for-length in term (or corrected to term) infants thereby distinguishing between wasting and global (but proportionate) growth faltering. Preterm infants should be plotted on the WHO chart by corrected age. An infant's corrected age (CA) is the number of weeks the infant was born preterm subtracted from the infant's chronologic age, thereby "correcting" the postnatal age for prematurity.[7] For example, a preterm infant who is born at 32 weeks' gestational age (GA) is born 8 weeks early (40 weeks full term − 32 weeks GA = 8 weeks). At a chronologic age of 12 weeks, this infant would have a CA of 4 weeks (12 weeks of age − 8 weeks preterm = 4 weeks CA). This infant's weight, length, and head circumference should therefore all be plotted at the 4-week position on the WHO curves.

NUTRITIONAL THERAPIES

Parent's own human milk is the preferred feeding for nearly all infants (see Chapter 6), but it is especially important in preterm infants for immunologic protection, intestinal maturation, and NEC prevention (when compared to formula). Enteral nutrition should generally begin in the first 24 to 48 hours of life.[8] The GA of the infant affects the decision to feed by mouth and/or gavage since suck/swallow/breathe coordination does not develop until 32 to 34 weeks' gestation (Table 35.6). Feeding initiation and advancement is based on clinical status with close attention to feeding tolerance. Most NICUs initiate feedings at "trophic" or "gut-priming" volumes of 10 to 20 mL/kg/d to stimulate gastrointestinal hormones, motility, and maturation,[8] followed by daily or twice daily 10 to 50 mL/kg feeding volume advancements until target volume is reached (typically 150-180 mL/kg/d) (Table 35.7). The youngest and smallest infants may receive gut-priming feeds for 1 to 5 days and advance feedings the slowest. However, a Cochrane review has found no evidence that slow feeding advancement reduces the risk of NEC.[9] Optimal timing for fortification is also not established; a wide range of fortification at 20 to 100 mL/kg has been studied.[10] The ability to achieve "full feeds" (goal feeds) is dependent on many factors, including maturity of the gastrointestinal tract, stomach capacity, and respiratory status (Table 35.7).

Fortification of human milk with human milk fortifiers (HMF) is recommended for all infants born less than 32 weeks GA or with a birth weight of less than 1500 g up until at least a late preterm PMA.[13,14] HMFs contain most macro- and micronutrients, but are particularly notable for their energy, protein, calcium, phosphorus, zinc, and vitamin A content. Bovine protein-based HMFs are available in different protein types (casein vs. whey), levels of hydrolysis (polymeric vs. partial vs. extensive), and protein content (low vs. high vs. standard). Human milk-based HMFs are also available. Generally, HMFs are added when tolerance to moderate volumes of human milk have been established (60-100 mL/kg), although NICU practices vary.[15] Further fortification may be required in the setting of poor growth or in instances of fluid restriction. A variety of macronutrient-specific additives (modulars) can be used to meet individualized

TABLE 35.6 ENTERAL FEEDING METHODS

Oral feeding

- Typically for infants >32-34 wk postmenstrual age
- Coordinated suck/swallow/breathe pattern is present.
- Respiratory rate <60 breaths/min with comfortable work of breathing
- Consider partial gavage feeding if infant takes >30 min/feed to prevent excess energy expenditure.
- Many preterm infants benefit from gradual transition from gavage to oral feeding.
- Lower flow bottle nipples may be helpful as preterm infants learn to feed.

Nasogastric/orogastric tube feeding

- All infants <32 wk GA, and older infants with ongoing poor suck/swallow/breathe coordination
- Respiratory rate >60 breaths/min
- Infants orally intubated or on NIPPV/CPAP/HFNC
- Feeds are typically intermittent/bolus feeds infused over 30-60 min and administered every 3 h.
- Continuous feeds may be used in cases of feeding intolerance or hypoglycemia.

Continuous transpyloric feeding

- Consider for infants with intolerance to gastric feeding, severe GER, and severe BPD/pulmonary hypertension who are at risk for aspiration.
- Placement of transpyloric tube can be more difficult than gastric tube placement.

Indications for gastrostomy tube feeding

- Typically for infants 40-44 weeks PMA who will be unable to sufficiently orally feed for several months
- May prevent oral aversion associated with long-term nasogastric tube feeding.

BPD, bronchopulmonary dysplasia; CPAP, continuous positive airway pressure; GA, gestational age; GER, gastroesophageal reflux; HFNC, high flow nasal cannula; NIPPV, noninvasive positive pressure ventilation.

TABLE 35.7 ENTERAL NUTRITION: FEEDING ADVANCEMENT AND GOALS FOR PRETERM INFANTS

Feeding initiation and advancement

- Initiate at and advance by 10-50 mL/kg/d based on weight, gestational age, and clinical status

TUBE FEEDINGS			
AGE	**INITIAL INFUSION**	**ADVANCEMENT**	**SUGGESTED TOLERATED RATE (JEJUNAL) OR GOAL (GASTRIC)**
CONTINUOUS JEJUNAL FEEDS[11]			
PRETERM			
<750 g[8]	10-20 mL/kg/d × 3 d	15-25 mL/kg/d	150-180 mL/kg/d
>750 g[12]	20-30 mL/kg/d	30 mL/kg/d	150-180 mL/kg/d
CONTINUOUS GASTRIC FEEDS			
PRETERM			
<750 g[8]	10-20 mL/kg/d × 3 d	15-25 g/kg/d	150-180 mL/kg/d
>750 g[12]	20-30 mL/kg/d	30 mL/kg/d	150-180 mL/kg/d

(continued)

TABLE 35.7 ENTERAL NUTRITION: FEEDING ADVANCEMENT AND GOALS FOR PRETERM INFANTS (*continued*)

BOLUS/INTERMITTENT GASTRIC FEEDS

PRETERM			
<750 g[8]	10-20 mL/kg/d divided into Q3-4 h feeds × 3 d	15-25 mL/kg/d divided into Q3 h feeds	150-180 mL/kg/d divided into Q3 h feeds
>750 g[12]	20-30 mL/kg/d divided into Q3 h feeds	30 mL/kg/d divided into Q3 h feeds	150-180 mL/kg/d divided into Q3 h feeds

Warning signs of feeding intolerance

- Increase in abdominal distention/girth
- Vomiting
- Bilious emesis
- Heme positive/frank blood in stools
- Reducing substances >0.5%
- Increase in apnea/bradycardia with feeds

Energy goal

- 110-130 kcal/kg/d
- Some infants may have increased needs up to 150 kcal/kg/d (BPD, SGA)

Protein goal

- 3.0-4.2 g protein/kg/d

Energy distribution

- Protein: 8%-12% calories
- Carbohydrate: 40%-55% calories
- Fat: 35%-50% calories

Calcium

- 120-230 mg/kg/d

Phosphorus

- 60-140 mg/kg/d

Multivitamin

- Infants receiving unfortified human milk or consuming <32 oz/d of infant formula should receive 400 IU (10 μg) daily of vitamin D.
- Infants receiving human milk with added HMF may not require multivitamin supplementation (depends on feeding volume).
- Infants receiving only human milk or human milk with added PDF do require vitamin D supplementation

Iron

- Preterm infants are born with low stores and are at risk for anemia.
- Initiate iron supplementation by 4-6 wk of age.
- Infant should generally be at full feeds (150 mL/kg/d at 24 kcal/oz.) prior to start of supplementation.

BPD, bronchopulmonary dysplasia; HMF, human milk fortifier; IU, international units; PDF, postdischarge formula; SGA, small for gestational age.

patient needs (Table 35.8). Chapter 16, has additional information on specific fortification and modular products. If parent's own human milk is not available, the use of pasteurized or irradiated donor human milk should be considered. Donor human milk is preferred for high-risk neonates, typically those less than 32 weeks PMA, less than 1500 g, with a history of NEC, or with congenital cardiac defects at risk of developing ischemic bowel.[14]

If human milk is not available, then preterm infant formula should be used. These formulas have been designed to match some of the developmental aspects of the preterm gastrointestinal tract, including relative exocrine pancreatic immaturity, lower lipase production, reduced bile acid pools, and lower lactase activity (Table 35.8). These formulas also contain higher concentrations of protein, electrolytes, vitamins, and minerals (especially calcium and phosphorus) to meet the demands of the preterm infant.

Preterm infants require supplementation with 2 to 4 mg/kg/d of elemental iron due to anemia of prematurity.[13,14] At a typical feeding volume of 150 mL/kg/d and energy density of 24 Cal/fl oz, most iron-fortified formulas provide 2.2 mg/kg/d; the iron content of human milk fortified with HMF needs to be calculated because iron content varies by HMF product. Supplementation with vitamin D is also routine with a minimum goal (feeds + supplementation) of 10 µg/d.[13] Higher dosing may be needed for infants with osteopenia of prematurity.

TABLE 35.8 ENTERAL NUTRITION IN PRETERM INFANTS: CHOICE OF FEEDING SUBSTRATE

Preterm infants require fortification of human milk (parent's own or donor).

- Volume of human milk required to meet nutrient needs is too high.
- Fat in human milk may adhere to the NGT/OGT tubing, which reduces available calories and fats.
- Degradation of bile salt-stimulating lipase in pasteurized donor human milk may limit fat absorption; concentration of heat-sensitive vitamins may also be reduced.

Human milk fortifiers (HMF)

- Indicated for the youngest, smallest infants; typically <34 weeks PMA and/or <2 kg when human milk is not available
- Hospital use only due to higher nutrient content that is not suitable for older infants taking larger feeding volumes
- Protein source can be:
  - Bovine or human milk based
  - Casein or whey predominant (if bovine based)
  - Polymeric, partially hydrolyzed, or extensively hydrolyzed
  - Low (0.3-0.35 g/5 mL), standard (0.42 g/5 mL), or high (0.5-0.56 g/5 mL) protein concentration
- Macronutrients cater to immature digestive function of preterm infants
  - Protein: may be hydrolyzed (bovine based)
  - Fat: medium-chain triglyceride predominant (bovine based)
  - Carbohydrate: reduced lactose (bovine based)
- Bovine-based fortifiers used in standardized recipes for 22 and 24 kcal/oz
- Human milk-based fortifiers used in standardized recipes for 24, 26, 28, 30 kcal/oz
- Additional vitamin D supplementation is required.
- Additional iron supplementation may be required.
- Most products are only available as a sterile liquid.

(continued)

TABLE 35.8 ENTERAL NUTRITION IN PRETERM INFANTS: CHOICE OF FEEDING SUBSTRATE *(continued)*

Preterm formulas

- Indicated for the youngest, smallest infants; typically <34 wk PMA and/or <2 kg when human milk is not available
- Hospital use only due to higher nutrient content that is not suitable for older infants taking larger feeding volumes
- Highest nutrient concentration formula, especially for protein, calcium, and phosphorus
- Available in 20, 24, 24 high protein and 30 kcal/oz RTF; can be mixed together to make additional energy densities
- Macronutrients cater to immature digestive function of preterm infants.
  - Protein: may have higher whey:casein ratio.
  - Fat: 40%-50% MCT oil
  - Carbohydrate: reduced lactose (40% or less)
- Additional vitamin D supplementation required.
- Only available as a sterile liquid

Preterm discharge formulas (transitional/postdischarge formulas)

- Indicated for late preterm infants (typically 34-37 wk PMA, >2 kg) until 3-6 mo corrected age (maximum 12 mo corrected age)
- Standard energy density is intermediate between preterm and term formulas at 22 kcal/oz; powder may be mixed >22 kcal/oz for infants with higher nutrient needs.
- Nutrient concentration is intermediate between preterm and term formulas; notably higher in protein, calcium, and phosphorus than term formulas.
- Macronutrients cater to the maturing digestive function of late preterm infants.
  - Protein: may have higher whey:casein ratio to aid in digestion
  - Fat: 20%-25% MCT oil
  - Carbohydrate: reduced lactose
- Additional vitamin D supplementation required for intake <770 mL/d at 22 kcal/oz
- Available as a powder or sterile liquid; powder may be added to fortify human milk

Human milk (See Chapter 6)

- Normative feeding for infants
- First choice feeding for preterm infants, but requires fortification to meet nutrient needs
- Donor human milk is recommended for infants <32 wk and/or <1500 g when parent's own milk is not available.

Standard term, cow's milk-based formulas (See Chapter 16)

- Indicated for term infants when human milk is not available or preterm infants >3-6 mo corrected age who are achieving adequate growth
- Not recommended for preterm infants; does not meet nutritional needs for energy, protein, vitamins, and minerals
- Macronutrient content mimics mature human milk and may be difficult for preterm infants to digest.
  - Protein: Most formulas mimic whey-to-casein ratio of mature human milk.
  - Fat: 0% MCT oil for mature infant digestive capability
  - Carbohydrate: lactose predominant for mature lactase activity in term infants
- Available as a powder, sterile liquid, or concentrate depending on the formula

Soy-based formulas (see Chapter 16)

- Not recommended for preterm infants
- Lower bioavailability of calcium and phosphorus due to soy phytates and higher levels of aluminum may have adverse effects on bone mineralization
- Indicated for galactosemia, secondary lactose intolerance
- Available as a powder, sterile liquid, or concentrate depending on the formula

TABLE 35.8 ENTERAL NUTRITION IN PRETERM INFANTS: CHOICE OF FEEDING SUBSTRATE (*continued*)

Therapeutic formulas (see Chapter 16)

- Includes rice starch-thickened, protein hydrolysate, free amino acid-based, altered mineral, or high MCT containing formulas
- Not recommended long-term for preterm infants due to suboptimal nutrient composition; if medically indicated may need to concentrate or provide additional protein and/or micronutrient supplementation
- Some only available as powders

Modulars (see Chapter 16)

- Used when increased energy/protein demands require further supplementation without additional micronutrients
- Fat, carbohydrate, and/or protein supplements may be added to human milk or formula if feeding does not meet infant needs.

EFA, essential fatty acids; MCT, medium-chain triglycerides; NGT, nasogastric tube; OGT, orogastric tube; PMA, postmenstrual age; RTF, ready-to-feed.

During periods when enteral nutrition is incomplete (such as in the first days after birth while enteral feeds are advancing) or is contraindicated (due to severe hemodynamic instability, NEC, or other congenital gastrointestinal anomalies) parenteral nutrition (PN) should be initiated. PN should begin within the first few hours of life for preterm infants born less than 32 weeks gestation or with a birth weight less than 1500 g to prevent catabolism and hypoglycemia secondary to limited glycogen stores. The PN solution should be advanced daily to provide recommended fluid and nutrient estimates (Table 35.5) while enteral feeding volumes are low. PN can then be weaned as enteral feeds advance to reach goal volumes and energy density.

Amino acid requirements in preterm infants are different both qualitatively and quantitatively from term infants and older children. Some amino acids, such as L-cysteine and taurine, are conditionally essential because preterm infants do not synthesize them in sufficient quantities as term infants do and can be added to PN. A specialized amino acid blend, designed to approximate the blood amino acid profile of the human milk-fed infant, is used for PN in the preterm infant. Extremely preterm and/or extremely low birth weight (ELBW) infants have increased rates of protein turnover. Therefore, they require higher protein intake than term infants to achieve ideal growth velocity and positive nitrogen balance.

For most preterm infants, a soybean- or mixed oil–based lipid solution is recommended as a calorically dense energy source as well as to supply the essential fatty acids (α-linolenic and linoleic acids).[16] Hypertriglyceridemia, fasting serum triglyceride level greater than 250 mg/dL, may occur in preterm infants due to reduced lipoprotein lipase activity[17]; treatment may require a dose reduction in the infusion of lipids or a cycled infusion (i.e., an infusion of the same volume over fewer hours). Patient-specific lipid emulsion recommendations continue to evolve as more research on newer-to-market mixed oil and 100% fish oil emulsions become available. For infants on PN long term (>3-4 weeks), fish oil lipid emulsion may be utilized as treatment for intestinal failure-associated liver disease (IFALD) or parenteral nutrition-associated cholestasis (PNAC). Alternatively, a reduced dose of soybean oil lipid emulsion may reduce the risks of IFALD while also providing an adequate amount of essential fatty acids to prevent and treat essential fatty acid deficiency. Mixed oil lipid emulsions should not be dose restricted because there is a higher risk of developing an essential fatty acid deficiency than with soybean oil lipid emulsions. Serum fatty acid profiles should be monitored in all infants receiving reduced dosing of soybean oil emulsions or goal dosing of mixed and fish oil lipid injectable emulsions, especially if enteral fat intake is minimal. When lipid emulsions are dose-restricted, high glucose infusion rates need to be tolerated to maintain adequate parenteral energy infusion (see also Chapter 17).

Protein, fat, and carbohydrate should be advanced while monitoring daily laboratory values until estimated needs are met (Table 35.5). Thereafter, weekly nutrition panels, which include serum chemistry profiles, liver biochemical tests, and a complete blood count, are used to evaluate the adequacy of the prescribed regimen. Macronutrients are calculated based on fluid volume as well as individual needs, which are assessed using energy expenditure equations and observed growth rates.

DISCHARGE PLANNING

Preterm infant formulas and HMFs are not available for home use due to their high nutrient concentrations designed to meet the needs of infants who take smaller feeding volumes. Close to hospital discharge, infants requiring nonhuman milk feedings should be transitioned to "postdischarge" formulas (PDF) or "transitional" formulas for home use. Studies suggest that compared to term formula, preterm infants–fed PDF demonstrate improved growth (weight, length, and head circumference).[18] Evidence is mixed on whether PDF may also benefit body composition, bone mineralization, and neurodevelopment.[18] Postdischarge formulas provide higher concentrations of energy, protein, vitamins, and minerals at a standard 22 kcal/oz dilution than term infant formulas (standard 20 kcal/oz.), but less than those in preterm infant formulas and human milk fortified with HMF (standard 24 kcal/oz.). Preterm infants receiving human milk may require additional nutrients from PDF as well. There is no optimal practice[18]; common methods include adding formula powder to pumped human milk, alternating moderately concentrated formula bottles with direct breastfeeding, or mostly direct breastfeeding with few highly concentrated formula "booster" bottles. PDF prescribed at higher than 22 kcal/oz and fortified human milk at any energy density require specialized mixing recipes. Referral to a community lactation consultant, Special Supplemental Food Program for Women, Infants, and Children (WIC), Early Intervention Program (EIP), and/or home-health nursing may be beneficial for assistance with feeding skills and weight checks. Additionally, the American Academy of Pediatrics[19] and countries throughout the world[20] recommend that preterm infants receive multidisciplinary follow-up care with attention to nutritional and neurodevelopmental needs.

REFERENCES

1. Ehrenkranz RA, Dusick AM, Vohr BR, et al. Growth in the neonatal intensive care unit influences neurodevelopmental and growth outcomes of extremely low birth weight infants. *Pediatrics*. 2006;117(4):1253-1261.
2. Cordova EG, Belfort MB. Updates on assessment and monitoring of the postnatal growth of preterm infants. *Neoreviews*. 2020;21(2):e98-e108.

3. Fenton TR, Kim JH. A systematic review and meta-analysis to revise the Fenton growth chart for preterm infants. *BMC Pediatr*. 2013;13(1):59.
4. Fenton TR, Elmrayed S, Alshaikh BN. Fenton third-generation growth charts of preterm infants without abnormal fetal growth: a systematic review and meta-analysis. *Paediatr Perinat Epidemiol*. 2025;39(6): 543-555.
5. Goldberg DL, Becker PJ, Brigham K, et al. Identifying malnutrition in preterm and neonatal populations: recommended indicators. *J Acad Nutr Diet*. 2018;118(9):1571-1582.
6. Vanek VW, Borum P, Buchman A, et al. ASPEN position paper: recommendations for changes in commercially available parenteral multivitamin and multi–trace element products. *Nutr Clin Pract*. 2012;27(4): 440-491.
7. Committee on Fetus and Newborn. Age terminology during the perinatal period. *Pediatrics*. 2004;114(5): 1362-1364.
8. Thoene M, Anderson-Berry A. Early enteral feeding in preterm infants: a narrative review of the nutritional, metabolic, and developmental benefits. *Nutrients*. 2021;13(7):2289.
9. Abiramalatha T, Thanigainathan S, Ninan B. Routine monitoring of gastric residual for prevention of necrotising enterocolitis in preterm infants. *Cochrane Database Syst Rev*. 2019;7:CD012937.
10. Bergner EM, Taylor SN, Gollins LA, Hair AB. Human milk fortification: a practical analysis of current evidence. *Clin Perinatol*. 2022;49(2):447-460.
11. Broekaert IJ, Falconer J, Bronsky J, et al. The use of jejunal tube feeding in children: a position paper by the Gastroenterology and Nutrition Committees of the European Society for Paediatric Gastroenterology, Hepatology, and Nutrition 2019. *J Pediatr Gastroenterol Nutr*. 2019;69(2):239-258.
12. Oddie SJ, Young L, McGuire W. Slow advancement of enteral feed volumes to prevent necrotising enterocolitis in very low birth weight infants. *Cochrane Database Syst Rev*. 2021;8(8):CD001241.
13. Meek JY, Noble L, Section on Breastfeeding. Policy statement: breastfeeding and the use of human milk. *Pediatrics*. 2022;150(1):e2022057988.
14. Darmstadt GL, Al Jaifi NH, Arif S, et al. New World Health Organization recommendations for care of preterm or low birth weight infants: health policy. *EClinicalMedicine*. 2023;63:102155.
15. Beggs MR, Bando N, Unger S, O'Connor DL. State of the evidence from clinical trials on human milk fortification for preterm infants. *Acta Paediatrica*. 2022;111(6):1115-1120.
16. Robinson DT, Calkins KL, Chen Y, et al. Guidelines for parenteral nutrition in preterm infants: the American Society for Parenteral and Enteral Nutrition. *J Parenter Enteral Nutr*. 2023;47(7):830-858.
17. Chan AP, Robinson DT, Calkins KL. Hypertriglyceridemia in preterm infants. *NeoReviews*. 2022;23(8): e528-e540.
18. Lucas A, Sherman J, Fewtrell M. Postdischarge nutrition in preterm infants. *NeoReviews*. 2022;23(8): e541-e557.
19. Committee on Fetus and Newborn. Hospital discharge of the high-risk neonate. *Pediatrics*. 2008;122(5): 1119-1126.
20. Seppänen AV, Barros H, Draper ES, et al. Variation in follow-up for children born very preterm in Europe. *Eur J Public Health*. 2024;34(1):91-100.

CHAPTER 36

Renal Disease

Chantelle Arentsen, Rachel Potvin, and Nicolle Quinn

Chronic kidney disease (CKD) is defined as abnormalities of kidney structure or function present for 3 or more months with implications for health. End-stage kidney disease (ESKD) is the final stage of CKD, where the kidneys are no longer functioning and renal replacement therapy (i.e., dialysis, renal transplant) is necessary to sustain life.[1] From 2016 to 2020, the primary cause of ESKD in children (0-17 years) was congenital anomalies of the kidney and urinary tract (CAKUT) followed by primary glomerular disease.[2]

In 2017, the Pediatric Renal Nutrition Taskforce (PRNT) was formed comprising international pediatric renal dietitians and pediatric nephrologists. The PRNT developed clinical practice recommendations (CPRs) as a guide for medical providers treating children with CKD stages 2-5 and those on dialysis (CKD2-5D). In addition to the PRNT practice recommendations, Table 36.1 lists valuable resources for the clinician regarding nutritional care for this patient population.

■ NUTRITION ASSESSMENT

Anthropometrics

A comprehensive nutrition assessment is crucial in identifying patients who would benefit from a nutrition intervention. After dietary intake assessment, the next step of the nutrition assessment focuses on anthropometrics: weight, length or height, head

TABLE 36.1 RESOURCES FOR THE CLINICIAN

- KDOQI Clinical Practice Guideline for Nutrition in Children with CKD (KDOQI): 2008 Update. National Kidney Foundation, *American Journal of Kidney Diseases*, Volume 53, Issue 3, S11-S104.
- Kidney Disease: Improving Global Outcomes (KDIGO): https://kdigo.org/guidelines/
- National Kidney Foundation (NKF): https://www.kidney.org/
- Pediatric Renal Dietitians of North America (PRONA): https://www.prona.info/
- Pediatric Renal Nutrition Taskforce: https://www.espn-online.org/nutrition-taskforce/
- DaVita Kidney Care: https://www.davita.com/
- NephCure: for Rare Kidney Diseases: https://nephcure.org/
- Renal Support Network: https://www.rsnhope.org/
- Academy of Nutrition and Dietetics (AND): https://www.eatright.org/
  - AND Renal Practice Group: https://www.renalnutrition.org/home
- National Kidney Disease Education Program (NKDEP) of the National Institute of Diabetes and Digestive and Kidney Diseases: https://www.niddk.nih.gov/health-information/community-health-outreach/information-clearinghouses/nkdep

circumference, and weight-for-length or body mass index (BMI).[3] See Chapter 2 for details. Growth should be assessed at least twice as often as recommended for healthy children for those with advanced CKD, comorbidities, risk factors for growth delay, and those who are not meeting their growth goals.[1] It is important to use the child's euvolemic (dry) weight when determining nutrition needs. Estimated dry weight is determined by a child's interdialytic weight gain (pre- and postdialysis weights), clinical assessment (blood pressure, edema), and laboratory studies (serum sodium and albumin levels).[1] The best indicator for malnutrition or obesity in children with CKD is BMI (or weight-for-length for children younger than age 2 years). Children with CKD tend to have higher fat-to-muscle ratio and reduced lean mass compared to healthy children. In addition, BMI may be a misleading metric of obesity in this population due to poor linear growth (and thus artificially higher BMI). Due to these limitations with BMI, mid-upper arm circumference with triceps skinfold is recommended as a measure of peripheral lean and fat mass.[3]

Energy

The suggested dietary intake (SDI) is recommended for assessing energy needs for children with kidney disease (Table 36.2) per the PRNT. For children with suboptimal weight gain (or slow linear growth related to inadequate intake), their energy prescription should be on the higher end of the SDI. For children who are overweight or obese, their energy prescription should be adjusted to promote appropriate rate of weight gain. It is important to not compromise the child's nutritional intake when making energy recommendations to ensure they are receiving a variety of vitamins, minerals, and balance of macronutrients.[4]

Protein

Similar to assessment of energy needs, the SDI is recommended for determining protein requirements (Table 36.2) per the PRNT. See Chapter 5 for additional pediatric nutritional requirements and recommendations. Protein intake at the lowest end of the SDI is considered the minimum safe amount, and protein intake should not be decreased below this level. Alternatively, protein intake at the higher end of the SDI is recommended for children who need to achieve better weight and height gain. For children receiving dialysis, protein requirements may need to be above the SDI to account for dialysate protein losses. For children receiving hemodialysis (HD), protein intake should be increased by at least 0.1 g/kg/d over estimated baseline needs. Protein losses are more significant for children receiving peritoneal dialysis (PD), so protein intake should be increased by at least 0.15 to 0.3 g/kg/d.[4]

Fluid

Children with CKD have similar basal fluid requirements when compared to healthy children. However, several factors play a role in determining a child's total fluid requirement. Children may require additional free water to avoid chronic intravascular depletion in the setting of polyuria (excessive urination). Fluid restriction may be indicated if oliguria (low urine output) or anuria (no urine output) is present to avoid complications of fluid overload. Fluid goals are based on blood pressure, volume status, urine output, and insensible losses.[5]

TABLE 36.2 ENERGY AND PROTEIN REQUIREMENTS FOR INFANTS, CHILDREN AND ADOLESCENTS WITH CKD2-5D AGED 0 TO 18 YEARS

SDI FOR ENERGY AND PROTEIN: BIRTH[a] TO 18 Y

MONTH	SDI[b] ENERGY (KCAL/KG/D)	SDI PROTEIN (G/KG/D)	SDI PROTEIN (G/D)
0	93-107	1.52-2.5	8-12
1	93-120	1.52-1.8	8-12
2	93-120	1.4-1.52	8-12
3	82-98	1.4-1.52	8-12
4	82-98	1.3-1.52	9-13
5	72-82	1.3-1.52	9-13
6-9	72-82	1.1-1.3	9-14
10-11	72-82	1.1-1.3	9-15
12	72-120	0.9-1.14	11-14

YEAR	SDI ENERGY (KCAL/KG/D)		SDI PROTEIN (G/KG/D)	SDI PROTEIN (G/D)
–	Male	Female		
2	81-95[c]	79-92[c]	0.9-1.05	11-15
3	80-82	76-77	0.9-1.05	13-15
4-6	67-93	64-90	0.85-0.95	16-22
7-8	60-77	56-75	0.9-0.95	19-28
9-10	55-69	49-63	0.9-0.95	26-40
11-12	48-63	43-57	0.9-0.95	34-42
13-14	44-63	39-50	0.8-0.9	34-50
15-17	40-55	36-46	0.8-0.9	Male: 52-65 Female: 45-49

CKD2-5D, chronic kidney disease stages 2-5 and those on dialysis; SDI, suggested dietary intake.
For children with poor growth, reference to the SDI for height age may be appropriate. Height age is the age that corresponds to an individual's height when plotted on the 50th percentile on a growth chart.
[a]Thirty-seven/40 weeks gestation. Premature infants have higher energy and protein requirements. The increased need for these and other particular nutrients (sodium, potassium, calcium, and phosphorus) must be balanced against the nutritional interventions to control the effects of CKD. This is outside the scope of this CPR.
[b]Suggested dietary intake (SDI) is based on the physical activity level (PAL) used by the international bodies: 1 to 3 year PAL 1.4; 4 to 9 year PAL 1.6; and 10 to 17 year PAL 1.8. Where guidelines have given a range of energy requirements for different levels of PAL, the lowest PAL has been taken for SDI energy in consideration that children with CKD are likely to have low activity levels.
[c]Scientific Advisory Committee on Nutrition (2011) Dietary Reference Values for Energy https://assets .publishing.service.gov.uk/government/uploads/system/uploads/attachment_data/528 Pediatr Nephrol (2020) 35:519–531file/339317/SACN_Dietary_Reference_Values_for_Energy.pdf
From Shaw V, Polderman N, Renken-Terhaerdt J, et al. Energy and protein requirements for children with CKD stages 2-5 and on dialysis-clinical practice recommendations from the Pediatric Renal Nutrition Taskforce. *Pediatr Nephrol*. 2020;35(3):519-531.

Electrolytes

Sodium

Monitoring of serum sodium concentration can be useful in assessing a child's fluid status. Hypernatremia may be an indication of dehydration or intravascular depletion of water. Conversely, hyponatremia may indicate excessive hydration, the syndrome of inappropriate antidiuretic hormone secretion (SIADH), inadequate intake, or deficiency. Urine sodium and urine creatinine can be useful to evaluate the kidneys' ability to filter blood. Urine sodium can help identify the cause of a high or low serum sodium level. Urine creatinine can assist with evaluating kidney function.[5] For children with salt-wasting diseases (i.e., obstructive uropathy, renal dysplasia), hyponatremia is common due to their inability to conserve sodium chloride. It is important to highlight that infants receiving PD are vulnerable to sodium losses due to their high ultrafiltration requirement per kilogram of body weight. Sodium supplementation in these cases is often required due to the low sodium content of breast milk and infant formula.[5] Table 36.3 highlights enteral nutrition products specific for patients with CKD, while Table 36.4 provides considerations for enteral feeding.

Potassium

Monitoring of serum potassium levels is important for children with CKD due to the prevalence of imbalances in potassium concentrations. Hyperkalemia may be present in children with excessive dietary potassium intake, decreased urine output, metabolic acidosis, constipation, medications, and inadequate dialysis. Hypokalemia may occur in children with renal tubular disorders, prolonged gastrointestinal losses (i.e., vomiting, diarrhea), and intensive dialysis regimens.[5] If serum potassium levels are outside of the normal range, dietary intake of potassium should be adjusted. Depending on the child's age, this can be achieved by manipulating formula composition, nutrition supplements, and food intake.[8] Sodium polystyrene sulfonate (SPS) is a medication used to treat hyperkalemia via sodium exchange. Pretreating (or decanting) breastmilk or formula with the powdered version of SPS is an effective treatment for hyperkalemia. However, it is important to closely monitor serum electrolytes (especially sodium, potassium, and calcium).[5]

Calcium and Phosphorus

It is crucial for children with CKD to have routine monitoring of serum calcium and phosphorus levels. The frequency of mineral evaluation depends on several factors, including trends, stage of CKD, changes in diet, dialysis, and medications. Adequate calcium and phosphorus intake is crucial to reduce the risk of metabolic bone disease. However, excessive intake of these minerals and decreased renal function may lead to nephrocalcinosis and vascular calcification.[9] Table 36.5 summarizes the SDI for calcium and phosphate in children with CKD2-5D. When a child presents with hyperphosphatemia or hyperparathyroidism, phosphorus intake should be limited to the SDI. Phosphate binder therapy may also be required to maintain blood concentrations within goal range. In cases of persistent hypophosphatemia, phosphorus intake should be increased to more than twice the SDI.[9] See Table 36.6 for a list of common nutrition-related medications and supplements used in children with CKD. Table 36.7 highlights nutritional and metabolic consequences of CKD.

TABLE 36.3 NUTRITIONAL PRODUCTS SPECIFIC FOR RENAL PATIENTS

PRODUCT	MANUFACTURER	POPULATION	PRODUCT INFORMATION
Similac PM 60/40	Abbott	0-12 mo	• Standard dilution: 20 kcal/oz • Nutritionally complete • 60:40 indicates whey-to-casein ratio • Low mineral content mimics human milk • Protein content: 2.2 g/100 mL • Powder
Kate Farms Renal Support	Kate Farms	1 y and older	• Standard dilution: 54 kcal/oz • Nutritionally complete • Plant-based/free of common allergens • Low mineral content • Protein content: 8 g/100 mL • Ready-to-feed
Renastart	Vitaflo	1 y and older	• Standard dilution: 30 kcal/oz • Not nutritionally complete • Low mineral content • Protein content: 7.5 g/100 mL • Powder
Renastep	Vitaflo	1 y and older	• Standard dilution: 60 kcal/oz • Not nutritionally complete • Low mineral content • Protein content: 4 g/100 mL • Ready-to-feed
Suplena	Abbott	4 y and older	• Standard dilution: 54 kcal/oz • Nutritionally complete • Low mineral content • Protein content: 4.5 g/100 mL • Ready-to-feed

Boost Breeze	Nestle	Ages 1-13 y	• Standard dilution: 30 kcal/oz • Not nutritionally complete • Low mineral content • Protein content: 3.6 g/100 mL • Ready-to-feed
Nepro	Abbott	Adult dialysis patients	• Standard dilution: 54 kcal/oz • Nutritionally complete • Low mineral content • Protein content: 8.1 g/100 mL • Ready-to-feed
Novasource Renal	Nestle	Adult dialysis patients	• Standard dilution: 60 kcal/oz • Nutritionally complete • Low mineral content • Protein content: 9.3 g/100 mL • Ready-to-feed
Ensure Clear	Abbott	Adults	• Standard dilution: 30 kcal/oz • Not nutritionally complete • Low mineral content • Protein content: 3.4 g/100 mL

TABLE 36.4 GENERAL CONSIDERATIONS FOR ENTERAL FEEDING

- Reduced oral intake (anorexia) in children with chronic kidney disease (CKD) or on dialysis is common due to several factors, including poor appetite, delayed gastric emptying, uremia, gastroesophageal reflux, and early satiety due to peritoneal dialysate fluids. Supplemental feedings can help increase energy intake and/or replace energy intake and fluids lost due to emesis.[6]
- Gastrostomy tube placement may benefit children with CKD if oral intake is poor and nutritional supplementation is needed for more than a few weeks.[6]
- Formula may need to be concentrated and/or supplemented with a carbohydrate/fat modular and/or liquid fat due to fluid restrictions or poor growth. Concentrated formulas have higher concentrations of micronutrients and electrolytes, which may require extra monitoring for some patients. Children receiving dialysis may need supplemental protein and/or potassium.[6,7]
- Blenderized tube feedings may be used in children with CKD or on dialysis.[6]
- Lab trends and growth should be closely monitored when formula composition is altered.[6]

TABLE 36.5 SUMMARY OF SUGGESTED DIETARY INTAKE FOR CALCIUM AND PHOSPHATE IN CHILDREN WITH CKD2-5D

AGE (Y)	SDI CALCIUM (MG)	SDI PHOSPHATE (MG)
0-< 4 mo	220	120
4-< 12 mo	330-540	275-420
1-3 y	450-700	250-500
4-10 y	700-1000	440-800
11-17 y	900-1300	640-1250

CKD2-5D, chronic kidney disease stages 2-5 and on dialysis; SDI, suggested dietary intake.
For children with poor growth, reference to the SDI for height age may be appropriate. This is the age that corresponds to their height when plotted at the 50th percentile on a growth chart.
From McAlister L, Pugh P, Greenbaum L, et al. The dietary management of calcium and phosphate in children with CKD stages 2-5 and on dialysis-clinical practice recommendation from the Pediatric Renal Nutrition Taskforce. *Pediatr Nephrol*. 2020;35(3):501-518.

TABLE 36.6 COMMON NUTRITION-RELATED MEDICATIONS AND SUPPLEMENTS IN CHILDREN WITH CKD

MEDICATION	CLINICAL INDICATION
Sodium polystyrene sulfonate (SPS)	Used to treat hyperkalemia via sodium exchange[5] Powdered formulation can be used to pretreat or "decant" formula.[7]
Calcium carbonate	If taken without meals, acts as a calcium supplement If taken with meals, acts as a phosphate binder[5]
Renvela	Noncalcium-based phosphate binder[5]
Sodium bicarbonate	Used to treat metabolic acidosis[5]

TABLE 36.6 COMMON NUTRITION-RELATED MEDICATIONS AND SUPPLEMENTS IN CHILDREN WITH CKD (*continued*)

MEDICATION	CLINICAL INDICATION
Ergocalciferol (vitamin D_2) or Cholecalciferol (vitamin D_3)	Used to treat vitamin D deficiency[5,7] Can improve PTH control[5]
Calcitriol	Active form of vitamin D used to treat low calcium levels Should not be used to treat vitamin D deficiency[7]
Water-soluble vitamins	Vitamin B and C complex with folic acid Recommended for all children receiving dialysis to replace losses of water-soluble vitamins[6]
Recombinant human growth hormone (rhGH)	Daily injection prescribed for growth failure[5]

CKD, chronic kidney disease; PTH, parathyroid hormone.

TABLE 36.7 NUTRITIONAL AND METABOLIC CONSEQUENCES OF CKD

PROBLEM	ETIOLOGY	TREATMENT
Metabolic acidosis	Renal tubular dysfunction leading to the kidneys: Inability to reabsorb bicarbonate Inability to generate bicarbonate Inability to excrete acid[10]	Alkalinizing medications: Sodium bicarbonate Sodium citrate
Salt wasting	Obstructive uropathy Renal dysplasia Tubulopathies[7]	Sodium supplementation
Renal osteodystrophy	Secondary hyperparathyroidism Hypocalcemia Calcitriol deficiency[8]	Decrease oral phosphorus intake (limit phosphate additives) Vitamin D supplementation Adequate calcium intake (SDI/age) Calcitriol Phosphorus binders

(*continued*)

TABLE 36.7 NUTRITIONAL AND METABOLIC CONSEQUENCES OF CKD (*continued*)

PROBLEM	ETIOLOGY	TREATMENT
Hyperkalemia	Decreased renal excretion Metabolic acidosis Constipation Medications (renin-angiotensin-aldosterone system inhibitors, calcineurin inhibitors, potassium-sparing diuretics, β-blockers)[11]	Limit foods with potassium additives. Limit dietary intake of higher potassium foods. Alter cooking method of potatoes, tuberous vegetables, and legumes (leaching, shredding, boiling, microwaving). Use of potassium-binding resin and decanting Correct acidosis
Growth failure	Growth hormone resistance Metabolic acidosis Inadequate energy intake Renal osteodystrophy Use of corticosteroids leading to suppression of growth hormone Salt wasting[7]	Growth hormone (rhGH) Alkalinizing medication to correct acidosis Adequate energy intake Adequate calcium and vitamin D Sodium supplementation
Hypertension	Renin-angiotensin-aldosterone system activation with increased angiotensin II formation Decreased sodium excretion due to nephron and tubular damage[7,11]	Limit sodium intake (limit added salt, processed foods, and fast food) Weight management Physical activity Antihypertensive medications
Fluid retention	Hypoperfusion of renal tissue leading to fluid and sodium retention Nephrotic syndrome Excessive fluid intake in the setting of prescribed fluid restriction[7,12,13]	Education on compliance with fluid restriction Limit foods liquid/semi-liquid at room temperature (ice cream, Jell-O, yogurt, gravy). Limit sodium intake.
Anemia	Reduced production of erythropoietin[14]	Erythropoietin (rHuEPO) Iron supplementation
Vitamin deficiencies (B vitamins and vitamin C)	Water-soluble vitamins lost in dialysate Low dietary intake[7,15]	Supplement with water-soluble vitamins
Hypervitaminosis A	Decreased urinary excretion Lack of dialytic removal[15]	Avoid vitamin A supplementation. Limit dietary intake to RDA/age.

TABLE 36.7 NUTRITIONAL AND METABOLIC CONSEQUENCES OF CKD (*continued*)

PROBLEM	ETIOLOGY	TREATMENT
Calcium oxalate stones	Hypercalciuria Hypocitraturia Hyperoxaluria Low fluid intake/low urine output High sodium intake Inadequate calcium intake Excessive protein intake Vitamin C supplementation[16]	Increase fluid intake Limit sodium intake Increase citrate intake (increase fruit and vegetable intake, limit nondairy animal protein) RDA/age for calcium Limit oxalate-rich foods if high urine oxalate. Avoid vitamin C supplements. Thiazide diuretics Potassium citrate

CKD, chronic kidney disease; RDA, recommended dietary allowance; SDI, suggested dietary intake.

■ PARENTERAL NUTRITION CONSIDERATIONS IN RENAL DISEASE

When patients with CKD are unable to maintain enteral nutrition support, parenteral nutrition (PN) may be indicated to provide adequate nutrition. A challenge when considering parenteral nutrition in the setting of acute or CKD is the common need to restrict fluid intake; hyperosmolar PN solutions and thus central venous access will likely be required.[16] See Chapter 17 for additional information on prescribing parenteral nutrition for children. For the CKD population, protein provision is typically higher due to losses during dialysis. It is recommended to start with a parenteral solution without added potassium, magnesium, and phosphorus and titrate these based on laboratory values. Since some micronutrients are excreted primarily through the kidneys, starting with a smaller dose of a multivitamin is recommended and following micronutrient levels closely.[5]

If the combination of oral and enteral intake is unable to meet a nonacute dialysis patient's energy needs, supplemental intra-dialytic parenteral nutrition (IDPN) may be indicated to improve nutritional status. IDPN has been shown to improve BMI in small, pediatric cohort studies when the cause is organic and not related to psychosocial causes of malnutrition.[7] IDPN is infused via the hemodialysis catheter during dialysis. IDPN consists of dextrose, amino acids, fat emulsion, and trace elements. It should not be used as a sole source of nutrition, but rather to supplement oral and/or enteral nutrition for the malnourished dialysis patient. By infusing during dialysis, the majority of amino acids are retained, and the IDPN fluid is removed during the ultrafiltration process. Hyperglycemia and hyperlipidemia are the primary potential adverse effects of IDPN and require routine monitoring.[7]

NUTRITIONAL CONSIDERATIONS IN THE POSTRENAL TRANSPLANT PATIENT

The transplant dietitian is a required member of the multidisciplinary transplant team and is involved in all stages of transplantation (pre-, peri-, and posttransplant) per the Centers for Medicare and Medicaid Services.[17] Transplantation is not an end to CKD or nutritional intervention, with the goal being to achieve normal growth, minimize side effects of immunosuppression medications, and adjust the nutrition regimen based on kidney function. Immediately postoperatively, there may be persistent electrolyte derangements, hyperglycemia, hypertension, and other side effects of newly introduced immunosuppression medication. Phosphorus supplementation may be indicated, as well as education on increasing phosphorus-rich foods in the diet to maintain safe levels due to an increase in urinary phosphorus excretion.[7]

Patients who take immunosuppression medication are at a higher risk for a foodborne illness. If they become ill, their symptoms could be more severe than a healthy individual, leading to hospitalization and potential death, according to food safety guidelines created by the United States Department of Agriculture (USDA). During the transplant hospital admission, education on food safety is imperative in addition to the importance of meeting fluid minimum, and long-term healthy eating.[5] Education should include how to handle and prepare food, focusing on the four basic steps for food safety: clean, separate, cook, and chill.[5] Education should also include the following: how to transport food safely, food storage guidelines, and how to become a better shopper.

Long-term complications from transplantation include obesity, dyslipidemia, and osteoporosis. Per the Kidney Disease Quality Outcomes Initiative, it is recommended renal transplant recipients receive 100% of the estimated energy requirement for age, using an adjusted body weight if indicated. Following a balanced diet, monitoring growth, laboratory values, and encouraging frequent physical activity will aid in achieving optimal outcomes.[7]

CONCLUSION

The nutritional management of a pediatric patient with CKD is complex and evolves over the course of the patient's lifespan and treatment course. Education over time ranges from formula preparation to dietary restrictions to food safety and healthy eating for life. The pediatric registered dietitian is a key member of the multidisciplinary team caring for children with kidney disease throughout the continuum of their disease process.

REFERENCES

1. Kidney Disease: Improving Global Outcomes (KDIGO) CKD Work Group. KDIGO 2024 clinical practice guideline for the evaluation and management of chronic kidney disease. *Kidney Int*. 2024;105(4S):S117-S314.
2. United States Renal Data System. ESRD among children and adolescents. In: *Annual Data Report: End Stage Renal Disease*. National Institutes of Health, National Institute of Diabetes and Digestive and Kidney Diseases; 2023.
3. Nelms CL, Shaw V, Greenbaum LA, et al. Assessment of nutritional status in children with kidney diseases-clinical practice recommendations from the Pediatric Renal Nutrition Taskforce. *Pediatr Nephrol*. 2021;36(4):995-1010.

4. Shaw V, Polderman N, Renken-Terhaerdt J, et al. Energy and protein requirements for children with CKD stages 2-5 and on dialysis-clinical practice recommendations from the Pediatric Renal Nutrition Taskforce. *Pediatr Nephrol*. 2020;35(3):519-531.
5. Pediatric Renal Dietitians of North America. Pediatric Renal Nutrition Pocket Guide. eds. Nelson P & Solan P. 1st ed. Morris Press; Kearney, NE USA, 2023
6. Nelms CL. Optimizing enteral nutrition for growth in pediatric Chronic Kidney Disease (CKD). *Front Pediatr*. 2018;6:214.
7. National Kidney Foundation. KDOQI clinical practice guideline for nutrition in children with CKD: 2008 update. *Am J Kidney Dis*. 2009;53(3):S11-S104.
8. Desloovere A, Renken-Terhaerdt J, Tuokkola J, et al. The dietary management of potassium in children with CKD stages 2-5 and on dialysis-clinical practice recommendations from the Pediatric Renal Nutrition Taskforce. *Pediatr Nephrol*. 2021;36(6):1331-1346.
9. McAlister L, Pugh P, Greenbaum L, et al. The dietary management of calcium and phosphate in children with CKD stages 2-5 and on dialysis-clinical practice recommendation from the Pediatric Renal Nutrition Taskforce. *Pediatr Nephrol*. 2020;35(3):501-518.
10. Capossela L, Ferretti S, D'Alonzo S, et al. Bone disorders in pediatric chronic kidney disease: a literature review. *Biology (Basel)*. 2023;12(11):1395.
11. Gallibois CM, Jawa NA, Noone DG. Hypertension in pediatric patients with chronic kidney disease: management challenges. *Int J Nephrol Renovasc Dis*. 2017;10:205-213.
12. Downie ML, Gallibois C, Parekh RS, Noone DG. Nephrotic syndrome in infants and children: pathophysiology and management. *Paediatr Int Child Health*. 2017;37(4):248-258.
13. Park MJ, Cho MH. Anemia in children with chronic kidney disease. *Child Kidney Dis*. 2023;27(2):82-88.
14. Anderson CE, Tuokkola J, Qizalbash L, et al. Assessment and management of vitamin status in children with CKD stages 2-5, on dialysis and post-transplantation: clinical practice points from the Pediatric Renal Nutrition Taskforce. *Pediatr Nephrol*. 2024;39(10):3103-3124.
15. Önal B, Kırlı EA. Pediatric stone disease: current management and future concepts. Turk Arch Pediatr. 2021;56(2):99-107.
16. American Society for Parenteral and Enteral Nutrition. *The ASPEN Pediatric Nutrition Support Core Curriculum*. 3rd ed. American Society for Parenteral and Enteral Nutrition; 2015.
17. Pieloch D, Friedman GG, DiCecco S, Ulerich L, Beer S, Hasse J. A standardized framework for transplant-specific competencies for dietitians. *Prog Transplant*. 2017;27(3):281-285.

APPENDIX 1

Conversion Tables (Approximate)

MASS/WEIGHT

1 ounce	=	28 grams
1/4 pound	=	0.11 kilograms
1/2 pound	=	0.23 kilograms
3/4 pound	=	0.34 kilograms
1 pound	=	0.45 kilograms
1 gram	=	0.036 ounces
1 kilogram	=	2.2 pounds

To convert ounces to grams, multiply by 28.
To convert grams to ounces, divide by 28.
To convert pounds to kilograms, multiply by 0.45.
To convert kilograms to pounds, multiply by 2.2.

LENGTH

1 inch	=	2.54 centimeters
1 foot	=	30.5 centimeters
1 yard	=	0.91 meters
1 mile	=	1.61 kilometers
1 millimeter	=	0.04 inches
1 centimeter	=	0.4 inches
1 meter	=	3.3 feet
1 meter	=	1.1 yard
1 kilometer	=	1093.7 yards
1 kilometer	=	0.62 miles
1 kilometer	=	3281 feet

To convert inches to centimeters, multiply by 2.54.
To convert centimeters to inches, multiply by 0.4.

AREA

1 square inch	=	6.5 square centimeters
1 square foot	=	0.0929 square meters
1 square yard	=	0.84 square meters
1 square centimeter	=	0.16 square inches
1 square meter	=	1.2 square yards
1 cubic foot	=	1728 cubic inches
1 cubic yard	=	27 cubic feet

LIQUID

1 teaspoon	=	5 milliliters		
1 tablespoon	=	15 milliliters		
1 fluid ounce	=	30 milliliters		
8 fluid ounces	=	236 milliliters		
16 fluid ounces	=	473 milliliters	=	1 pint
32 fluid ounces	=	946 milliliters	=	1 quart
128 fluid ounces	=	3785 milliliters	=	1 gallon
1 milliliter	=	0.03 fluid ounces		
1 liter	=	1000 milliliters	=	1.06 quarts

To convert milliliters to ounces, divide by 30.
To convert ounces to milliliters, multiply by 30.

TEMPERATURE

	CELSIUS (CENTIGRADE)	FAHRENHEIT
Water freezes	0 °C	32 °F
Room temperature	22 °C	72 °F
Body temperature	37 °C	98.6 °F
Water boils	100 °C	212 °F

To convert Fahrenheit to Celsius, subtract 32, multiply by 5, and divide by 9.
To convert Celsius to Fahrenheit, multiply by 9, divide by 5, and add 32.

ENERGY

1 kilojoule (kJ)	=	0.239 kilocalorie
1 kilocalorie (kcal)	=	4.190 kilojoules

To convert kilocalories to kilojoules, multiply the kcal value by 4.2.

NITROGEN TO PROTEIN

1 gram of nitrogen	=	6.25 grams of Protein

INTERNATIONAL UNIT (IU) EQUIVALENTS

1 IU vitamin E	=	0.67 mg d-α-tocopherol (natural form)
1 IU vitamin E	=	0.45 mg dl-α-tocopherol (synthetic)
1 IU vitamin A	=	0.3 µg retinol or RAE (retinol activity equivalents)
1 IU vitamin A	=	0.6 µg supplemental β-carotene
1 IU vitamin D	=	0.025 µg cholecalciferol

MILLIEQUIVALENT-MILLIGRAM CONVERSION TABLE

MINERAL ELEMENT	CHEMICAL SYMBOL	ATOMIC WEIGHT	VALENCE
Bicarbonate	HCO_3	61	1
Calcium	Ca	40	2
Chlorine	Cl	35.4	1
Magnesium	Mg	24.3	2
Phosphorus	P	31	2
Phosphate	PO_4	95	3
	HPO_4	96	2
	H_2PO_4	97	3
Potassium	K	39	1
Sodium	Na	23	1
Sulfur	S	32	2
Sulfate	SO_4	96	2
Zinc	Zn	65.4	2

Milliequivalents = (Milligrams/Atomic Weight) × Valence

To convert milligrams to milliequivalents, divide the milligrams by the atomic weight and multiply by the valence.

Example: Convert 2000 mg sodium to mEq of sodium

$$2000 \div 23 \times 1 = 87 \text{ mEq sodium}$$

To convert milliequivalents to milligrams, multiply the milliequivalents by the atomic weight and divide by the valence.

Example: Convert 20 mEq sodium to mg sodium

$$20 \times 23 \div 1 = 460 \text{ mg sodium}$$

MILLIEQUIVALENTS FOR SELECTED SALTS

SALT	mEq/GRAM SALT	mg SALT/MEQ
Ammonium chloride	18.7	53.5
Calcium acetate	12.7	78.7
Calcium carbonate	20	50
Calcium chloride	14	73
Calcium glubionate	3.2	312.5
Calcium gluconate	4	224
Calcium gluceptate	4.1	244
Calcium lactate	6	154
Magnesium chloride	9.8	102
Magnesium oxide	49.7	20
Magnesium sulfate	8.2	122
Potassium acetate	10	98
Potassium bicarbonate	10	100
Potassium chloride	13	75
Potassium citrate	9	108
Potassium gluconate	4.3	233
Potassium iodide	6	166
Sodium acetate	7.3	137
Sodium bicarbonate	12	84
Sodium chloride	17	58.8
Sodium citrate	10	98
Sodium iodide	7	150
Sodium lactate	9	112
Zinc sulfate	7	144

CONVERSION TABLE FOR SODIUM/SODIUM CHLORIDE

QUANTITY	mEq SODIUM	mg SODIUM	mg SODIUM CHLORIDE
1/8 teaspoon salt	13	300	750
¼ teaspoon salt	26	600	1500
½ teaspoon salt	52	1200	3000
¾ teaspoon salt	78	1800	4500
1 teaspoon salt	104	2400	6000

CLINICAL CHEMISTRY SI CONVERSION FACTORS

	CONVENTIONAL UNITS	CONVERSION FACTOR (MULTIPLY)	SI UNITS
Alkaline phosphatase	IU/L	1	U/L
Alanine aminotransferase	U/L	1	U/L
Albumin	g/dL	10	g/L
Ammonia (NH_4)	µg/dL	0.5872	µmol/L
Aluminum	ng/mL	0.0371	µmol/L
Aspartate aminotransferase	U/L	1	U/L
Bilirubin	mg/dL	17.1	µmol/L
Calcium	mg/dL	0.25	mmol/L
Carbon dioxide	mEq/L	1	mmol/L
Chloride	mEq/L	1	mmol/L
Cholesterol	mg/dL	0.026	mmol/L
Copper	µg/dL	0.16	µmol/L
Creatinine	mg/dL	88.4	µmol/L
Glucose	mg/dL	0.055	mmol/L
Iron, total	µg/dL	0.179	µmol/L
Magnesium	mEq/L	0.5	mmol/L
Osmolality	Osm/kg	1	mmol/L
Phosphorus	mg/dL	0.323	mmol/L
Potassium	mEq/L	1	mmol/L
Protein, total	g/dL	10	g/L
Sodium	mEq/L	1	mmol/L
Triglycerides	mg/dL	0.011	mmol/L

APPENDIX 2

Drug-Nutrition Interactions

	NUTRITIONAL CONSIDERATIONS	POSSIBLE GASTROINTESTINAL SIDE EFFECTS	POSSIBLE EFFECTS ON LAB VALUES	COMMENTS/RECOMMENDATIONS
Antiarthritic				
Abatacept (Orencia)	Infusion contains maltose May be present in human milk	Nausea Abdominal pain Dyspepsia Diverticulitis of the gastrointestinal tract (rare, severe)	May result in falsely ↑ blood glucose levels with dehydrogenase pyrroloquinoline quinone or glucose dye-oxidoreductase testing methods on the day of infusion	
Adalimumab (Humira)		Nausea Abdominal pain	↑ Cholesterol ↑ Alk phos	
Anakinra (Kineret)		Vomiting Gastroenteritis Constipation	↑ GGT ↑ Serum transferase ↑ Cholesterol	*Hepatitis reported in postmarketing* studies
Baricitinib (Olumiant)	Administer with or without food Not known if present in breast milk	Abdominal pain Nausea Esophageal candidiasis Weight gain	↑ ALT, AST ↑ GGT ↑ HDL ↑ LDL ↑ Cholesterol ↑ Triglycerides ↑ Creatinine	Gastrointestinal perforation reported in postmarketing studies Tablets may be dispersed and administrated orally or via GT, NGT, or OGT If tablets are crushed, use proper control measures (e.g., ventilated enclosure) or personal protective equipment (i.e., N95 respirator) The manufacturer indicates that dispersed tablets are stable in water for up to 4 h

Certolizumab Pegol (Cimzia)	May be present in breast milk	Nausea/diarrhea Intestinal obstruction Abdominal pain	↑ Serum transaminases Falsely elevated aPTT	
Etanercept (Enbrel)	May be present in breast milk	Diarrhea Gastroenteritis	↑ Serum transaminases, 2-3 times the upper limit of normal	
Golimumab (Simponi)		Constipation Nausea	↑ALT, AST	
Anticoagulants				
Coumarins: Warfarin (Coumadin)	Vitamin K antagonist Concomitant use of warfarin with vitamin K may decrease anticoagulant effects; consistent intake of vit K essential High doses of vit A, E, or C may alter prothrombin time Considered compatible with breastfeeding	Nausea/vomiting/diarrhea Hemorrhage Anorexia Dysgeusia	Increased bleeding time	Breastfed infants may be more sensitive to warfarin due to low amounts of vit K in breast milk Herbal teas, tonka beans, melilot, and woodruff contain natural coumarins and will ↑ warfarin effects Fried or boiled onions may ↑ drug effect by ↑ fibrinolytic activity
Rivaroxaban (Xarelto)	May be present in breast milk May contain lactose	Gastroenteritis Vomiting Abdominal pain Gastrointestinal hemorrhage Cholestasis Jaundice	↑ Serum transaminases (>3 × ULN) May prolong aPTT	

(continued)

	NUTRITIONAL CONSIDERATIONS	POSSIBLE GASTROINTESTINAL SIDE EFFECTS	POSSIBLE EFFECTS ON LAB VALUES	COMMENTS/RECOMMENDATIONS
Antidiabetic				
Acarbose (Precose)	Take with first bite of each main meal Do not take with pancreatic Enzymes	Abdominal pain Diarrhea Flatulence	↓ Fasting glucose ↓ Postprandial glucose ↓ HCT ↓ HbA1c ↑ ALT, AST	Titrate dose to ↓ GI side effects
Semaglutide (Ozempic, We-govy, Rybelsus)	Oral: Administer ≥30 min before the first food/beverage or medications of the day with ≤4 oz of plain water only, eating 30-60 min after the dose	Abdominal pain Constipation Nausea/vomiting/diarrhea Decreased appetite Cholelithiasis Flatulence Gastritis Gastroenteritis Dysgeusia	Hypoglycemia ↑ ALT ↑ Amylase ↑ Lipase ↓ HbA1c	May require dose reduction of insulin and/or insulin secretagogues to avoid hypoglycemia *May increase serum concentration of* Levothyroxine Semaglutide slows gastric emptying, which may alter absorption of other medications GI effects tend to occur during dose escalation and decrease over time

Antidiarrheals				
Loperamide (Imodium)	Administer with plenty of clear fluids to prevent dehydration May be present in breast milk	Abdominal pain Constipation Nausea	QT prolongation	Oral solution may contain propylene glycol Oral solution may contain sorbitol which can exacerbate diarrhea in short bowel syndrome Use with caution in patients with hepatic impairment due to reduced first-pass metabolism; monitor for signs of CNS toxicity
Antihistamine Drugs				
Cyprohepta-dine (Periactin)	Appetite stimulant Increased weight gain and growth rate Administration with food increases drug bioavailability Not known if present in breast milk	Xerostomia Nausea/vomiting/diarrhea Abdominal pain Increased appetite	May interfere with response to diagnostic antigen skin tests ↑ Amylase ↓ Fasting glucose	
Diphen-hydramine (Benadryl)	May increase appetite and increase weight gain	Nausea/vomiting/diarrhea Anorexia Constipation Dry mucous membranes Epigastric discomfort Xerostomia Thrombocytopenia	May suppress the wheal and flare reactions to skin test antigens	

(*continued*)

	NUTRITIONAL CONSIDERATIONS	POSSIBLE GASTROINTESTINAL SIDE EFFECTS	POSSIBLE EFFECTS ON LAB VALUES	COMMENTS/RECOMMENDATIONS
Loratadine (Claritin)	Administer without regard to meals Food increases bioavailability May increase appetite May administer oral disintegrating tablet with or without water Some products may contain phenylalanine and/or sodium May be present in breast milk	Abdominal pain Altered salivation Anorexia Constipation Dysgeusia Dyspepsia Flatulence Gastritis Hiccups Nausea/vomiting/diarrhea Stomatitis Xerostomia	Abnormal liver function tests May interfere with response to diagnostic antigen skin tests	May decrease maternal serum prolactin concentrations when administered prior to the establishment of lactation
Anti-Infective Drugs				
Antibiotics, General	Some antibiotics are folate and B_{12} antagonists	Nausea/vomiting/diarrhea Lactase deficiency	Anemia	Decreased synthesis of vitamin K by gut microflora Depletion of gut microflora can also lead to dysbiosis that can alter the digestion and absorption of nutrients

Aminoglycosides	Increased urinary excretion of potassium and magnesium May also deplete sodium and calcium	Decreased appetite Nausea/vomiting Increased salivation	↑ BUN ↑ ALT, AST ↑ LDH ↑ Bilirubin ↓ Calcium ↓ Magnesium ↓ Potassium ↓ Sodium	
Amoxicillin, Amoxicillin/clavulanic acid (Augmentin)	Take with food to reduce GI upset May be present in breast milk	Nausea/vomiting/diarrhea Incidence of diarrhea higher with Augmentin vs. amoxicillin alone Mucocutaneous candidiasis	Amoxicillin/clavulanic acid will result in high urine concentrations of amoxicillin May result in false (+) when testing for the presence of glucose in the urine using the Clinitest, Benedict solution, or Fehling solution Glucose tests based on enzymatic glucose oxidase reactions (e.g., Clinistix) may be used	Suspension may be mixed with milk, fruit juice, water, ginger ale, or cold drinks; administer dose immediately after mixing
Aztreonam (Azactam)	May be present in breast milk	Nausea/vomiting/diarrhea	↑ ALT, AST ↑ Creatinine Prolonged PT, PTT	
Cephalosporins	Possible nephrotoxicity with vitamin K deficiency	GI mucosa damage Vomiting Diarrhea	Prolonged PT ↓ Potassium	

(*continued*)

	NUTRITIONAL CONSIDERATIONS	POSSIBLE GASTROINTESTINAL SIDE EFFECTS	POSSIBLE EFFECTS ON LAB VALUES	COMMENTS/RECOMMENDATIONS
Chloramphenicol (Chloromycetin)	Take on an empty stomach Decreased protein synthesis Increased need for riboflavin, B_6, B_{12} May be present in breast milk	Vomiting Diarrhea Stomatitis Enterocolitis Glossitis	Anemia	
Clindamycin (Cleocin)	Grapefruit juice may increase serum concentrations Take with a full glass of water to avoid esophageal irritation May be present in breast milk	Nausea/vomiting/diarrhea Esophagitis Pseudomembranous colitis	↑ LFTs	
Clofazimine (Lamprene)	Administer with meals or milk to maximize absorption May be present in breast milk	Constipation, abdominal pain Nausea/vomiting/diarrhea Anorexia GI bleeding Dysgeusia	↑ Glucose	Capsules must be swallowed whole and should not be opened
Dapsone	Do not administer with alkaline foods or antacids (may decrease dapsone absorption) Administer with meals if GI upset occurs	Vomiting Anorexia Abdominal pain Pancreattis	↑ Potassium ↓ Albumin ↑ ALT, alk phos ↑ LDH ↑ Bilirubin	

Fosfomycin (Monurol)	May be administered without regard to meals May be present in breast milk	*Clostridioides difficile*-associated diarrhea Nausea/vomiting/diarrhea Abdominal pain Anorexia Constipation Flatulence Xerostomia Cholestatic jaundice Hepatic necrosis	↓ Phosphorus ↓ Magnesium ↓ Potassium ↑ Sodium ↑ ALT	Each gram of IV fosfomycin contains ~0.32 g of sodium Always mix with 3-4 oz (90-120 mL) cool water before ingesting; do not administer in its dry form or mix with hot water
Linezolid (Zyvox)	Concurrent use of linezolid and foods or beverages containing large quantities of tyramine may result in a significant pressor response Administer with or without food	Nausea/diarrhea Dyspepsia Oral moniliasis Tongue discoloration Localized abdominal pain Constipation Pseudomembranous colitis	↑ ALT May cause lactic acidosis ↑ Lactate dehydrogenase ↑ Amylase ↑ Lipase	Patients receiving linezolid and tyramine-containing foods or beverages should be monitored for significant blood pressure increases Avoid foods containing large amounts of tyramine (e.g., aged cheese, sour cream, red wine); <100 mg/meal

(continued)

	NUTRITIONAL CONSIDERATIONS	POSSIBLE GASTROINTESTINAL SIDE EFFECTS	POSSIBLE EFFECTS ON LAB VALUES	COMMENTS/RECOMMENDATIONS
Macrolides: Azithromycin, Clarithromycin, Erythromycin	Rate and extent of GI absorption may be altered depending upon the formulation Azithromycin: Food does not affect bioavailability of the tablet formulation, immediate release oral suspension, or the 1 g suspension regimen; ↑ absorption of extended-release suspension when given with a high-fat meal Clarithromycin: Food delays rate, but not extent, of absorption; food increases extended-release clarithromycin AUC by ~30% relative to fasting conditions Erythromycin: Serum levels may be altered if taken with food (formulation-dependent)	Abdominal pain Cramping Nausea/vomiting/diarrhea Stomatitis Dyspepsia	False (+) urinary catecholamines, 17-hydroxycorticosteroids, 17-ketosteroids May elevate hepatic enzymes	Do not crush enteric coated or delayed release products Azithromycin: Immediate release suspension and tablet may be taken without regard to food; extended-release suspension should be taken on an empty stomach (at least 1 h before or 2 h following a meal) Clarithromycin: Immediate release tablets and oral suspension may be given with or without meals, may be taken with milk; extended-release tablets should be taken with food Erythromycin: Avoid milk and acidic beverages 1 h before or after a dose; administer after food to decrease GI discomfort
Metronidazole (Flagyl)	Food decreases peak drug concentration May administer with food to minimize GI upset	Nausea/vomiting/diarrhea Metallic taste Xerostomia Furry tongue	False (−)/decreased AST levels May interfere with AST, ALT, triglycerides, glucose, and LDH testing	Disulfiram reaction with alcohol

Moxifloxacin	Multivitamins/Minerals (with ADEK, Folate, Iron) may decrease the serum concentration by decreasing the absorption of orally administered moxifloxacin Administer at least 2 h before or 6 h after the dose of a multivitamin that contains polyvalent cations (e.g., calcium, iron, magnesium, selenium, zinc) Administer without regard to meals It is not known if moxifloxacin is present in breast milk	Nausea/vomiting/diarrhea Abdominal pain Constipation Abdominal distension/distress Flatulence Gastritis Gastroenteritis GERD Anorexia/decreased appetite Dysgeusia Xerostomia	↑ Chloride ↑ Ionized calcium ↑ Serum albumin ↓ Potassium ↑ ALT Altered amylase and lipase levels Hypoglycemia
Neomycin (Mycifradin)	Decreased absorption of fat, MCT, vitamins A, D, K, B_{12}, sodium, glucose, lactose, sucrose, xylose; may also deplete β-carotene, calcium, iron, magnesium, potassium Administer without regard to meals It is not known if neomycin is excreted into breast milk	Nausea/vomiting/diarrhea Colitis Candidiasis Inactivation of bile salts GI mucosal damage Decreased activity of disaccharidases Lipase inhibition Malabsorption syndrome (with prolonged therapy)	↑ BUN, creatinine

(continued)

	NUTRITIONAL CONSIDERATIONS	POSSIBLE GASTROINTESTINAL SIDE EFFECTS	POSSIBLE EFFECTS ON LAB VALUES	COMMENTS/RECOMMENDATIONS
Penicillins	Administer with water on an empty stomach (1 h before or 2 h after meals) May take with food to ↓ GI upset Increased urinary potassium excretion May inactivate B_6 Food ↓ drug absorption	Decreased appetite Diarrhea	↓ Potassium False (+) or (−) urinary glucose determined using Clinitest, positive Coombs' (direct) False (+) urinary serum proteins	
Quinolones	Dairy-containing foods, mineral supplements, calcium fortified juices decrease drug concentrations Administer 2 h after meals May take with food to ↓ GI upset May increase caffeine concentrations	Nausea/vomiting/diarrhea GI bleeding Abdominal pain Anorexia Pseudomembranous colitis Dyspepsia	Anemia ↑ ALT, AST, alk phos ↑ BUN, creatinine	Ciprofloxacin—oral suspension **not** suitable for enteral feeding tubes
Sulfonamides	Decreased synthesis of folic acid, B vitamins, vitamin K Decreased iron absorption Increased urinary excretion of vitamin C Presence of food delays but does not ↓ absorption	Decreased appetite Nausea/vomiting Stomatitis Pseudomembranous colitis Abdominal pain	↑ Potassium False (+) protein in urine, false (+) urine glucose with Clinitest	Avoid large amounts of vitamin C or acidifying agents (cranberry juice) to prevent crystalluria

Tetracyclines	Chelate divalent ions Decreased absorption of calcium, iron, magnesium, zinc, amino acids Increased urinary excretion of vitamin C Absorption of tetracycline hydrochloride ↓ by 50% when taken with milk/dairy products Take on empty stomach 1 h before/2 h after dose Avoid milk/dairy products, polyvalent ions within 2-3 h of dose	Nausea/vomiting/diarrhea Anorexia Stomatitis Glossitis Antibiotic-associated pseudomembranous colitis Esophagitis Oral candidiasis	↑ BUN ↑ Bilirubin ↑ ALT, AST, alk phos False (–) urine glucose with Clinistix False (+) urine glucose using Clinitest	Doxycycline and minocycline may be given without regard to meals but best to avoid concurrent administration with milk/dairy products
Trimethoprim (Trimpex, TMP)	Decreased folate concentrations	Nausea/vomiting/diarrhea Epigastric distress Glossitis	Anemia ↑ ALT, AST, alk phos ↑ BUN, creatinine	Leucovorin may be given until normal hematopoiesis is restored
Antifungals				
Amphotericin B (Fungizone)	Possible nephrotoxicity with increased urinary excretion of potassium and magnesium	Decreased appetite Nausea/vomiting Steatorrhea Diarrhea with oral formulation	↓ Potassium ↓ Magnesium ↑ BUN, creatinine	Monitor potassium, magnesium, supplementation usually necessary

(continued)

	NUTRITIONAL CONSIDERATIONS	POSSIBLE GASTROINTESTINAL SIDE EFFECTS	POSSIBLE EFFECTS ON LAB VALUES	COMMENTS/RECOMMENDATIONS
Caspofungin (Cancidas)	It is not known if caspofungin is present in breast milk	Nausea/vomiting/diarrhea Abdominal pain Anorexia Mucosal inflammation	↓ Potassium ↑ Calcium ↑ Cr ↑ ALT, AST, alk phos ↑ Bilirubin	
Fluconazole (Diflucan)	Food delays time of peak absorption but has no effect on total amount of drug absorbed May be present in breast milk	Mild-moderate GI upset Nausea/vomiting/diarrhea Abdominal pain Xerostomia	↓ Potassium ↑ Cholesterol ↑ Triglycerides ↑ AST, ALT, alk phos	When administering via feeding tube, hold enteral nutrition
Flucytosine (Ancobon)	May take with food; food ↓ rate but not extent of absorption Magnesium or aluminum salts delay rate of absorption It is not known if flucytosine is present in breast milk	Nausea/vomiting/diarrhea Enterocolitis	↑ BUN, creatinine ↑ ALT, AST, alk phos ↑ CK, LDH False ↑ in serum creatinine values if Ektachem analyzer used	
Griseofulvin (Grisactin, Fulvicin)	High fat foods ↑ absorption rate It is not known if griseofulvin is excreted in breast milk	Nausea/vomiting/diarrhea Oral thrush GI upset Anorexia	False (+) urinary VMA levels ↑ ALT, AST ↑ Bilirubin	

Itraconazole (Sporanox)	Food ↑ absorption of capsule formulation Hypochlorhydria may ↓ absorption Grapefruit juice ↓ itraconazole AUC by 30% Absorption ↑ when taken with a cola beverage	Nausea/vomiting/diarrhea Abdominal pain Anorexia	↓ Potassium ↑ ALT, AST, alk phos ↑ LDH ↑ Triglyceride	Formulations are not interchangeable Take capsules with food Take oral solution on an empty stomach
Ketoconazole (Nizoral)	Food ↑ rate and extent of absorption Administration with an acidic beverage (cola, citrus juice) enhances absorption Take with food to ↓ GI upset May be present in breast milk	Nausea/vomiting/diarrhea Abdominal discomfort GI bleeding	↑ ALT, AST, alk phos	
Micafungin (Mycamine)	It is not known if micafungin is present in breast milk	Nausea/vomiting/diarrhea Mucosal inflammation Constipation Anorexia Dyspepsia	↓ Potassium ↓ Magnesium ↓ Calcium Hypoglycemia Hyperglycemia ↑ Sodium ↑ ALT, AST, alk phos	

(continued)

	NUTRITIONAL CONSIDERATIONS	POSSIBLE GASTROINTESTINAL SIDE EFFECTS	POSSIBLE EFFECTS ON LAB VALUES	COMMENTS/RECOMMENDATIONS
Posaconazole (Noxafil)	Adequate posaconazole absorption from GI tract and subsequent plasma concentrations are dependent on food for efficacy	Nausea/vomiting/diarrhea Anorexia Abdominal pain Constipation Dyspepsia	↑ALT, AST, alk phos ↑ Bilirubin Hyperglycemia ↓ Potassium ↓ Magnesium ↓ Calcium	Immediate release suspension: Must be administered during or within 20 min of a full meal or oral liquid nutritional supplement; alternatively, may be given with an acidic carbonated beverage Delayed-release tablets: Administer with food when possible, but may be given with or without food
Voriconazole (Vfend)	High-fat meals reduce extent of absorption Take 1 h before or 1 h after *meals*	Nausea/vomiting Anorexia Constipation Abdominal pain	↑ ALT, AST, alk phos ↑ Bilirubin ↓ Potassium ↓ Magnesium ↑ Creatinine	Enteral tube feedings may decrease oral absorption; may hold tube feedings for 1 h before and 1 h after a voriconazole dose
Antihelmintics				
Albendazole (Albenza)	Bioavailability increased when taken with a fatty meal May be present in breast milk	Nausea/vomiting Abdominal pain	↑ LFTs	For systemic infections, coadministration with a high-fat meal to increase absorption; for intraluminal infections, give on an empty stomach
Ivermectin (Stromectol)	Bioavailability ↑ 2.5-fold when administered following a high-fat meal Take on an empty stomach with water May be present in breast milk	Nausea/diarrhea/vomiting Abdominal pain Anorexia Constipation	↑ ALT, AST	

Mebendazole (Vermox)	Food ↑ drug absorption Administer with food May be present in breast milk	Nausea/vomiting/diarrhea Abdominal pain Anorexia	Transient abnormalities in LFTs	
Miltefosine (Impavido)	Administer with food to decrease GI distress It is not known if miltefosine is present in breast milk	Nausea/vomiting/diarrhea Abdominal pain ↓ appetite Abdominal distention Constipation Dysphagia Flatulence Melena	↑ LFTs ↑ Bilirubin ↑ Creatinine	Ensure adequate fluid intake during treatment to prevent dehydration
Praziquantel (Biltricide)	Grapefruit juice may ↑ the serum concentration of praziquantel Administer tablets with water during meals	Nausea Abdominal distress Anorexia	↑ LFTs	Tablets should be promptly swallowed whole (do not chew) to avoid bitter taste May crush the tablets and mix in a variety of liquids (e.g., orange juice, honey) to reduce the bitter taste Administer 30 min before or 2 h after a meal when treating tapeworm infections

(*continued*)

	NUTRITIONAL CONSIDERATIONS	POSSIBLE GASTROINTESTINAL SIDE EFFECTS	POSSIBLE EFFECTS ON LAB VALUES	COMMENTS/RECOMMENDATIONS
Antimalarials				
Artemether/ Lumefantrine (Coartem)	Administer with a full meal for best absorption It is not known if artemether or lumefantrine are present in breast milk Grapefruit Juice may increase serum concentration of Artemether and Lumefantrine	Nausea/vomiting/ diarrhea Abdominal pain Anorexia	QT prolongation	Patients should be encouraged to take with a meal as soon as food can be tolerated; patients who remain averse to food during treatment should be closely monitored as the risk of recrudescence increases
Chloroquine phosphate (Aralen)	Administer with food to decrease GI distress May be present in breast milk	Nausea/vomiting/ diarrhea Anorexia Stomatitis Weight loss	↓ Glucose has been reported ↑ Liver enzymes	Bitter taste may be masked by mixing with chocolate syrup
Hydroxy-chloroquine (Plaquenil)	Food increases bioavailability Administer with food to decrease GI distress May be present in breast milk	Nausea/vomiting/ diarrhea Anorexia Abdominal cramps	↑ALT, AST ↑ Bilirubin ↑ PT Anemia	
Primaquine phosphate	Administer with food to decrease GI distress May be present in breast milk	Nausea/vomiting Abdominal cramps Anorexia	Anemia	Drug has bitter taste

Pyrimethamine (Daraprim)	↓ Serum folate concentrations Administer with food to decrease GI distress May be present in breast milk	Anorexia Abdominal cramps Vomiting/diarrhea Atrophic glossitis	Anemia	Leucovorin may be given until normal hematopoiesis is restored
Sulfadoxine and Pyrimethamine (Fansidar)	↓ Serum folate concentrations Take with meals	Anorexia Gastritis Glossitis Vomiting/diarrhea	↑ALT, AST Anemia	Leucovorin may be given until normal hematopoiesis is restored
Antiprotozoals				
Atovaquone (Mepron)	Food increases bioavailability Must administer with food It is not known if atovaquone is present in breast milk	Nausea/vomiting/diarrhea Abdominal pain Constipation Anorexia Oral candidiasis Pancreatitis	↓ Sodium ↑ Amylase	Patients who cannot take with meals or have chronic diarrhea or GI problems at risk for drug malabsorption and treatment failure
Nitazoxanide (Alinia)	Food increases AUC Administer with food May be present in breast milk	Nausea/vomiting/diarrhea Abdominal pain GERD		
Paromomycin (Humatin)	Administer with food Poorly absorbed when given orally	Nausea/vomiting/diarrhea Abdominal cramps Enterocolitis (secondary) Steatorrhea Heartburn		

(continued)

	NUTRITIONAL CONSIDERATIONS	POSSIBLE GASTROINTESTINAL SIDE EFFECTS	POSSIBLE EFFECTS ON LAB VALUES	COMMENTS/RECOMMENDATIONS
Antiretrovirals				
Protease Inhibitors				
Atazanavir (Reyataz)	Administer with food Bioavailability ↑ when taken with food May be present in breast milk Garlic may decrease serum concentrations	Nausea/vomiting/diarrhea	↑ Cholesterol ↑ Amylase ↑ Bilirubin ↑ Lipase	May cause redistribution of fat (e.g., buffalo hump, peripheral wasting with increased abdominal girth, cushingoid appearance)
Fosamprenavir (Lexiva)	Tablets may be taken with or without food Children should take oral suspension *with* food; adults should take oral suspension *without* food Garlic may decrease serum concentrations	Nausea/vomiting/diarrhea Abdominal pain May cause transaminase elevations, hepatitis, and/or exacerbate preexisting hepatic dysfunction	↑ ALT, AST, alk phos ↑ *Bilirubin* ↑ Triglycerides ↑ Total cholesterol Hyperglycemia ↑ Lipase	Take tablets with food if taken with ritonavir May be administered without regard to food if not taken with ritonavir May cause redistribution of fat (e.g., buffalo hump, peripheral wasting with increased abdominal girth)
Indinavir (Crixivan)	Take on empty stomach; if GI upset a problem, take with light meals or other liquids ↓ Absorption when given with high amounts of protein or fatty foods Grapefruit juice ↓ AUC by 26% Garlic may decrease serum concentrations	Nausea/vomiting/diarrhea Abdominal pain Metallic taste Pancreatitis	↑ ALT, AST, alk phos ↑ Bilirubin ↑ Triglycerides Hyperglycemia (rare)	Ensure adequate hydration May administer with food if taken in combination with ritonavir If coadministered with didanosine, give at least 1 h apart on an empty stomach

Lopinavir and Ritonavir (Kaletra)	Solution should be taken with food Tablet may be taken with or without food It is not known if fosamprenavir is present in breast milk Garlic may decrease serum concentrations	Nausea/vomiting/diarrhea Abdominal pain Altered taste Weight loss	↑ ALT, AST, alk phos ↑ Bilirubin ↑ GGTP ↑ Triglycerides ↑ Amylase ↑ Lipase Hypercholesterolemia Hyperglycemia Alterations in sodium (↑↓)	Solution: Must administer with food; if using didanosine, take didanosine 1 h before or 2 h after lopinavir/ritonavir Tablet: swallow whole, do not break, crush, or chew; may be taken with didanosine when taken without food
Nelfinavir (Viracept)	Food ↑ absorption May be present in breast milk Garlic may decrease serum concentrations	Nausea/vomiting/diarrhea Abdominal pain Anorexia Dyspepsia Epigastric pain Mouth ulceration GI bleeding Pancreatitis	↑ALT, AST, alk phos, Hyperlipemia Hyperuricemia ↑ Glucose Anemia	Powder formulation contains 11.2 mg phenylalanine per gram powder Do not administer with acidic foods or juices (results in bitter taste)
Ritonavir (Norvir)	Administer with food to ↑ absorption May cause avitaminosis Garlic may decrease serum concentrations	Nausea/vomiting/diarrhea Taste perversion Abdominal pain Pancreatitis	↑ Triglycerides ↑ Cholesterol ↑ Creatine phosphokinase Hyperglycemia (rare) ↑ ALT, AST, alk phos Alterations in potassium (↑↓) ↑ Amylase ↑ GGT ↑ Bilirubin	Liquid formulations tastes unpleasant, reserve use for tube fed patients or mix with chocolate milk or nutritional supplement Solution contains ethanol and propylene glycol; not recommended for use with polyurethane feeding tubes (potential incompatibility), but may be used with silicone and polyvinyl chloride (PVC) feeding tubes

(continued)

	NUTRITIONAL CONSIDERATIONS	POSSIBLE GASTROINTESTINAL SIDE EFFECTS	POSSIBLE EFFECTS ON LAB VALUES	COMMENTS/RECOMMENDATIONS
Tipranavir (Aptivus)	Coadministration with ritonavir is required Garlic may decrease serum concentrations	Nausea/vomiting/diarrhea Abdominal pain Weight loss Dehydration Taste perversion Pancreatitis	↑ Triglycerides ↑ Cholesterol ↑ Amylase ↑ Lipase↑ALT, AST ↑ GGT ↑ Bilirubin	Administer with ritonavir capsules or solution without regard to meals; administer with ritonavir tablets with meals Capsule contains dehydrated ethanol Oral solution formulation contains vitamin E; additional vitamin E supplements should be avoided May cause redistribution of fat (e.g., buffalo hump, peripheral wasting with increased abdominal girth, cushingoid appearance) May cause facial wasting
Nucleoside and Nucleotide Reverse Transcriptase Inhibitors				
Abacavir (Ziagen)	Food does not affect AUC May be present in breast milk	Nausea/vomiting/diarrhea Anorexia Pancreatitis Abdominal pain Pancreatitis	Mild hyperglycemia Hypertriglyceridemia Lactic acidosis ↑ Amylase	Fat redistribution and accumulation have been reported

Emtricitabine (Emtriva)	May be administered with or without food May be present in breast milk	Nausea/vomiting/diarrhea Abdominal discomfort Gastroenteritis	↑ CPK ↑ Amylase ↑ Lipase ↑ Triglycerides ↑ Glucose ↑ ALT, AST, alk phos ↑ Bilirubin Anemia	May cause redistribution of fat
Lamivudine (Epivir, 3TC)	Food may ↓ rate of absorption and peak serum concentrations, but does not significantly change the AUC May be present in breast milk	Nausea/vomiting/diarrhea Feeding problems Abdominal discomfort Pancreatitis Anorexia Stomatitis	↑ ALT, AST ↑ Bilirubin ↑ Amylase ↑ Glucose ↑ Lipase	May cause fat redistribution and accumulation
Stavudine (Zerit, d4T)	Take without regard to food Food ↓ peak serum concentrations by 45%, bioavailability not changed Some products may contain sucrose May be present in breast milk	Nausea/vomiting/diarrhea Abdominal pain Anorexia Pancreatitis	↑ ALT, AST ↑ Bilirubin ↑ Lipase Hyperglycemia Hyperlipidemia	Capsule may be opened and dispersed in a small amount of water

(continued)

	NUTRITIONAL CONSIDERATIONS	POSSIBLE GASTROINTESTINAL SIDE EFFECTS	POSSIBLE EFFECTS ON LAB VALUES	COMMENTS/RECOMMENDATIONS
Tenofovir Disoproxil Fumarate (Viread)	Administer with meals to improve absorption High-fat meals ↑ oral bioavailability May be present in breast milk	Nausea/vomiting/diarrhea Flatulence Anorexia Pancreatitis	↑ LFTs ↓ Phosphorus ↑ Amylase	Powder should be mixed with 2-4 oz of soft and swallowed immediately (avoids bitter taste)
Zidovudine (Retrovir, AZT, ZDV)	Folate/B_{12} deficiency increases zidovidine-associated myelosuppression May take with food Rate of absorption and peak serum concentration may ↓ when taken with food May be present in breast milk	Nausea/vomiting/diarrhea Anorexia Abdominal pain Pancreatitis Dysgeusia	↑ AST, alk phos ↑ LDH Anemia Lactic acidosis	Take capsules while in upright position to ↓ risk of esophageal ulceration Syrup is strawberry flavored May cause fat redistribution and *accumulation*
Reverse Transcriptase Inhibitor (Non-nucleoside)				
Doravirine (Pifeltro)	Administer with or without food It is not known if doravirine is present in breast milk	Nausea/diarrhea Abdominal pain	↑ Lipase ↑ ALT, AST, alk phos ↑ Bilirubin ↑ Creatinine ↑ LDL	

Efavirenz (Sustiva)	Take with water on an empty stomach preferred Avoid high-fat/high-caloric meals; high fat/high caloric meals ↑ AUC and peak concentration and may ↑ adverse effects May be present in breast milk	Nausea/vomiting/diarrhea Abdominal pain	↑ Triglycerides ↑ Amylase Hypercholesterolemia ↑ LFTs ↑ HDL ↑ ALT, AST	Take with water on an empty stomach preferred Tastes peppery (grape jelly may be used to improve taste) Tablets should not be broken; some clinicians recommend opening capsules and adding to liquid or food for patients that cannot swallow capsules, however this is not recommended because no pharmacokinetic data are available
Etravirine (Intelence)	Take after meals Food increases absorption of etravirine by ~50% May be present in breast milk	Nausea/diarrhea	↑ Triglycerides ↑ Cholesterol ↑ LDL Hyperglycemia ↑ ALT, AST	Central redistribution of body fat May disperse tablets in glass of water; stir well prior to drinking and rinse glass several times to ensure administration of complete dose Do not use carbonated beverages or warm (>40 °C) water
Nevirapine (Viramune)	Can be given without regard to food May be present in breast milk	Nausea/vomiting/diarrhea Abdominal pain	↑ LFTs ↑ Triglycerides ↑ HDL ↑ GGT ↑ ALT, AST ↑ Amylase Most cases of nevirapine-associated hepatic toxicity occur during the first 12 wk of therapy; about one-third of cases occur after 12 wk of treatment; in some cases, patients present with nonspecific prodromal signs or symptoms of hepatitis and rapidly progressed to hepatic failure	Central redistribution of body fat Extended-release tablets must be swallowed whole and not crushed, chewed, or divided

(*continued*)

	NUTRITIONAL CONSIDERATIONS	POSSIBLE GASTROINTESTINAL SIDE EFFECTS	POSSIBLE EFFECTS ON LAB VALUES	COMMENTS/RECOMMENDATIONS
Rilpivirine (Edurant)	Administer with a normal- to high-calorie meal; absorption increased by ~40% when taken with a normal to high-caloric meal Administration with a protein supplement drink alone does not increase absorption May be present in breast milk	Abdominal discomfort/ pain ↓ Appetite Nausea/vomiting/ diarrhea	↑ Cholesterol ↑ LDL ↑ Triglycerides ↑ ALT, AST ↑ Bilirubin ↑ Creatinine	May cause redistribution of fat
Entry and Fusion Inhibitors				
Enfuvirtide (Fuzeon)	It is not known if enfuvirtide is present in breast milk	Diarrhea/nausea Weight loss Abdominal pain ↓ Appetite, anorexia Pancreatitis Xerostomia	↑ Transaminases ↑ CPK	
CCR5 Antagonist				
Maraviroc (Selzentry)	Can be given with or without food; absorption somewhat reduced with ingestion of a high-fat meal It is not known if maraviroc is present in breast milk	Abdominal pain Altered appetite Constipation Vomiting ↓Gastric motility	↑ Transaminases ↑ Bilirubin ↑ Amylase	

Integrase inhibitor				
Cabotegravir (Apretude, Vocabria)	Administer with a meal at same time daily Absorption increased 14% with high-fat meal (compared to fasting) It is not known if cabotegravir is present in breast milk	Nausea/vomiting/diarrhea Abdominal distress ↓ Appetite Flatulence May cause weight gain	↑ Lipase ↑ ALT, AST ↑ Creatinine Hypercholesterolemia ↑ Triglycerides	
Dolutegravir (Tivicay)	May be administered without regard to meals Iron, zinc, and selenium supplements may decrease serum concentration of dolutegravir May be present in breast milk	Nausea/vomiting Abdominal pain/distress Flatulence Hepatitis May cause weight gain	↑ Lipase Hyperglycemia ↑ ALT, AST Hyperbilirubinemia ↑ Triglycerides Hypercholesterolemia ↑ HDL ↑ LDL ↑ Creatinine	Take at least 2 h before or 6 h after supplements containing iron or calcium; alternatively, dolutegravir and supplements containing calcium or iron can be taken together with food
Raltegravir (Isentress)	May be administered without regard to meals; however, clinically insignificant variability in absorption exists depending on meal type May be present in breast milk	Nausea/diarrhea	↑ CPK ↑ Amylase ↑ Lipase ↑ ALT, AST, total bilirubin	Chewable tablets contain phenylalanine
Capsid Inhibitors				
Lenacapavir (Sunlenca)	Administer with or without food It is not known if lenacapavir is present in breast milk	Nausea	↑ Creatinine Hyperglycemia ↑ ALT, AST Hyperbilirubinemia	

(continued)

	NUTRITIONAL CONSIDERATIONS	POSSIBLE GASTROINTESTINAL SIDE EFFECTS	POSSIBLE EFFECTS ON LAB VALUES	COMMENTS/RECOMMENDATIONS
Post-Attachment Inhibitor				
Ibalizumab (Trogarzo)	It is not known if ibalizumab is present in breast milk	Nausea/diarrhea	↑ Serum glucose ↑ Uric acid ↑ Lipase ↑ Direct/total bilirubin ↑ Creatinine	
gp120-Attachment Inhibitor				
Fostemsavir (Rukobia)	Administer with or without food It is not known if fostemsavir is present in breast milk	Nausea/vomiting/diarrhea Abdominal pain Dysgeusia Dyspepsia	QT prolongation ↑ Lipase ↑ LDL ↑ Uric acid ↑ Triglycerides Hypercholesterolemia Hyperglycemia ↑ Direct/total bilirubin ↑ CPK ↑ ALT, AST (Hepatoxicity has been associated with antiretroviral combination therapy, particularly among patients coinfected with hepatitis B virus (HBV) and/or hepatitis C virus (HCV.)	Swallow tablets whole; do not chew, crush, or split tablets

CYP3A Inhibitor				
Cobicistat (Tybost)	Administer with food and at the same time as other coadministered antiretroviral agents It is not known if cobicistat is present in breast milk	Jaundice Ocular icterus Nausea/vomiting Abdominal pain	False elevations in serum creatinine Hyperbilirubinemia ↑ Amylase ↑ Lipase ↑ GGT ↑ ALT, AST ↑ HDL ↑ LDL ↑ Triglycerides, Hypercholesterolemia ↑ Creatinine Vomiting Abdominal pain	May inhibit tubular secretion of creatinine without affecting actual renal glomerular function
Antitubercular Agents				
Capreomycin	It is not known if capreomycin is present in breast milk		Hypocalcemia Hypokalemia Hypomagnesemia ↑ BUN, creatinine	
Cycloserine (Seromycin)	May administer without regard to meals B_6 antagonist ↓ absorption of calcium, magnesium, vitamin B_{12} Decreased folate utilization and vitamin K synthesis May increase B_{12} and folate requirements May be present in breast milk		Anemia ↑ ALT, AST	Some neurotoxic effects may be prevented or lessened by pyridoxine supplementation

(continued)

	NUTRITIONAL CONSIDERATIONS	POSSIBLE GASTROINTESTINAL SIDE EFFECTS	POSSIBLE EFFECTS ON LAB VALUES	COMMENTS/RECOMMENDATIONS
Ethambutol (Myambutol)	May deplete copper and zinc Take with food to ↓ GI upset	Nausea/vomiting Abdominal pain Anorexia	↑ Uric acid levels Abnormal LFTs	
Ethionamide (Trecator)	Neurotoxic effects may be prevented or relieved by the coadministration of pyridoxine May be taken with or without meals Separate the administration of ethambutol and mineral supplements by at least 2 h to avoid interactions and ensure proper absorption of the supplements	Nausea/vomiting/diarrhea Abdominal pain Anorexia Excessive salivation Metallic taste Stomatitis Weight loss	Hypoglycemia ↑ Bilirubin ↑ LFTs	
Isoniazid	Administer on an empty stomach (1 h before or 2 h after meals) with water Administration with food significantly reduces bioavailability May cause pellagra May decrease folic acid absorption and alters pyridoxine metabolism	Epigastric discomfort Nausea/vomiting Pancreatitis Jaundice	↑ ALT, AST Hyperglycemia Metabolic acidosis Hyperbilirubinemia	If unable to swallow tablets, may crush tablet and mix in a soft food or liquid, or starch-based pudding administered as a slurry

	Increase dietary intake of folate, niacin, and magnesium Isoniazid has weak monoamine oxidase inhibiting activity and may potentially inhibit tyramine metabolism May inhibit diamine oxidase resulting in headache, sweating, palpitations, flushing, diarrhea, itching, wheezing, dyspnea, or hypotension if taken with histamine-containing foods May be present in breast milk		
Pyrazinamide	May take without regard to food May be present in breast milk	Nausea/vomiting Anorexia Hepatoxicity	Hyperuricemia ↑ Serum iron
Rifabutin (Mycobutin)	High-fat meal may decrease the rate but not extent of drug absorption Take with food to ↓ GI upset It is not known if rifabutin is present in breast milk	Nausea/vomiting/diarrhea Anorexia Dyspepsia Abdominal pain Dysguesia Flatulence Jaundice	↑ LFTs

(continued)

	NUTRITIONAL CONSIDERATIONS	POSSIBLE GASTROINTESTINAL SIDE EFFECTS	POSSIBLE EFFECTS ON LAB VALUES	COMMENTS/RECOMMENDATIONS
Rifampin	Take on empty stomach. Food may decrease or delay amount of drug absorbed May be present in breast milk	Nausea/vomiting/ diarrhea Anorexia Stomatitis May discolor teeth	↑ LFTs Inhibits standard assay used to assess serum B_{12} and folate	
Antivirals				
Acyclovir (Zovirax)	May administer with food; food does not appear to impact absorption May be present in breast milk	Nausea/vomiting/ diarrhea Anorexia	↑ LFT ↑ BUN, creatinine ↑ Bilirubin ↑ Transaminases	
Amantadine (Symmetrel)	Administer without regard to food May be present in breast milk	Nausea/vomiting/ diarrhea Xerostomia Anorexia Constipation	↑ LFTs ↑ BUN, creatinine ↑ Bilirubin	
Cidofovir (Vistide)	It is not known if cidofovir is present in breast milk	Nausea/vomiting/ diarrhea Anorexia Pancreatitis	Metabolic acidosis ↑ LFTs ↑ BUN, creatinine ↓Serum bicarbonate	

Famciclovir (Famvir)	May take with food to ↓ GI upset Rate of absorption and/or conversion to penciclovir and peak concentration are ↓ with food, bioavailability not affected It is not known if famciclovir is present in breast milk	Nausea/vomiting/diarrhea Constipation Anorexia Abdominal pain Cholestatic jaundice	Abnormal hepatic function tests
Foscarnet (Foscavir)	It is not known if foscarnet is present in breast milk	Nausea/vomiting/diarrhea Cachexia Constipation Increased thirst Weight loss Abdominal pain Aphthous stomatitis Dysgeusia Dyspepsia Dysphagia Melena Pancreatitis Xerostomia	Hypocalcemia/low ionized calcium Hyper/hypophosphatemia Hypomagnesemia Hypokalemia Abnormal albumin-globulin ratio Acidosis Hyponatremia ↑ LDH ↑ Alk phos ↑ LFTs

(continued)

	NUTRITIONAL CONSIDERATIONS	POSSIBLE GASTROINTESTINAL SIDE EFFECTS	POSSIBLE EFFECTS ON LAB VALUES	COMMENTS/RECOMMENDATIONS
Ganciclovir (Cytovene)	Administer with food High-fat meal ↑ AUC It is not known if ganciclovir is present in breast milk Some products may contain sodium	Nausea/vomiting/diarrhea Pancreatitis Anorexia Dysgeusia Dyspepsia Dysphagia Eructation Weight loss	↑ LFTs ↑ BUN, creatinine	Do not open capsules or crush tablets
Oseltamivir (Tamiflu)	May be administered without regard to meals Administer with food to ↓ GI upset May be present in breast milk	Nausea/vomiting/diarrhea Pseudomembranous colitis	Abnormal hepatic function tests	Administer with food to ↓ GI upset Capsules may be opened and mixed with sweetened liquid (e.g., chocolate syrup)
Valacyclovir (Valtrex)	May be taken with or without food Administer with food to ↓ GI upset Valacyclovir is rapidly metabolized to acyclovir. Following administration of valacyclovir, acyclovir is present in breast milk; unchanged valacyclovir has not been detected in breast milk	Nausea/vomiting/diarrhea Abdominal pain	↑ ALT, AST, alk phos	Maintain adequate hydration

Valganciclovir (Valcyte)	Take with food Coadministration with a high-fat meal increased AUC by 30% It is not known if ganciclovir or valganciclovir are present in breast milk	Nausea/vomiting/ diarrhea Abdominal pain Constipation Dyspepsia ↓ Appetite	Hyperglycemia ↑ Potassium ↓ Calcium ↓ Magnesium ↓ Phosphorus ↑ ALT, AST	Take with food
Miscellaneous Anti-Infective Agents				
Clofazimine (Lamprene)	Food ↑ extent of absorption Administer with meals/milk to maximize absorption and reduce GI side effects May be present in breast milk	Nausea/vomiting/ diarrhea Abdominal pain Constipation Bowel obstruction GI bleeding Dysgeusia	Hyperglycemia	
Methenamine (Hiprex, Mandelamine)	Administer with food Foods/diets which alkalinize urine pH > 5.5 ↓ activity of methenamine Cranberry juice can be used to acidify urine and ↑ activity of methenamine	Nausea/vomiting/ diarrhea Abdominal cramping Anorexia Stomatitis	Albuminuria ↑ AST, ALT ↓ Urine pH	Ensure patient is properly hydrated Some products may contain tartrazine

(*continued*)

	NUTRITIONAL CONSIDERATIONS	POSSIBLE GASTROINTESTINAL SIDE EFFECTS	POSSIBLE EFFECTS ON LAB VALUES	COMMENTS/RECOMMENDATIONS
Nitrofurantoin (Furadantin, Macrodantin)	Food ↑ total amount absorbed Administer with food or milk to decrease adverse effects Cranberry juice or other urine acidifiers enhance drug action May be present in breast milk	Nausea/vomiting/diarrhea Anorexia Pancreatitis Abdominal pain Constipation	Anemia ↑ AST, ALT	
Pentamidine (Pentam)	It is not known if pentamidine is present in breast milk	Nausea/vomiting/diarrhea Metallic taste Pancreatitis Anorexia Dyspepsia Xerostomia	Anemia ↑ *Potassium* Hypo/hyperglycemia ↓ Magnesium ↓ Calcium ↑ BUN, creatinine ↑ Hepatic enzymes	
Antihyperlipidemics				
Alirocumab (Praluent)	It is not known if alirocumab is present in breast milk	Diarrhea	↑ Serum transaminases ↓ LDL-C	Lipid profile (fasting or nonfasting) before initiating treatment Fasting lipid profile should be rechecked 4-12 wk after initiation and every 3-12 mo thereafter For patients undergoing LDL apheresis, may be administered without regard to the timing of apheresis

Cholestyramine (Questran)	Administer before meals Decreased absorption of fat, MCT, fat-soluble vitamins, B_{12}, iron, folate, calcium, glucose, xylose, electrolytes To minimize binding, administer vitamins/minerals 1 h before or 4-6 h after cholestyramine Due to lack of systemic absorption, cholestyramine is not expected to be present in breast milk	Constipation Nausea Anorexia Weight changes Abdominal distention	↑ Triglyceride ↑ ALT, AST, alk phos ↑ Phosphorus ↑ Chloride ↓ Cholesterol ↓ LDL ↓ Calcium ↓ Potassium ↓ Sodium	
Colesevelam (Welchol)	Administer with meals ↓ Absorption fat-soluble vitamins Chronic use may be associated with bleeding problems due to hypoprothrombinemia from vitamin K deficiency Due to lack of systemic absorption, colesevelam is not expected to be present in breast milk	Nausea Abdominal pain Constipation Dyspepsia Pancreatitis	↑ Triglyceride	To avoid GI distress, do not take in dry form

(continued)

	NUTRITIONAL CONSIDERATIONS	POSSIBLE GASTROINTESTINAL SIDE EFFECTS	POSSIBLE EFFECTS ON LAB VALUES	COMMENTS/RECOMMENDATIONS
Colestipol	↓ Absorption fat-soluble vitamins, iron May bind to B_{12}-intrinsic factor complex May require folic acid, iron supplements Administer vitamins or mineral supplements, at least 1 h before or 4 h after colestipol Due to lack of systemic absorption, colestipol is not expected to be present in breast milk	Anorexia Abdominal distention Nausea/vomiting/diarrhea Constipation	Transient ↑ ALT, AST ↑ Alk phos	
Ezetimibe (Zetia)	May be taken without regard to meals Administer >2 h before or >4 h after bile acid sequestrants May be present in breast milk	Hepatotoxicity Hepatocellular hepatitis Cholestatic hepatitis Autoimmune hepatitis-like syndrome Abdominal pain Cholecystitis Cholelithiasis Nausea Pancreatitis	↓ total cholesterol ↓ LDL ↓ Apolipoprotein B ↓ Non-HDL cholesterol Elevated transaminases (≥3 × ULN)	Before starting treatment, patients should be placed on a standard cholesterol-lowering diet for 6 wk and continue diet during drug therapy

HMG-CoA Reductase Inhibitors ("Statins")				
Atorvastatin, Cerivastatin, Lovastatin, Fluvastatin, Pravastatin, Simvastatin	Depletes coenyzme Q10 Food ↑ drug absorption Serum drug levels may↑ when taken with grapefruit juice	Abdominal pain Constipation Nausea/vomiting/ diarrhea Dyspepsia Flatulence Regurgitation Xerostomia Anorexia Pancreatitis	Abnormal thyroid function tests ↑ LFTs ↑ CPK	Risk of myopathy and/or rhabdomyolysis is ↑ with daily intake of large quantities of grapefruit juice (>1 quart/day)
Gemfibrozil (Lopid)	↓ Coenzyme Q10, Vitamin E Administer 30 min prior to breakfast and dinner It is not known if gemfibrozil is present in breast milk	Epigastric pain Xerostomia Anorexia Constipation Abdominal pain Flatulence Nausea/vomiting	↑ ALT, AST, ↑ CPK ↑ LDH	
Antiarrhythmics				
Amiodarone (Cordarone)	Food increases rate and extent of oral absorption; high-fat meals can increase AUC; grapefruit juice increases oral absorption May be present in breast milk	Nausea/vomiting Constipation Anorexia Xerostomia Pancreatitis	↑ Ammonia ↑ LFTs ↑ Bilirubin ↑ Triglycerides Hyperglycemia	

(continued)

	NUTRITIONAL CONSIDERATIONS	POSSIBLE GASTROINTESTINAL SIDE EFFECTS	POSSIBLE EFFECTS ON LAB VALUES	COMMENTS/RECOMMENDATIONS
Digoxin (Lanoxin)	Meals containing high fiber or bran or foods high in pectin may decrease digoxin absorption Avoid natural licorice May be present in breast milk	Nausea/vomiting/diarrhea Feeding intolerance Abdominal pain Anorexia	↑ Potassium ↓ Magnesium	Increased risk of digoxin toxicity in patients who are ↓ potassium, ↓ magnesium
Flecainide (Tambocor)	Dairy products (milk, formula, yogurt) may interfere with drug absorption Clearance of flecainide may be decreased in patients with strict vegan diets due to urine pH >8 May be present in breast milk	Nausea Xerostomia Metallic taste		Avoid concurrent administration with milk or milk-based formulas; monitor serum drug concentrations and decrease the dose when milk consumption ↓ Monitor serum concentrations closely with any changes in milk or milk-based formula consumption; dose adjustments may be necessary
Verapamil (Calan)	Grapefruit juice ↑ serum concentrations Can be administered with or without food May be present in breast milk	Constipation Nausea/diarrhea Abdominal discomfort Gingival hyperplasia Xerostomia Paralytic ileus (nonobstructive)	↑ LFTs	

Antihypertensives				
ACE inhibitors: Benazepril, Captopril, Enalapril, Lisinopril	Administer on empty stomach Food decreases the rate but does not significantly decrease the extent of absorption Limit salt substitutes or potassium-rich diet May deplete zinc	Nausea/diarrhea Ageusia	↓ Glucose ↑ Potassium	May result in a loss of sense of smell and taste Avoid natural licorice, which causes sodium and water retention and increases potassium loss
Calcium channel blockers: Amlodipine (Norvasc), Nifedipine (Procardia)	Grapefruit juice increases oral absorption Administer without regard to food Administer with low fat foods to minimize flushing	Nausea/vomiting/diarrhea Constipation Abdominal pain Dysphagia Xerostomia Weight changes Gingival hyperplasia	↑ LFTs	Administer without regard to food Avoid natural licorice products
Hydralazine (Apresoline)	Inactivates B_6 Administer with food Food enhances bioavailability May be present in breast milk	Nausea/vomiting/diarrhea Constipation Paralytic ileus Anorexia	↓ Hgb ↓ WBC	Avoid natural licorice

(continued)

	NUTRITIONAL CONSIDERATIONS	POSSIBLE GASTROINTESTINAL SIDE EFFECTS	POSSIBLE EFFECTS ON LAB VALUES	COMMENTS/RECOMMENDATIONS
Methyldopa (Aldomet)	Increased need for B_{12}, folate May be administered without regard to food May be present in breast milk	Nausea/diarrhea Colitis Liver disorders Xerostomia "Black" tongue Constipation Cholestasis	Anemia ↑ BUN ↑ ALT, AST, alk phos ↑ Bilirubin ↑ Sodium ↑ Potassium	May be administered without regard to food
Anti-Inflammatory Agents				
Salicylates	Administer with food to ↓ GI upset Increased vitamin C requirements Possible iron deficiency May ↓ serum folate levels	Nausea/vomiting/diarrhea GI bleeding	Proteinuria Increased bleeding time Interferes with Gerhardt test, VMA determinators, 5-HIAA, and xylose tolerance tests	Limit curry powder, paprika, licorice Fresh fruits containing vitamin C may displace drug from binding sites, resulting in increased urinary excretion of aspirin
Celecoxib (CeleBREX)	May be administered without regard to meals Peak concentrations are delayed and AUC ↑when taken with a high-fat meal May be present in breast milk	Nausea/vomiting/diarrhea Abdominal pain Dyspepsia Gastroesophageal reflux Flatulence GI bleeding Anorexia Stomatitis Pancreatitis	↑ ALT, AST Hypoglycemia ↓ Sodium	

Ibuprofen (Motrin, Advil)	May deplete folate Administer with food to ↓ GI upset May be present in breast milk	Nausea/vomiting/diarrhea GI bleeding Heartburn Dyspepsia	Acidosis	Some products may contain phenylalanine and/or potassium
Indomethacin (Indocin)	Decreased absorption of amino acids, glucose, xylose May deplete iron, folate May be present in breast milk	Nausea/vomiting/diarrhea Constipation Dyspepsia GI bleeding Epigastric pain Anorexia Weight gain	↑ Potassium ↓ Vitamin C Anemia ↓ Glucose (iv form)	
Ketorolac (Toradol)	High-fat meals may delay time to peak by approximately 1 h and decrease peak level Administer with milk to ↓ GI upset May be present in breast milk	Dyspepsia Nausea/vomiting/diarrhea GI pain Constipation	↑ LFTs ↑ Potassium ↓ Sodium	

(continued)

	NUTRITIONAL CONSIDERATIONS	POSSIBLE GASTROINTESTINAL SIDE EFFECTS	POSSIBLE EFFECTS ON LAB VALUES	COMMENTS/RECOMMENDATIONS
Corticosteroids: Hydrocortisone, Methylprednisolone, Prednisone, Prednisolone, Betamethasone, Dexamethasone	↑ Protein catabolism, ↓ glucose tolerance, accelerated vitamin D metabolism, ↑ sodium and water retention, ↓ absorption and ↑ excretion of potassium, zinc, vitamin C, calcium, and phosphorus ↑ B_6 and folate requirements Possible growth suppression and impaired wound healing May be present in breast milk	Increased appetite Xerostomia Dysgeusia Peptic disease Vomiting/diarrhea Weight gain	↑ Glucose ↑ Triglyceride ↑ Cholesterol ↑ Sodium ↓ Potassium ↓ Calcium ↓ T4 ↓ Uric acid ↓ Zinc ↑ Prealbumin	
Budesonide (Entocort EC)	Administration of capsules with a high-fat meal delays peak concentration, but does not alter the extent of absorption	Nausea/vomiting Abdominal pain Anorexia Diarrhea Dyspepsia Flatulence Gastroenteritis Glossitis Intestinal obstruction	↓ Potassium Dyslipidemia	Grapefruit juice may double systemic exposure of orally administered budesonide; avoid grapefruit juice when using oral capsules Swallow whole; do not crush or chew caps

	May be present in breast milk	Oral candidiasis Taste perversion Tongue edema Weight gain Xerostomia		May cause redistribution of body fat
5-aminosalicyclic acid derivatives: Balsalazide, Mesalamine, Olsalazine, Sulfasalazine	Folate depletion Take with food May be present in breast milk	Abdominal pain Cramps Flatulence Anorexia Gastritis Dyspepsia, Nausea/ vomiting/diarrhea Constipation Hemorrhoids Anorexia Weight loss	↑ ALT, AST ↑ Triglycerides ↑ Amylase ↑ GGT ↑ LDH	Consider folate supplementation Balsalazide: May cause staining of teeth or tongue when sprinkled on food
Sulfasalazine (Azulfidine)	Impairs folate absorption Increase dietary iron intake Administer after meals or with food May be present in breast milk	Nausea/vomiting/ diarrhea Anorexia Pancreatitis	↑ LFTs	Consider folate supplementation

(continued)

	NUTRITIONAL CONSIDERATIONS	POSSIBLE GASTROINTESTINAL SIDE EFFECTS	POSSIBLE EFFECTS ON LAB VALUES	COMMENTS/RECOMMENDATIONS
Antineoplastic Drugs				
Asparaginase (Elspar)	It is not known if asparaginase is present in breast milk	Nausea/vomiting Abdominal cramps Pancreatitis Anorexia	↓ Albumin ↑ Uric acid ↑ Ammonia Hyperglycemia ↓ Thyroxine ↑ Bilirubin Hypercholesterolemia Hypertriglyceridemia ↑ Hepatic enzymes ↑ Lipase	
Carboplatin (Paraplatin)	May be present in breast milk	Nausea/vomiting/diarrhea Anorexia Hemorrhagic colitis Mucositis Metallic taste Constipation	↓ Calcium ↓ Magnesium ↓ Potassium ↓ Sodium ↑ BUN, creatinine ↑ Alk phos ↑ AST	

Cyclophosphamide (Cytoxan)	May be present in breast milk	Anorexia Nausea/vomiting Mucosal injury Dysgeusia	Anemia ↑ Uric acid ↓↑Potassium Hyperuricemia ↓ Sodium Positive Coombs ↑ LDH ↑ Glucose ↑ LFTs		Maintain high fluid intake Take with food only if GI distress occurs
Dactinomycin (Cosmegen)	Decreased absorption of calcium, iron and fat It is not known if dactinomycin is present in breast milk	Anorexia Nausea/vomiting/diarrhea Stomatitis	↓ Calcium Hyperuricemia ↑ LFTs		
Fluorouracil (5-FU)	Do not eat 2 h before or after administration Increased need for B_1 Malabsorption of glucose, xylose It is not known if fluorouracil is present in breast milk	Severe nausea/vomiting/diarrhea GI bleeding Anorexia Stomatitis Esophagitis	Anemia ↓ Albumin ↑ ALT, alk phos ↑ Bilirubin ↑ LDH		Increase dietary intake of thiamine Use of acidic solutions to dilute fluorouracil for oral use may result in precipitation of drug and ↓ absorption Maintain adequate hydration
Hydroxyurea (Hydrea)	Supplemental administration of folic acid is recommended Hydroxyurea may mask development of folic acid deficiency May cause vitamin D deficiency	Nausea/vomiting/diarrhea Anorexia Constipation Gastrointestinal irritation Mucositis Pancreatitis Stomatitis Weight gain	↑ LFTs ↑ BUN, creatinine ↑ GGT		

(continued)

	NUTRITIONAL CONSIDERATIONS	POSSIBLE GASTROINTESTINAL SIDE EFFECTS	POSSIBLE EFFECTS ON LAB VALUES	COMMENTS/RECOMMENDATIONS
Imatinib (Gleevec)	Should be taken with food and a large glass of water to decrease gastrointestinal irritation Avoid grapefruit juice (may increase imatinib plasma concentration) May be present in breast milk	Nausea/vomiting/diarrhea Abdominal pain Anorexia Weight gain Dyspepsia Constipation Growth suppression Increase appetite	↓ Potassium ↑ ALT, AST, alk phos ↑ Creatinine Hyperglycemia ↓ Calcium ↓ Albumin ↑ Bilirubin ↓ LDH Hypercalcemia Hypomagnesemia Hypophosphatemia	
Methotrexate (MTX)	Folate antagonist Milk-rich foods may decrease absorption ↓ absorption of fat, B_{12}, lactose, carotene, cholesterol May be present in breast milk	GI mucosal injury Anorexia Nausea/vomiting/diarrhea Stomatitis	Anemia ↑ Uric acid ↑ ALT ↑ Bilirubin	Milk-rich foods may decrease absorption Folate may decrease drug response
Cytoprotectives				
Amifostine (Ethyol)	It is not known if amifostine is present in breast milk	Nausea/vomiting/diarrhea Metallic taste Hiccups	↓ Calcium ↓ Magnesium	

Dexrazoxane (Zinecard)	↑ Urinary excretion of iron, zinc, calcium It is not known if dexrazoxane is present in breast milk	Nausea/vomiting/diarrhea Abdominal pain Anorexia Constipation	↓ Sodium ↓ Calcium ↓ Zinc ↑ Iron ↑ Amylase ↑ Triglycerides ↑ ALT, AST, alk phos ↑ Bilirubin ↑ LDH	
Leucovorin	Contraindicated in patients with pernicious anemia secondary to B_{12} deficiency May be present in breast milk	Nausea/diarrhea Anorexia		
Mesna (Mesnex)	It is not known if mesna is present in breast milk	Nausea/vomiting/diarrhea Dysguesia	↓ Potassium ↑ Serum transaminases False (+) urinary ketones with Chemstrip, Multistix, or Labstix May result in false-positive reactions in Tillman reagent-based urine screening tests for ascorbic acid	Dilute well prior to oral administration to ↓ sulfur odor; dilute 1:1 to 1:10 in carbonated cola drinks, fruit juice or in milk; most palatable in chilled grape juice
Antirheumatic				
Abatacept (Orencia)	May be present in breast milk	Nausea/diarrhea Abdominal pain Dyspepsia	May cause false ↑ glucose with some testing methods	Avoid *Echinacea* (has immunostimulant properties) Abatacept for IV infusion contains maltose

(continued)

	NUTRITIONAL CONSIDERATIONS	POSSIBLE GASTROINTESTINAL SIDE EFFECTS	POSSIBLE EFFECTS ON LAB VALUES	COMMENTS/RECOMMENDATIONS
Autonomic Drugs				
Anticholinergics, General	Decreased absorption of electrolytes, iron; increased absorption of monosaccharides	Nausea/vomiting Constipation Xerostomia		Increase hydration and fiber intake to minimize adverse effects
Anticonvulsants				
Phenobarbital, Phenytoin/fosphenytoin, Primidone	To ensure consistent absorption, administer at same time with regards to meals Vitamin D deficiency; osteomalcia, ↓ absorption of folate, B_{12}; ↑ vitamin K catabolism; may also deplete biotin Increases the hepatic metabolism of vitamin D to inactive compounds and reduces calcium absorption Dietary requirements for vitamins D, K, C, B_{12}, folate may be increased with chronic use High doses of pyridoxine may decrease effects of phenobarbital, pentobarbital May be present in breast milk	Nausea/vomiting/diarrhea Altered taste	↑ Alk phos ↓ Calcium ↓ Magnesium ↓ Folate ↓ B_{12} ↓ vitamins K, B_6, C, D ↓ Sodium (neonates) Megaloblastic anemia	Tube feedings ↓ phenytoin bioavailability

Carbamazepine (Tegretol)	Grapefruit juice increases the oral bioavailability by 40% High-fat meals may increase rate of absorption and reduce time to peak levels of extended-release product but do not effect AUC Administer with food to ↓ GI upset May be present in breast milk	Nausea/vomiting/diarrhea Abdominal cramps Xerostomia Glossitis	↓ Sodium ↑ LFTs ↑ GGT ↑ Alk phos
Ethosuximide (Zarontin)	Folate requirements may be increased Administer with food to ↓ GI upset May be present in breast milk	Nausea/vomiting Anorexia Abdominal pain Hiccups	Abnormal hepatic function tests
Felbamate (Felbatol)	Administer with food to ↓ GI upset May be present in breast milk	Nausea/vomiting/diarrhea Anorexia Constipation Dyspepsia Weight loss Buccal mucous membrane swelling Pancreatitis	↑ LFTs ↓ Potassium ↓ Sodium ↑ LDH

(continued)

	NUTRITIONAL CONSIDERATIONS	POSSIBLE GASTROINTESTINAL SIDE EFFECTS	POSSIBLE EFFECTS ON LAB VALUES	COMMENTS/RECOMMENDATIONS
Gabapentin (Neurontin)	Food slightly increases rate and extent of drug absorption; ↑ AUC May be present in breast milk	Nausea/vomiting Constipation Dyspepsia Weight gain	False (+) urine protein with Multistix Hyperglycemia Hyponatremia	Content of capsule bitter tasting May administer immediate release without regards to meals
LamoTRIgine (LaMICtal)	Food has no effect on absorption May be present in breast milk	Nausea/vomiting Dyspepsia Abdominal pain Xerostomia Constipation Weight loss Anorexia Flatulence Weight gain	Hyperglycemia	Lamictal XR: May be given without regard to meals; swallow whole; do not chew, crush, or cut Lamictal chewable/dispersible tablets: May be chewed, dispersed in water or diluted fruit juice, or swallowed whole
LevETIRAcetam (Keppra)	Food may delay, but does not affect the extent of absorption May be taken without regard to meals May be present in breast milk	Nausea/vomiting/diarrhea Anorexia Constipation	Hypokalemia Hyponatremia	

TiaGABine (Gabitril)	Food reduces the rate but not the extent of absorption Take with food It is not known if tiagabine is present in breast milk	Nausea/vomiting/diarrhea Abdominal pain ↑ Appetite Gingivitis Mouth ulceration Stomatitis Weight gain/loss	Hypercholesteremia Hyperglycemia	
Valproic acid (Depacon, Depakene, Depakote)	May deplete carnitine and folate May administer with food to ↓ GI upset Do not administer tablet with milk May be present in breast milk	Nausea/vomiting/diarrhea Dyspepsia Constipation Pancreatitis Weight gain Taste perversion	↑ Ammonia ↓ Carnitine False (+) urine ketones ↑ ALT, AST	Swallow delayed release capsules whole; do not crush, break, or chew Do not administer with carbonated drinks
Vigabatrin (Sabril)	May be given without regard to meals May be present in breast milk	Nausea/vomiting/diarrhea Weight changes Constipation Abdominal pain Dyspepsia	↓ ALT, AST	

(continued)

	NUTRITIONAL CONSIDERATIONS	POSSIBLE GASTROINTESTINAL SIDE EFFECTS	POSSIBLE EFFECTS ON LAB VALUES	COMMENTS/RECOMMENDATIONS
Zonisamide (Zonegran)	May deplete biotin, B_1, B_2, niacin, pyridoxine, B_{12}, vitamin K May be present in breast milk	Nausea/vomiting/ diarrhea Anorexia Abdominal pain Dyspepsia Weight loss Constipation Xerostomia Taste perversion	↑ Alk phos ↑ Transaminases ↑ LDH ↑ BUN, creatinine Metabolic acidosis	
Psychotherapeutic Agents				
Alprazolam (Xanax)	High-fat meals eaten <2 h before dose of an extended-release tablet may increase peak concentrations by 25% Note: Doses given immediately after a high-fat meal may increase time to peak concentration; extent of absorption and AUC not impacted by food May be present in breast milk	Xerostomia Constipation Nausea/vomiting/ diarrhea May increase or decrease appetite	↑ Bilirubin ↑ ALT, AST	Extended-release tablet: Do not crush, break or chew extended-release tablet Immediate-release tablet: Administer with food to ↓ GI upset Caffeine antagonizes effects Orally disintegrating tablets may contain phenylalanine

Aripiprazole (Abilify)	May be taken with or without food May be present in breast milk	Anorexia ↑ Salivation Nausea/vomiting Constipation ↑ Weight, primarily w/baseline BMI < 23	↓ HDL Hypercholesterolemia ↑ LDL cholesterol ↑ Triglycerides Hyperglycemia Abnormal hepatic function tests	May be taken with or without food Some products may contain phenylalanine Oral solution contains fructose 200 mg and sucrose 400 mg/mL
BuPROPion (Wellbutrin; Zyban)	May be taken without regard to meals May be present in breast milk	Nausea/vomiting/diarrhea Weight loss Xerostomia Constipation Abdominal pain Flatulence Anorexia ↑ Appetite Taste perversion Dyspepsia Dysphagia	Hyponatremia	Extended-release tablets should be swallowed whole; do not crush, chew, or divide Insoluble shell of the extended-release tablet may remain intact during GI transit and is eliminated in the feces
BusPIRone (BuSpar)	Food may delay oral absorption, decrease the first-pass metabolism, increase oral bioavailability Grapefruit juice may greatly increase buspirone concentrations It is not known if buspirone is present in breast milk	Nausea/vomiting/diarrhea Flatulence Xerostomia	↑ Prolactin ↑ ALT, AST	

(continued)

	NUTRITIONAL CONSIDERATIONS	POSSIBLE GASTROINTESTINAL SIDE EFFECTS	POSSIBLE EFFECTS ON LAB VALUES	COMMENTS/RECOMMENDATIONS
Phenothiazines: Chlorpromazine, Prochlorperazine, Thioridazine, Thiothixene	Interferes with riboflavin metabolism, ↓ B_{12} absorption, ↑ riboflavin elimination and depletion Increase dietary riboflavin Administer with food to ↓ GI upset	Constipation Increased appetite and weight Xerostomia	↑ Cholesterol, ↑ Bilirubin False (+) for PKU, amylase, urophyrins, urobilinogen	Dilute oral concentrate solution in juice before administration (undiluted oral chlorpromazine concentrate may precipitate in tube feeding)
Diazepam (Valium)	Grapefruit juice significantly increases bioavailability May be present in breast milk	Nausea Constipation Hiccups Salivation changes	False (−) urinary glucose with Clinistix or Diastix ↑ ALT, AST ↑ Alk phos	Limit caffeine intake
Imipramine, Amitriptyline	May increase need for riboflavin Administer with food to ↓ GI upset May be present in breast milk	Nausea/vomiting/diarrhea Constipation Increased or decreased weight Altered taste	Increased or decreased glucose	

Selective Serotonin Reuptake Inhibitors (SSRIs): Citalopram (CeleXA), Fluoxetine (Prozac), Paroxetine (Paxil)	Administer with food to ↓ GI upset May cause decreased growth (smaller increases in weight and height in children and adolescents) Tryptophan supplements may ↑ CNS and GI adverse effects	Nausea/diarrhea Xerostomia Anorexia Dyspepsia Constipation Weight loss Anorexia Flatulence Gastritis	↓ Glucose ↓ Sodium	
Haloperidol (Haldol)	Administer with food to ↓ GI upset Drug will precipitate if oral concentrate mixed with coffee or tea May be present in breast milk	Xerostomia Constipation Nausea/vomiting/diarrhea Dyspepsia Hypersalivation Weight gain	↓↑ Glucose ↓ Sodium ↓ Magnesium ↑ Prolactin	Dilute oral concentrate with >2 oz water or acidic beverage
Lithium (Eskalith, Lithobid)	Decreased calcium uptake by bones May inhibit magnesium dependent enzymes Administer with food to ↓ GI upset Alters glucose tolerance May be present in breast milk	Nausea/vomiting/diarrhea ↑ appetite Xerostomia	↑ Magnesium ↑ Glucose ↑ Calcium ↓ Sodium	Avoid changes in sodium content; ↓ in sodium can ↑ lithium toxicity

(continued)

	NUTRITIONAL CONSIDERATIONS	POSSIBLE GASTROINTESTINAL SIDE EFFECTS	POSSIBLE EFFECTS ON LAB VALUES	COMMENTS/RECOMMENDATIONS
Cerebral Stimulants				
Atomoxetine (Strattera)	High-fat meal decreases the rate, but not the extent of absorption May be administered without regard to food It is not known if atomoxetine is present in breast milk	Weight loss Xerostomia Nausea/vomiting Abdominal pain ↓ Appetite Flatulence Constipation Dyspepsia Growth suppression (weight/height)		Swallow whole with water or other liquids; do not crush, chew, or open capsule
Dextroamphetamine (Dexedrine)	Acidic foods, juices, or vitamin C may decrease GI absorption May be present in breast milk	Appetite suppression Weight loss Growth suppression Nausea/vomiting/diarrhea Xerostomia Metallic taste		
Methylphenidate (Ritalin)	Food may increase oral absorption Administer 30-45 min before a meal May be present in breast milk	Decreased appetite Depression of height and weight Nausea/vomiting/diarrhea	↑ ALT ↑ Bilirubin	

Sedatives				
Barbiturates	Increased excretion of vitamin C; ↓ absorption of B_1; may also deplete calcium and biotin; may increase the metabolism of vitamins D and K; folate and vitamin D deficiency High doses of pyridoxine may decrease drug effect Dietary requirements of Vit B_{12}, C, D, K, folate and calcium may be increased with prolonged use May be present in breast milk	Nausea/vomiting/diarrhea Taste perversion	↑ Alk phos ↓ Calcium ↓ Magnesium ↓ Folate ↓ B_{12} ↓ Vitamins K, B_6, C Megaloblastic anemia	
Electrolytes and Water Balance Drugs				
Diuretics				
Acetazolamide (Diamox)	Avoid natural licorice (causes Na+ and water retention, ↑ excretion of potassium) Administer with food to ↓ GI upset May be present in breast milk	GI irritation Anorexia Nausea/vomiting Xerostomia Melena Dysguesia Metallic taste Black stools May cause growth retardation	↓ Potassium ↓ Sodium ↑ Glucose Abnormal hepatic function tests Hyperchloremic metabolic acidosis May cause false (+) for urinary protein with Albustix, Labstix, Albutest	Do not crush or chew long-acting capsules Tablet may be crushed and mixed with chocolate or cherry syrup to mask bitter taste of drug Some products may contain sodium

(continued)

	NUTRITIONAL CONSIDERATIONS	POSSIBLE GASTROINTESTINAL SIDE EFFECTS	POSSIBLE EFFECTS ON LAB VALUES	COMMENTS/RECOMMENDATIONS
Amiloride (Midamor)	Avoid natural licorice (causes Na+ and water retention, ↑excretion of potassium) and salt substitutes Food decreases absorption by 30% Administer with food or meals to avoid GI upset It is not known if amiloride is present in breast milk	Nausea/vomiting/diarrhea Abdominal pain Appetite changes GI bleeding Heartburn Dyspepsia Flatulence Xerostomia Constipation	May alter LFTs ↑ Potassium Hyperchloremic metabolic acidosis	
Bumetanide (Bumex), Furosemide (Lasix)	↑ Excretion of magnesium, calcium, potassium, zinc ↓ Carbohydrate tolerance Administer with food	Nausea/vomiting/diarrhea Anorexia Xerostomia	↓ Calcium ↓ Magnesium ↓ Potassium ↓ Chloride ↑ Glucose ↑ BUN ↑ Uric acid	Avoid use of salt substitutes
Metolazone (Zaroxoyln)	Administer with food May be present in breast milk	Abdominal bloating GI irritation Bitter taste Nausea/vomiting	↓ Sodium ↓ magnesium ↓ Potassium ↓ Chloride	Avoid natural licorice

		Anorexia Xerostomia Pancreatitis	↑ Glucose Hyperuricemia ↑ Creatinine	
Spironolactone (Aldactone)	Potassium sparing; avoid diets high in potassium ↑ Calcium excretion Administer with food Food increases the bioavailability May be present in breast milk	Nausea/vomiting/diarrhea Anorexia Gastritis Cramping GI bleeding	↑ Potassium ↑ BUN, creatinine ↑ Magnesium ↑ Uric acid ↓ Sodium ↓ Chloride ↓ Calcium	Avoid natural licorice
Thiazides	↑ Excretion of potassium, magnesium, zinc, riboflavin ↓ Calcium excretion Administer with food Glucose intolerance May be present in breast milk	Nausea/vomiting/diarrhea Constipation Anorexia Cramping	↑ Uric acid ↑ Calcium ↓ Potassium ↓ Magnesium ↓ Chloride ↓ Bicarbonate ↓ Phosphorus ↑↓ Glucose	Avoid natural licorice
Triamterene (Dyrenium)	Potassium sparing; avoid salt substitutes and diets high in potassium Administer with food It is not known if triamterene is present in breast milk	Nausea/vomiting/diarrhea Xerostomia	Abnormal LFTs ↑ Potassium ↓ Sodium ↓ Magnesium ↑ Chloride ↑ Uric acid	

(continued)

	NUTRITIONAL CONSIDERATIONS	POSSIBLE GASTROINTESTINAL SIDE EFFECTS	POSSIBLE EFFECTS ON LAB VALUES	COMMENTS/RECOMMENDATIONS
Gastrointestinal Drugs				
Antacids				
Aluminum hydroxide	↑ Calcium absorption Can form insoluble salts with dietary phosphorus; may cause hypophosphatemia ↓ Absorption of vitamins A, C; inactivates B_1 Considered compatible with breastfeeding	Constipation Anorexia Nausea/vomiting Bezoar or fecalith formation	↓ Magnesium ↓ Phosphorus	
Magnesium hydroxide	Considered compatible with breastfeeding	Diarrhea Abdominal cramps	↑ Magnesium	Take with water
Sodium bicarbonate	Concurrent administration with iron may ↓ iron absorption Administer 1-3 h after meals Prolonged and excessive consumption of calcium/dairy products can cause high calcium concentrations (i.e., milk-alkali syndrome) Found in breast milk	Gastric distention Flatulence	↓ Potassium ↓ Calcium ↑ Sodium ↑ Osmolality Metabolic alkalosis	

Antihyperammonemic Agents				
Lactulose (Cephulac, Chronulac)	Contraindicated in galactose restricted diets Administer with juice/milk It is not known if lactulose is present in breast milk	Nausea/vomiting/ diarrhea Constipation	↓ Ammonia	
Sodium phenylbutyrate (Buphenyl)	Administer with food, feedings Do not mix with acidic beverages (e.g., cola, fruit juices) as drug may precipitate It is not known if sodium phenylbutyrate is excreted in breast milk	Anorexia Abnormal taste Nausea/vomiting Weight gain Abdominal pain	↑ Cholesterol ↓ Ammonia ↓ Potassium ↑ Sodium ↑ Chloride ↑ Phosphorus ↓ Albumin ↑ LFTs ↑ Bilirubin Alkalosis	Suspension: Do not administer via NG or gastrostomy tube (use powder)
Cathartics				
Bisacodyl (Dulcolax)	↓ Absorption of glucose Administer on empty stomach; do not administer within 1 h of ingesting milk or dairy products (causes GI irritation) It is not known if bisacodyl is present in breast milk	Nausea/vomiting/ diarrhea Abdominal cramps Rectal burning	↓ Potassium ↓ Calcium	

(continued)

	NUTRITIONAL CONSIDERATIONS	POSSIBLE GASTROINTESTINAL SIDE EFFECTS	POSSIBLE EFFECTS ON LAB VALUES	COMMENTS/RECOMMENDATIONS
Docusate sodium	Alters intestinal absorption of water and electrolytes It is not known if docusate is present in breast milk	Diarrhea Abdominal cramping Intestinal obstruction Throat irritation	↑ Glucose ↓ Potassium	Administer liquid (not syrup) with milk/juice to mask bitter taste
Magnesium sulfate	↓ Nutrient absorption May be present in breast milk	↑ Intestinal transient time Nausea/vomiting/diarrhea	↑ Magnesium	
Mineral oil	May ↓ absorption of fat-soluble vitamins; impairs calcium, carotene, and phosphorus absorption	Decreased weight Anorexia Nausea/vomiting/diarrhea Abdominal cramps Anal itching	↓ β carotene	Nonemulsified mineral oil May be taken on an empty stomach; emulsified mineral oil may be administered with meals and is more palatable
Phosphate enema (Fleet)	May deplete calcium, magnesium, potassium, sodium	Abdominal pain Nausea	↑ Phosphorus ↓ Potassium	Mixture of sodium phosphate salts: Monobasic sodium phosphate monohydrate: 19 g Dibasic sodium phosphate heptahydrate: 7 g

Antisecretory Agents				
H2 antagonists: Cimetidine (Tagamet), Famotidine (Pepcid)	↓ B_{12}, may deplete zinc Limit xanthine containing foods and beverages May be present in breast milk	Nausea/vomiting/diarrhea Constipation Loss of sense of smell and taste Mild diarrhea Xerostomia Dysguesia Anorexia	↑ ALT, AST ↑ BUN, creatinine	
Proton pump inhibitors: Esomeprazole (Nexium), Lansoprazole (Prevacid), Omeprazole (Prilosec) Pantoprazole (Protonix)	↓ B_{12} Absorption is decreased up to 50% when taken with food May be present in breast milk	Nausea/vomiting/diarrhea Abdominal pain Constipation Fatulence Dyspepsia Dysphagia Epigastric pain Mellena Anorexia Dysgeusia Taste perversion Taste loss	↓ Sodium Hyperuricemia ↑ LFTs ↑↓ Glucose Hyperlipemia ↓ Calcium ↓ Potassium ↓ Magnesium	For G/NG tube administration, dissolve in an acidic fluid For NJ/J tube administration, dissolve in a basic fluid Do not crush or chew capsule/tablet contents May increase the risk of bone fracture

(continued)

	NUTRITIONAL CONSIDERATIONS	POSSIBLE GASTROINTESTINAL SIDE EFFECTS	POSSIBLE EFFECTS ON LAB VALUES	COMMENTS/RECOMMENDATIONS
Sucralfate (Carafate)	↓ Absorption of fat-soluble vitamins Take on empty stomach Aluminum salt may accumulate in renal failure It is not known if sucralfate is present in breast milk	Nausea/diarrhea Constipation Gastric discomfort Xerostomia	↑ Aluminum (in renal failure) ↑ Glucose	Avoid administration via feeding tubes; increases risk of bezoar formation
Octreotide (Sandostatin)	May ↓ absorption of dietary fats May ↓ vitamin B_{12} Administer injections between meals to ↓ GI side effects May be present in breast milk	Nausea/vomiting/diarrhea Abdominal pain Constipation Flatulence Xerostomia Dyspepsia Steatorrhea Biliary sludge Pancreatitis	↓↑ Glucose ↑ LFTs	
Hormones and Synthetic Substitutes				
Oral contraceptives	↓ Absorption of water-soluble vitamins; ↓ magnesium, ↓ zinc ↑ copper absorption	Nausea/vomiting ↑↓ weight Bloating	Megaloblastic anemia ↑ Glucose ↑ Triglyceride ↑ Vitamin A ↑ Vitamin E	

			↑ Iron ↑ Copper ↑ Alk phos ↑ Bilirubin ↓ Folate ↓ Calcium ↓ Magnesium ↓ B_6 ↓ B_{12} ↓ Zinc
Danazol	Food delays time to peak levels *High-fat meal increases* plasma concentration Contraindicated in breast feeding patients	Nausea/vomiting Appetite changes Constipation Pancreatitis Weight gain	Glucose intolerance ↓ HDL ↑ LDL
Immunosuppressants			
Azathioprine (Imuran)	Administer with food May be present in breast milk	Nausea/vomiting/diarrhea Anorexia Stomatitis Pancreatitis Steatorrhea	False ↑ creatinine

(*continued*)

	NUTRITIONAL CONSIDERATIONS	POSSIBLE GASTROINTESTINAL SIDE EFFECTS	POSSIBLE EFFECTS ON LAB VALUES	COMMENTS/RECOMMENDATIONS
Cyclosporine (Neoral, SandImmune, Gengraf)	Grapefruit and grapefruit juice may affect cyclosporine metabolism (↑ cyclosporine levels) May be present in breast milk	Nausea/vomiting/diarrhea Abdominal discomfort Anorexia Hiccups Weight loss	↓ Magnesium ↑ Potassium Hyperuricemia ↑ BUN, creatinine ↑ Triglycerides (with IV form) ↑ Glucose	To improve palatability, dilute with milk, chocolate milk, orange juice, apple juice, stir well and drink at once Do not allow to stand, rinse glass with diluent to ensure entire dose is taken
Mycophenolate (CellCept)	Food decreases Cmax by 40% Take on an empty stomach to decrease variability; however, may be taken with food if necessary in stable renal transplant recipients It is not known if mycophenolate is present in breast milk	Nausea/vomiting/diarrhea Constipation Abdominal pain Dyspepsia Anorexia	↓↑ Potassium ↑ Cholesterol ↓ Phosphorus ↑ Glucose	Do not open contents of capsule or crush tablets
Everolimus (Afinitor)	May be administered with or without food To reduce variability, take consistently regarding food Avoid grapefruit and grapefruit juice May be present in breast milk	Nausea/vomiting/diarrhea Constipation Abdominal pain Biliary obstruction Cholangitis Cholestasis Decreased appetite	Hypercholesterolemia Hyperglycemia Hyperkalemia Hypokalemia Hypomagnesemia Hypophosphatemia Hypocalcemia Hyponatremia	

		Dyspepsia Dysphagia Epigastric distress Flatulence Gastritis Gastroenteritis Gastroesophageal reflux disease Gingival hyperplasia Ascites	↑ LFTs ↑ Alk phos ↑ Bilirubin	
Sirolimus (Rapamune)	Should be administered consistently (with or without food) to minimize variability Avoid grapefruit juice; may ↓ clearance Ingestion with high-fat meals ↓ peak concentrations but ↑ AUC It is not known if sirolimus is present in breast milk	Nausea/diarrhea Constipation Abdominal pain Weight loss Pancreatitis	↑ Triglycerides ↑ Cholesterol ↑↓ Calcium ↑ Phosphorous Hyper/hypoglycemia ↓ Potassium ↓ Magnesium ↓ Sodium ↑ LDH	Do not crush, split, or chew tablets Solution should be mixed with at least 2 oz of water or orange juice; no other liquids should be used for dilution
Tacrolimus (Prograf, FK506)	Give on empty stomach Food decreases rate and extent of absorption Grapefruit may ↑ serum tacrolimus May be present in breast milk	Nausea/vomiting/diarrhea Constipation Dyspepsia Pancreatitis	↓ Magnesium ↑ Potassium ↑ BUN, creatinine ↑ Glucose ↑ Calcium	

(continued)

	NUTRITIONAL CONSIDERATIONS	POSSIBLE GASTROINTESTINAL SIDE EFFECTS	POSSIBLE EFFECTS ON LAB VALUES	COMMENTS/RECOMMENDATIONS
			↑ALT, AST, GGT ↑ LDH ↑ Cholesterol Acidosis ↓ Bicarbonate ↓ Iron	
Antiasthmatics				
Albuterol (Proventil, *Ventolin*)	It is not known if albuterol is present in breast milk	GI upset Xerostomia Nausea/vomiting Heartburn Unusual taste	↓ Potassium Metabolic acidosis ↑ Glucose ↑ ALT, ↑ AST Hyperglycemia	Caffeinated beverages may increase albuterol's side effects
Aminophylline/ Theophylline	Food does not impact absorption High protein, low carbohydrate meals and charcoal broiled meats will decrease theophylline levels May be present in breast milk	GI upset GI reflux Nausea/vomiting/ diarrhea Abdominal pain Cramping	↑ Uric acid ↑ Glucose ↑ Free fatty acids ↑ Total cholesterol ↑ HDL ↑ HDL/LDL ratio	Limit intake of charcoal broiled meats, caffeinated beverages Maintain consistent intake of protein and carbohydrates
Terbutaline	May be present in breast milk	Nausea/vomiting Dysguesia	↓ Potassium ↑ Glucose ↑ CPK	

Zafirlukast (Accolate)	Should be taken on an empty stomach (1 h before or 2 h after meals) Food ↓ absorption by 40% May be present in breast milk	Nausea/vomiting/diarrhea	↑ ALT ↑ Bilirubin	
Chelating Agents				
Deferoxamine (Desferal)	When taken with high doses of vitamin C, patients may develop impaired cardiac function, which is reversible upon discontinuation of vitamin C supplements It is not known if deferoxamine is present in breast milk	Abdominal discomfort, diarrhea, nausea/vomiting Growth suppression	↑ ALT, AST	Avoid vitamin C in patients with preexisting cardiac failure; start vitamin C supplementation only after the first month of deferoxamine; do not exceed vitamin C doses of 50 mg/d in children <10 y of age, 100 mg/d in older children, 200 mg/d in adults
Deferasirox (Exjade)	Administer at same time each day on an empty stomach, 30 min before meals Bioavailability increased variably when taken with food It is not known if deferasirox is present in breast milk	Nausea/vomiting/diarrhea Abdominal pain	↑ ALT ↑ Bilirubin	Do not chew or swallow whole tablets Completely disperse tablets in water, orange juice, or apple juice; rinse remaining residue with more fluid and drink
Dimercaprol	Dimercaprol may enhance the nephrotoxic effect of iron salts It is not known if dimercaprol is present in breast milk	Nausea/vomiting Salivation May cause burning sensation to lips and mouth	False (+) ketones	

(continued)

	NUTRITIONAL CONSIDERATIONS	POSSIBLE GASTROINTESTINAL SIDE EFFECTS	POSSIBLE EFFECTS ON LAB VALUES	COMMENTS/RECOMMENDATIONS
Edetate calcium disodium	Do not breast feed until blood lead levels <40 µg/dL	Nausea/vomiting/diarrhea Abdominal cramps Anorexia	↓ Magnesium ↓ Potassium ↑ Calcium ↓ Zinc Hyperuricemia ↓ Alk phos	
Penicillamine	Administer on an empty stomach 1 h before or 2 h after meals and at least 1 h apart from other drugs, milk, antacids, iron-containing products, and zinc-containing products Iron and zinc may decrease drug effectiveness; for Wilson disease: ↓ copper in diet; for lead toxicity: ↓ calcium in diet Maternal use of penicillamine may decrease copper and zinc concentrations in breast milk	Nausea/vomiting Oral lesions Epigastric pain Dysgeusia Ageusia Pancreatitis Sore throat Weight gain	↓ Iron ↓ Glucose False (+) ketones ↑ Alk phos	

Succimer	Administer with fruit juice to mask odor It is not known if succimer is present in breast milk	Nausea/vomiting/diarrhea Anorexia Metallic taste Breath may smell of sulfur Sore throat	↑ ALT, AST, alk phos ↑ Cholesterol Falsely ↓ CPK Falsely ↓ uric acid False (+) urine ketones with Ketostix)	Ensure adequate hydration Capsules may be opened and sprinkled on soft foods
Trientine	Administer at least 1 h before or 2 h after meals and at least 1 h apart from any drug, food, or milk; may be taken closer to meals if needed to improve adherence Food, dairy products, or other sources of polyvalent cations will be chelated by trientine It is not known if trientine is present in breast milk	Abdominal pain Change in bowel habits (e.g., abnormal stools, constipation, soft stools) Alopecia Colitis Gastritis	↓ iron	
5-HT3 Receptor Antagonists				
Dolasetron, Granisetron, Ondansetron	Administer without regard to meals Food slightly increases the extent of absorption Not known if present in milk	Taste perversion Diarrhea Abdominal pain Constipation Dyspepsia Anorexia	↓ Potassium ↑ ALT, AST ↑ Bilirubin	

(continued)

	NUTRITIONAL CONSIDERATIONS	POSSIBLE GASTROINTESTINAL SIDE EFFECTS	POSSIBLE EFFECTS ON LAB VALUES	COMMENTS/RECOMMENDATIONS
Replacement Solutions/Mineral Supplements				
Calcium salts	High calcium intake interferes with phosphorus absorption; may also interfere with iron absorption Caffeine may decrease calcium absorption and increase calcium excretion Do not give orally with bran, whole grain cereals, or foods high in oxalates (will ↓ calcium absorption) Present in breast milk	Nausea/vomiting Constipation Xerostomia	↑ Amylase ↑ Calcium ↓ Phosphorus ↓ Magnesium	Oral dosage forms should be administered with meals to be effective when treating hyperphosphatemia
Cysteine	May chelate copper in parenteral nutrition solutions Present in breast milk	Nausea	Hyperammonemia, Metabolic acidosis	
Fluoride	Do not administer with milk Magnesium, aluminum, and calcium containing supplements may decrease fluoride absorption Present in breast milk	GI upset Nausea/vomiting		Some products contain tartrazine which may cause allergic reactions

Iron salts	Administer with water or juice for maximal absorption Milk, cereals, fiber, eggs, tea, coffee decrease iron absorption Concurrent administration with >200 mg vitamin C per 30 mg elemental iron will increase absorption of oral iron Present in breast milk	GI irritation Epigastric pain Nausea/vomiting Constipation	False (+) guaiac test ↑ LFTs ↑ GGT	Liquid preparations may stain the teeth Do not administer with milk or dairy products
Magnesium salts	High magnesium intake may impair calcium absorption; may also decrease phosphorus absorption Present in breast milk	Nausea/vomiting/diarrhea Ileus	↑ Magnesium ↑ Potassium ↑ Calcium ↓ Phosphorus	Lemon juice may be added to the magnesium sulfate solution to improve the taste
Potassium chloride	↓ Absorption of B_{12} Administer with food Present in breast milk	Nausea/vomiting/diarrhea Abdominal pain GI lesions	↑ Potassium ↑ Chloride ↓ Sodium	
Phosphorus	High intake decreases magnesium absorption Administer with food to ↓ diarrhea Avoid giving with oxalate or phytate-containing foods Present in breast milk	Nausea/vomiting/diarrhea Flatulence	↑ Phosphorus ↓ Calcium ↓ Magnesium ↑ Potassium with potassium salts ↑ Sodium with sodium salts	

(continued)

	NUTRITIONAL CONSIDERATIONS	POSSIBLE GASTROINTESTINAL SIDE EFFECTS	POSSIBLE EFFECTS ON LAB VALUES	COMMENTS/RECOMMENDATIONS
Sodium chloride	Administer with full glass of water Present in breast milk	Nausea/vomiting	↑ Sodium ↑ Chloride Metabolic acidosis	
Zinc salts	Coffee, foods high in phytate, and dairy products ↓ zinc absorption Avoid foods high in calcium or phosphorus Administer with food if GI upset occurs Present in breast milk	Nausea/vomiting Indigestion		
Ascorbic acid (Vitamin C)	Increases iron absorption, impairs copper absorption, and impairs cyanocobalamin absorption Present in breast milk	Nausea/vomiting/ diarrhea Heartburn	False (+) urinary glucose with cupric sulfate reagents False (–) urinary glucose with glucose oxidase method False (–) with amine dependent occult blood test	
Cyanocobalamin	Use in folic acid-deficient patients may improve folate-deficient megaloblastic anemia and obscure true diagnosis Administer intranasal product at least 1 h before or after ingestion of hot foods or liquids; hot foods can cause nasal secretions that can result in medication loss	Diarrhea	↓ Potassium	

	Hematologic response antagonized by chloramphenicol Present in breast milk			
Folic acid	May be administered without regard to meals Hematologic response antagonized by chloramphenicol Large doses may mask the hematologic effects of B_{12} deficiency, obscuring diagnosis of pernicious anemia May interfere with zinc absorption Present in breast milk	GI upset Bitter taste		Not contained in oral liquid vitamin products due to stability issues
Niacin	Should be taken with meal; low-fat meal if treating hyperlipidemia Concomitant administration with hot drinks or food will increase flushing or pruritus Present in breast milk	Nausea/vomiting/diarrhea GI upset Heartburn Anorexia	↑ Glucose Hyperuricemia ↓ Phosphorus Abnormal LFTs False (+) urine glucose with Benedict reagent	Avoid hot drinks around the time of niacin dose
Vitamin A	Administer with food or milk Mega doses may interfere with iron, iodine, copper, and calcium absorption; can also interfere with absorption of ascorbic acid, Vitamins K, D, E Vitamin A requirements are increased in breastfeeding women	Vomiting/diarrhea Gingivitis seen with long term use	↑ Bilirubin ↑ ALT, AST, alk phos	

(continued)

	NUTRITIONAL CONSIDERATIONS	POSSIBLE GASTROINTESTINAL SIDE EFFECTS	POSSIBLE EFFECTS ON LAB VALUES	COMMENTS/RECOMMENDATIONS
Vitamin D	May be administered without regard to meals Reduced intake impairs calcium and phosphorus absorption and utilization The amount in breast milk does not correlate with serum levels in the infant and the vitamin D content of human milk is not enough to meet the recommended intake for a nursing infant	Nausea/vomiting Constipation Anorexia Xerostomia Metallic taste Weight loss	↑ Calcium ↑ Cholesterol	
Vitamin E	Inhibits the reticulocyte and hemoglobin response to iron May administer with or without food Vitamin E breast milk concentrations decrease over time and are highest immediately postpartum	Nausea/diarrhea Intestinal cramps	↑ Cholesterol ↑ Triglycerides ↑ Creatinine kinase	
Vitamin K	May be administered with or without food Vitamin K absorption ↓ when taken with Olestra-containing foods	Dysgeusia	↑ Bilirubin seen in neonates	

Miscellaneous Agents				
Allopurinol (Zyloprim)	Administer after meals with plenty of fluid Increases risk of kidney stone formation when taken with large doses of Vitamin C Present in breast milk	GI irritation Dyspepsia Nausea/vomiting/ diarrhea Abdominal pain Gastritis	Elevated hepatic enzymes Hyperbilirubinemia ↑ Calcium ↑ Glucose ↓ Potassium ↓ Sodium Lactic acidosis	
Biguanides: Metformin (Glucophage)	May deplete Coenzyme Q10 Folic acid, B_{12} Administer with a meal (to decrease GI upset) Present in breast milk	Nausea/vomiting/ diarrhea Anorexia Flatulence Abdominal discomfort Constipation Heartburn Metallic taste Dyspepsia	↓ Glucose Lactic acidosis	
Colchicine	↓ Absorption of B_{12}, vitamin A, folate, potassium, fat, sodium, nitrogen, lactose Administer without regard to meals Grapefruit juice may increase colchicine serum concentrations	Intestinal mucosal damage Nausea/vomiting/ diarrhea Constipation GI bleeding Steatorrhea	↑ AST, alk phos ↓ B_{12} ↓ Vitamin A ↓ Cholesterol	Maintain adequate fluid intake

(continued)

	NUTRITIONAL CONSIDERATIONS	POSSIBLE GASTROINTESTINAL SIDE EFFECTS	POSSIBLE EFFECTS ON LAB VALUES	COMMENTS/RECOMMENDATIONS
Clonidine (Catapres)	May be administered without regard to meals Present in breast milk	Nausea/vomiting/diarrhea Abdominal pain Anorexia Constipation Parotid gland pain Parotitis Pseudo-obstruction Taste perversion Throat pain Weight gain Xerostomia	Hyperglycemia (transient) Abnormal hepatic function tests (mild; transient)	May be administered without regard to meals Swallow extended-release formulations whole; do not crush or chew
Diazoxide (Proglycem)	Administer on an empty stomach 1 h before or 1 h after meals Present in breast milk	Nausea/vomiting/diarrhea Abdominal pain Anorexia Ileus Pancreatitis Pancreatic necrosis Taste loss (transient)	↑ AST, alk phos Hyperglycemia Sodium retention	

Endothelin Antagonist: Bosentan (Tracleer)	Food does not affect bioavailability May be administered with or without food	Weight gain	↑ ALT, AST	Avoid grapefruit and grapefruit juice
GuanFACINE (Tenex)	Do not administer with high-fat meal It is not known if guanfacine is present in breast milk	Nausea/vomiting/diarrhea Abdominal pain ↓ Appetite Constipation Stomach discomfort Xerostomia Weight gain		Swallow extended-release tablet whole with water, milk, or other liquid; do not crush, break, or chew Extended-release formulation: high-fat meal ↑ peak concentration and AUC
Isotretinoin (Accutane)	Food or milk ↑ bioavailability Vitamin A supplements increase toxic effects It is not known if isotretinoin is present in breast milk	Xerostomia Anorexia Nausea/vomiting IBS Acute pancreatitis	↑ Triglycerides ↑ ALT, AST, alk phos ↑ Glucose ↑ Calcium ↓ HDL ↑ Cholesterol Hyperuricemia ↑ LDH ↑LDL	

(continued)

	NUTRITIONAL CONSIDERATIONS	POSSIBLE GASTROINTESTINAL SIDE EFFECTS	POSSIBLE EFFECTS ON LAB VALUES	COMMENTS/RECOMMENDATIONS
Sevelamer (Renvela)	Reduced levels of folic acid, and vitamins D, E, and K may occur Take with meals May reduce maternal absorption of fat soluble vitamins and folic acid; supplementation may be needed	Abdominal pain Flatulence Constipation	↑ Calcium Metabolic acidosis	Tablets must be swallowed whole; do not crush, chew, or break
Sildenafil (Revatio, Viagra)	Present in breast milk Administer tablets without regard to meals at least 4-6 h apart Grapefruit juice may increase serum levels/toxicity of orally administered sildenafil	Diarrhea Dyspepsia	↑ LFTs ↑ ↓ Glucose ↑ Sodium	Avoid grapefruit juice
Levodopa	High protein diets may ↓ efficacy of levodopa Administer with food Avoid foods high in pyridoxine content Present in breast milk	Nausea/diarrhea Constipation Anorexia GI bleeding Xerostomia	↑ Homocysteine ↑ Serum bilirubin ↑ LDH	

Levothyroxine (Synthroid)	Administer on empty stomach Iron supplements increase thyroid requirements Limit intake of goitrogenic foods Dietary fiber may decrease absorption	Diarrhea Weight loss Abdominal cramps ↑ Appetite		
Orlistat (Xenical)	Reduces the absorption of Vitamins D and E and β-carotene Administer during or up to 1 h after each main meal containing fat Separate dose by at least 2 h from multivitamin containing fat-soluble vitamin It is not known if orlistat is present in breast milk	Gastric discomfort Nausea Fatty/oily stool Diarrhea	Increased levels of urinary oxalate	Patients should be advised to adhere to dietary guidelines Gastrointestinal adverse events may increase if taken with a diet high in fat (>30% total daily calories from fat)
Paricalcitol (Zemplar)	Administer with or without food It is not known if paricalcitol is present in breast milk	Nausea/vomiting/diarrhea GI bleeding Constipation Abdominal pain Dyspepsia Xerostomia	Hypoglycemia Alterations in calcium status ↑ Potassium In predialysis patients, paricalcitol may increase serum creatinine	Excessive vitamin D administration may lead to over suppression of PTH, hypercalcemia, hypercalciuria, hyperphosphatemia

(continued)

	NUTRITIONAL CONSIDERATIONS	POSSIBLE GASTROINTESTINAL SIDE EFFECTS	POSSIBLE EFFECTS ON LAB VALUES	COMMENTS/RECOMMENDATIONS
Teduglutide (Gattex)	It is not known if teduglutide is present in breast milk It is not known if teduglutide is present in breast milk	Fluid retention Abdominal distention Abdominal pain Nausea/vomiting Cholecystitis ↓ Appetite Flatulence Intestinal obstruction Intestinal stenosis Pancreatic pseudocyst Colonic or rectal polyp Cholangitis Cholelithiasis Pancreatitis	↑ Serum bilirubin ↑ Alk phos ↑ Amylase ↑ Lipase	Teduglutide may increase absorption of oral medications Treatment discontinuation may result in fluid and electrolyte imbalance; carefully monitor fluid/electrolyte status

ALT, alanine transaminase; aPTT, activated partial thromboplastin time; AST, aspartate aminotransferase; AUC, Area Under the Curve; BUN, blood urea nitrogen; CNS, central nervous system; CPK, creatine phosphokinase; GERD, gastroesophageal reflux disease; GGT, Gamma-Glutamyl Transferase; GI, gastrointestinal; GT, Gastric tubes; HCT, hematocrit; HDL, high-density lipoprotein; IV, intravenous; LDH, lactate dehydrogenase; LDL, low-density lipoprotein; LFT, Liver Function Tests; MCT, medium-chain triglyceride; NGT, nasogastric tubes; OGT, orogastric tubes; PT, prothrombin time; PTT, partial thromboplastin time; ULN, upper limit of normal

APPENDIX 3

Growth Charts

Kristen J. Slusher

The WHO growth standards should be used for healthy infants and children from birth to 2 years of age and the CDC growth charts should be used for children 2 to 20 years of age. WHO/CDC growth charts are included in this appendix.

Anthropometric assessment of the nutritional status of patients with genetic and other medical conditions can be difficult using the standard WHO and CDC charts. To better evaluate the growth patterns in these populations, specialized weight and height curves for several syndromes have been published. The following table includes references for these specialized growth charts, along with website addresses for those that are available electronically.

Specialized Growth Charts[a]

CONDITION	REFERENCE	STANDARD	ONLINE ACCESS (IF AVAILABLE)
Achondroplasia	Neumeyer L, Merker A, Hagenäs L. Clinical charts for surveillance of growth and body proportion development in achondroplasia and examples of their use. *Am J Med Genet A*. 2021;185(2):401-412.	0-48 mo: • Length/height- and weight-for-age • Head circumference-for-age 0-20 y: • BMI-for-age • Waist circumference-for-age • Foot length-for-age 2-20 y: • Sitting height- and sitting height / height ratio-for-age • Arm span- and leg length (SILL)-for-age 4-20 y: • Height- and weight-for-age	https://www.achondroplasia-growthcharts.com/
Brachmann (Cornelia) deLange Syndrome	Kline AD, Barr M, Jackson LG. Growth manifestations in the Brachmann-de Lange syndrome. *Am J Med Genet*. 1993;47(7):1042-1049.	Birth to 36 mo: • Length- and weight-for-age 2-18 y: • Height- and weight-for age Birth to 18 y: • Head circumference-for-age	https://www.cdlsusa.org/wp-content/uploads/2018/10/growth-charts-boy.pdf https://www.cdlsusa.org/wp-content/uploads/2018/10/growth-charts-girl.pdf

Cerebral Palsy (quadriplegia)	Krick J, Murphy-Miller P, Zeger S, Wright E. Pattern of growth in children with cerebral palsy. *J Am Diet Assoc*. 1996;96(7):680-685. Carr LJ, Reddy SK, Stevens S, Blair E, Love S. Definition and classification of cerebral palsy. *Dev Med Child Neurol*. 2005;47(8):508-510.	Birth to 10 y: • Stature- and weight-for age • Weight-for-stature 2-20 y Groups 1-5: • Height- and weight-for-age • BMI-for-age	https://doi.org/10.1016/S0002-8223(96)00188-5 https://www.lifeexpectancy.org/articles/GrowthCharts/All.pdf
Down Syndrome	Zemel BS, Pipan M, Stallings VA, et al. Growth charts for children with Down syndrome in the United States. *Pediatrics*. 2015;136(5):e1204-e1211.	Birth to 36 mo: • Length/height- and weight-for-age • Weight-for-length • Head circumference 2-20 y: • Height- and weight-for-age • Head circumference	https://www.cdc.gov/birth-defects/hcp/down-syndrome-growth-charts/index.html
Marfan Syndrome	Erkula G, Jones KB, Sponseller PD, Dietz HC, Pyeritz RE. Growth and maturation in Marfan syndrome. *Am J Med Genet*. 2002;109:100-115.	0-36 mo: • Height- and weight-for-age 2-18 y: • Weight-for-height	
Myelomeningocele	Ekvall SW, Ekvall VK, eds. Appendix 2. In: *Pediatric Nutrition in Chronic Diseases and Development Disorders: Prevention, Assessment, and Treatment*. 2nd ed. Oxford University Press; 2005:403-404.	0-20 y: • Height- and weight-for-age	
Noonan Syndrome	Witt DR, Keena BA, Hall JG, Allanson JE. Growth curves for height in Noonan syndrome. *Clin Genet*. 1986;30(3):150-153. Isojima T, Sakazume S, Hasegawa T, et al. Growth references for Japanese individuals with Noonan syndrome. *Pediatr Res*. 2016;79(4):543-548.	0-20 y: • Length/height- and weight-for- age	http://jspe.umin.jp/medical/files_chart/NSGC_boy_eng.pdf http://jspe.umin.jp/medical/files_chart/NSGC_girl_eng.pdf

(*continued*)

CONDITION	REFERENCE	STANDARD	ONLINE ACCESS (IF AVAILABLE)
Prader-Willi Syndrome	Butler MG, Meaney FJ. Standards for selected anthropometric measurements in Prader-Willi syndrome. *Pediatrics*. 1991;88(4):853-860. Butler MG, Sturich J, Lee J, et al. Growth standards of infants with Prader-Willi syndrome. *Pediatrics*. 2011;127(4): 687-695. Butler MG, Lee J, Manzardo AM, et al. Growth charts for non-growth hormone treated Prader-Willi syndrome. *Pediatrics*. 2015;135(1):e126-e135. Butler MG, Lee J, Cox DM, et al. Growth charts for Prader-Willi syndrome during growth hormone treatment. *Clin Pediatr*. 2016;55(10), 957-974.	0-22 y: • Head length-for-age • Head breadth-for-age • Hand length-for age • Middle finger length-for-age • Palm length-for-age • Hand breadth-for-age • Foot length-for-age • Foot breadth-for-age • Triceps skinfold-for-age • Subscapular skinfold-for-age ***Non-Growth Hormone-Treated*** 0-36 mo: • Weight-for-age • Length-for-age • Head circumference-for-age • BMI-for-age • Weight/length-for-age 3-18 y: • Weight-for-age • Length-for-age • Head circumference-for-age • BMI-for-age	https://pmc.ncbi.nlm.nih.gov/articles/PMC6712978/pdf/nihms-1046733.pdf https://ipwso.org/information-for-medical-professionals/pws-growth-charts/

		Growth Hormone-Treated 0-36 mo: • Height- and weight-for-age 0-18 y: • Head circumference-for-age • Weight/height-for-age 3-18 y: • Height- and weight-for-age • BMI-for-age	
Sickle Cell Disease	Thomas PW, Singhal A, Hemmings-Kelly M, Serjeant GR. Height and weight reference curves for homozygous sickle cell disease. *Arch Dis Child.* 2000;82(3):204-208.	Birth to 18 y: • Height- and weight-for-age	
Silver-Russell Syndrome	Tanner JM, Lejarraga H, Kameron N. The natural history of the Silver-Russell syndrome: a longitudinal study of 39 cases. *Pediatr Res*. 1975;9:611-623.	2-19 y: • Height and height velocity (includes periods of treatment with human growth hormone)	
Turner Syndrome	Lyon AJ, Preece MA, Grant DB. Growth curve for girls with Turner syndrome. *Arch Dis Child.* 1985;60(10):932-935.	2-19 y: • Height-for-age (girls)	https://www.sbp.com.br/fileadmin/user_upload/sbp/2024/janeiro/23/Sindrome_de_Turner.pdf
Williams Syndrome	Morris CA, Demsey SA, Leonard CO, Dilts C, Blackburn BL. Natural history of Williams syndrome: physical characteristics. *J Pediatr*. 1988;113(2):318-326.	0-18 y: • Height-for-age	

[a]Unless otherwise specified, charts are available for both girls and boys.

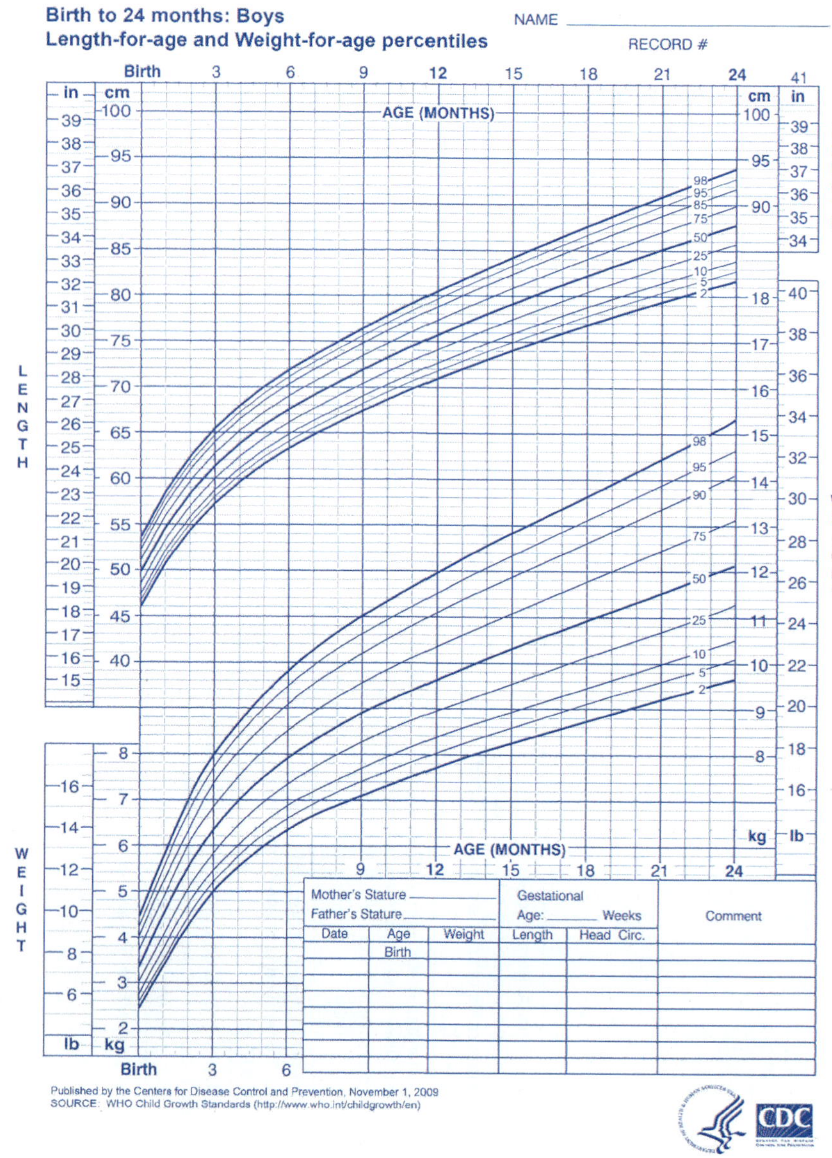

■ **Figure A3.1** Birth to 24 months: boys length-for-age percentiles and weight-for-age percentiles.

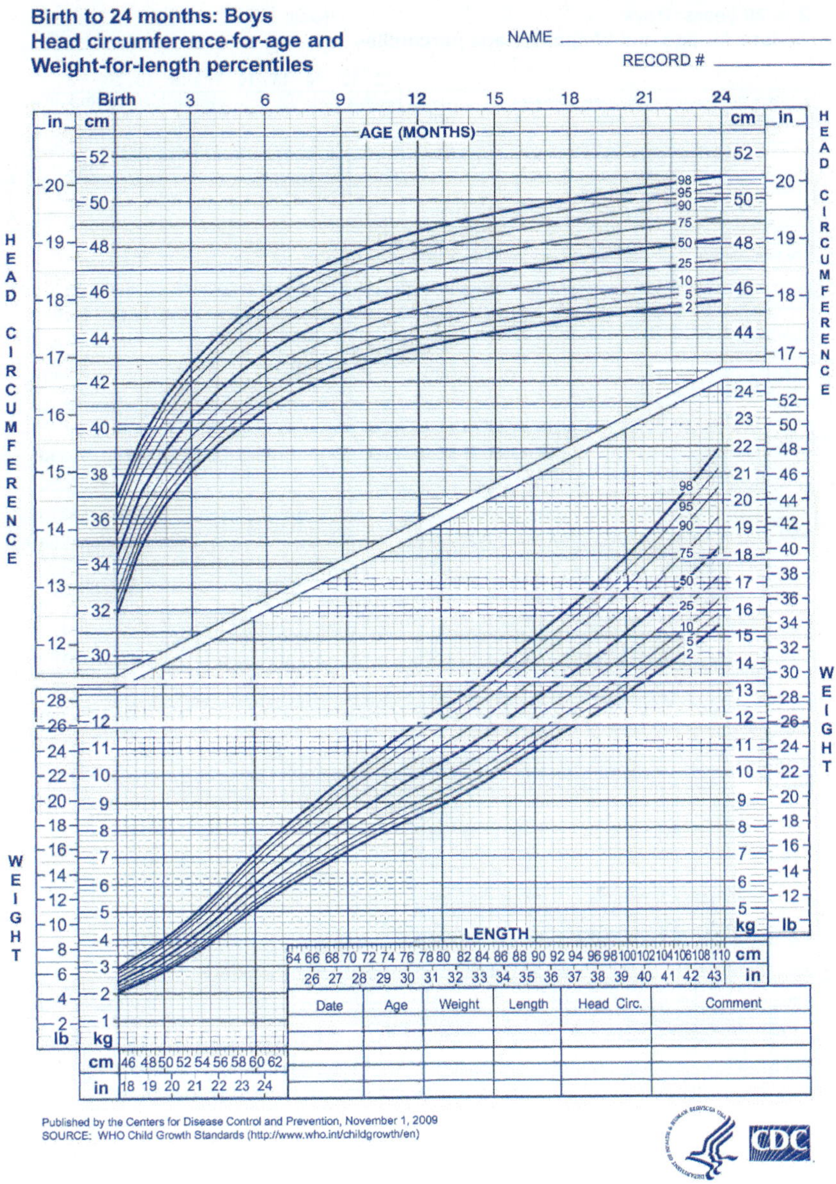

Figure A3.2 Birth to 24 months: boys weight-for-length percentiles and head circumference-for-age percentiles.

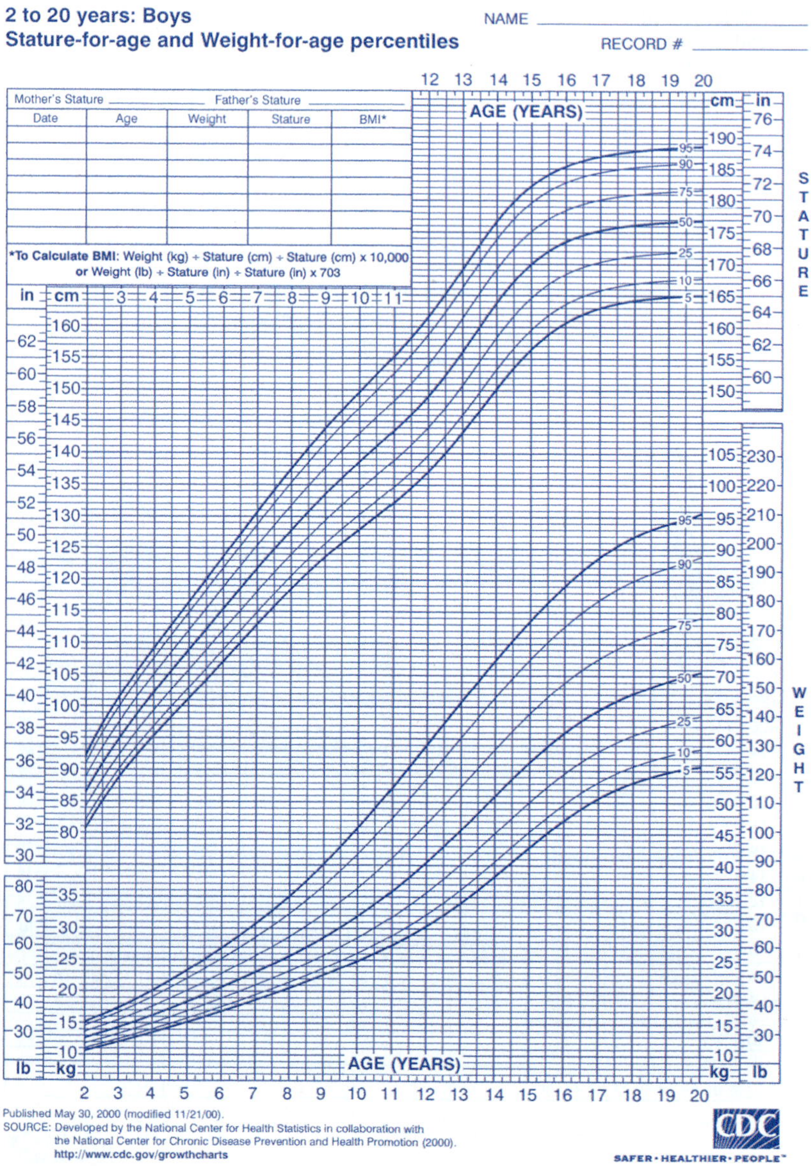

■ **Figure A3.3** 2 to 20 years: boys stature-for-age and weight-for-age.

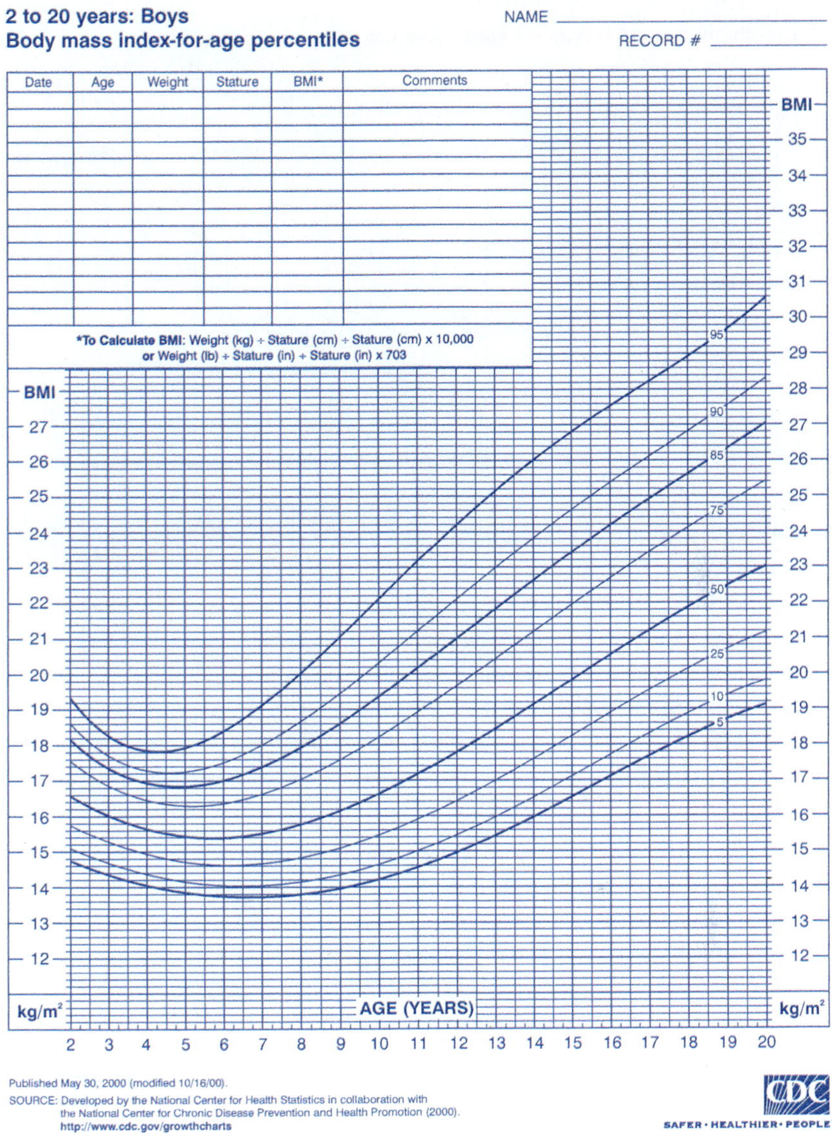

Figure A3.4 2 to 20 years: boys BMI-for-age.

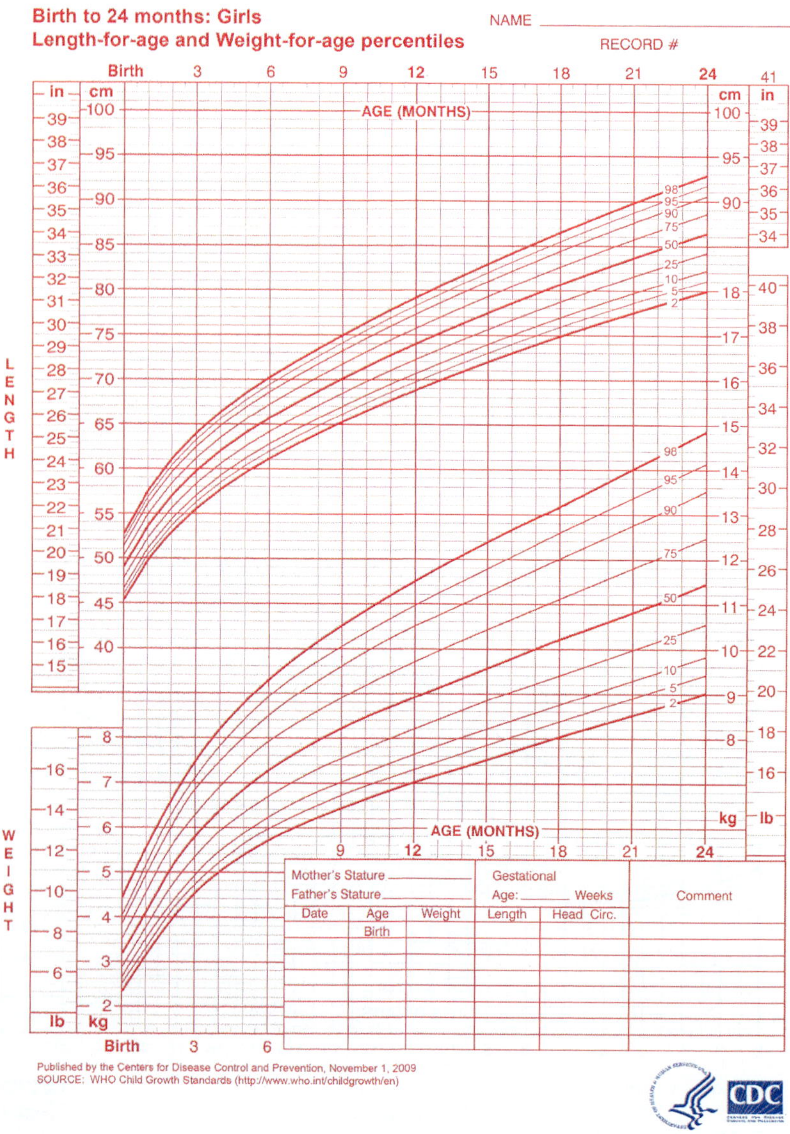

Figure A3.5 Birth to 24 months: girls length-for-age percentiles and weight-for-age percentiles.

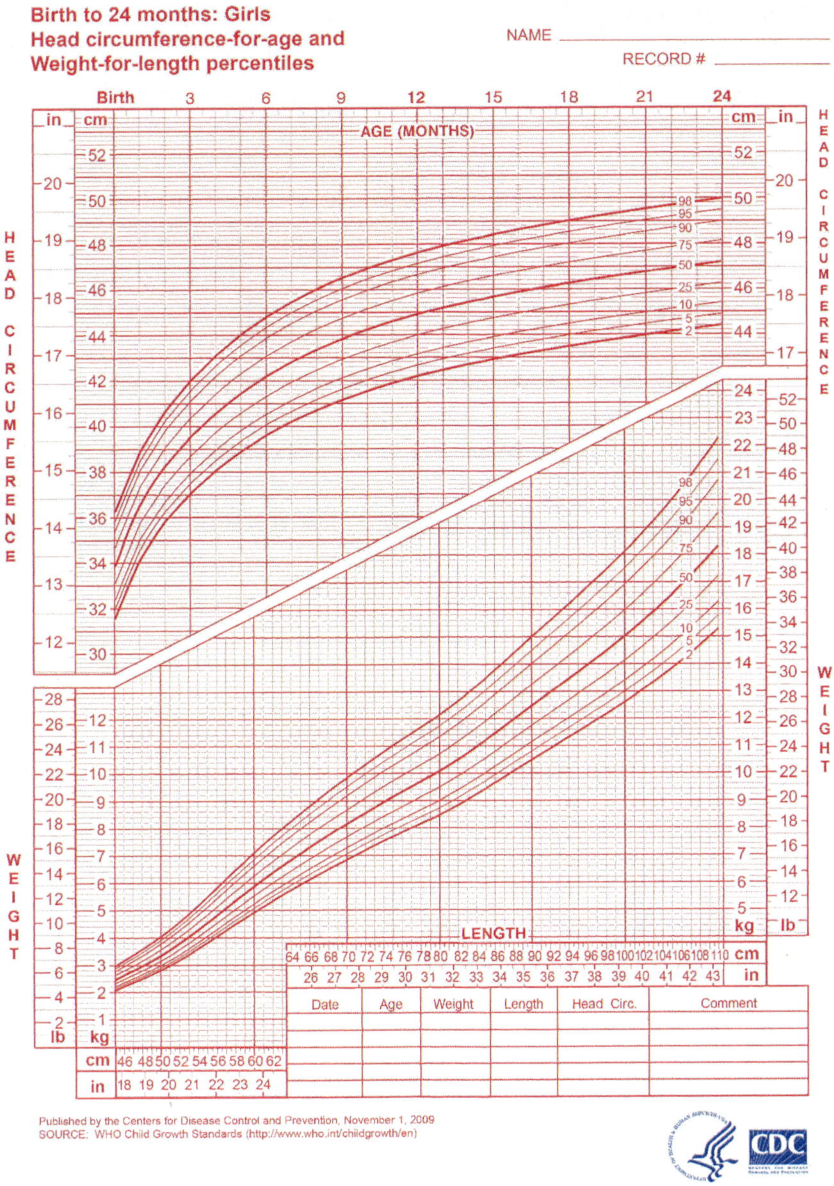

Figure A3.6 Birth to 24 months: girls weight-for-length percentiles and head circumference-for-age percentiles.

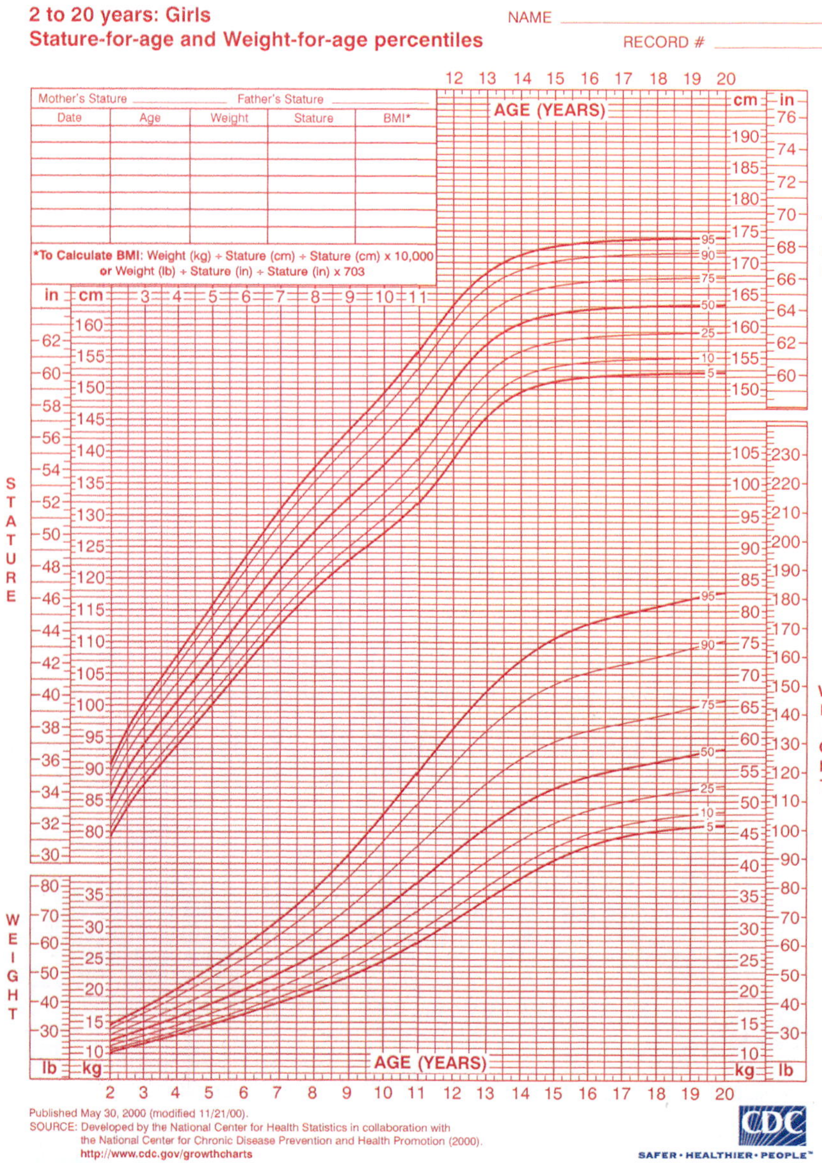

Figure A3.7 2 to 20 years: girls stature-for-age and weight-for-age.

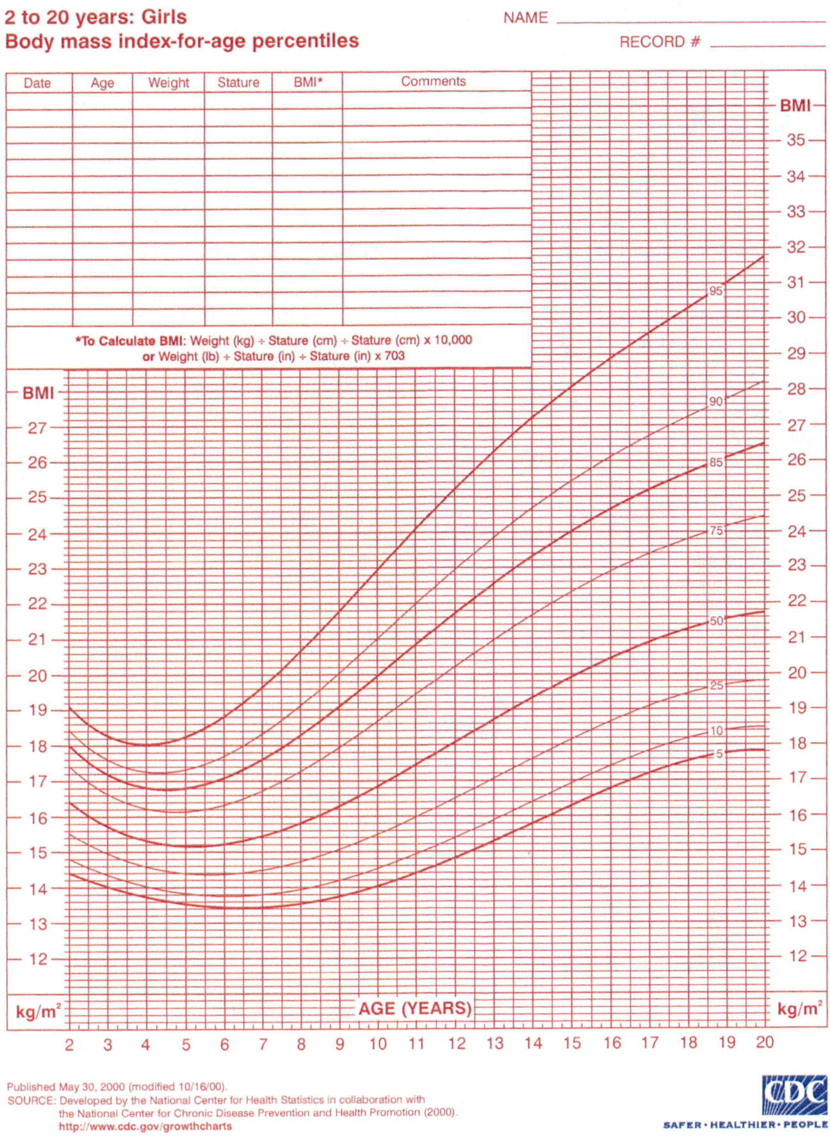

■ **Figure A3.8** 2 to 20 years: girls BMI-for-age.

Index

Note: Page numbers followed by *f* refer to figures; page numbers followed by *t* refer to tables.